Two week loan

S

Please return on or before the last
date stamped below.
Charges are made for late return.

13/09/05		

IS 239/0799

INFORMATION SERVICES PO BOX 430, CARDIFF CF10 3XT

Interindividual Variability in Human Drug Metabolism

Interindividual Variability in Human Drug Metabolism

Edited by

G. M. Pacifici
Associate Professor of Pharmacology
University of Pisa
Italy

O. Pelkonen
Professor of Pharmacology
University of Oulu
Finland

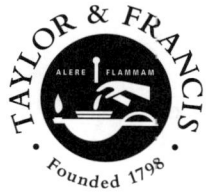

London and New York

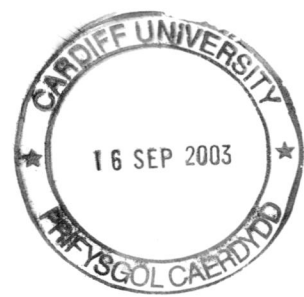

First published 2001 by Taylor & Francis
11 New Fetter Lane, London EC4P 4EE

Simultaneously published in the USA and Canada
by Taylor & Francis Inc,
29 West 35th Street, New York, NY 10001

Taylor & Francis is an imprint of the Taylor & Francis Group

© 2001 Gian Maria Pacifici and Olavi Pelkonen

Typeset in Sabon and Gill Sans by Exe Valley Dataset Ltd, Exeter
Printed and bound in Great Britain by St Edmundsbury Press,
Bury St Edmunds, Suffolk

British Library Cataloguing in Publication Data
A catalogue record for this book is available
from the British Library

Library of Congress Cataloging in Publication Data
Interindividual variability in human drug metabolism / edited by Gian Maria
Pacifici, Olavi Pelkonen.
  p.; cm.
  Includes bibliographical references and index.
    1. Drugs—Metabolism.   2. Biochemical variation.   I. Pacifici, Gian Maria.
  II. Pelkonen, R. O. (R. Olavi)
    [DNLM: 1. Pharmaceutical Preparations—metabolism.   2. Drug Therapy—
adverse effects.   3. Drug Toxicity.   4. Variation (Genetics).   QV 38 I598 2001]
RM301.55.I56 2001
615'.7—dc21   00–066798

ISBN 0–7484–0864–9

Contents

Tables

Figures

Contributors

D. J. Back is Professor of Pharmacology at the University of Liverpool, England. He is a past editor of the *British Journal of Clinical Pharmacology* and author or co-author of more than 300 articles on pharmacokinetics and drug interactions.

J. Benítez is Professor of Pharmacology and Clinical Pharmacology in the Department of Pharmacology at the University of Extremadura, Spain. He has published over 100 papers, mostly in the field of pharmacogenetics, and is co-editor of *Clinical Pharmacology in Psychiatry*. He sits on the editorial boards of several journals.

L. Bertilsson is a Professor in the Department of Clinical Pharmacology at the Karolinska Institute, Huddinge University Hospital, Sweden. He has published more than 250 articles and is on the editorial board of *Clinical Pharmacology and Therapeutics*, *Clinical Drug Investigation*, and *Pharmacogentics*.

P. Bonnabry is Chief Pharmacist at the University Hospital in Geneva, Switzerland. His research interests include the quality assurance of drug prescription and dispensation, and the prediction of drug metabolism interactions.

A. R. Boobis is Professor of Biochemical Pharmacology in the Section on Clinical Pharmacology and Deputy Director of the Health Toxicology Unit at Imperial College School of Medicine, London. His main research interests are in the human P450 system and mechanistic toxicology. He has published over 150 papers, numerous invited chapters and reviews, and regularly presents at international conferences.

B. Burchell is Professor of Medical Biochemistry and Head of the Department of Molecular and Cellular Pathology at the University of Dundee, Scotland. He is President of the European Society of Biochemical Pharmacology and has published more than 200 articles.

J. A. Carrillo is Associate Professor of Pharmacology in the Department of Pharmacology at the University of Extremadura, Spain. He has extensively investigated genetic and environmental factors implicated in the distribution of drug-metabolising enzymes in man.

M. J. Coffey is a Postdoctoral Research Fellow at the Wales Heart Research Institute, Department of Pharmacology, Therapeutics and Toxicology, University of Wales College of Medicine, Cardiff, Wales.

M.-L. Dahl is Professor of Clinical Medicine at Uppsala University, Sweden. Her research interests include psychotropic drug metabolism, interindividual and interethnic drug metabolism, and the clinical implications of polymorphic drug metabolism in psychiatry.

P. Dayer is Head of the Division of Clinical Pharmacology at the University Hospital in Geneva, Switzerland. He is co-author of a number of articles on the computer-based prediction of drug metabolism interactions.

B. Ethell is a Scientific Officer and Research Assistant in the Department of Molecular and Cellular Pathology, University of Dundee, Scotland.

K. Findlay holds a Degree in Pharmacology and has recently received a PhD from the University of Dundee, Scotland. She is currently Trainee Study Director at Inveresk Research International, Scotland.

M. Furlanut is Professor of Pharmacology and Director of the Institute of Clinical Pharmacology and Toxicology at the University of Udine, Italy. His research interests include pharmacokinetics, and the toxicology of drugs, including psychotropic and anticancer drugs.

G. Gatti is Lecturer in Pharmacology at the University of Pavia, Italy. Her interests include pharmacokinetics, drug interaction, drug metabolism, and therapeutic drug monitoring. She is the author of over 100 publications in these fields.

S. E. Gibbons is a Research Associate in the Department of Pharmacology and Therapeutics at the University of Liverpool. Her research interests include therapeutic drug monitoring of the antiretroviral agents used in the treatment of HIV infection and drug–drug interactions amongst these agents.

R. Hume is Professor of Developmental Medicine at the University of Dundee, Scotland. He is the author of more than 170 articles for leading scientific journals.

M. Ingelman-Sundberg is Professor of Molecular Toxicology at the Karolinska Institutet, Stockholm, Sweden. He is on the editorial boards of several journals and has written a large number of articles on clinical pharmacology, molecular genetics and molecular toxicology.

G. Jedlitschky is a Postdoctoral Research Fellow in the Division of Tumour Biochemistry DFKZ, Heidelberg, Germany.

A.-S. Johansson is a PhD student in the Department of Biochemistry at Uppsala University, Sweden. Her research interests include glutathione transferases, their polymorphisms in man and their role in preventing cancer and other degenerative diseases.

W. Kalow is Professor Emeritus in the Department of Pharmacology at the University of Toronto, Canada. His work has helped to establish pharmocogenetics as a specific field of pharmacology and human genetics, and he is editor of *The Pharmacogenetics of Drug Metabolism* (1992) and *Pharmacogenomics* (in press). His current interest is the development of a simplified method of measuring the genetic component in variable drug responses.

S. H. Khoo is a Consultant Physician at the Royal Liverpool University Hospital and a Senior Lecturer in Pharmacology and Therapeutics at the University of Liverpool. His research interests include optimisation of antiretroviral therapy and pharmacological reasons for virologic failure.

U. Klotz is Senior Research Assistant and Lecturer in Pharmacology and Toxicology at the Dr Margarete-Fischer-Bosch-Institute of Clinical Pharmacology in Stuttgart, Germany. He is on the editorial boards of several journals and has written over 300 articles and nine books.

P. Kremers is head of a research laboratory on drug metabolism and biochemical toxicology in the Institute of Pathology at the University of Liege, Belgium. His research interests include drug metabolism and the development of biomarkers to study the effects of environmental pollutants. He has published more than 130 articles.

H. K. Kroemer is Professor and Chairman of the Department of Pharmacology at the University Hospital, Ernst Moritz Arndt University, Greifswald, Germany. His research interests include drug metabolism, oncology and cardiovascular disease.

T. Leemann was Chief Pharmacist at the University Hospital in Geneva, Switzerland. He is co-author of a number of articles on the computer-based prediction of drug metabolism interactions.

G. N. Levy is Senior Research Scientist in the Department of Pharmacology at the University of Michigan, USA. His field of teaching and research is pharmacogenetics with a particular interest in the role of genetic polymorphisms in modulating risk of cancer and other diseases.

B. Mannervik holds a chair in the Department of Biochemistry at Uppsala University, Sweden. His major research interests are the design and engineering of proteins, biochemical toxicology and cancer, the bio-chemistry of glutathione, experimental design and mathematical model-ling, and general enzymology. He has published more than 350 articles on biochemistry.

G. M. Pacifici is Associate Professor of Pharmacology in the Department of Neurosciences at the University of Pisa, Italy. Since 1971 he has worked continuously on the metabolism of drugs in humans and has published over 150 articles on the subject in leading scientific journals. In 1980 he established a bank of human tissues, which is continuously being developed and expanded, and in 1983 obtained a PhD in Clinical Pharmacology from the Karolinska Institute in Stockholm. He is co-editor (with G. N. Fracchia) of *Advances in Drug Metabolism in Man,* published in 1995.

O. Pelkonen is Professor of Pharmacology in the Medical Faculty of the University of Oulu, Finland. His research interests include xenobiotic metabolism in humans and the role of *in vitro* drug metabolism in the development of pharmaceuticals. He has published over 150 articles mainly on drug metabolising enzymes.

E. Perucca is Associate Professor of Medical Pharmacology at the University of Pavia, Italy. His special interests are pharmacokinetics, therapeutic drug monitoring and clinical trial methodology. He is the author of over 350 publications and is on the editorial boards of several journals.

A. Rane is Professor of Clinical Pharmacology at the Karolinska Institutet, Huddinge University Hospital, Stockholm, Sweden.

A. M. Rossi is the Senior Scientist and Co-ordinator of the Laboratory of Molecular Genetics in the Department of Human and Environmental Sciences at the University of Pisa, Italy. Her main interest has focused on the role of xenobiotic metabolism in modulating the induction of genetic damage at gene and chromosome level following environmental or experimental exposure. She is the author of many articles in the field.

J. Sievering is a computer scientist at the University of Geneva, Switzerland. He is co-author of a number of articles on the computer-based prediction of drug metabolism interactions.

D. Smith is a Technician in the Department of Molecular and Cellular Pathology at the University of Dundee. She is currently studying for a MSc in Biological Sciences.

M. Soars obtained a BSc from the University of Warwick, England, in 1998 and is currently studying for a PhD at the University of Dundee, Scotland.

E. Spina is Associate Professor of Neuropsychopharmacology in the Institute of Pharmacology at the University of Messina, Italy. His main interest is clinical neuropsychopharmacology and drug metabolism. He is the author of more than 90 articles for journals in this field.

W. W. Weber is Professor Emeritus (Active) in the Department of Pharmacology at the University of Michigan, Ann Arbor, USA. His field of teaching and research is pharmacogenetics.

R. Weinshilboum is Professor of Molecular Pharmacology and Experimental Therapeutics and Internal Medicine at the Mayo Medical School in Rochester, Minnesota, USA. His major area of research has been the pharmacogenetics of drug metabolism, with a focus on methylation and sulfation.

G. Wu is a pharmacokinetic modelling expert working for the Novartis company in Switzerland. He is the author of many articles in the field.

L. Yan is a Research Fellow in the Oncology Centre at the Johns Hopkins Medical Institute, Baltimore, USA. Her particular research interest is the pharmacogenetics of phase II enzymes.

Foreword

This volume is devoted to factors determining interindividual variability in drug metabolism in humans, which is one of the main factors that regulates the steady-state plasma concentrations of drugs and hence their clinical effects. Differences between patients in dose requirements are thus to a great extent dependent on corresponding difference in rates of drug metabolism. In clinical practice these differences are seldom known or assessed quantitatively before the dose is decided. This is in sharp contrast to the situation with drugs that are excreted unchanged by the kidney and whose clearance is quantitatively related to kidney function, which often is known to the clinician. Dose dependent adverse reactions and some therapeutic failures should theoretically be possible to avoid by individualised dosage schedules. Research aiming to explore the mechanisms involved in interindividual variability in drug metabolism has therefore a great potential to improve the quality of drug therapy.

This research field was initiated already in the early 1960s by the late B. B. Brodie who outlined the perspectives in his famous Sollman Award lecture 'Of mice, microsomes and man' (1963). Since then, numerous symposia have been published and recent research summarised in many excellent books, recent examples being *Pharmacogenetics of Drug Metabolism* (Kalow 1992) and *Advances in Drug Metabolism in Man* (Pacifici and Fracchia 1955).

This volume outlines the most recent advances in the field, with much emphasis on genetic factors causing interindividual and interethnic differences in drug metabolism and hence drug response. The individual contributions convincingly demonstrate that there is a steady progress in this research. This is most evident in the understanding of the regulation of different drug metabolising enzymes and in documenting interindividual differences in the metabolism of various groups of drugs. The progress is much slower in demonstrating the clinical utility of all this new knowledge, such as the usefulness in patient care of phenotyping and genotyping procedures to predict drug metabolic rates and, indirectly, the outcome of drug therapy. This is to some extent explained by the complexities of modern drug therapy (drugs with active metabolites, frequent and sometimes chaotic combination therapy and drug interactions) and the possible existence of genetic variability in drug-receptor interactions. This complexity should not discourage researchers regarding the clinical significance of their work but rather serve as a stimulus to prove their case in controlled clinical trials of the role of drug metabolic variations for the outcome of drug therapy.

Folke Sjöqvist, MD, PhD, FRCP
Professor of Clinical Pharmacology
Stockholm, January 2001

References

Brodie, B. B. (1964) 'Of mice, microsomes and man', *The Pharmacologist* **6**: 12–26.

Kalow, W. (1992) *Pharmacogenetics of Drug Metabolism*, Pergamon Press, New York.

Pacifici, G. M. and Fracchia, G. N. (1995) *Advances in Drug Metabolism in Man*, European Commission, D6 XII-Science Research and Development.

Chapter I

Genetic factors that cause variability in human drug metabolism

W. Kalow

When considering human pharmacogenetics, most physicians and most investigators are thinking most of the time of monogenic variants which change the therapeutic or toxic response to one or more pharmacologically active agents.

In contrast to the sharply definable monogenic inheritance, there is also multigenic inheritance. This is measured in terms of heritability, and its causes are mostly not defined. Unusual drug responses at the edges of frequency distribution curves may represent either kind of variation.

This introductory survey chapter will enumerate principles by quoting examples, many of which will be described in greater detail in later chapters in this book.

Categories of genetic variation

Monogenic variants

Monogenic variation means replacement of one nucleotide with another in a given stretch of DNA. Such variation may be silent, i.e. without affecting amino acid composition. In many cases, even the exchange of an amino acid has no noticeable effect upon the function of a protein. We will ignore these possibilities. In pharmacogenetics, the concern is mutations that affect the response to drugs or toxicants.

In family studies, monogenic variants are generally characterised by Mendelian inheritance, which implies – if recessive – the existence of homozygotes and heterozygotes. The term "polymorphism" should not be indiscriminately applied to these variants. Polymorphism indicates by strict terminology a high frequency of a monogenic variant. This is of some importance since there can be fundamental differences in the formative histories of polymorphic and of rare variants.

A polymorphic locus is one at which the most common allele has a frequency of more than 0.01; it means that at least 2% of the population must be heterozygous at that locus (Harris, 1980). This is a population frequency far too high to be a fresh mutation; it must be a variant resulting from an old mutation which is maintained in the population either by being functionally neutral (Kimura and Ohta, 1973) or by "balanced polymorphism" (Ford, 1971). This latter term means that the gene is maintained in the population because a disadvantage of the homozygous carriers of the variant is balanced by an advantage with improved survival of the heterozygotes. No such rule applies to rare variants which might represent fresh mutations that could be genetic disasters.

The clearest graphical representation of a polymorphic variation is a bimodal frequency distribution of the variable trait. The clearest genetic indication is the full establishment of the responsible allelic change of DNA composition.

The occurrence of variant drug-metabolising enzymes is clearly a major cause of the variability of drug metabolism (Kalow, 1962, 1992, 1997; Price Evans, 1993; Weber, 1997). Allelic structural variants of drug-metabolising enzymes are best known from their direct effects upon metabolic capacity, but they may also affect this capacity indirectly by changing the enzyme stability or the responsiveness to inducers or inhibitors.

Continuous or multigenic variations

It is common to note some differences of pharmacokinetics or pharmacodynamics between people without any concern for the cause or causes. The more careful the observation, the more clear is an ever-present lack of consistency either of the drug action, or of the activity of drug-metabolising enzymes (Clark, 1937). A pharmacological use of this reliable variation is made by determining the ED50, the median effective dose, that is, the dose of a drug that produces a defined effect in 50% of a population.

Structural variation of enzymes is only one of the genetic causes of metabolic individuality. There is variable gene expression (Lander, 1999), which may lead to variable formation of the gene product, the protein. There may be genetically variable enzyme destroyers, stabilisers, transcription enhancers and repressors, inducers, inhibitors, or regulators. Drug metabolism may be affected by transport systems or by the protein binding of drugs; both may regulate the access to drug-metabolising enzymes. We will attempt here to register at least some of these different possibilities.

This ever-present variation shows graphically as a normal frequency distribution curve, a Gauss curve (Vogel and Motulsky, 1986). The underlying variation may be called multifactorial on the assumption that both genetic and environmental factors contribute to it.

Comparisons between pairs of identical and fraternal twins have traditionally been used to distinguish between the genetic and environmental components contributing to this overall variation (Vesell, 1992). The genetic component is usually defined as multigenic and measured in terms of heritability. Since drug effects may come and go, twin studies can be replaced in pharmacology by giving the drug a few times to each person in a group of people, and by statistically comparing inter- and intra-individual variability (Kalow et al., 1999).

Consider the observation of a difference between normal distribution curves observed in different populations or under different circumstances. Such differences are traditionally evaluated by comparing the means and by calculating the statistical significance of the difference. However, this kind of data interpretation can be misleading in pharmacology. It may be more accurate and pharmacologically more useful to compare the edges of histograms or frequency distribution curves, rather than the means (Kalow and Bertilsson, 1994). The outliers in drug response (i.e. persons without response or with a toxic response) represent usually the edges of distribution curves.

Virtually nobody ever asks about the nature of the variants which determine the magnitude of the standard deviation (SD) or of the derived coefficient of variation (CV). This lack of questioning reflects an unspoken understanding that very numerous diverse and perhaps undefinable factors may contribute to the variation.

By strict definition, multigenic means that at least three genes are involved. Often the number of genes or of environmental controllers is uncertain, i.e. an enzyme activity is measured without definition of the controlling factors.

Combinations of monogenic and multigenic variation

Multifactorial variation usually penetrates even monogenically controlled enzyme activity. For example, even persons homozygous for wild-type CYP2D6 ("extensive metabolisers") do not all have uniform CYP2D6 activity. This may represent differences in enzyme expression, but other causes may be hormonal variations, variable formation of inducers, inhibitors, or stimulants of enzyme activity.

In case of transition between monogenic and multigenic variations, the smooth pattern of multigenic variation may be distorted by a monogenic variant that more or less affects the measured parameter. Graphically, such cases may show up as distortions of the normal Gauss curve. Because of the frequent clinical importance of the variability of drug effects, such deviations are traditionally investigated in pharmacology by testing for non-linearity of probit plots, an old device (Finney, 1952). A newer method to show such deviations is the use of NTV plots (Endrenyi and Patel, 1991). Yue et al.(1997) gave examples to show that old-style histograms should not be neglected.

Monogenic variants of drug-metabolising enzymes

Absence of enzyme activity

The term "poor metabolizer" was devised to indicate a lack of enzymatic activity of CYP2D6 (Mahgoub *et al.*, 1977). Subsequently, this lack has been found to be due to different molecular causes (Daly *et al.*, 1996). There may be frameshift mutations as in *CYP2D6*3, CYP2D6*6A, CYP2D6*6B, CYP2D6*13, CYP2D6*16*, splicing defects as in *CYP2D6*4A, *4B, *4C, *4D, CYP2D6*11*, gene deletion as in *CYP2D6*5*, the presence of a stop codon as in *CYP2D6*8*, or an inactivating insertion as in *CYP2D6*15*.

Furthermore, as shown in the overview paper by Daly *et al.* (1996), the variants *CYP2D6*4A* and *CYP2D6*4B*, are typically seen in Europe and carry seven or six, respectively, nucleotide changes; of these six or seven changes, only one has been found in Africa, only three in Japan, and the same three and an additional one also in China. On the other hand, each of these populations carry changes seen nowhere else. From the evolutionary perspective, it is interesting to note that the G→C change at nucleotide 4628 is seen in all populations and thus must be older than the 150,000-year-old departure of *Homo sapiens* from Africa. The other mutations must be comparatively young, affecting only more recently separated populations.

Although the pharmacogenetics of the P450 cytochrome CYP2D6 have been more intensely investigated than those of other proteins of that class, CYP2D6 is not unique. For instance, the S-mephenytoin hydroxylase, now designated CYP2C19, is known to have nine functionally inactive variants numbered from *CYP2C19*2A* to *CYP2C19.8* (CYP Home Page, 2000). There are ten different single base-pair substitutions of which one (991A→G) occurs seven times while five occur only once. Several substitutions create aberrant splice sites, one a premature stop codon, one a missing initiation codon (Goldstein and De Morais, 1994). Some of these variants have been shown to occur with different frequencies in different populations, for example in Japanese and Caucasians (Inoue *et al.*, 1997). It is usually so that ethnically distinct populations show different allele frequencies (Kalow and Bertilsson, 1995).

The principles, shown here by quoting experiences with CYP2D6 and CYP2C19, are general and may be seen also in other enzymes.

Altered enzyme function

A change of amino acid in or near the active center of an enzyme may lead to alterations of K_m or of k_{cat}, the binding constant or the turnover number. V_{max} variations are ambiguous in that they may indicate changes of k_{cat} and thereby of enzyme function, or they may reflect changes of enzyme concentration by one or more of several factors. The latter possibility will be discussed in a subsequent section.

K_m variants may alter enzyme specificity, that is, the degree of enzymatic deficiency may vary with the substrate. One of the earliest examples is the variant of butyrylcholinesterase which was originally referred to as "atypical plasma cholinesterase" (Kalow, 1962) which has Gly in place of Asp 70 (Lockridge, 1992). This variant has a 200-fold increase of K_m for the muscle relaxant succinylcholine without change of V_{max}, causing the failure to metabolise the drug under clinical conditions (Kalow, 1959). The same variant binds o-nitrophenyl butyrate with normal K_m, while many substrates that carry one positive charge show an approximate ten-fold K_m elevation (Masson et al., 1997).

By contrast, the K-variant of butyrylcholinesterase which is characterised by a 539 Ala→Thr change, is described as showing an approximate 30% reduction of V_{max} with all substrates (Bartels et al., 1992); it probably represents a k_{cat} variation.

In a recent study in this laboratory, the glucuronyl transferase UGT2B7 with a 268 Tyr→His substitution was the subject of investigation. It showed a two-fold K_m elevation and a ninety-fold k_{cat} reduction when oxazepam was substrate, while there were no changes from the wild-type enzyme when ketoprofen was the substrate (Patel, 1997).

As described above, there are many variants of the P450 cytochrome CYP2D6 which are characterised by reduced activity (Marez et al., 1997; CYP Home Page, 2000). Woolhouse et al. (1985) investigated CYP2D6 in a Ghanaian population of 154 subjects and reported a correlation of $r=0.47$ between the rates of metabolism of debrisoquine and sparteine, two substrates known to be metabolised by CYP2D6; an equivalent study in Europe had yielded a correlation coefficient of $r=0.91$. While there were no detailed kinetic data, these results strongly suggest the occurrence of different relative substrate specificities by the predominant forms of the enzyme in the two populations. This interpretation is consistent with observations in Zimbabwe (Masimirembwa et al., 1996), and also with comparisons between Swedes and Chinese (see Chapter 2).

Alteration of enzyme stability

The discovery of the genetic variation of glucose-6-phosphate dehydrogenase (G-6-pD) provides an interesting history (Luzzatto and Mehta, 1995). During World War II, American soldiers in tropical countries received primaquine for prophylaxis against malaria; only black soldiers responded to this treatment, sometimes with a hemolytic reaction. After the war, the reason was found to be a deficiency of G-6-pD (Carson et al., 1956), a deficiency affecting only some populations because it conveyed resistance to malaria (Motulsky, 1960). It became an important point that the deficiency was often temporary: in people of African descent, the hemolytic reaction tended to disappear over time in spite of continued primaquine application (Beutler, 1993). The reason became clear when it was found that the enzyme was genetically unstable. That is, the enzyme located in red blood cells deteriorated with ageing of the cells. Hemolysis meant destruction of the older cells and their replacement by young ones. The young cells contained enough fresh G-6-pD to make the symptoms disappear. Subsequently, it was found that G-6-pD deficiency in Italians was much more serious; it did not represent enzyme deteriation with red cell ageing but formation of a deficient enzyme. G-6-pD is now known to have perhaps as many as 400 variants.

Enzyme stability is often not specifically investigated. In addition, lack of enzyme stability may represent peculiar problems. For instance, Primo-Parmo et al. (1997) described a variant of butyrylcholinesterase called BChE115D that deteriorates in vitro on freezing and thawing, but is of normal persistence in vivo.

Different responsiveness to inducer or regulator

Sachse et al. (1998) recently reported a C→A variant in the first intron of the CYP1A2 gene; the variation affected the enzyme inducibility by cigarette smoke but not the activity of the uninduced enzyme.

There are currently four known variants of the P450 CYP1A1 (Cascorbi et al., 1996). Of these, the m2 variant, an A→G change at nucleotide 4889, shows higher activity than the wild-type, suggesting an elevation of enzyme concentration due to an improved response to enzyme induction.

Polymorphic variation of N-acetyltransferase type 2 (NAT2) has been known since 1957. On the basis of kinetic studies, Jenne (1965) described slow acetylation as being due to low concentration of a normally functioning enzyme. In 1990, Grant et al. confirmed this view by reporting that slow acetylators had low concentrations of immunoreactive N-acetyltransferase protein. This could be assumed to be defective transcription. More recently, Weber and Vatsis (1995) described studies of hepatic tissue preparations and of heterologous mammalian expression systems for NAT2. They listed eleven nucleotide changes in the human enzyme. They suggested that 'slow' acetylation of isoniazid and sulphamethazine by variant NAT2 proteins thus far examined may be due to impaired efficiency in translation of mutant NAT2 mRNA and to enhanced degradation of mutant NAT2 protein. It may be that different variants of NAT2 do not have a uniform cause for their slow enzymatic activity, but the interesting fact remains that there are mutations of the enzyme which lead to the production of fewer molecules.

Instability of messenger mRNA can be responsible for limited enzyme formation. An example of such a mechanism causing a human disease is β-thalassemia (Lim et al., 1992), but there are no well-documented examples in human pharmacogenetics. If an enzyme is insufficiently formed, it may not be easy to determine whether the fault is in the structure of the enzyme or the regulator.

Gene duplication or multiplication

Gene duplication may lead to excessive enzyme formation and thereby to rapid metabolic function. Detailed accounts of duplication and multiplication of the CYP2D6 gene has come from Sweden in recent years (Johansson et al., 1993). There is a high frequency of this mutation in North Africa (Aklillu et al., 1996; McLellan et al., 1997). African population admixture in Spain obviously accounts for a greater frequency of this variation in Spain than in Sweden.

The quoted examples represent duplication of a normal enzyme due to the wild-type gene. One must expect the possibility of duplication also of variant genes.

Regulatory and other alternate variants

There may be monogenic variants affecting drug metabolism due to mutations in systems other than the drug-metabolising enzymes themselves. Best known are the regulatory variants; these and some other monogenic variants will be quoted in this section. At the same time, many of the modifying variations may not reflect mutations of known genes, but may also arise from multigenic factors.

Regulatory variants that alter enzyme formation

Genetic variation in mice of the aryl hydrocarbon receptor (AHR) has been known for many years through the work of Nebert (1979, 1988). He and his collaborators have shown the fundamental importance of this system for cancer investigations and other topics. These findings became of great interest for investigators of humans when it was found that cigarette smoke causes the induction of the P450 cytochromes CYP1A1 and CYP1A2 via the AHR system, and that smoking and lung cancer are related. In 1973, Kellermann et al. reported human genetic differences in an AHR induction response, but several subsequent investigators could not confirm this finding. In 1995, Kawajiri et al. in Japan found a high frequency of an Arg→Lys change at codon 554 in the AHR, a change showing large interethnic differences with infrequent ocurrence in European populations (Wong et al., 1998) – but this mutation does not appear to affect the induction of CYP1A1. It remains to be seen whether the variant has some of the other functions of AHR, such as induction of other enzymes.

Induction of drug-metabolising enzymes by phenobarbital has been widely investigated in rats but much less so in humans. Chronic exposure to high doses of phenobarbital caused hepatocellular adenomas in rats and mice, but not in humans (Whysner *et al.*, 1996). Vesell and Page showed in 1969, with the help of a twin study, that there was genetic control of phenobarbital induction in humans. Phenobarbital controls RNA expression. Other drugs can do the same; it means an important new principle is established (Bailey, 1998).

Endogenous inducers and inhibitors

Glucocorticoids are known inducers of the steroid forming and metabolising P450 cytochromes of the C17 and C21 families, but also of the important drug-metabolising CYP3A4 (Hashimoto *et al.*, 1993). Person-to-person variation of CYP3A4 is more extensive than that of other cytochromes; very recently, a structural enzyme variant has been discovered (CYP Home Page, 2000), but there is usually a normal distribution of enzyme activity. Since there are various genetic conditions that may affect glucocorticoid formation (Donohoue *et al.*, 1995), this might affect CYP3A4 levels.

Cytochrome CYP3A4 does not only occur in liver but also in the intestinal wall, where its activity may affect drug absorption (Benet *et al.*, 1996). The regulations of CYP3A4 concentration in liver and gut are independent of each other, proving that it is not the CYP3A4 structure, but that there must be at least two different elements able to regulate its formation.

Shively and Vesell (1975) found 11-hydroxycorticoids in several subjects 42% higher at 6 a.m. than at 2 p.m., but the half-lives of both, acetaminophen and phenacetin, were shorter in the afternoon than in the morning. They did not test for any causative relationship between the steroid level and the half-lives.

Caffeine is metabolised much faster by children than by adults (Lambert *et al.*, 1990), but this age difference is not visible in liver samples derived from adults and children (unpublished observation). The principal enzyme determining caffeine elimination is CYP1A2 (Kalow and Tang, 1993). One may assume that the *in vivo* metabolic difference is due to inhibition of CYP1A2 by steroid hormones while the inhibition is not noticed in the diluted microsomal preparations used *in vitro*. Support for this hypothesis comes from the fact that the children's rate of caffeine metabolism decreases at puberty, that the metabolic rate is lower in women taking oral contraceptives (Kalow and Tang, 1991), and that the rate decreases drastically during pregnancy (Bologa *et al.*, 1991).

Drug-binding proteins

Both human serum albumin ("Alb") and α_1-acid glycoprotein ("AAG") are genetically variable transport proteins. Kragh-Hansen *et al.* (1989) reported, for instance, that Alb Canterbury (313 Lys→Asn) and Alb Parklands (365 Asp→His) showed much reduced binding of warfarin, salicylate, and diazepam. Hervé *et al.* (1996) distinguished between the A variant of AAG and the mixture of the F1 and S variants of AAG; they reported, for example selective binding of methadone to the A variant and of dipyridamole to the F1–S mixture, while other drugs showed various degrees of preferences. Any variable binding of drugs in plasma must be expected to account for some person-to-person differences in the functional properties of a drug, perhaps by altering access to enzymes or receptors.

Trans-membrane transport systems

P-glycoproteins are widely distributed in the body. They represent, for example, the blood–brain barrier. In the gastrointestinal epithelial layer, they regulate the entry of drugs; they may counter-transport invading drugs (Hunter *et al.*, 1993) by acting as an ATP-dependent efflux pump, and thereby function as part of the absorption barrier in the intestine. By diminishing absorption, they diminish hepatic drug metabolism and also local drug metabolism by intestinal cytochromes (as, for example, by CYP3A4). Genetic alterations of P-glycoprotein that cause altered substrate affinities have been discussed in 1997 by Chen *et al.*, by Ma *et al.* and by Taguchi *et al.*, and by Ramachandra *et al.* in 1996.

P-glycoprotein also conveys the multidrug resistance which is clinically often disturbing in anticancer therapy (Arts *et al.*, 1999). Overexpression of the *mdr-1* gene forming the glycoprotein P-170, typically affects anthracyclines, vinca alkaloids, epipodophyllotoxins and taxol (Ling, 1997). It is an interesting finding that a P-glycoprotein, apparently identical with that in humans, accounts for some forms of multiple drug resistance in bacteria (Van Veen *et al.*, 1998).

Conclusions

All pharmacologists, and most professionals, including physicians and representatives of pharmaceutical companies, are aware of genetic variations of numerous drug-metabolising enzymes. These variations include mutations that cause absence or functional alterations of enzyme activity, and in some cases enhanced activity due to gene duplication. Much less investigated are transcriptional, translational, hormonal, or other regulatory or inhibitory variants that determine enzyme formation and function, including enzyme stability. Many of these variants may be monogenic and thereby clearly definable, but we cannot afford to neglect multigenic variations that are also capable of producing outliers in terms of drug response. In fact, most of the ever-present variations of drug response, exemplified by the term ED50, must be multifactorial.

It is a peculiar fact that most of the pharmacogenetic variants in humans affect drug metabolism rather than targets of drug action. At the present time, it is not clear whether this prominence of metabolic variation expresses the history of analytical developments, or whether it represents an aspect of human evolution.

References

Aklillu, E., Persson, I., Bertilsson, L., Johansson, I., Rodrigues, F. and Ingelman-Sundberg, M. (1996) 'Frequent distribution of ultrarapid metabolizers of debrisoquine in an Ethiopian population carrying duplicated and multiduplicated functional CYP2D6 alleles', *J. Pharmacol. Exp. Ther.* 78: 441–6.

Arts, H. J., Katsaros, D., De Vries, E. G., Massobrio, M., Genta, F., Danese, S., Arisio, R., Scheper, R. J., Kool, M., Scheffer, G. L., Willems, P. H., Van De Zee, A. G. and Suurmeijer, A. J. (1999) 'Drug resistance-associated markers P-glyco-protein, multidrug resistance-associated protein 2, and lung resistance protein as prognostic factors in ovarian carcinoma', *Clin. Cancer Res.* 5: 2798–2805.

Bailey, D. (1998) 'Pharmacogenomics – it's not just pharmacogenetics', *Curr. Opin. Biotechnol.* 6: 595–601.

Bartels, C. F., Jensen, F. S., Lockridge, O., Vanderspek, A. F. L., Rubinstein, H. M., Lubrano, T. and Ladu, B. N. (1992) 'DNA mutation associated with the human butyrylcholinesterase K-variant and its linkage to the atypical variant mutation and other polymorphic sites', *Am. J. Hum. Genet.* 50: 1086–103.

Benet, L. Z., Kroetz, D. L. and Heiner, L. B. (1996) 'Pharmacokinetics: the dynamics of drug absorption, distribution, and elimination', in Goodman and Gilman's, *The Pharmacological Basis of Therapeutics*, ed. by J. G. Hardman *et al.*, McGraw-Hill, Inc., New York, p. 14.

Beutler, E. (1993) 'Study of glucose-6-phosphate dehydrogenase: history and molecular biology', *Am. J. Hematol.* 42: 53–8.

Bologa, M., Tang, B., Klein, J., Tesoro, A. and Koren, G. (1991) 'Pregnancy-induced changes in drug metabolism in epileptic women', *J. Pharmac. Exp. Therap.* 257: 735–40.

Carson, P. E., Flanagan, C. L., Iokes, C. E. and Alving, A. S. (1956) 'Enzymatic deficiency in primaquine-sensitive erythrocytes', *Science* 124: 484–5.

Cascorbi, I., Brockmoller, J. and Roots, I. (1996) 'A C4887A polymorphism in exon 7 of human CYP1A1: population frequency, mutation linkages, and impact on lung cancer susceptibility', *Cancer Res.* 56: 4965–9.

Chen, G., Duran, G. E., Steger, K. A., Lacayo, N. J., Jaffrezou, J. P., Dumontet, C. and Sikic, B. I. (1997) 'Multidrug-resistant human sarcoma cells with a mutant P-glycoprotein, altered phenotype, and resistance to cyclosporins', *J. Biol. Chem.* 272: 5974–82.

Clark, A. J. (1937) *General Pharmacology, Handbuch Der Experimentellen Pharmakologie*, Verlag Von Julius Springer, Berlin, Volume 4, pp. 1–228.

CYP Home Page (2000) http://www.imm.ki.se/CYPalleles/(updated 15 February, 2000).

Daly, A. K., Brockmoller, J., Broly, F., Eichelbaum, M., Evans, W. E., Gonzalez, F. J., Huang, J. D., Idle, J. R., Ingelman-Sundberg, M., Ishizaki, T., Jacqz-Aigrain,

E., Meyer, U. A., Nebert, D. W., Steen, V. M., Wolf, C. R. and Zanger, U. M. (1996) 'Nomenclature for human CYP2D6 alleles', *Pharmacogenetics* **6**: 193–201.

Donohoue, P. A., Parker, K. and Migeon, C. J. (1995) 'Congenital adrenal hyperplasia', in C. R. Scriver, A. L. Beaudet, W. S. Sly and D. Valle (eds), *The metabolic and molecular bases of inherited disease*, McGraw-Hill, Inc., New York, pp. 2929–66.

Endrenyi, L. and Patel, M. (1991) 'Evaluation of two assumptions: single straight line, and single normal distribution', *Trends in Pharmacol. Sci.* **12**: 293–6.

Finney, D. J. (1952) *Probit Analysis. A Statistical Treatment of the Sigmoid Response Curve*, Cambridge University Press, Cambridge.

Ford, E. B. (1971) *Ecological Genetics*, Chapman & Hall, London.

Goldstein, J. and De Morais, S. (1994) 'Biochemistry and molecular biology of the human CYP2C subfamily', *Pharmacogenetics* **4**: 285–99.

Grant, D. M., Morike, K., Eichelbaum, M. and Meyer, U. A. (1990) 'Acetylation pharmacogenetics. The slow acetylator phenotype is caused by decreased or absent arylamine N-acetyltransferase in human liver', *J. Clin. Invest.* **85**: 968–72.

Harris, H. (1980) *The Principles of Human Biochemical Genetics*, Elsevier, Amsterdam.

Hashimoto, H., Toide, K., Kitamura, R., Fujita, M., Tagawa, S., Itoh, S. and Kamataki, T. (1993) 'Gene structure of CYP3A4, an adult-specific form of cytochrome P450 in human livers, and its transcriptional control', *Eur. J. Biochem.* **218**: 585–95.

Hervé, F., Duche, J. C., D'Athis, P., Marche, C., Barre, J. and Tillement, J. P. (1996) 'Binding of disopyramide, methadone, dipyridamole, chlorpromazine, lignocaine and progesterone to the two main genetic variants of human α_1-acid glycoprotein: evidence for drug-binding differences between the variants and for the presence of two separate drug-binding sites on α_1-acid glycoprotein', *Pharmacogenetics* **6**: 403–15.

Hunter, J., Jepson, M. A., Tsuruo, T., Simmons, N. L. and Hirst, B. H. (1993) 'Functional expression of P-glycoprotein in apical membanes of human intestinal Caco-2 cells. Kinetics of vinblastine secretion and interaction with modulators', *J. Biol. Chem.* **268**: 14991–7.

Inoue, K., Yamazaki, H., Imiya, K., Akasaka, S., Guengerich, F. P. and Shimada, T. (1997) 'Relationship between CYP2C9 and 2C19 genotypes and tolbutamide methyl hydroxylation and S-mephenytoin 4'-hydroxylation activities in livers of Japanese and Caucasian populations', *Pharmacogenetics* **7**: 103–13.

Jenne, J. W. (1965) 'Partial purification and properties of the isoniazid transacetylase in human liver. Its relationship to the acetylation of p-aminosalicylic acid', *J. Clin. Invest.* **44**: 1992–2002.

Johansson, I., Lundqvist, E., Bertilsson, L., Dahl, M. L., Sjoqvist, F. and Ingelman-Sundberg, M. (1993) 'Inherited amplification of an active gene in the cytochrome P450 CYP2D locus as a cause of ultrarapid metabolism of debrisoquine', *Proc. Natl. Acad. Sci.* **90**: 11825–9.

Kalow, W. (1959) 'The distribution, destruction and elimination of muscle relaxants', *Anesthesiology* **20**: 505–18.

Kalow, W. (1962) *Pharmacogenetics. Heredity and the Response to Drugs*, W. B. Saunders Company, Philadelphia.

Kalow, W. (ed.) (1992) *Pharmacogenetics of Drug Metabolism*, Int. Encycl. Pharmacol. Therap. Sect. 137, Pergamon Press, Inc., New York.

Kalow, W. (1997) 'Pharmacogenetics in biological perspective', *Pharmacol. Rev.* **49**: 369–79.

Kalow, W. and Bertilsson, L. (1994) 'Interethnic factors affecting drug response', *Adv. Drug Res.* **25**: 1–59.

Kalow, W. and Tang, B. K. (1991) 'Use of caffeine metabolite ratios to explore CYPlA2 and xanthine oxidase activities', *Clin. Pharmacol. Ther.* **50**: 508–19.

Kalow, W. and Tang, B. K. (1993) 'The use of caffeine for enzyme assays: a critical appraisal', *Clin. Pharmacol. Ther.* **53**: 503–14.

Kalow, W., Ozdemir, V., Tang, B.-K., Tothfalusi, L. and Endrenyi, L. (1999) 'The science of pharmacological variability: an essay', *Clin. Pharmacol. Ther.* **66**: 445–7.

Kawajiri, K., Watanabe, J., Eguchi, H., Nakachi, K., Kiyohara, C. and Hayashi, S. (1995) 'Polymorphisms of human Ah receptor gene are not involved in lung cancer', *Pharmacogenetics* **5**: 151–8.

Kellermann, G., Shaw, C. R. and Luyten-Kellermann, M. (1973) 'Aryl hydrocarbon hydroxylase indicibility and bronchogenic carcinoma', *New Engl. J. Med.* **289**: 934–7.

Kimura, M. and Ohta, T. (1973) 'Mutation and evolution at the molecular level', *Genetics* **73**: 19–35.

Kragh-Hansen, U., Brennan, S. O., Galliano, M. and Sugita, O. (1989) 'Binding of warfarin, salicylate, and diazepam to genetic variants of human serum albumin with known mutations', *Molecular Pharmacology* **37**: 238–42.

Lambert, G. H., Schoeller, D. A., Humphrey, H. E. B., Kotake, A. N., Lietz, H., Campbell, M., Kalow, W., Spielberg, S. P. and Budd, M. (1990) 'The caffeine breath test and caffeine urinary metabolite ratios in the Michigan cohort exposed to polybrominated biphenyls: a preliminary study', *Environmental Health Perspectives* **89**: 175–81.

Lander, E. S. (1999) 'Array of hope', *Nature Genetics* **21** (Suppl): 3–4.

Lim, S. K., Sigmund, C. D., Gross, K. W. and Maquat, L. E. (1992) 'Nonsense codons in human b-globin mRNA results in the production of mRNA degradation products', *Mol. Cell. Biol.* **12**: 1149–61.

Ling, V. (1997) 'Multidrug resistance: molecular mechanisms and clinical relevance', *Cancer Chemotherapy & Pharmacology* **40**: 3–8.

Lockridge, O. (1992) 'Genetic variants of human serum butyrylcholinesterase influence the metabolism of the muscle relaxant succinylcholine', in M. Kalow (ed.) *Pharmacogenetics of Drug Metabolism*, Int. Encycl. Pharmacol. Therap. Sect. 137, Pergamon Press, New York, pp. 15–50.

Luzzatto, L. and Mehta, A. (1995) 'Glucose 6-phosphate dehydrogenase deficiency', in C. R. Scriver, A. L. Beaudet, W. S. Sly and D. Valle (eds) *The Metabolic and Molecular Bases of Inherited Disease*, Vol. 111, McGraw-Hill, Inc., New York, pp. 3367–98.

Ma, J. F., Grant, G. and Melera, P. W. (1997) 'Mutations in the sixth trans-membrane domain of P-glycoprotein that alter the pattern of cross-resistance also alter sensitivity to cyclosporin A reversal', *Mol. Pharmacol.* **51**: 922–30.

McLellan, R. A., Oscarson, M., Seidegard, J., Price Evans, D. A. and Ingelman-Sundberg, M. (1997) 'Frequent occurrence of CYP2D6 gene duplication in Saudi Arabians', *Pharmacogenetics* **7**: 187–91.

Mahgoub, A., Dring, L. G., Idle, J. R., Lancaster, R. and Smith, R. L. (1977) 'Polymorphic hydroxylation of debrisoquine in man', *Lancet* 2: 584–6.

Marez, D., Legrand, M., Sabbagh, N., Lo Guidice, J. M., Spire, C., Lafitte, J. J., Meyer, U. A. and Broly, F. (1997) 'Polymorphism of the cytochrome P450 CYP2D6 gene in a European population: characterization of 48 mutations and 53 alleles, their frequencies and evolution', *Pharmacogenetics* 7: 193–202.

Masimirembwa, C. M., Hasler, J. A., Bertilsson, L., Johansson, I., Ekberg, O. and Ingelman-Sundberg, M. (1996) 'Phenotype and genotype analysis of debrisoquine hydroxylase (CYP2D6) in a black Zimbabwean population. Reduced enzyme activity and evaluation of metabolic correlation of CYP2D6 probe drugs', *Eur. J. Clin. Pharmacol.* 51: 117–22.

Masson, P., Legrand, P., Bartels, C. F., Froment, M. T., Schopfer, L. M. and Lockridge, O. (1997) 'Role of aspartate 70 and tryptophan 82 in binding of succinyldithiocholine to human butyrylcholinesterase', *Biochemistry* 36: 2266–77.

Motulsky, A. G. (1960) 'Metabolic polymorphisms and the role of infectious diseases in human evoulation', *Hum. Biol.* 32: 28.

Nebert, D. W. (1979) 'Genetic differences in the induction of monooxygenase activities by polycylic aromatic compounds', *Pharmac. Ther.* 6: 395–417.

Nebert, D. W. (1988) 'The 1986 Bernard B. Brodie Award lecture. The genetic regulation of drug-metabolizing enzymes', *Drug Metab. Dispos.* 16: 1–8.

Patel, M. (1997) 'Genetic variability of an uridine-diphosphoglucuronosyl-trans-ferase: UGT2B7', University of Toronto, PhD Thesis.

Price Evans, D. A. (1993) *Genetic Aspects of Drug Therapy,* Cambridge University Press, Cambridge, pp. 1–655.

Primo-Parmo, S. L., Lightstone, H. and La Du, B. N. (1997) Characterization of an unstable variant (BChE 115D) of human butyrylcholinesterase', *Pharmaco-genetics* 7: 27–34.

Ramachandra, M., Ambudkar, S. V., Gottesman, M. M., Pastan, I. and Hrycyna, C. A. (1997) 'Functional characterization of a glycine 185–to-valine substitution in human P-glycoprotein by using a vaccinia-based transient expression system', *Mol. Biol. Cell.* 7: 1485–98.

Sachse, C., Brockmoller, J., Bauer, S., Cascorbi, I. and Roots, I. (1998) 'A novel C→A polymorphism in intron 1 of CYP1A2 is correlated with higher inducibility by smoking and is a potential risk factor for bladder cancer', poster at the 12th International Symposium on Microsomes and Drug Oxidations, Montpellier (France) July 20–24.

Shively, C. A. and Vesell, E. S. (1975) 'Temporal variations in acetaminophen and phenacetin half-life in man', *Clin. Pharmacol. Ther.* 18: 413–24.

Taguchi, Y., Morishima, M., Komano, T. and Ueda, K. (1997) 'Amino acid sub-stitutions in the first transmembrane domain (TM1) of P-glycoprotein that alter substrate specificity', *FEBS Lett.* 413: 142–6.

Van Veen, H. W., Callaghan, R., Soceneantu, L., Sardini, A., Konings, W. N. and Higgins, C. F. (1998) 'A bacterial antibiotic-resistance gene that complements the human multidrug-resistance P-glycoprotein gene', *Nature* 391: 291–5.

Vesell, E. S. (1992) 'Pharmacogenetic perspectives gained from twin and family studies', in W. Kalow (ed.) *Pharmacogenetics of Drug Metabolism,* Int. Encycl. Pharmacol. Therap. Sect. 137, Pergamon Press, New York, pp. 843–63.

Vesell, E. S. and Page, J. G. (1969) 'Genetic control of the phenobarbital-induced shortening of plasma antipyrine half-lives in man', *J. Clin. Invest.* 48: 2202–9.

Vogel, F. and Motulsky, A. G. (1986) *Human Genetics. Problems and Approaches,* Springer-Verlag, Berlin, pp. 1–807.

Weber, W. W. (1997) *Pharmacogenetics,* Oxford University Press, Oxford, New York.

Weber, W. W. and Vatsis, K. P. (1995) 'Human N-acetyltransferases: genetic polymorphism and metabolic profiles of the major isoforms', in G. M. Pacifici and G. N. Fracchia (eds) *Advances in Drug Metabolism in Man,* European Commission, Luxembourg, pp. 353–405.

Whysner, J., Ross, P. M. and Williams, G. M. (1996) 'Phenobarbital mechanistic data and risk assessment: enzyme induction, enhanced cell proliferation, and tumor promotion', *Pharmacol. Ther.* 71: 153–91.

Wong, J. M. Y., Harper, P. A., Meyer, U. A., Bock, K. W., Mörike, K., Lagueux, J., Ayotte, P., Tyndale, R. F., Sellers, E. M., Manchester, D. K. and Okey, A. B. (2001) 'Ethnic variability in the allelic distribution of human aryl hydrocarbon receptor condon 554 and assessment of variant receptor function in vitro', *Pharmacogenetics* 11: 85–94.

Woolhouse, N. M., Eichelbaum, M., Oates, N. S., Idle, J. R. and Smith R. L. (1985) 'Dissociation of co-regulatory control of debrisoquin/phenformin and sparteine oxidation in Ghanaians,' *Clin. Pharmacol. The.* 37: 512–21.

Yue, Q. Y., Iselius, L. and Sawe, J. (1997) 'Indices and graphical approaches for the detection of interindividual and interethnic variations in codeine metabolism', *Br. J. Clin, Pharmacol.* 44: 239–44.

Chapter 2

Interethnic differences in drug disposition and effects

L. Bertilsson and W. Kalow

Abbreviations

ADH, alcohol dehydrogenase; ALDH, aldehyde dehydrogenase; CYP, member of the cytochrome P450 family of enzymes; EM, extensive metaboliser, (phrase originally coined to describe normal metabolism of debrisoquine); G-6-pD, glucose-6-phosphate dehydrogenase; MR, metabolic ratio, defined as the ratio parent drug/metabolite in urine, indicating phenotype; NAT2, N-acetyltransferase type 2; NAT1, N-acetyltransferase type 1; PM, poor metaboliser (phrase originally coined to describe deficient metabolism of debrisoquine); RFLP, restriction fragment length polymorphism; PCR, polymerase chain reaction.

Historical introduction

Serious attention to interethnic or interracial differences in drug response started with the rise of pharmacogenetics: during the second world war, primaquine hemolysis was observed in the US army; it occurred mostly in black soldiers. Studies after the war revealed the cause of the drug-induced hemolysis to be a genetic deficiency of glucose-6-phosphate dehydrogenase (G-6-pD) (Carson *et al.*, 1956). Later, the racial differences could be explained by an association between G-6-pD deficiency and ability to survive Falciparum malaria; that is, the deficiency conveyed a biological advantage in malaria-infested countries and therefore accumulated in such countries (Vulliamy *et al.*, 1992). Another early observation was the distinction between genetically slow and fast acetylators of isoniazid (Bonicke and Reif, 1953; Hughes *et al.*, 1954) and the realisation that the proportion of slow acetylators varied widely between human populations (Evans, 1992). In short, the fact that there could be interracial or interethnic differences in drug response on a genetic basis has been well established since the 1950s. However, the occurrence of such differences was perceived as something exceptional.

In later years, among physicians it was mostly the psychiatrists who emphasised ethnic differences in drug response, and who registered geographical differences in the standard doses of various antipsychotic drugs (Griffith, 1977; Katz, 1979; Comas-Diaz and Jacobsen, 1991). Such differences were often labeled with terms that tended to discount genetic factors (e.g. cross-cultural, transcultural).

During the past few decades, immigration has turned the city of Toronto in Canada into one with an ethnically mixed population. When testing student volunteers at the University of Toronto in studies of the metabolism of amobarbital and of debrisoquine, interethnic differences of metabolic pathways showed up as incidental observations (Kalow, 1982 a, b). These observations became a signal beacon and stimulated searches for other interethic differences in drug metabolism and response. The term "pharmacoanthropology" was applied as being neutral in respect to nature-nurture questions, and as emphasising science rather than politics (Kalow 1984 a, b; 1992 a, b).

Whatever terminology may be finally chosen to circumscribe the topic, pertinent observations have greatly increased during recent years, and the international pharmaceutical industry, as well as many regulatory agencies, pay increasing attention to interethnic variation in pharmacologic and toxic response characteristics (Hahn, 1992; Holloway and Yam, 1992; Persidis, 1998).

The review articles of the topic by Kalow (1991), Wood and Zhou (1991), Kudzma (1992), and Kalow and Bertilsson (1994) present many examples. The review by Johnson (1997) specialises in discussions of mechanism-related ethnic differences like active transport, blood flow, and protein binding, besides metabolism. There are two specialised books (Kalow *et al.*, 1986, and Lin *et al.*, 1993). A volume entitled *Pharmacogenetics of Drug Metabolism* (Kalow, 1992b) contains many accounts of differences of drug-metabolising enzymes between populations.

The purpose of this review is to present the background and general principles of pharmacoanthropology. This is to be followed by an overview of documented cases with emphasis on the most instructive and best investigated examples. We did not attempt to establish a complete registry of cases.

The fundamental factors that may create interethnic differences in drug response

Clearly genetic factors

Pharmacogenetics

Most variations classified as pharmacogenetic deal with variants definable as monogenic on the basis of either DNA data, biochemical studies, observations in families or kinships, or of non-normal frequency distributions in a population.

Pharmacogenetics accounts for the currently most important aspect of pharmacoanthropology, namely the part that deals with allelic variants of substantial frequency, that is, polymorphic, monogenic variants. Besides the malaria-associated occurrence of glucose-6-phosphate-dehydrogenase deficiency (G-6-pD), the great majority of such variants are found among drug-metabolising enzymes. A case in point is the deficiency of the debrisoquine/sparteine oxidase, i.e. of "CYP2D6" by modern designation (see, The CYP2D6 polymorphism).

Person-to-person variation of these xenobiotic-metabolising enzymes is prominent, and many allelic variants have high frequencies. It is an important observation that allele frequencies usually differ between the races. A recent count showed thirty-one drug-metabolising enzymes to be genetically variable within a population; mostly Caucasian (European) populations were tested. Of these variable enzymes, twenty-seven (81%) also showed interethnic differences in allele frequency; most comparisons were with Asian populations (Kalow, unpublished).

Interethnic differences in allele frequency have two consequences (Kalow, 1991; 1992b). One way is simple and straightforward: if the allele causes formation of, for example, an enzyme variant that represents a deficiency, the proportion of persons with this deficiency tend to differ between populations. For instance, homozygotes for CYP2D6 deficiency, who are detectable by their inability to hydroxylate debrisoquine, represent about 7% of the population in Europe, but less than 1% in East Asia (see, The CYP2D6 polymorphism). The second consequence is frequently overlooked: the presence of deficiency homozygotes implies that there must be heterozygotes, i.e. persons with one functional and one deficiency gene who might have on average half the full enzyme activity. As individuals, these may not be reliably detectable by functional tests, but a population of heterozygotes is likely to average half the full enzyme activity. It follows from the Hardy–Weinberg law that the heterozygotes are always much more frequent than the deficiency homozygotes (i.e. if the allele frequencies are $p+q=1$, the genotype frequencies are $p^2+2pq+q^2=1$). Hence the presence of the heterozygotes may noticeably lower the average enzyme activity of a population. Considering populations with 7% and 1% deficiency homozygotes, the heterozygote frequencies would be 39% and 18%, respectively.

This review will mostly deal with these relatively common, interethnic differences of allele frequency that represent monogenic, often polymorphic, variants; the reason is that they have been best investigated. However, as will be discussed under Nature/Nurture problems below, there are also clearcut interethnic differences of multifactorial nature.

Population genetics

Drug developers and regulating bodies have yet to work out in which populations a new drug may require new testing. To illustrate the problem, one may ask, for example, whether a drug developed in Britain needs re-evaluation for use in Poland or in Greece or in North Africa, or to what extent a drug evaluation in Beijing would be valid for Taiwan, Japan, or Thailand. This is a principally unsolved problem with implications which affect the testing of minorities within a country, particularly in countries with many immigrants such as the USA and Canada (Holloway and Yam, 1992). However, China also has fifty-five minorities which make up approximately 67 million people (Etler, 1992). The thorough study of Czeizel *et al.* (1991) defined ten ethnic groups with some pharmacogenetic implications within present-day Hungary.

Obvious differences have been used throughout the ages to distinguish human populations. First, there are differences in appearance such as skin color, body size, or facial characteristics. A second big divider is language. Third, there are cultural differences such as different religions, or customs which have independently evolved as a consequence of geography. Such differences, or the sum of several such differences, have been the basis for the traditional divisions between human races, or ethnic groups. This has changed with the entry of genetics into anthropology.

During the past few decades, studies of origin and classification of human populations have been shaped prominently by the work of the geneticists Nei (1987) and Cavalli-Sforza *et al.* (1988). Both have based their population studies on counts of numerous gene freqencies. Cavalli-Sforza used these to measure genetic distances between forty-two different human populations. The comparison between these populations led to 1,722 measurements of genetic distance between two populations, each measurement presented in the form of a best estimate and its range of error. He condensed this vast array of data into a representation of nine clusters of genetically close populations, as shown in Figure 2.1. This Figure represents similar conclusions as those reached by Nei, except that Nei (1987) envisioned a much shorter separation time between southeast Asians and the natives of New Guinea and Australia.

One interesting feature of this tree is the relatively early separation between southeast Asian and northeast Asian populations. This is important since most Chinese are of the southeast Asian group, while Korean and Japanese populations belong to the northeast Asian branch. However, the most important characteristic is the early separation of the sub-Sahara African populations from all other populations. Thus the genetic distance between any of the sub-Saharan African population on the one hand, and Europeans and Asians on the other, is very much larger than between any other population groups. It should mean that when investigating African populations for pharmacogenetic variability, there are bound to be

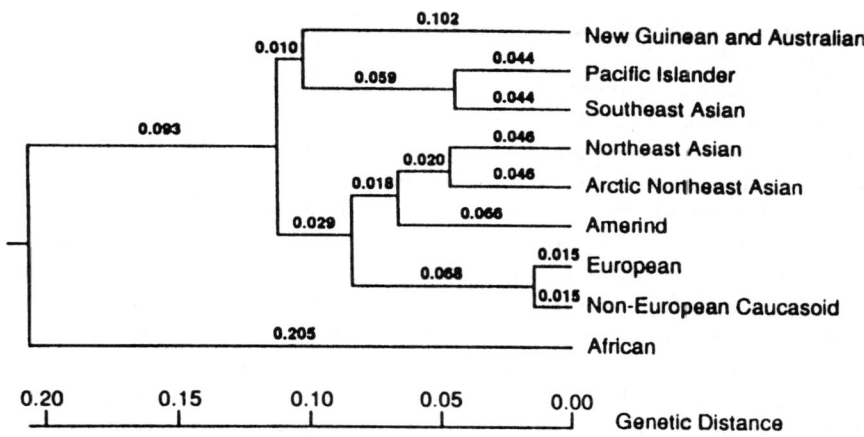

Figure 2.1 Linkage tree depicting data for nine major human populations. Condensed data from a linkage tree constructed originally for forty-two populations on the basis of 120 measured allele frequencies. The abscissa indicates genetic distances, reflecting separation times; the separation between African (sub-Saharan) and non-African populations took place about 100,000 years ago, that between South Asians and Australians about 55,000, that between Caucasoids and North-East Asians approximately 43,000 years ago.
From Figure 2.3.3 and Table 2.5.1 by Cavalli-Sforza et al. (1994).

surprises. It also means that for drugs to be introduced into Africa, there is a special need for safety investigations. This is a topic in which economic and scientific interests could clash.

Nature/nurture problems

Within populations, family and twin studies usually permit a distinction between genetic and environmental causes of interindividual differences (Vesell, 1992), but these methods are usually not available for the classification of interethnic differences. The use of DNA-based methods is therefore mandatory to study the genetic component in interethnic differences. It is not surprising that recombinant methodology is more and more used in the pharmaceutical industry for the study of those interethnic differences which have their origin in pharmacogenetics.

However, it is worth keeping in mind that population differences in drug response may reflect a complex situation. For instance, it has long been known that hypertensive disease is much more frequent in urban Blacks as compared with most Whites (Freis, 1986). The magnitude of the genetic contribution to this difference tends to be masked by covariables (Winkleby et al., 1988). The racially different therapeutic drug responses might reflect differences in causative pathology of the disease rather than inherent racial differences of pharmacological responsiveness (Aviv and Aladjem, 1990).

An instructive example of a decision analysis considering ethnicity and gender has been presented by Jordan *et al.* (1991) before using isoniazid for tuberculosis treatment. Here, as in other cases, ethnicity is one of several factors that may have to be weighed against each other.

Within populations, the vast majority of interindividual differences in drug response or metabolism with normal or near-normal frequency distributions is registered in terms of standard deviation – without any attempt to find the cause or causes of such variation, or without the more modest attempt to measure the heritability of such variation. However, variations which are left undefined when studying a single population may give rise to a mean difference when two or more populations are studied, thereby calling for an explanation. A case in point is the glucuronidation of codeine which shows unremarkable normal variation (Figure 2.2) in both Swedes and Chinese (Yue and Säwe, 1992). However, the average glucuronidation of codeine differs sufficiently between Chinese and Swedes (Yue and Säwe, 1992) to be likely of clinical significance. Kalow *et al.* (1998,

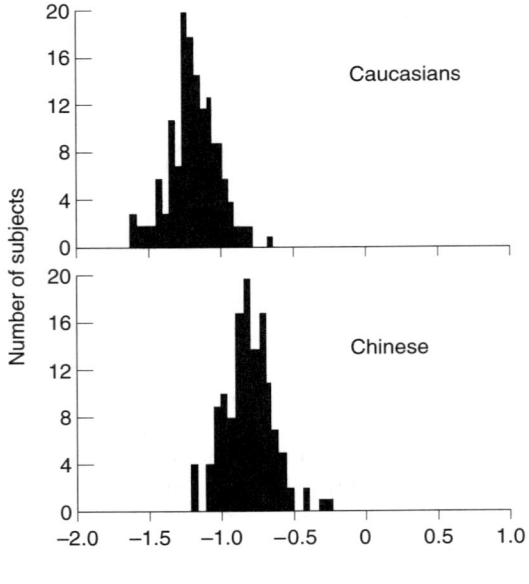

Figure 2.2 Frequency distributions of the log MRs for codeine glucuronidation (codeine/glucuronide) in 149 Caucasians and 133 Chinese.
Reprinted from Yue *et al.*, 1989b with permission of the copyright holder, Blackwell Scientific Publisher, Ltd., Oxford.

1999) are therefore investigating a new method that seems to facilitate an assessment of the genetic component in many cases of Gaussian variation; in essence, the method consists in comparing the inter- and intraindividual magnitudes of variation.

It has been pointed out before (Kalow 1991, 1992b) that a difference between population averages in drug response may be epidemiologically significant even if the difference is relatively small in comparison to the scatter of data within each population. The reason is the likely lack of overlap between the edges of the two distribution curves (Figure 2.3). In other words, the number of subjects represented by curve segments above or below a certain critical value may grossly differ between the two curves; hence the proportion of subjects suffering from side-effects of a drug may differ substantially between such populations.

Person-to-person variation of a drug effect within each of two populations may register as mostly heritable – and yet one must consider the possibility that an average difference between these populations may be due to different climate or different customary food. Thus, heritability data in one population must be considered unreliable as an indicator of the

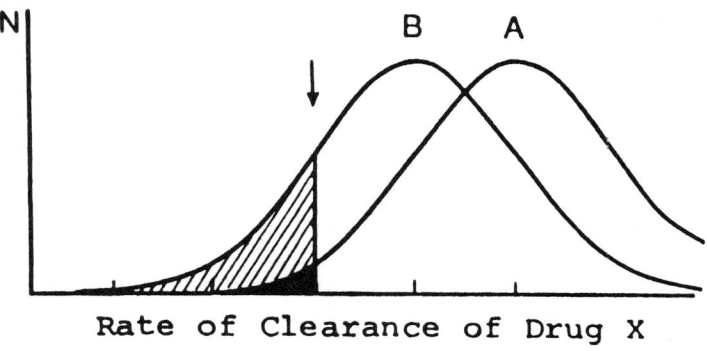

Figure 2.3 The edge effect of different averages. The hypothetical curves A and B represent normal frequency distributions for the elimination capacity of drug X in two populations; the abscissa registers the rate of drug clearance, the ordinate indicates the number of subjects who show a particular rate of clearance. The arrow indicates the critical rate below which the drug causes toxicity. Curves A and B have identical standard deviations but their means are one standard deviation apart. That is, the difference between the means is small compared with the range of variation within each population. Therefore, such differences are often neglected. The arrow is located two and one standard deviations below the means of A and B, respectively. These data imply that approximately 2% of population A (black area) and 16% of population B (shaded plus black area) would suffer toxicity from the standard dose of drug X. The eight-fold difference would grow substantially with the shift of the arrow towards lower values on the abscissa.

cause of an interethnic difference. A practical means to circumvent some of this difficulty is to study members of the same population in different environments, e.g., Indians living in Bombay and in London, or Chinese in China and in Sweden, or Blacks in rural or urban Africa.

Emphasis on environmental factors

In the four following brief sections, we will merely cite some environmental factors which are known to affect drug response, and which, therefore, by their presence or absence might create population differences.

Climate

Climatic differences dictate the availability of different foods – thereby asserting an indirect effect of climate. Both cold acclimation or adjustment to hot surroundings go along with numerous physiological adaptations. These geographically determined differences of food (Velazquez and Bourges, 1984) or temperature (Schönbaum and Lomax, 1993) might be reflected in different pharmacological and toxicological responses to some drugs. However, systematic studies of climate-caused population differences in drug response seem to be missing.

Nutrition and lifestyle

Starvation, malnutrition, and protein deficiency – all are able to cause differences in drug disposition (Anderson et al., 1986). However, these leading factors can be assessed with relative ease and their effects discounted when the task is to compare populations for innate drug-metabolising capacities. There are inborn errors of nutrient metabolism (Rosenberg, 1984; Walcher and Kretchmer, 1993; Motulsky, 1996) which might directly or indirectly affect responsiveness to drugs or toxins. Interethnic differences are well known for lactose tolerance (Nei and Saitou, 1986) and for the fish-odor syndrome (Dolphin et al., 1997).

Induction of drug-metabolising enzymes by smoking is a well-established fact. It has been shown recently that the amount smoked is affected by the activity of the polymorphic P450 cytochrome CYP2A6 (Pianezza et al., 1998). Since the deficiency of CYP2A6 shows interethnic variability (Fernandez-Salguero et al., 1995), cigarette use will almost certainly differ between populations, causing the concentration of inducible drug-metabolising enzymes to vary. Enzyme induction by certain foods (Okey, 1992), or inhibition of such enzymes by drugs, contraceptives, environmental toxicants, or foods (e.g., naringenin in grapefruit) (Fuhr et al., 1993) could cause population differences in drug metabolism which may be difficult to assess, particularly if the modifying sources are obscure.

Health

Comparisons betweeen populations in different states of health will be medically important and may serve as a means to study the effects of a disease, but such comparisons would not contribute to any assessment of innate differences in responsiveness to drugs. For instance, we have never seen the average capacity for caffeine metabolism by CYP1A2 as low as in a group of children in Zimbabwe from an area with much bilharziosis (Masimirembwa *et al.*, 1995).

A situation of special interest may be encountered if the incidence or severity of a disease differs between populations. A case in point is the association between exposure to malaria and the occurrence of G-6-pD deficiency. This deficiency in turn may cause drug-induced hemolysis, an effect virtually limited to malaria-exposed populations. There are many genetic factors which affect susceptibility to infectious disease. In most cases, it is unknown whether these factors differ between populations and whether they might alter any response to a drug or toxicant.

Cultural factors

Today, most psychiatrists have come to recognise the existence of pharmacogenetic factors that may cause interethnic differences in response to neuroleptic and antidepressant drugs, as evident in the book by Lin *et al.* (1993). In addition there is in psychiatry a rich literature on cultural factors that may affect the nature, frequency, and persistence of mental disorders, and that may also influence toxic and therapeutic responses to drugs (e.g., Lefley, 1990). An example is the need for a practising psychiatrist to consider and to utilise the family setting of a patient in order to achieve success with a particular drug therapy. This need differs much between societies in which family and clan associations are differently valued; hence, neglect of family factors may cause therapeutic failure more readily in some than in other populations.

Other differences are reflected in attitudes towards disease and cure. Cost and inconvenience, as well as expectations, may affect both compliance and perception of benefit of a therapy. One should not forget that elements of witchcraft in drug therapy are ancient. They are real. Modern man talks about placebo effects instead of witchcraft.

The evolving body of knowledge: differences in drug metabolism

The cytochrome P450 system

General aspects of the CYP superfamily

The cytochrome P450 (CYP) superfamily of enzymes has over 100 different isozymes in mammals (see Gonzalez, 1992). These enzymes use oxygen to transform lipophilic compounds to more hydrophilic substances, which are mostly prone to phase II conjugation reactions. Both endo- and exogenous substances may be substrates for various CYP isozymes. In humans more than thirty CYP enzymes have been demonstrated. Reviews on various aspects of this important group of enzymes are available (Gonzalez, 1992; several chapters in Kalow, 1992b; Kalow and Bertilsson 1994; Ingelman-Sundberg *et al.*, 1999). We will here focus our attention on two polymorphic enzymes CYP2D6 ("debrisoquine/sparteine hydroxylase") and CYP2C19 ("S-mephenytoin hydroxylase"), where we have gained pronounced information of interethnic differences in the activity of these enzymes.

The CYP2D6 polymorphism

INTERETHNIC DIFFERENCES IN THE PM PHENOTYPES

Maghoub *et al.* (1977) and Tucker *et al.* (1977) found that hydroxylation of the antihypertensive drug debrisoquine is polymorphic in nature. In independent studies, Eichelbaum *et al.* (1979) showed that the oxidation of sparteine also is polymorphic. Initially the metabolic reaction was thought to be an N-oxidation, but it was later found to be a C-hydroxylation followed by dehydration. Several studies in Caucasians have shown that poor metabolisers (PMs) of debrisoquine are also PMs of sparteine and a close correlation between the metabolic ratios (MRs) of the two drugs was found ($r_s=0.91$; $n=38$; $p<0.001$; Eichelbaum *et al.*, 1982). In contrast, Woolhouse *et al.* (1985) found in Ghana that PMs of debrisoquine were extensive metabolisers (EMs) of sparteine. Masimirembwa *et al.* (1996a) found a similar discrepancy between the two CYP2D6 substrates debrisoquine and metoprolol in Zimbabweans. The reason for the difference between Caucasians and Africans in this respect remains to be elucidated.

The incidence of PMs of debrisoquine has been investigated in many populations, in most of them with a fairly small number of subjects (see Eichelbaum and Gross, 1992). Among 1,011 Swedish Caucasians, sixty-nine (6.28%) were found to be PMs of debrisoquine (Table 2.1 and Figure 2.4) (Bertilsson *et al.*, 1992). This incidence is very similar to what has been shown for other European (see Alván *et al.*, 1990) and American (Nakamura *et al.*, 1985) Caucasian populations.

Four different Chinese nationalities, i.e., Han, Mongolian, Wei, and Zang, were phenotyped with debrisoquine by Professor Lou and associates in Beijing (Bertilsson *et al.*, 1992). The incidence of PMs was very low in all four populations (1.8, 0.78, 0.65 and 1.48%, respectively) and the distributions of MRs were similar. Figure 2.4 (upper panel) shows the combined data from 695 Chinese obtained from these four groups (Bertilsson *et al.*, 1992). Seven (1.01%) were PMs using the antimode of

Table 2.1 Incidence of PMs of debrisoquine (MR>12.6) and of S-mephenytoin (S/R ratio >0.9) in a Chinese and a Swedish population

Hydroxylation polymorphism	Chinese subjects		Swedish subjects		
	PM/total	%	PM/total	%	p
Debrisoquine	7/695	1.01	69/1011	6.82	<0.0001
S-mephenytoin	20/137	14.6	16/488	3.28	<0.0001

Notes
Reproduced by permission from Bertilsson *et al.* (1992).

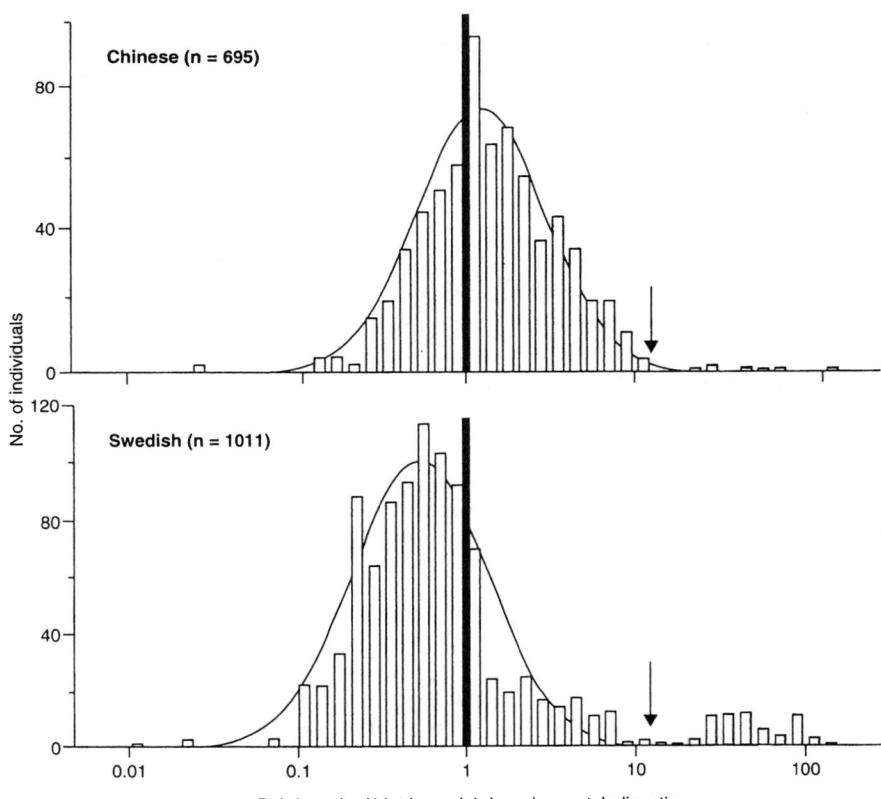

Figure 2.4 Distribution of the urinary debrisoquine/4-hydroxydebrisoquine metabolic ratio (MR) in 695 Chinese and 1,011 Swedish healthy subjects. The arrows indicate MR=12.6, the antimode between EM and PM. A line is drawn at MR=1. Most Chinese EM have MR>1, while most Swedish EM have MR<1. Reproduced by permission from Bertilsson *et al.* (1992).

MR = 12.6 obtained from Caucasian populations. A similarly low incidence of PM has been demonstrated in studies of Japanese (Nakamura *et al.*, 1985) and Koreans (Sohn *et al.*, 1991).

It is apparent in Figure 2.4 that the distribution of the MR of Chinese EMs is shifted to the right compared with Swedish EMs (Kolmogorov-Smirnov test; $p < 0.01$; Bertilsson *et al.*, 1992). Most Swedes have MR < 1, whereas the opposite is true for Chinese subjects. These results show that the mean rate of hydroxylation of debrisoquine is lower in Chinese EMs compared with Caucasian EMs.

INTERETHNIC DIFFERENCES IN CYP2D6 ALLELES CAUSING DECREASED ENZYME ACTIVITY

The gene encoding the CYP2D6 enzyme has been localised to chromosome 22 (Eichelbaum *et al.*, 1987). Using restriction fragment length polymorphism (RFLP) analysis after hydrolysis with the *Xba*I restriction enzyme, Skoda *et al.* (1988) identified two mutant alleles reflected by 11.5 and 44 kb fragments which were present in the PM phenotype. The 11.5 kb fragment had a deletion of the entire *CYP2D6* gene (Gaedigk *et al.*, 1991), while the 44 kb fragment contains an inserted pseudogene (Heim and Meyer, 1992). A 29 kb fragment was linked both to mutated and unmutated alleles. With allele specific-PCR (polymerase chain reaction) amplification Heim and Meyer (1990) could distinguish the "wild-type" 29 kb fragment from those with point mutations called A ("frame shift mutation") and B ("splicing mutation"). The A, B and deletion alleles are now termed *CYP2D6*3*, *4* and *5*, respectively (Daly *et al.*, 1996). In Caucasians the *CYP2D6*4* accounts for more than 75% of the mutant *CYP2D6* alleles (Broly *et al.*, 1991; Dahl *et al.*, 1992). The *4* allele is almost absent in Chinese and this is the reason for the low incidence of 1% PM in this population compared with 7% in Caucasians. The occurrence of the gene deletion (*CYP2D6*5*) is very similar, i.e., about 5% in Caucasians, Orientals and Black Africans. This shows that this is a very old mutation, which occurred before the separation of the three major human races 100–150,000 years ago (see Figure 2.1).

The right shift of the distribution of MR in Chinese EMs shown in Figure 2.4 was puzzling ever since the first study was performed in Chinese (Lou *et al.*, 1987). First we thought that there were differences between debrisoquine analytical methods used in Beijing and Stockholm, but this could be excluded. In a series of molecular genetic investigations (Yue *et al.*, 1989a; Johansson *et al.*, 1991), we could finally show that 51% of Chinese *CYP2D6* alleles contain a C188T causing a Pro34Ser amino acid substitution (Johansson *et al.*, 1994). This gives an unstable enzyme with decreased catalytic activity. As shown in Figure 2.5 the presence of this C188T mutation causes the right shift among the investigated 152 Koreans (Roh *et al.*, 1996a). The frequency of this allele *CYP2D6*10* is about 50%

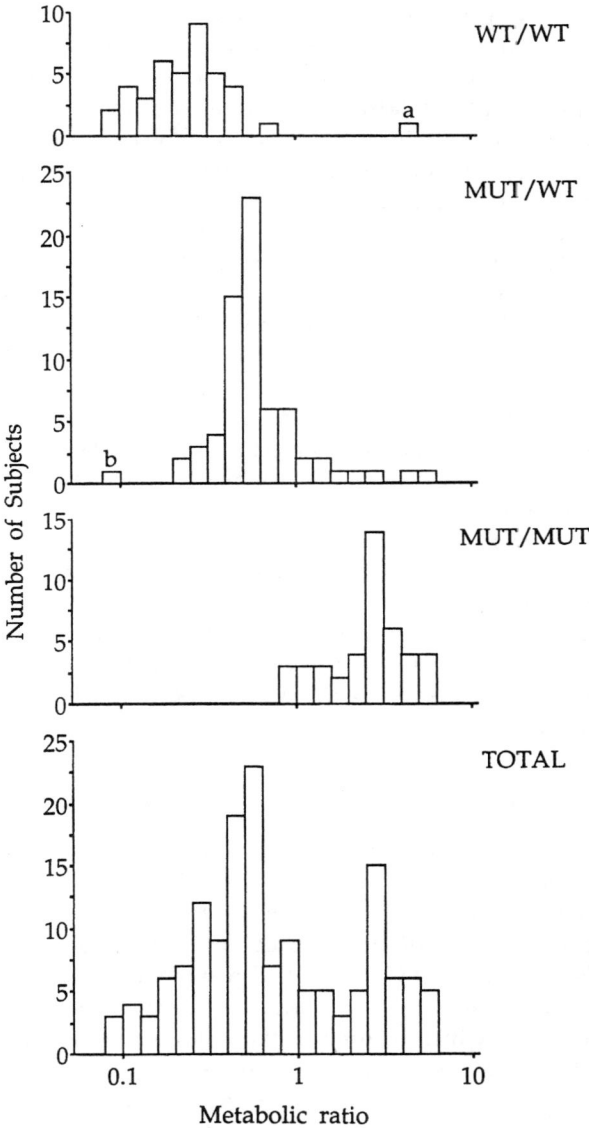

Figure 2.5 Distribution of the debrisoquine metabolic ratio in three genotype groups related to *CYP2D6*10* allele and in the total population of 152 Korean subjects. WT/WT, subjects homozygous for the wt allele (no $C^{188}{\to}T$ mutation) (n=40); MUT/WT, subjects heterozygotes (n=69); MUT/MUT, subjects homozygous for the *CYP2D6*10* allele (n=43); a, subject with an *Eco*RI fragment with a length between 9.4 kb and 12.1 kb, indicative of a new variant of *CYP2D6* gene; b, subject with a 12.1 kb *Eco*RI haplotype, indicative of the *CYP2D6*2X2* allele. Reproduced by permission from Roh *et al.* (1996a).

and similar among Chinese, Japanese and Koreans. Wang *et al.* (1993) found very similar results in Chinese living in Taiwan.

In studies on the hydroxylation of debrisoquine in Black Zimbabweans, Masimirembwa *et al.* (1996b) found a right shift in the MR of EM similar to that found in Orientals. A mutated allele was subsequently identified and *CYP2D6*17* encodes an enzyme with decreased activity. Among Black Africans, the frequency of this allele is 34% in Zimbabweans (Masimirembwa *et al.*, 1996b), 17% in Tanzanians (Wennerholm *et al.*, 1999) and 9% in Ethiopians (Aklillu *et al.*, 1996).

There are thus population-specific *CYP2D6* alleles with the *4 in Caucasians encoding no enzyme and the *10 and *17 alleles in Orientals and Africans, respectively, encoding an enzyme with decreased activity. In Caucasians and Orientals a close geno- and phenotype relationship has been demonstrated in several studies. Wennerholm *et al* (1999) have recently shown, when excluding subjects with *CYP2D6*3, *4, *5, *6, *10* and *17, that the debrisoquine MR is higher (lower CYP2D6 activity) in black Tanzanians compared with Swedish and Korean healthy subjects (Roh *et al.*, 1996a). In the three respective groups, subjects with MR >1 comprised 41, 7 and 0% of the EM populations with *CYP2D6*1 or *2 only. Novel mutations causing decreased CYP2D6 activity in Tanzanians were investigated, but not found. Wennerholm *et al.* (1999) discuss possible environmental factors which could cause this decreased activity: inhibition by food constituents, downregulation by cytokines or interferon as a consequence of common infections, etc.

ULTRARAPID METABOLISM CAUSED BY CYP2D6 GENE DUPLICATION/AMPLIFICATION

The problems in treating PMs of debrisoquine with various drugs have been discussed many times over the years (see Eichelbaum and Gross, 1992). Much less attention has been given to patients at the other extreme of the distribution of MR, i.e. the ultrarapid hydroxylators. Some years ago, Bertilsson *et al.* (1985) described a woman with depression having an MR of debrisoquine of 0.07, who had to be treated with 500 mg of nortriptyline daily, which is three to five times the recommended dose. The molecular basis for the ultrarapid hydroxylation in this patient and in another who had to be treated with megadoses of clomipramine was later demonstrated (Bertilsson *et al.*, 1993). These patients had an XbaI 42 kb fragment containing two different functionally active *CYP2D6* genes in the *CYP2D* locus causing extra enzyme to be expressed. The same year a father and his daughter and son with twelve extra copies of the *CYP2D6* gene were described (Johansson *et al.*, 1993). This is the first demonstration of an inherited amplification of an active gene coding for a drug-metabolising enzyme. These subjects were ultrarapid hydroxylators of debrisoquine with MR 0.01–0.02. The 12.1 kb fragment obtained by

*Eco*RI RFLP analysis corresponds to the presence of a duplicated *CYP2D6*2* gene in the *CYP2D* locus (Johansson *et al.*, 1993). There are also a few examples of duplicated *CYP2D6*1* and **4* alleles (Bernal *et al.*, 1999).

The frequency of subjects having duplicated/multiduplicated genes has been shown to be 1–2% in a Swedish population (Dahl *et al.*, 1995), 3.6% in Germans (Sachse *et al.*, 1997), 10% in Northern (Bernal *et al.*, 1999) and 7% in Southern Spain (Agundez *et al.*, 1995) and as high as 29% in Black Ethiopians (Aklillu *et al.*, 1996) and 20% in Saudi Arabians (McLellan *et al.*, 1997). There is thus a European-African north-south gradient in the incidence *CYP2D6* gene duplication. The high incidence among Ethiopians and Saudi Arabians indicates that the high frequency in Spain may have an ancestry in the Arabian conquest in the Mediterranean area (Bernal *et al.*, 1999). The high frequency of duplicated genes among the Arabs might be the result of a dietary pressure favoring the preservation of duplicated *CYP2D6* genes because of the ability of the enzyme to metabolise plant toxins including alkaloids (McLellan *et al.*, 1997).

European subjects with *CYP2D6* gene duplication have been shown to be ultrarapid metabolisers of debrisoquine with MR usually between 0.01 and 0.15 (Dahl *et al.*, 1995; Bernal *et al.*, 1999). In Black Ethiopians, however, subjects with multiple *CYP2D6* genes have higher MR usually between 0.1 and 1 (Aklillu *et al.*, 1996). These subjects thus do not have the ultrarapid metabolism of debrisoquine demonstrated for Caucasians with multiple genes. This might be due to environmental factors in Africa causing a decreased CYP2D6 activity as discussed for Tanzanians (Wennerholm *et al.*, 1999).

SUBSTRATES OF CYP2D6 AND INTERETHNIC DIFFERENCES IN THEIR METABOLISM

Since the discovery of the polymorphic metabolism of debrisoquine/sparteine during the 1970s, several important drugs have been shown to be metabolised by CYP2D6 (Eichelbaum and Gross, 1992). Table 2.2 shows some of these drugs. Substrates of CYP2D6 are all lipophilic bases. Koymans *et al.* (1992) have developed a computer-based model of the active site of the enzyme. This model may be able to predict novel substrates for CYP2D6.

Whether a drug is metabolised by CYP2D6 or not may be investigated in many different ways both *in vitro* and *in vivo*. To establish the quantitative importance of the enzyme for the total metabolism of the drug, *in vivo* studies need to be performed. We will here give two examples with nortriptyline and haloperidol. The tricyclic antidepressant nortriptyline was one of the first clinically important drugs to be demonstrated to be metabolised by CYP2D6 (Bertilsson *et al.*, 1980; Mellström *et al.*, 1981) (Table 2.2). These studies were performed in panels of healthy subjects and

Table 2.2 Some drugs whose metabolism is catalysed by the CYP2D6 enzyme, i.e. the debrisoquine/sparteine hydroxylase

β-Adrenoceptor blockers	Antidepressants	Neuroleptics
Metoprolol	Amitriptyline	Haloperidol
Propranolol	Clomipramine	Perphenazine
Timolol	Desipramine	Risperidone
	Fluoxetine	Thioridazine
Antiarrythmic drugs	Fluvoxamine	Zuclopenthixol
Encainide	Imipramine	
Flecainide	Mianserine	*Miscellaneous*
Perhexiline	Nortriptyline	Codeine
Propafenone	Paroxetine	Debrisoquine
Sparteine		Dextromethophan
		Perhexiline
		Phenformin

the results have been confirmed *in vivo* in patients and *in vitro* using human liver microsomes. In a recent study by Dalén *et al.* (1998), nortriptyline was given as a single oral dose to twenty-one healthy Swedish Caucasian subjects with different genotypes. As shown in Figure 2.6 there is a decrease in the plasma concentration of nortriptyline from subjects with no functional *CYP2D6* genes (5PM with the *CYP2D6*4/*4* genotype), to those with 1, 2 and 3 (gene duplication) functional genes (five in each group). Plasma concentrations of nortriptyline were extremely low in one subject with 13 *CYP2D6* genes. This is the son in the family mentioned above (genotype *CYP2D6*2x13/*4*). The plasma concentrations of the formed metabolite 10–hydroxynortriptyline show the opposite pattern, i.e., highest concentrations in the subject with thirteen genes and lowest in PM (Figure 2.6). As depicted in Figure 2.7 there was a close relationship between the clearance of nortriptyline and the debrisoquine MR in these Caucasian subjects. This study clearly demonstrates the impact of the detrimental *CYP2D6*4* allele, as well as the duplication/amplification of the *CYP2D6*2* gene on the metabolism of the two drugs debrisoquine and nortriptyline (Dalén *et al.*, 1998).

Yue *et al.* (1998) investigated the influence of the Asian specific *CYP2D6*10* allele on nortriptyline disposition in Chinese subjects living in Sweden. The protocol was identical to that of Dalén *et al.* (1998) in Caucasians. Five subjects in each group with the genotypes *CYP2D6*1/*1*, *CYP2D6*1/*10* and *CYP2D6*10/*10* i.e. with 0, 1 and 2 *10 alleles were given a single oral dose of notriptyline. Figure 2.8 shows the relationship between nortriptyline clearance and debrisoquine MR in these fifteen Chinese subjects. There was a clear decrease of the CYP2D6 activity by the *CYP2D6*10* allele as measured by both debrisoquine and nortriptyline disposition. The Chinese subjects with *CYP2D6*10/*10* (Figure 2.8) have, compared with Caucasian PM with the genotype *CYP2D6*4/*4*, a higher mean nortriptyline clearance (0.80 versus 0.32 l/h/kg) and

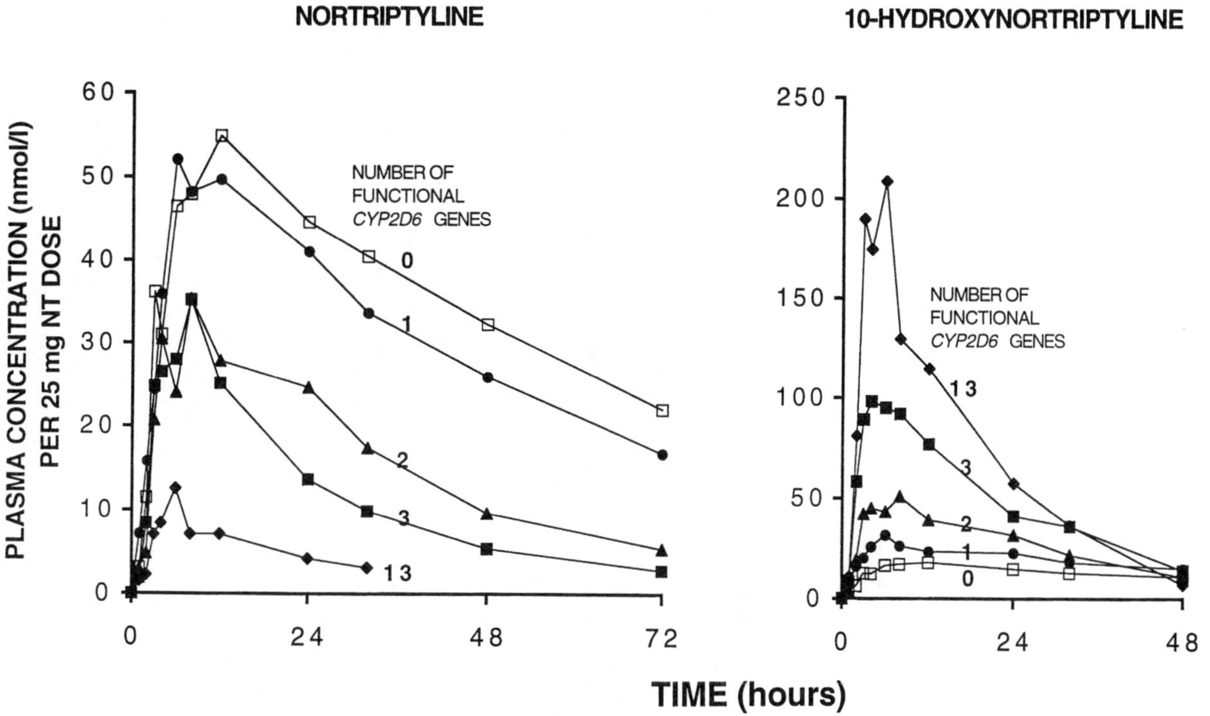

NORTRIPTYLINE

10-HYDROXYNORTRIPTYLINE

NUMBER OF
FUNCTIONAL
CYP2D6 GENES

0
1
2
3
13

NUMBER OF
FUNCTIONAL
CYP2D6 GENES

13
3
2
1
0

250

200

150

100

50

0

60

50

40

30

20

10

0

PLASMA CONCENTRATION (nmol/l)
PER 25 mg NT DOSE

0   24   48   72

0   24   48

TIME (hours)

Figure 2.6 Mean plasma concentrations of nortriptyline and 10-hydroxynortriptyline in different genotype groups after a single oral dose of nortriptyline. The numerals close to the curves represent the number of functional *CYP2D6* genes in each genotype group. In groups with 0–3 functional genes there are five subjects in each group. There is only one subject with thirteen functional genes. Reproduced by permission from Dalén *et al.* (1998).

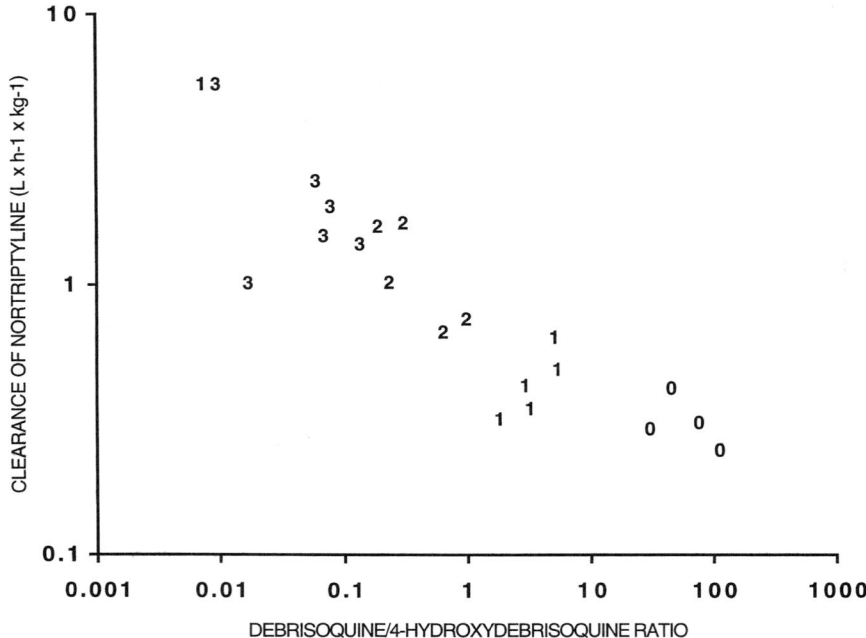

Figure 2.7 Relation between apparent oral plasma clearance of nortriptyline and the debrisoquine metabolic ratio for twenty subjects ($r_S = -0.89$; $p = 0.0001$). Numerals represent the number of functional genes in each subject. Reproduced by permission from Dalén *et al.* (1998).

lower debrisoquine MR (<12 and >12, respectively) (Figure 2.7). These studies show that the Asian *CYP2D6*10* allele encodes an enzyme with decreased activity. This effect is less pronounced than the Caucasian-specific *CYP2D6*4* allele which codes for no enzyme at all. Genotyping of *CYP2D6* may be a useful tool to predict the pharmacokinetics of CYP2D6 substrates in individual patients. It should, however, be remembered that there are population-specific alleles.

Desipramine, a tricyclic antidepressant similar to nortriptyline, is also hydroxylated by CYP2D6 (Bertilsson and Åberg-Wistedt, 1983). Rudorfer *et al.* (1984) gave a single oral dose of desipramine to sixteen Caucasian and fourteen Chinese healthy subjects. The mean total plasma clearance of desipramine was higher in Caucasians than in Chinese (123 and 74 l/h, respectively; $p < 0.05$). The difference was also significant when clearance was based on body weight. Although the investigated populations were of limited size, the study of Rudorfer *et al.* (1984) and other studies reviewed by Lin *et al.* (1991) indicate that Chinese metabolise antidepressants more slowly than do Caucasians. This fits with the right shift of the debrisoquine MR in Chinese compared with Caucasians (Figure 2.4), which is due to the

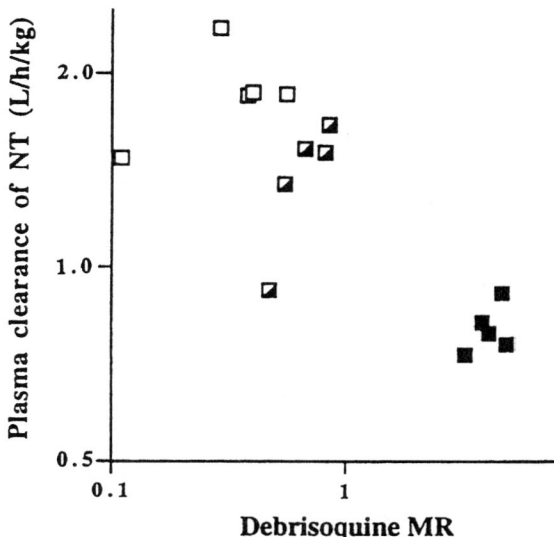

Figure 2.8 Relationship between the oral plasma clearance of nortriptyline after a single oral 25 mg dose and the debrisoquine metabolic ratio (MR) ($r_S = -0.71$; $p<0.01$) in three different genotypic Chinese groups with five subjects in each group. Solid squares, homozygous *CYP2D6*10*; half-solid squares, heterozygous *CYP2D6*1/*10*; open squares, homozygous *CYP2D6*1*. Reproduced by permission from Yue et al. (1998).

frequent occurrence of the *CYP2D6*10* in Oriental populations (Figure 2.5). Recently, Morita *et al.* (2000) showed a pronounced influence of the *CYP2D6*10* allele on the steady-state plasma levels of nortriptyline and its 10-hydroxy metabolite in Japanese patients. This explains at least partly why Orientals are generally treated with lower doses of antidepressants compared with Caucasians (Lou, 1990).

Llerena *et al.* (1992) gave single oral doses of haloperidol to a panel of six EMs and six PMs of debrisoquine (Figure 2.9). PMs eliminated haloperidol significantly slower than EMs, the mean plasma half-life being longer (29.4 and 16.3 h, respectively; $p<0.01$) and the mean clearance lower (1.16 and 2.49 L/h/kg, respectively; $p<0.05$) (Llerena *et al.*, 1992). In a clinical study involving eight Caucasian patients with schizophrenia treated with depot haloperidol (as the decanoate), the dopamine D2 receptor occupancy was determined by positron emission tomography 1 and 4 weeks after intramuscular injection of the drug (Nyberg *et al.*, 1995). One of the patients was genotypically a PM of debrisoquine. Of the group, he had the highest plasma concentration of haloperidol and also the highest D2 receptor occupancy.

Two studies from Hirosaki in Japan (Suzuki *et al.*, 1997; Mihara *et al.*, 1999) have shown a relationship between increased haloperidol plasma

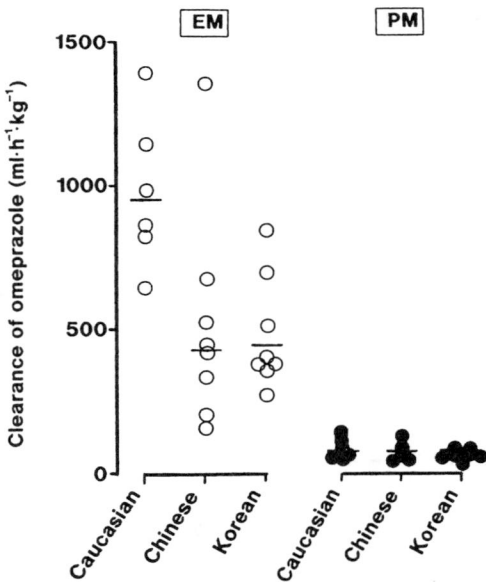

Figure 2.9 Individual oral clearance estimates of omeprazole observed in Caucasian (Swedish), Chinese, and Korean healthy subjects belonging to extensive metaboliser (EM) and poor metaboliser (PM) phenotypes of S-mephenytoin. Each subject received a single oral 20 mg dose of omeprazole. The horizontal lines indicate the geometric mean value in each of the groups. The clearance of omeprazole was significantly ($p < 0.001$) different between the EM and PM phenotypes in all three ethnic groups. However, among the three EM groups, the clearance was significantly higher in the Caucasian group than in the Chinese ($p < 0.05$) and Korean ($p < 0.01$) groups.
Reproduced by permission from Ishizaki *et al.* (1994).

concentrations and the presence of *CYP2D6*10* (and *5) alleles in Japanese patients treated with oral doses of haloperidol. The dose used was 12 mg daily. In a recent study in Korea (Roh *et al.*, 2001) a relationship between haloperidol concentration and *CYP2D6* genotype was established in patients receiving less than 20 mg daily, but not in patients receiving higher doses. We believe that the high affinity–low capacity CYP2D6 is the predominant enzyme at low concentrations/doses of haloperidol, while the low affinity–high capacity CYP3A4 becomes more important at higher doses. We could thus conclude that at least at low doses haloperidol is metabolised by CYP2D6. The metabolic pathway of haloperidol catalysed by CYP2D6 is presently not known. Also other neuroleptics such as perphenazine, risperidone, thioridazine and zuclopenthixol are metabolised by CYP2D6 (Bertilsson and Dahl, 1996).

Lin and Finder (1983) noted that the dosage of neuroleptics used in Asians is lower than that used in Caucasians. Later it was shown that

Chinese had 52% higher plasma concentration of haloperidol than US non-Asian (White and Black) patients given a fixed dose of oral haloperidol (Potkin *et al.*, 1984). Patients in the two populations were matched for sex and body weight. Similarly, Lin *et al.* (1988) showed that Asian healthy volunteers had higher serum haloperidol concentrations than did a matched group of Caucasians after both oral and intramuscular single doses. Furthermore, Asians had a more prominent serum prolactin response to haloperidol than Caucasians which, however, was not fully accounted for by the difference in kinetics between the two ethnic groups (Lin *et al.*, 1988). This indicates that both pharmacokinetic and dynamic factors contribute to the difference in response to neuroleptics between Caucasians and Asians.

ENDOGENOUS SUBSTRATES OF CYP2D6

In addition to differences in the metabolism of several drugs (Table 2.2) between the phenotypes of debrisoquine hydroxylation, there are differences between EMs and PMs in personality shown in Swedish (Bertilsson *et al.*, 1989a) and Spanish (Llerena *et al.*, 1993) healthy subjects. This indicates that CYP2D6 may also metabolise endogenous substances important for central nervous system function. This enzyme is also present in the human brain, although the activity is lower than in the liver (Kalow and Tyndale, 1992). There might be an association between a dopamine transporter and the brain CYP2D6 (Niznik *et al.*, 1990; Kalow and Tyndale, 1992), suggesting a role of the dopamine system in the brain as part of the CYP2D6-personality relationship. Brøsen *et al.* (1993) found evidence that PMs of debrisoquine develop side-effects to neuroleptics more easily than EMs (discussed by Llerena *et al.*, 1993). This gives further evidence for a relationship between CYP2D6 and dopamine neurotransmission in the brain. Possibly this might be part of the ethnic differences in sensitivity to neuroleptics indicated by Lin *et al.* (1988).

The CYP2C19 polymorphism

ETHNIC DIFFERENCES IN CYP2C19

Mephenytoin is an old anticonvulsant that has now been replaced by drugs such as phenytoin and carbamazepine. It is a racemic drug and the S-enantimer is rapidly hydroxylated in the 4-position while the R-enantiomer is slowly N-demethylated (for review see Wilkinson *et al.*, 1992). It was found that about 3% of Caucasians had a very slow hydroxylation of S-mephenytoin (Küpfer and Preisig, 1984; Wedlund *et al.*, 1984). EMs of S-mephenytoin eliminate the S-enantiomer rapidly. About 1 day after the intake of racemic drug, the S/R ratio in urine will be close to zero in EMs and about one in PMs (Sanz *et al.*, 1989). The S-mephenytoin hydroxylase is CYP2C19 (Wrighton *et al*, 1993; Goldstein *et al*, 1994). In Caucasians the 3% incidence of PMs of S-mephenytoin varies very little between studies (see Alván *et al*., 1990; Wilkinson *et al*., 1992). Several studies (Jurima *et al*., 1985; Nakamura *et al*., 1985; Horai *et al*., 1989) have shown that the incidence of PMs in Japanese is much higher (18–23%). In Chinese (17.4% found by Horai *et al*., 1989; 14.6% found by Bertilsson *et al*., 1992; Table 2.1) and in Koreans (12.6%; Sohn et al., 1992b; Roh et al., 1996a) there is a distinctly increased incidence of PMs of S-mephenytoin compared with Caucasians.

De Morais *et al*. (1994a, b) demonstrated the two major alleles of *CYP2C19* causing the PM phenotype. The *CYP2C19*2* (m_1) is present in Asians and Caucasians in about the same frequency. The presence of the *3* (m_2) in Asians is the cause of the increased incidence of PM of S-mephenytoin in this part of the world. It is interesting to note that there is an increased incidence of the *CYP2D6*2* allele on Vanuatu and other Pacific islands causing the presence of more than 70% PM on many of the islands (Kaneko *et al*., 1999).

When twenty-two Caucasian PM of S-mephenytoin and/or omeprazole were genotyped for *CYP2C19*2* and *3*, forty-two of the forty-four mutated alleles could be accounted for (Chang *et al*., 1995) (Table 2.3). Similarly, thirty-one of thirty-two Korean PM were homozygous for mutated alleles (Roh *et al*., 1996b). In a recent study in Tanzanians (Herrlin *et al*., 1998) a fairly poor relationship was found between CYP2C19 geno- and phenotype. There was, on the other hand, a fairly close relationship between the phenotypes using the two probes mephenytoin and omeprazole. In parallel to what was discussed above for CYP2D6, the activity of CYP2C19 might be decreased by environmental factors in Tanzania and other parts of Africa. There might be a generally decreased drug metabolism capacity in Africa as Masimirembwa *et al*. (1995) also found in Zimbabwean children, who metabolised the CYP1A2 substrate caffeine very slowly.

Table 2.3 Allele frequency of *CYP2C19* in Black African (Tanzanian), Caucasian (Swedish) and Oriental (Korean) poor metabolisers (PM) of S-mephenytoin and/or omeprazole

Population	PM (n)	CYP2C19 allele (%)			Reference
		*1	*2	*3	
Caucasian	22	4.5	93.2	2.3	Chang et al. (1995)
Oriental	32	1.6	67.2	31.3	Roh et al. (1996b)
African	8[a]	18.8	75.0	6.3	Herrlin et al. (1998)

Notes
CYP2C19*1 is defined as not *2 or *3.
[a] These eight were phenotyped with mephenytoin. Also in other subjects phenotyped with omeprazole there was a discorcordance between geno- and phenotype, i.e., the percentage CYP2C19*1 in these PM was high.

SUBSTRATES OF CYP2C19

The list of drugs that have been shown to be substrates of CYP2C19 (Table 2.4) is much shorter than that of CYP2D6 (Table 2.2). The reason might be that the latter enzyme has been much more investigated than the former. While CYP2D6 metabolises only lipophilic bases, substrates of CYP2C19 could be acids (e.g. mephenytoin), bases (e.g. propranolol) or neutral substances (e.g. diazepam). Imipramine (Skjelbo *et al.*, 1991) and propranolol (Ward *et al.*, 1989) are both hydroxylated by CYP2D6 and N-dealkylated by CYP2C19. The antimalarial proguanil is bioactivated to cycloguanil by CYP2C19 (Ward *et al.*, 1991) and the authors suggest that the antimalarial effect is absent or impaired in PMs of S-mephenytoin. If so, the effect of this drug might be less in Orientals and possibly also in Black patients compared with Caucasians.

INTERETHNIC DIFFERENCES IN THE DISPOSITION OF DIAZEPAM

Inaba *et al.* (1985) showed that diazepam is an inhibitor of the hydroxylation of S-mephenytoin in human liver microsomes. When diazepam was given as a single oral dose to a panel of EMs and PMs of S-mephenytoin in Sweden the disposition was slower in PMs compared with EMs (Bertilsson *et al.*, 1989b). The mean half-life was more than doubled in PMs compared with EMs (88.3 and 40.8 h, respectively). A subsequent study was then performed by Zhang *et al.* (1990) in Beijing. Chinese EMs and PMs of S-mephenytoin were given a single oral dose of diazepam and the plasma samples were analysed in Sweden. To our surprise there was neither a difference in the plasma clearance nor in half-life between EMs and PMs in these Chinese subjects. The mean half-lives in Chinese EMs and PMs (85.1 and 88.3 h) were long and similar to the Caucasian PMs (88.3 h). In a study performed in Koreans, Sohn *et al.* (1992b) found a longer mean half-life and lower clearance in PMs compared with EMs of S-mephenytoin. These three studies thus show that the plasma clearance of diazepam is higher in EMs compared with PMs among Caucasians and Koreans, but not among Chinese.

We (Bertilsson and Kalow, 1993) suggested that among the eight Chinese EM most were heterozygotes causing a relatively low clearance of diazepam, which was not significantly different from that found in the PM.

Table 2.4 Examples of drugs whose metabolism is catalysed by CYP2C19, i.e. the S-mephenytoin hydroxylase (see Wilkinson *et al.* 1992)

Carisoprolol	S-Mephenytoin
Citalopram	Moclobemide
Clomipramine	Omeprazole
Diazepam and demethyldiazepam	Proguanil
Imipramine	Propranolol

The high incidence of mutated *CYP2C19* alleles among Chinese should theoretically indicate that 4.4 of the eight EM should be heterozygotes. By chance seven of the eight had low clearance of diazepam and might be heterozygotes (Bertilsson and Kalow, 1993). These studies were performed before genotyping techniques were available (de Morais *et al.*, 1994a, b).

Diazepam is to a major extent demethylated to an active metabolite (about 60%), which in itself is a registered drug in certain countries (Bertilsson *et al.*, 1989b). Demethyldiazepam is to a major part hydroxylated to oxazepam. In the first study on diazepam disposition in Caucasian EMs and PMs of S-mephenytoin, the demethyl metabolite was also administered on a separate occasion (Bertilsson *et al.*, 1989b). In PMs compared with EMs, its mean clearance was lower (5.0±0.9 and 11.0±0.8 ml/min, respectively; $p<0.0001$) and the half-life longer (128±23 and 59±17 h, respectively; $p<0.0001$). In the studies on Chinese (Zhang *et al.*, 1990) and Koreans (Sohn *et al.*, 1992b), demethyldiazepam was not given *per se*, but the plasma concentrations of this metabolite were measured after the diazepam dose. The mean half-lives were longer in PMs than in EMs in both Chinese (161±37 (SD) and 116±29h, respectively; $p<0.02$) and Koreans (213±11 (S.E.M.) and 96±11 h, respectively; $p<0.001$). These results indicate that both the formation of demethyldiazepam from diazepam and its disappearance by hydroxylation are catalysed by CYP2C19 and that there are pronounced interethnic differences in both metabolic reactions.

INTERETHNIC DIFFERENCES IN OMEPRAZOLE METABOLISM

Omeprazole is a proton pump blocker used to treat peptic ulcer disease and reflux esophagitis. It is completely metabolised by, for example, C-hydroxylation and oxidation of the sulphoxide group to a sulphone. Most subjects eliminate the drug with a half-life of 0.5–1.0 h, while a few percent have longer half-lives (Andersson *et al.*, 1990a). Slow metabolisers of omeprazole had significantly slower metabolism of diazepam than did rapid metabolisers (Andersson *et al.*, 1990a). Since diazepam metabolism had been shown to be associated with the hydroxylation of S-mephenytoin in Caucasians (Bertilsson *et al.*, 1989b), a study was performed, which showed that four slow metabolisers of omeprazole were all PMs of S-mephenytoin (Andersson *et al.*, 1990b). The five investigated rapid metabolisers of omeprazole were all EMs of S-mephenytoin. Thus both omeprazole and diazepam are metabolised by CYP2C19. This explains why the two drugs interact in rapid metabolisers of omeprazole (EMs of S-mephenytoin), but not in slow metabolisers (PMs of S-mephenytoin) (Andersson *et al.*, 1990a). In PMs there is no CYP2C19 enzyme for which diazepam and omeprazole could compete.

EMs and PMs of S-mephenytoin were selected from phenotyped healthy subjects at Karolinska Institutet, Sweden and Beijing Medical University,

China (Andersson *et al.*, 1992). They were given a single 20 mg oral dose of omeprazole and plasma concentrations of parent drug and hydroxy and sulphone metabolites were determined in plasma during 10 h after drug intake. In both Chinese and Swedes the AUC (area under the plasma concentration versus time curve) for parent drug was higher in PM than in EM. For hydroxy-omeprazole it was the opposite showing that this metabolite is formed by CYP2C19 (Andersson *et al.*, 1992). The sulphone metabolite is not formed by this enzyme, but by CYP3A4 (Andersson *et al.*, 1993; Böttiger *et al.*, 1997).

In an independent study in Koreans, Sohn *et al.*, (1992a) showed that PMs of S-mephenytoin had a slow 5-hydroxylation of omeprazole compared with EMs. The disposition of omeprazole in Koreans seems to be very similar to that in Chinese reported by Andersson *et al.* (1992). Ishizaki *et al.* (1994) compared the disposition of omeprazole in the three populations studied (Figure 2.9). The clearance of omeprazole was higher in EM than in PM of S-mephenytoin in all three populations *(p<0.001)*. It is interesting to note that the clearance was higher in Swedish EM than in Chinese EM *(p<0.05)* and Korean EM *(p<0.01)*. This is probably due to the high frequency of heterozygotes in Oriental EM compared with Caucasian EM (compare the discussion with diazepam above). These studies point not only to a higher incidence of PM but also to heterozygotes among Orientals compared with Caucasians.

EFFECTS OF OMEPRAZOLE IN RELATION TO CYP2C19 GENOTYPE

In a study on healthy Swedish Caucasian subjects given 20 mg of omeprazole daily for 8 days, a very pronounced meal-induced gastrin release was recorded both in subjects with one and two mutated *CYP2C19* alleles compared with very rapid omeprazole metabolisers (Chang *et al.* 1995). Similar results were obtained in twenty-five Caucasian patients with acid related disease, in whom omeprazole had more pronounced effect on plasma gastrin in heterozygous EM compared with homozygous EM after 8 days of treatment with increase from day 0 to day 8 of 157% and 16%, respectively *(p=0.002)* (Sagar *et al.*, 2000). Among the heterozygotes the gastrin increase was more pronounced in the *H. pylori* positive (226%) compared with *H. pylori* negative patients (80%) *(p=0.02)*. In the same twenty-five patients omeprazole treatment for 8 days caused a more pronounced increase of 24-h intragastric pH in heterozygotes compared with homozygous EM with median pH at day 8 of 5.5 and 3.1, respectively *(p<0.0001)*. As the frequency of PM is low in Caucasians, only two of the twenty-five patients were PM. In these two patients both the gastrin release and increase in pH were similar or more pronounced than the effects seen in heterozygotes. These studies in healthy subjects (Chang *et al.*, 1995) and in patients (Sagar *et al.*, 2000) show that 20 mg omeprazole daily has a pronounced and similar effect on pH and gastrin release in PM and heterozygotes compared with subjects with two functional alleles. In Asia, where both the frequency of PM and heterozygotes is higher than in Caucasians, more pronounced mean effects of 20 mg of omeprazole daily would be seen than in Europe. This is, however, a hypothesis and needs to be proven.

Furuta *et al.* (1998) showed a close relationship between the *CYP2C19* genotype and the cure rate of *H. pylori* infection and peptic ulcer in 62 Japanese patients treated with omeprazole and amoxicillin. The mean cure rates for *H. pylori* infection in patients with 0, 1 and 2 mutated *CYP2C19* alleles were 28.6, 60 and 100%, respectively. Similar results were recently presented in another Japanese study (Tanigawara *et al.*, 1999).

PRONOUNCED DIFFERENCES IN THE DISPOSITION OF CLOMIPRAMINE BETWEEN JAPANESE AND SWEDISH PATIENTS

Clomipramine is a tricyclic antidepressant causing potent serotonin uptake inhibition (Träskman *et al.*, 1979). It is metabolised to desmethyl-clomipramine to a major extent by CYP2C19 (Nielsen *et al.*, 1994). As this metabolite is a potent noradrenaline uptake inhibitor (Träskman *et al.*, 1979), treatment with clomipramine gives a combined effect on the serotonin and noradrenaline neuronal systems. We have compared plasma concentrations of clomipramine and its N-desmethyl metabolite in 108 Japanese and 174 Swedish patients on long-term treatment with clomi-pramine (Shimoda *et al.*, 1999). Most of the Japanese *(n=96)* and a minority of Swedish patients *(n=43)* were treated with benzodiazepines. When combining all populations (Japanese, Swedes, with and without benzodiazepines) in a linear multiple regression, clearance of clomipramine was correlated with ethnic group *(p<0.00001)* and age *(p<0.00005)*, but it was uncorrelated with gender, body weight, and administration of benzodiazepines. The clearance of clomipramine was three to four-fold higher in Swedish compared with Japanese patients at a similar age (Shimoda *et al.*, 1999). This pronounced difference is most probably related to the lower mean CYP2C19 activity in Asians compared with Caucasians. It was also found that the plasma concentration ratio between parent drug clomipramine and desmethylmetabolite was twice as high in Japanese compared with Swedish patients (Shimoda *et al.*, 1999). This implicates a more pronounced serotonergic than noradrenergic neuronal effect in Japanese than Swedish patients.

The N-acetyltransferases

As mentioned in the introductory paragraph, the polymorphism of N-acetyltransferase (NAT) and the evidence for its interethnic variability are discoveries of the 1950s (Bonicke and Reif, 1953; Hughes *et al.*, 1954) and are thereby a backbone of pharmacogenetics. Since that time, numerous population studies have been conducted; exhaustive documentations based on various phenotyping procedures have been compiled by Weber (1987) and Evans (1992). The more recent development of genotyping procedures is extending and refining the traditional concepts.

The first investigations concerned the capacity for metabolism of the antituberculous drug, isoniazid. It was found that the primary metabolism was acetylation, that the difference represented a monogenic trait, that the slow acetylation capacity was recessively inherited, and that the tested populations of Caucasians could be divided into almost equal numbers of fast and slow acetylators (Weber, 1987; Evans, 1992). Later, the most commonly used test drug became sulfamethazine and recently, caffeine has found increasing use (see Kalow and Tang, 1993); altogether, Evans (1992) listed sixty publications containing a variety of phenotyping methods. Besides isoniazid, important drugs that have been clinically affected by this polymorphism include procainamide, hydralazine, dapsone, and salicylazo-sulfapyridine (SASP). However, research interest has currently shifted from effects of the polymorphism upon the fate of specific drugs towards associations between acetylator status and certain forms of cancer. There is a measurable excess of bladder cancer in slow acetylators exposed to arylamines, and a tendency for an increase of colorectal cancer in rapid acetylators (Evans, 1992).

Phenotype frequencies have been tested worldwide over a period of three to four decades in different populations and may be rounded and briefly summarised as follows: the percentage of slow acetylators is in Europe almost 60%, in Africa about 50%, in Japan and China about 15%, in the South Pacific close to 12%, and in many other populations around 50% (see Table 2.5 for genotype frequencies as calculated from

Table 2.5 N-acetyltransferase (NAT2) polymorphism: frequency of the slow acetylator gene (q) in different populations as established by functional tests

Population	Number of studies	Values of q	
		Mean	Range
Eskimo	4	0.23	0.00–0.46
South Pacific (Islands)	5	0.35	0.11–0.80
East Asian[a]	14	0.37	0.25–0.49
N and S American Indian	10	0.50	0.29–0.67
Africa[b]	19	0.71	0.48–0.95
Central & Western Asian	22	0.74	0.44–0.87
European	50	0.75	0.55–0.86

Notes
Data condensed from Evans (1992).
[a] Korean, Chinese, Japanese.
[b] Except Kung population, who have q=0.18.

phenotypes). In Canadian Inuit (Eskimos), slow acetylators make up only about 5% of the population; these data imply that about 60% of the Inuit, but only 5% of Europeans are homozygous fast acetylators. This high level of activity of a large part of the Inuit population called for use of a high dose of isoniazid in a slow-release preparation for antituberculous treatment (Jeanes et al., 1972).

It is now clear that there are two spatially separated genes on chromosome 8 (pter-q11) which have single exons and which produce the acetyltransferases referred to as NAT1 and NAT2 (Blum et al. 1991; Grant et al., 1991; Grant, 1993). The polymorphic enzyme which selectively metabolises isoniazid and the other substrates mentioned above is NAT2 (Grant et al., 1991). NAT1 selectively metabolises p-aminobenzoic acid (PABA) and p-aminosalicylic acid (PAS). The carcinogenic arylamines tend to be metabolised by both NAT1 and NAT2 – an important point for future cancer studies. Other clinical considerations regarding the variability of both enzymes have been discussed by Spielberg (1996).

Grant et al. (1997) have listed fifteen structural variants of NAT2. The nomenclature system has been described by Vatsis et al. (1995). Four of the enzymes (NAT2*4, NAT2*12A, NAT2*12B and NAT2*13) produce the rapid acetylator phenotype, nine are slow, and two are too new to be known. The fifteen variants can be accounted for by seven nucleotide substitutions which occur singly or in combination. Four of the variants occur frequently enough to explain about 95% of the acetylation poly-morphism in different populations. Here we will be concerned only with these common ones which are produced by the rapid NAT2*4, and the slow variants NAT2*5B, NAT2*6A, and NAT2*7B. They have been used to compare populations (Deguchi et al., 1990; Blum et al., 1991; Hickman and Sim, 1991; Vatsis et al., 1991).

The wild-type allele called "NAT2*4" which occurs in at least 98% of rapid acetylators, and its base pair positions are the standard of reference. NAT2*5B is assessed by testing for the C→T change at position 481; there are two variants but in practice, this C 481T change reveals the presence of NAT2*5B. The second slow acetylator variant (NAT2*6A) with two base pair changes is caught by testing G→A at 590, and the third (NAT2*7B) by measuring G→A at 857. Old names for NAT2*5B are S1A, M1 and r_3, for NAT2*6A are S2, M2 and r_2, and for NAT2*7B are S3, M3 and r_1, respectively.

Slow acetylation may represent a change of V_{max}, K_m, or decreased stability (Grant et al., 1997).

Table 2.6 gives a compilation of recent gene counts obtained by various investigators in different populations; some of the data allow a direct comparison with the older but much more massive phenotype counts shown in Table 2.5. Comparable overall frequencies of the slow acetylator genes can be seen in Caucasians and in East Asians; phenotyping and genotyping

Table 2.6 Frequencies of (%) wild-type (wt) and three slow acetylator alleles of NAT2 in different populations

Measured base pair shift *	Allele designation	Caucasians[b,e,f]	U.S. Hispanics[e]	U.S. Blacks[e]	U.S. Korean[e]	Chinese[c,e]	Japanese[a]	Australian Aboriginal[d]
Genes tested (n)		674	296	192	196	308	172	88
wt	4	27.9	58.8	38.5	66.3	54.6	68.6	47.7
481 CT	5B	41.6	26.7	19.9	3.0	6.6	0	2.2
590 GA	6A	28.7	18.2	14.9	19.4	28.2	24.4	21.6
857 GA	7B	1.6	13.9	3.7	11.2	10.6	7.0	40.9
Frequency of slow acetylator genes (q) **		0.72	0.59	0.59	0.34	0.45	0.31	0.65

Notes

*The change at base pair position 481 is associated with a shift at 341 plus a shift at 803 in 98% of cases. The changes at base pair 590 and at base pair 857 are mostly associated with a shift at 282.

**The square of the gene frequencies in the last row gives an indication of the proportion of slow acetylators in a population.

The information in this table is compiled from data by [a]Deguchi et al., 1990; [b]Graf et al., 1992; [c]Hayes et al., 1993; [d]Ilett et al., 1993; [e]Lin et al., 1993; [f]Meyer U.A. (unpublished observations).

did indeed produce similar counts. The strikingly new information in Table 2.6 is the distinction between three slow acetylator genes. Particularly S1 predominates in Caucasians while it occurs infrequently in Orientals. It is the relative lack of the S1 alleles that accounts for the low frequency of slow acetylators in East Asia, where slow acetylation is usually due to the S2 allele (Grant, 1993).

It may be worth noting that, considering only the four acetylator genes shown in Table 2.6, a slow acetylator may represent any one of nine genotypes. A rapid acetylator may be one of four kinds of heterozygotes or a homozygote for the wild-type gene. A biochemical puzzle lies in the fact that the low enzyme activity of slow acetylators does not appear to be a matter of a slow reaction velocity, but of low enzyme concentration (Grant *et al.*, 1990; Blum, 1991). The mechanism remains to be explored. Another remarkable fact is that the base pair change C→T at 481 which seems to be functionally important (Grant, 1993) does not produce an alteration of amino acids; perhaps the change affects the process of transcription or translation.

A recent paper describes fifteen genetic variants of NAT1 (Hughes *et al.*, 1998). Only nine had been quoted by Grant *et al.* (1997) and thirteen by Lin *et al.* (1998). However, ethnic data do not yet seem to be available.

Esterases

The two human esterases for which there are extensive pharmacogenetic data are butyrylcholinesterase (plasma cholinesterase) and paraoxonase (human serum paraoxonase/arylesterase).

Butyrylcholinesterase

The first genetic variant of butyrylcholinesterase (BChE) was identified in 1956, designated "atypical cholinesterase", and characterised as a high K_m variant (Kalow and Genest, 1957). This was one of the first examples of pharmacogenetics (Kalow, 1962, 1988), and since there was an easy method to identify this variant in a small sample of plasma, numerous populations (Whittaker, 1986) totaling approximately 100,000 subjects have been screened for the presence of this variant. Other variants were discovered later as described by Lockridge (1992), and the molecular basis of all except some extremely rare variants has been elucidated in recent years (La Du, 1995).

There is a single copy of the gene *BCHE* for butyrylcholinesterase. It is located on chromosome 3 in region 3q21–25. Biochemically, the "atypical" or A variant is characterised by resistance to inhibitors like dibucaine; it represents the amino acid alteration 70 Asp→Gly (Masson *et al.*, 1997). DNA data have shown that there are two F-variants (243 Thr→Met and

390 Gly→Val) in Caucasian populations (Jensen *et al.*, 1995) which show reduced inhibition by sodium fluoride; in addition, a 330 Leu→Ile variant was fluoride resistant in Japan (Sudo *et al.*, 1997). There are at least twelve "silent" or S variants without or with only minimal enzyme activity (Primo-Parmo *et al.*, 1996b). All these convey functional cholinesterase deficiency with possible clinical consequences. A special variant, perhaps without clinical effect, is the K variant (named for Kalow by Rubinstein *et al.*, 1978) with amino acid change 539 Ala→Thr. This mutation reduces enzyme activity by about one third without affecting affinities. It occurs in linkage disequilibrium with the A variant, i.e., the 70 Asp→Gly mutation tends to be accompanied by the 539 Ala→Thr mutation (Gaffney and Campbell, 1994). In addition, there are some extremely rare variants with functional deficiency. There are about twenty different genetic variants of this enzyme (Jensen *et al.*, 1995).

Since the A and F variants can be detected by functional tests also in heterozygotes, their gene frequencies have been repeatedly calculated. Listings covering about 75,000 subjects have been compiled by Whittaker (1986). An abbreviated list covering different populations is shown in Table 2.7. On average, the highest allele frequencies of the A variant were found in Europe and India, but exceptionally high frequencies of 0.0473 and 0.0755 occurred in the Jews of Iraq and Iran, respectively. The silent phenotype is present in about 1:10,000,000 Caucasians but there were accumulations of cases in Alaska and in the Vysyas of Andhra Pradesh (India). About 1% of Caucasians (Jensen *et al.*, 1996) and 0.4% of Japanese (Shibuta *et al.*, 1994) are homozygous for the K variant which thereby is the most frequently encountered cholinesterase variant.

Deficiency of butyrylcholinesterase activity prolongs the effects of succinylcholine, a usually very short acting muscle relaxant used in anes-

Table 2.7 Frequencies of atypical and fluoride variants of butyrylcholinesterase

Population	No. of subjects	Gene frequencies	
		$E_1{}^a$	$E_1{}^f$
Europeans	35,770	0.0170	0.0021
Africans	6,467	0.0046	0.0135
Orientals	2,422	0.0002	0.0004
Asian Indians[a]	1,564	0.0150	0.0180
Oceania indigenous populations	3,020	0.0108	0.0
American aboriginal populations[a]	6,689	0.0039	0.0

Notes

$E_1{}^a$, and $E_1{}^f$ represent the genes for atypical and fluoride-resistant cholinesterase variants, respectively. The frequencies are mainly based on determinations of heterozygotes. Data are extracted from tabulations of Whittaker (1986) who quoted 78 references in her Tables, involving $E_1{}^a$ measurements in almost 75,000 subjects.

[a] An accumulation of cases of the silent allele occurred in the Vysyas of Andhra Pradesh and in lower Yukon and Alaskan villages.

thesia, sometimes causing fatalities (Kalow and Gunn, 1957; Lockridge, 1992). There are indications that serious toxicities of cocaine may be associated with cholinesterase deficiency (Hoffman *et al.*, 1992, Schwartz and Johnson, 1996); injections of butyrylcholinesterase have been recommended to treat cocaine poisoning (Gorelick, 1997; Mattes *et al.*, 1997).

Paraoxonase (PON1)

Paraoxon is the biologically active metabolite of parathion, an insecticide of the class of organophosphates. Paraoxonase (PON1) is a calcium-dependent enzyme in human plasma which on the basis of inhibition characteristics has long been classified as an A-esterase (Aldridge, 1953). The variant discovered by Krisch in 1968 is slow in metabolising paraoxon but has normal activity towards phenylacetate; it is therefore often referred to as "paraoxonase/arylesterase" (La Du, 1992). It is the member of a family of which the genes *PON1* and *PON2* are located on human chromosome 7 (Primo-Parmo *et al.*, 1996a). Potential functions of PON1 have been enumerated by Mackness *et al.* (1998); these include a suspected role of genetic variants in the development of atherosclerosis and coronary heart disease, as reported in both Caucasian and Japanese populations (Sanghera *et al.*, 1998). Human paraoxonase activity is a clinically important determinant of the toxicity of paraoxon or other organophosphates; the question of the importance of this variant for Gulf War Syndrome has therefore been raised (Mackness *et al.*, 1997).

Paraoxonase type 1 is now known to have two polymorphisms. The variant discovered by Krisch in 1968 represents the change 192Arg/Gln (Adkins *et al.*, 1993). The variant 55Leu/Met is well described by Leviev *et al.* (1997). Most interethnic data refer to the 1968 discovery, whereby the wild type and the mutant are called B and A variants. Frequency distribution curves of paraoxonase activity tend to be bimodal whereby the low-activity mode represents the homozygotes for the A variant. The variants are distinguished (Eckerson *et al.*, 1983) not only by their level of enzymatic activity but also by qualitative features such as substrate selectivity, opposing response to Na^+ in the presence of Ca^{2+}, and response to inhibition by chlorpromazine.

The ratio of the hydrolysis rates of paraoxon and phenylacetate is the best phenotypic criterion to distinguish the two allelic variants of paraoxonase (Eckerson *et al.*, 1983). The B-type hydrolyses paraoxon about five times faster than does the A-type but there are obviously some extraneous factors that can affect enzyme activity. The superiority of this ratio over the simple measurements of paraoxon hydrolysis was impressively demonstrated in a study of a Sudanese population (La Du and Adkins, 1986). The ratio showed a trimodal distribution compatible with the Hardy–Weinberg law, while paraoxonase activity by itself seemed to be almost normally distributed.

Most worldwide population data (Figure 2.10) are based on measurements of only paraoxon hydrolysis (Playfer *et al.*, 1976; Diepgen and Geldmacher-v. Mallinckrodt, 1986). In many populations, quoted gene frequencies are undoubtedly estimates. In Caucasians, both phenotyping methods have always given consistent results (La Du, 1992). Ten independent studies of a total of 9,166 subjects indicated a gene frequency of 0.72 with a range from 0.60 to 0.76 for the low-activity allele. In the Sudan, that frequency was 0.484. In other words, in the Sudan about a quarter of the population had the low-activity variant of paraoxonase while this is the variant of about half of the Caucasians. A study from Singapore (Roy *et al.*, 1991) indicated gene frequencies of the rapid variant of 0.86 in Chinese and 0.96 in Filipinos. Carro-Ciampi *et al.* (1983) using the method of Smolen *et al.* (1982) found the slow genotype in forty-two of eighty-two Caucasians, but in only four of sixty-seven Inuit (Eskimos) and in four of fifty-seven native Indians from northern Canada (Figure 2.11).

Thus, paraoxonase activity divides European populations into about half with slow and half with rapid activity but everywhere else, the slow variant appears to be the more rare. One can only speculate on any toxicological or medical consequences which these differences may have.

Alcohol-metabolising enzymes

In the current context, we will use the term "alcohol" not in its chemical sense in which there are many different alcohols with various (often poorly investigated) metabolic fates. This overview will be confined to the variable elements of ethanol metabolism.

Ethanol is mainly metabolised by alcohol dehydrogenase (ADH) to acetaldehyde which in turn is oxidised by aldehyde dehydrogenase (ALDH) to acetic acid (Figure 2.12). Genetic variation of alcohol dehydrogenase was discovered in 1964 by von Wartburg *et al.*, that of aldehyde dehydrogenase in 1978 by Harada, Agarwal and Goedde. In the years since these discoveries, both variations have become targets of many investigations, and topics of specialised books (Goedde and Agarwal, 1987; Crabbe and Harris, 1991; Weiner *et al.*, 1997). While aldehyde dehydrogenase genotypes have been known for many years to influence drinking behavior and alcohol-induced liver damage, the clinical significance of alcohol dehydrogenase variants is still unraveling. In addition, alcohol dependence is influenced by factors other than the dehydrogenases (Ferguson and Goldberg, 1997; Reich *et al.*, 1998).

Alcohol dehydrogenase (ADH)

There are seven different ADH classes (gene families) which are expressed in different but overlapping sets of tissues (Edenberg *et al.*, 1996). Here we will be concerned only with class I ADH, consisting of three genes *ADH1*,

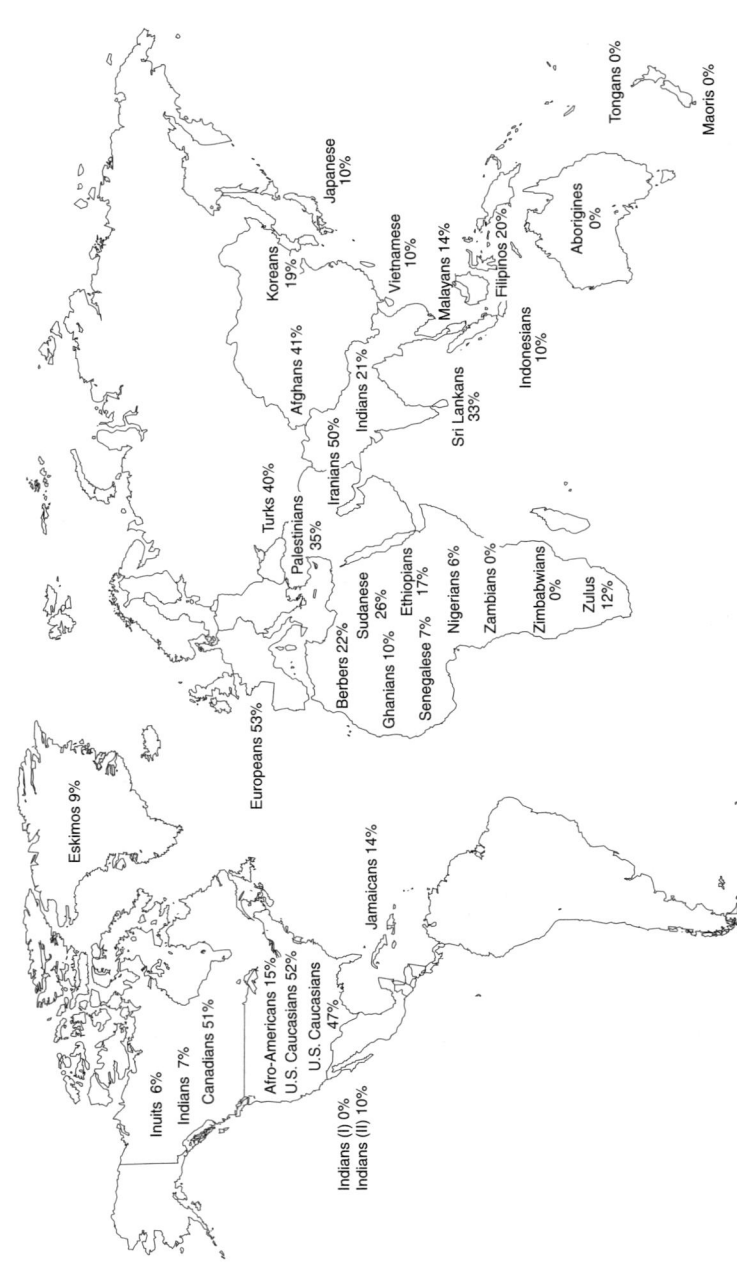

Figure 2.10 Worldwide distribution of paraoxonase polymorphism. The percentage of individuals with low serum paraoxonase in population samples from various ethnic groups throughout the world. First compiled from Playfer *et al.*, 1976; Carro-Ciampi *et al.*, 1983; Eckerson *et al.*, 1983b; Geldmacher-v. Mallinckrodt and Diepgen, 1988. The figure presented here is as supplemented and modified by La Du (1992), with permission of the author and the copyright holder, Pergamon Press.

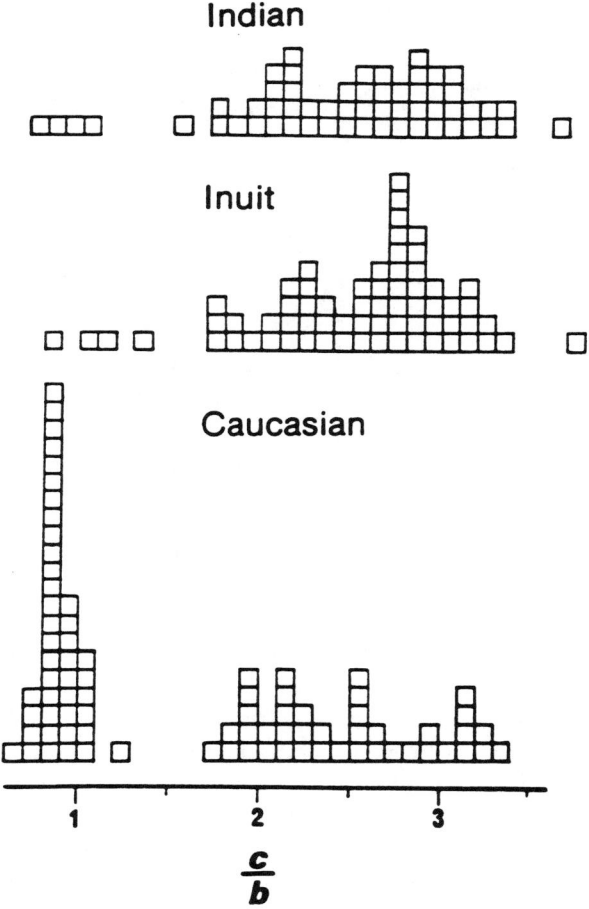

Figure 2.11 Paraoxonase phenotyping ratio c/b. Paraoxon hydrolysis rates b were measured in the presence of 5×10^{-3} M $CaCl_2$, and c in 5×10^{-3} M $CaCl_2$ plus 5×10^{-1} M NaCl. Each square represents one individual. The data below c/b = 1.5 indicate the homozygotes with the A variant for low paraoxonase activity. This Figure is from Carro-Ciampi *et al.* (1983) with permission of the publisher, Canadian J. Physiol. and Pharmacol.

ADH2, and *3DH3,* located on chromosome 4 between 4q21 and 4q24. Their products are referred to as alpha, beta, and gamma ADH, respectively (Jornvall and Hoog, 1995). All these dehydrogenases are expressed in adult liver, beta and gamma also in kidney.

The ADH class I molecules are dimers, composed of two subunits. They may be homodimers composed of alpha/alpha, beta/beta, gamma/gamma units or they are the heterodimers alpha/beta, alpha/gamma, and beta/

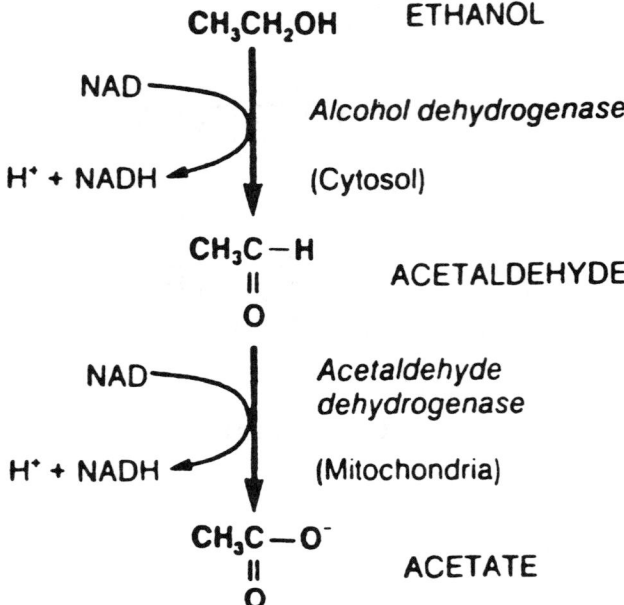

Figure 2.12 The first two steps of ethanol metabolism.

gamma. There is genetic variation of the beta and gamma subunits. There are three beta variants beta1, beta2, and beta3. If for instance somebody is heterozygous having beta1 and beta2, the ADH is expected to consist of the following ten dimers formed by random association: alpha/alpha, beta1/beta1, beta1/beta2, beta2/beta2, gamma/gamma; alpha/beta1, alpha/beta2, alpha/gamma, beta1/gamma, and beta2/gamma. If this person were also heterozygous at the *ADH3* locus to produce gamma1 and gamma2 subunits, his or her alcohol dehydrogenase should consist of eighteen different dimers. Because of these complexities, population comparisons are best made on the basis of allele frequencies (Table 2.8).

The three subunits alpha or ADH1, beta or ADH2, and gamma or ADH3, are structurally similar. Each consists of 374 amino acids (Bosron and Li, 1986). In the context of ethnic comparisons, the most important difference is between the "typical" subunit beta1 which is predominant in Caucasians and the "atypical" beta2 subunit which is prominent in Orientals. The occurrence of beta3 in American Blacks is a comparatively new observation. In position 47, beta1 contains arginine, beta2 histidine, beta3 glycine (Hurley *et al.*, 1994). PCR tests are available which distinguish between these subunits. The ARG to HIS mutational difference causes profound functional alterations in that the "atypical" (beta2) variant is the better catalyst (Hurley *et al.*, 1990). Table 2.9 gives a summary of the

Table 2.8 Frequency of ADH alleles in different populations

ADH$_2$^{I}	β_I	β_2	β_3	γ^I	γ^2
White American	>95%	<5%	<5%	50%	50%
White European	90	10	<5	60	40
Japanese	35	65	<5	95	5
Black American	85	<5	15	85	15

Note
From Crabb and Harris (1981), with permission of authors and publisher.

Table 2.9 Kinetic properties of human ADH isoenzymes in ethanol oxidation

Constant	$\alpha\alpha$	$\alpha\alpha$	$\beta_1\beta_1$	$\beta_2\beta_2$	$\gamma^I\gamma^I$	$\gamma^2\gamma^2$
K_m, NAD$^+$ (μM)	13	7.4	180	712	7.9	8.7
K_m, ethanol (μM)	4.2	0.049	0.94	36	1.0	0.63
K_i, NAD$^+$ (μM)	32	90	340	2,300	–	–
V_{max} (min)	27	9.2	400	300	87	35
pH optimum	10.5	10.5	8.5	7.0	10.5	10.5

Note
Adapted from Burnell and Bosron (1989).

kinetic constants which determine the rate of ethanol oxidation by the heritable homodimers under experimental conditions. Thus *in vitro*, depending on the choice of conditions, beta$_2$ oxidises ethanol several times as fast as does beta$_1$ while beta$_3$ may be less efficient than beta$_1$. The functional differences between the two gamma alleles are comparatively small.

However, if the re-oxidation of NADH to cofactor NAD is the rate-limiting step of ethanol oxidation *in vivo* (Suddendorf, 1989), the different capabilities of alcohol dehydrogenase may not be fully reflected in the elimination rate of ethanol. There are also the possibilities that the effect of the variants depends on ethanol concentration, or that beta$_2$ causes an initial spurt of ethanol oxidation in Orientals which is not seen in Caucasians who have the beta$_1$ allele and in Blacks who have the beta$_3$ allele. Nevertheless, functional clarification of these problems has been provided by recent comparative genotyping of alcoholics and non-alcoholics. Studies in Chinese (Thomasson *et al.*, 1991; Shen *et al.*, 1997) and in Japanese (Higuchi, 1994; Tanaka *et al.*, 1996), supported by meta-analysis (Whitfield, 1997), indicated significantly reduced frequencies of beta$_2$ and gamma$_1$ in alcoholics, besides the aldehyde dehydrogenase deficiency (see below). It means that the high rate of ethanol conversion to the toxic and unpleasant acetaldehyde reduces ethanol consumption, particularly if acetaldehyde is slowly metabolised.

In short, the interethnic differences in the structure of alcohol dehydrogenase appear to have sufficient effects upon the fate of ethanol to be one of the determinants of alcoholism. Furthermore, one should not exclude the possibility that variation of alcohol dehydrogenase matters for the fate of endogenous (Strasser *et al.*, 1996; Kedishvili *et al.*, 1996) or exogenous substrates (Kassam *et al.*, 1989; Burnell and Bosron, 1989). Ethanol is also metabolised by CYP2E1, but this enzyme is quantitatively less important than the alcohol dehydrogenases (Maezawa *et al.*, 1995).

Aldehyde dehydrogenase

Traditionally established as being of clinical significance is variation of the mitochondrial aldehyde dehydrogenase referred to as ALDH2 (Goedde and Agarwal, 1992). There are additional and different aldehyde dehydro-genases which are cytosolic enzymes and which seem to be also relevant in the present context (Ambroziak and Pietruzko, 1993), but this review will be confined to ALDH2, the best investigated enzyme of this group. Virtually all recent studies of alcoholism in Asians include data on ALDH2. The gene for this enzyme is located on chromosome 12 (Vasiliou, 1997). ALDH2 occurs mostly in liver and kidney and takes the form of a tetramer which consists normally of four identical subunits.

This tetrameric composition is important. There is an inactive genetic variant of ALDH2 which represents a point mutation. Glutamic acid at the 14th position from the C-terminus is substituted in the deficient enzyme by lysine (Hempel *et al.*, 1985). Even if the tetramer contains only one genetically inactive subunit, the whole tetramer is inactive. This means that there is enzyme deficiency even in the heterozygote, or in other words, ALDH2 deficiency is inherited as a dominant trait (Singh *et al.*, 1989)! Most published population comparisons therefore simply list the percentages of deficiency subjects.

Goedde and Agarwal (1992) list test results from twenty-nine different populations and a total of 3,248 subjects. The data can be summarised (Table 2.10) by the statements that Central Asian, East Asian, and South-East Asian populations showed deficiencies in the order of 30 to 50%. The deficiency was absent in European, Near-East, and African populations. North American Indians showed deficiency rates of 2–5%, South American Indians of 40–45%. O'Dowd *et al.* (1990) have shown that the functional enzyme deficiency in South American Indians must be due to a different mutation than the deficiency in Asians. This observation raises interesting questions regarding the biological significance of the mitochondrial alde-hyde dehydrogenase.

The clinical importance of ALDH2 deficiency for alcohol ingestion rests on the chemical reactivity and therefore toxicity of the ethanol-derived substrate acetaldehyde. If the enzymatic removal of acetaldehyde is not fast enough, ethanol intake tends to cause facial flushing and a drop in blood pressure with tachycardia (Higuchi *et al.*, 1992), i.e., effects which are perceived as an unpleasant sensation. The unpleasantness, or even an embarrassed reaction to the visual flushing, have been deterrents of excessive

Table 2.10 Distribution of ALDH2 isozyme deficiency in different populations

Population	Sample size	% deficiency in ALDH2
Orientals		
Ainu	80	20
Chinese		
Han	120	45
Korean (Mandschu)	209	25
Mongolian	198	30
Zhuang	106	25
Indonesians	30	39
Japanese	184	44
Koreans (South)	75	27
Phillipinos	110	13
Thais (North)	110	8
Vietnamese	138	53
South American Indians		
Atacameños (Chile)	133	43
Shuara (Ecuador)	99	42
North American Indians		
Navajo (New Mexico)	56	2
Sioux (North Dakota)	90	5
Mexican Indians		
Mestizo (Mexico City)	43	4
Caucasians and Blacks		
Asian Indians	50	0
Egyptians	260	0
Fangs	37	0
Germans	300	0
Hungarians	177	0
Israelis	77	0
Kenyans	23	0
Liberians	184	0
Matyo	106	0
Romai	84	0
Sudanese	40	0
Turks	65	0

Note
Reprinted from Goedde and Agarwal (1986), with the permission of the authors and the copyright holder, Alan R. Liss, New York.

ethanol consumption and thereby of alcoholism. In Japan, however, the deterrent effect of these sensations has been claimed to be gradually diminishing (Hasumura and Takeuchi, 1991).

G-6-pD deficiency

Glucose-6-phosphate dehydrogenase is a large structure with many genetic variants – perhaps more than any other human protein (Yoshida and

Beutler, 1986; Luzzatto, 1986; Beutler, 1993; Luzzatto and Mehta, 1989). Some of these variants are rare, some are polymorphic, i.e. frequent in at least one population. The rare ones tend to be rare because they generate disease in the form of chronic hemolytic anemia. The polymorphic ones tend to be symptomless unless a drug or an infection overwhelms the protective function of the enzyme; persons with, for example, the A or the Mediterranean variants may go through life without ever realising that they have G-6-pD deficiency. Approximately one tenth of the world population has one or other of the approximately 300 different variants of G-6-pD; however, the incidence of the polymorphic variants differs grossly between populations.

G-6-pD is an almost ubiquitous cytosolic enzyme which catalyses the first step in the hexose monophosphate pathway (Luzzatto and Mehta, 1989). Its most essential function is to produce the NADPH required to maintain the concentration of reduced glutathione (GSH) in the face of oxidative stress. GSH together with catalase and glutathione peroxidase represent the defense against hydrogen peroxide, and this is particularly true in red blood cells. Hydrogen peroxide is often a byproduct arising during drug oxidation. Therefore, some drugs tend to produce destruction of the red cells, that is hemolysis, in case of G-6-pD deficiency.

The G-6-pD classes I to V (Table 2.11) represent a WHO-accepted classification of the variants which pertains mostly to their hemolytic potential. The class I deficiencies cause the serious hereditary blood disorder called "chronic nonspherocytic hemolytic anemia" (CNSHA); it is by necessity a rare disorder caused by non-polymorphic variants. Classes II and III are responsible for the hemolytic anemias which may be initiated by certain drugs or by infection. These are the classes with liberal representation of polymorphic variants. Class IV indicates normal G-6-pD as, for

Table 2.11 Summary of G-6-pD variants

Class	Number of G-6-pD variants		
	Polymorphic	Rare	Total
I	0	83	83
II	49	109	158
III	22	74	96
IV	14	43	57
V	0	2	2
Total	85	311	396

Notes
Class I variants are associated with nonspherocytic hemolytic anemia. Class II variants are severely deficient, with less than 10% residual activity. Class III variants are moderately deficient, with 10–60% of normal residual activity. Class IV variants have nearly normal or normal activity (60–150% of normal). Class V variants have increased activity compared with normals.
Adapted from Luzzato and Mehta (1989).

example, the B+ and the A+ alleles. Class V consists of a few variants with greater than normal activity; they do not cause pathology.

The gene *Gd* producing G-6-pD is located on the X chromosome at Xq28 (Beutler, 1990). It means that the deficiency is sex-linked. Males either do or do not have the deficiency, but females with their two X chromosomes may be heterozygous; within a population, it is mostly the males who show the deficiency. In females during early embryogenesis, each cell eliminates at random one of the two X chromosomes so that in heterozygotes, approximately half the cells are normal and the other half are G-6-pD deficient. Epidemiological data indicate that the protective effect of G-6-pD deficiency against malaria operates mostly via the heterozygous females. (The random elimination of X chromosomes, so that they either do or do not have the deficiency variant, represents a natural labeling of cells which has been utilised, for example, in cancer research.)

On the basis of geographical correlations and of various *in vitro* studies, we must accept as an established fact that G-6-pD deficiency favors survival of Falciparum malaria (Vulliamy *et al.*, 1992). Thereby, the polymorphic forms of the deficiency variants tend to accumulate in malaria-exposed populations. This explains the large ethnic and racial differences in the occurrence of G-6-pD deficiency. However, the mechanism of the malaria protection is complex (Usanga and Luzzatto, 1985) and still not fully understood (Vulliamy *et al.*, 1992). It probably involves a sufficient survival time of particularly the malaria-infected heterozygous infant girls to allow them to develop immunological defenses against malaria. This could mean that after puberty, their better state of health might render them more fertile than their less protected sisters.

Since the occurrence of G-6-pD deficiency, of sickle cell anemia, and of thalassemia, all seem to be related to the incidence of malaria, combinations of these traits are not uncommon.

Figure 2.13 gives an indication of the worldwide frequency distribution of G-6-pD variants. Table 2.12 provides a functional description of some selected variants listed by Luzzatto and Mehta (1989). The WHO classes give an indication of the ranges of clinical significance which the different variants may have. Listed are the kinetic alterations which may lead to clinical enzymopathy. There are no variants without enzyme activity; they are probably not compatible with life and are eliminated *in utero* (Beutler 1993).

Many of the polymorphic variants have in common that they are unstable enzymes which lose activity over time. It means that cells with a rapid turnover in the body contain recently formed and therefore active G-6-pD molecules. Red blood cells with their 4-month lifespan gradually lose more or less of their G-6-pD activity. In consequence, the G-6-pD deficiency may affect the red blood cells without noticeably affecting other tissues. Since the red cell is the target of the malaria parasite, G-6-pD

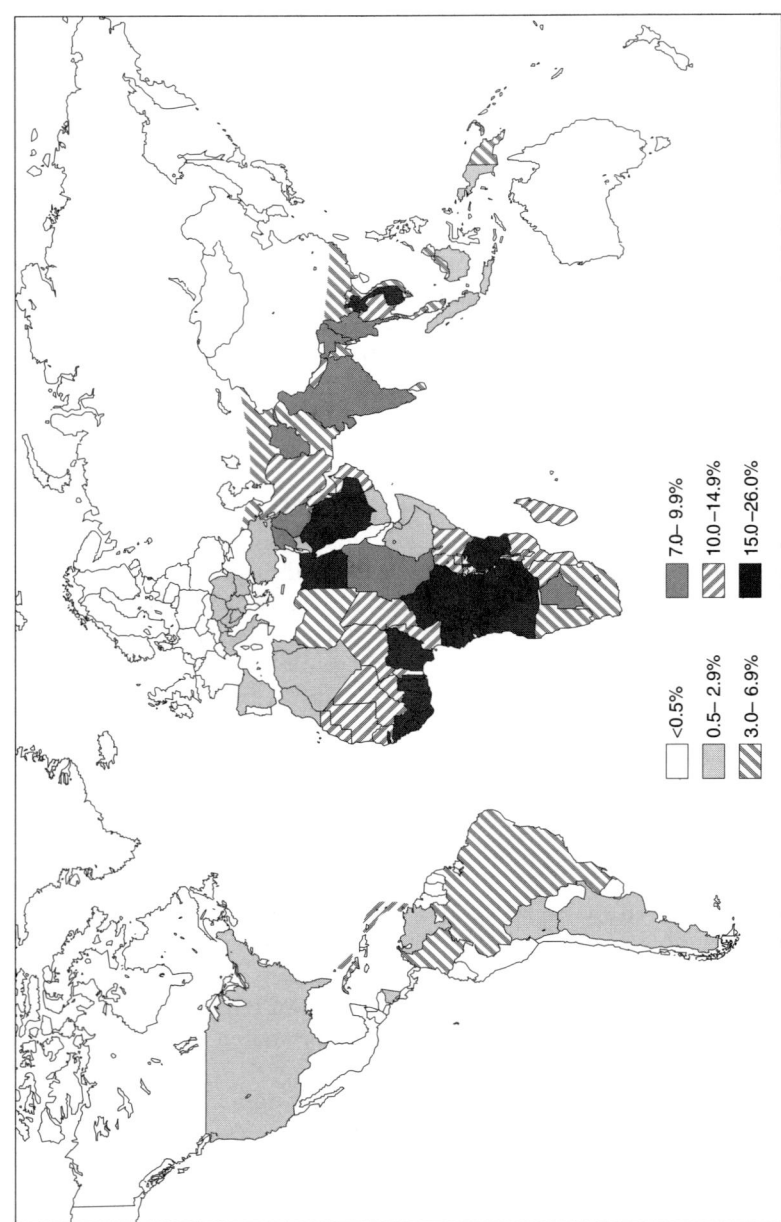

Figure 2.13 World distribution of G-6-pD deficiency. The values shown by the different shadings are frequencies in the populations of the various countries of G-6-pD-deficient males (which are also gene frequencies, since the gene is X-linked). The map has been assembled by Luzzatto and Mehta (1989) and is reproduced with permission of the authors and McGraw-Hill.

Table 2.12 Kinetic properties of some representative G-6-pD variants which are not associated with chronic hemolytic anemia

Variant	Activity (% of normal)	K_m (μM) G6P	K_m (μM) NADP	Inhibition by NADPH[a]	WHO class
B+ (normal)	100	50–70	2.9–4.4	1.38	4
A+	80	Normal	Normal	1.2	4
A–	8–20	Normal	Normal	0.62	3
Union	<3	8–12	3.6–5.2	0.22	2
Markham	1.5–10	4.4–6.3	–	0.375	2
Mediterranean	<5	19–26	1.2–1.6	0.4	2

Notes
[a]Ratio of K_m and K_I at pH 7.3. Variants with higher values are more sensitive to NADPH inhibition.
Adapted from Yoshida (1986).

deficiency can have a protective effect against malaria without necessarily disturbing general health.

To date, most of the approximately 300 variants counted as being different have been distinguished from each other by functional tests and by electrophoretic mobility. If a variant is thought to represent a new discovery, it is not necessarily an easy matter to decide via enzyme tests whether the same variant has been identified elsewhere already. Difficulties of G-6-pD classification by testing red blood cells arise because the amount of blood that can be taken from any individual is limited, the blood is likely collected because the G-6-pD activity is low, and the enzyme may have suffered some deterioration during shipment to the laboratory. These difficulties are avoided by using DNA-based tests for classification. The use of such tests has already eliminated several erroneous distinctions between variants and on the other hand has revealed distinct entities where none were thought to be (Beutler, 1993). Furthermore, molecular genetics has started to give new insight into some broad aspects of G-6-pD variation.

The entire *Gd* gene consists of 20,114 bp (base pairs) with 13 exons; there are 1548 bp in the coding sequence. By summer 1992, about forty different mutations had been identified (Beutler, 1993). Some of the polymorphic variants contain more than one mutation, and certain mutations are common to several variants. All except three of the known mutations produce enzyme alterations. One of the three silent mutants turned out to be an interesting marker: it is at nucleotide 1311.

Beutler (1992, 1993) in his overviews has provided some important generalisations:

The normal (wild-type) G-6-pD as observed commonly in the northern hemisphere is referred to as B+. In Africa, a variant called A+ is very common; today, about 20% of the X-chromosomes in American Blacks contain A+. It has about the same enzymatic activity as B+, but has higher electrophoretic mobility because aspartate replaces asparagine due to a A→G mutation at nucleotide (nt) 376 (Hirono and Beutler, 1988). The G-6-pD deficiency typical of Blacks is A-; this has always one amino acid substitution in addition to the mutation which characterises A+. The most common second mutation in A− is G→A at nt 202. However, there may be mutations at nt 680 or nt 968 instead. Thus, at the molecular level, there are three A− variants instead of one. On the other hand, a few separately recorded variants were at first erroneously thought to be distinct from A−. In any case, all African deficiency variants are descendants of A+ (Kay et al., 1992).

One of the more common variants in the Orient is G-6-pD Canton which has a mutation at nt 1376 (Beutler, 1993); the same mutation turned out to be present in three other variants which had been thought to be independent. An equivalent situation occurred in Europe. G-6-pD Mediterranean is characterised by a C→T substitution at nt 563. The four variants formerly distinguished as G-6-pD Cagliari, Dallas, Birmingham and Sassari turned out to be identical with G-6-pD Mediterranean.

However, there is a peculiar observation in that virtually all persons from Southern Europe and the Near East who have G-6-pD Mediterranean also have the noncoding mutation at nt 1311. In addition, this noncoding mutation is common in the area and present in 20% of the Mediterranean population. Since subjects from India with G-6-pD Mediterranean did not have the 1311 mutation, Beutler (1992) suggested that G-6-pD Mediterranean arose as independent mutations in Europe and in India.

The main pathological effects of G-6-pD deficiency are neonatal jaundice and hemolysis. Neonatal jaundice can be due to overproduction or undersecretion of bilirubin and thus can have many causes, but the likelihood of its occurrence is much enhanced in the presence of G-6-pD deficiency. Neonatal jaundice on the basis of G-6-pD deficiency is a relatively prominent problem in China and in Greece. The prevalence of G-6-pD deficiency in the Chinese and Malayan population of Singapore is in the order of 1.4%, but about 25% of newborns with jaundice have the deficiency. The relative magnitude of these figures varies. In Greece with an adult deficiency rate of slightly less than 5%, the rate is about 15% of cases with neonatal jaundice. Such population differences are compatible with the recently provided evidence by Kaplan et al. (1997) that it is the combination of deficiencies of G-6-pD and of glucuronyltransferase UDPGT1 (Gilbert syndrome) that causes neonatal jaundice.

Drug-induced hemolysis in G-6-pD deficiency generally requires enzymatic drug oxidation. Hence variability in drug oxidation may cause variability of the hemolytic response. A case in point has been the demonstration that the sulfonamides dapsone and promizole cause hemolysis only in persons with the double weakness of G-6-pD deficiency and genetically slow acetylation capacity (Brewer, 1986); the slow acetylation of these drugs increases their oxidative metabolism. A much investigated but not yet fully understood double defect must be the cause of favism, the hemolytic episode occurring in some Mediterranean people after eating fava beans; favism occurs only in persons with G-6-pD deficiency but not in all persons with this deficiency (Kattamis, 1986). It seems that the fate of the glycoside divicine, a component of the fava bean, varies metabolically or immunologically between persons.

Conclusions

It seems to be a fair notion that there is a rising interest in the differences of drug response that have been observed between the human races. Among the several factors that account for the increasing interest are the new opportunities of physicians in many urban centers to treat refugees and members of minorities. In the pharmaceutical industry with global sales programs, regional peculiarities in drug dosage or any accumulation of adverse reactions need to be known. Students of anthropology, population genetics, or molecular genetics see the opportunity for new observations.

Acknowledgements

The studies in the authors' laboratories reviewed here have been supported by the Medical Research Council of Canada (MT-4763), the Swedish Medical Research Council (3902), the EU Biomed1 (CT94–1622), Biomed2 (BMH4– CT96–0291) and Karolinska Institutet.

References

Adkins, S., Gan, K. N., Mody, M. and La Du, B. N. (1993) 'Molecular basis for the polymorphic forms of human serum paraoxonase/arylesterase: glutamine or arginine at position 191, for the respective A or B allozymes', *Am. J. Hum. Genet.* 52: 598–608.

Agúndez, J. A. G., Ledesma, M. C., Ladero, J. M. and Benitez, J. (1995) 'Prevalence of *CYP2D6* gene duplication and its repercussion on the oxidative phenotype in a white population', *Clin. Pharmacol. Ther.* 57: 265–9.

Aklillu, E., Persson, I., Bertilsson, L., Johansson, I., Rodriguez, F. and Ingelman-Sundberg. M. (1996) 'Frequent distribution of ultrarapid metabolizers of debrisoquine in an Ethiopian population carrying duplicated and multiduplicated functional CYP2D6 alleles', *J. Pharmacol. Exp. Ther.* 278: 441–6.

Aldridge, W. N. (1953) 'Serum esterases. II. An enzyme hydrolyzing diethyl p-nitrophenyl phosphate (E600) and its identity with the A-esterase of mammalian sera', *Biochem. J.* 53: 117–24.

Alván, G., Bechtel, P., Iselius, L. and Gundert-Remy, U. (1990) 'Hydroxylation polymorphisms of debrisoquine and mephenytoin in European populations', *Eur. J. Clin. Pharmacol.* 39: 533–7.

Ambroziak, W. and Pietruszko, R (1993) 'Metabolic role of aldehyde dehydrogenase', in H. Weiner, R. Lindahl, D. W. Crabb and T. G. Flynn (eds) *Enzymology and Molecular Biology of Carbonyl Metabolism 4,* New York: Plenum Presss, pp. 5–15.

Anderson, K. E., Conney, A. H. and Kappas, A. (1986) 'Nutrition as an environmental influence on chemical metabolism in man', in W. Kalow, H. W. Goedde and D. P. Agarwal (eds) *Ethnic Differences in Reactions to Drugs and Xenobiotics*, New York: Alan R. Liss, pp. 39–54.

Andersson, T., Cederberg, C., Edvardsson, G., Heggelund, A. and Lundborg, P. (1990a) 'Effect of omeprazole treatment on diazepam plasma levels in slow versus normal rapid metabolisers of omeprazole', *Clin. Pharmacol. Ther.* 47: 79–85.

Andersson, T., Miners, J. O., Veronese, M., Tassaneeyakul, W., Tassaneeyakul, W., Meyer, U. A. and Birkett, D. J. (1993) 'Identification of human liver cytochrome P450 isoforms mediating omeprazole metabolism', *Br. J. Clin. Pharmacol.* 36: 521–30.

Andersson, T., Regårdh, C. G., Dahl-Puustinen, M. L and Bertilsson, L. (1990b) 'Slow omeprazole metabolizers are also poor S-mephenytoin hydroxylators', *Ther. Drug. Monit.* 12: 415–6.

Andersson, T., Regårdh, C. G., Lou, Y. C., Zhang, Y., Dahl, M. L. and Bertilsson, L. (1992) 'Polymorphic hydroxylation of S-mephenytoin and omeprazole metabolism in Caucasian and Chinese subjects', *Pharmacogenetics* 2: 25–31.

Aviv, A. and Aladjem, M. (1990) 'Essential hypertension in blacks: epidemiology, characteristics, and possible roles of racial differences in sodium, potassium, and calcium regulation', *Cardiovascular Drugs & Therapy* 4 (Suppl. 2): 335–42.

Bernal, M. L., Sinues, B., Johansson, I., McLellan, R. A., Wennerholm, A., Dahl, M. L., Ingelman-Sundberg, M. and Bertilsson, L. (1999) 'Ten percent of North Spanish individuals carry duplicated or triplicated CYP2D6 genes associated with ultrarapid metabolism of debrisoquine', *Pharmacogenetics* 9: 657–60.

Bertilsson, L. and Åberg-Wistedt, A. (1983) 'The debrisoquine hydroxylation test predicts steady-state plasma levels of desipramine', *Br. J. Clin. Pharmacol.* 15: 388–90.

Bertilsson, L., Åberg-Wistedt, A., Gustafsson, L. L. and Nordin, C. (1985) 'Extremely rapid hydroxylation of debrisoquine – a case report with implication for treatment with nortriptyline and other tricyclic antidepressants', *Ther. Drug. Monit.* 7: 478–80.

Bertilsson, L., Alm, C., de las Carreras, C., Edman, G., Schalling, D. and Widén, J. (1989a) 'Debrisoquine hydroxylation polymorphism and personality', *Lancet* I: 555.

Bertilsson, L. and Dahl, M. L. (1996) 'Polymorphic drug oxidation: relevance to the treatment of psychiatric disorders', *CNS Drugs* 5: 200–23.

Bertilsson, L., Dahl, M. L., Sjöqvist, F., Åberg-Wistedt, A., Humble, M., Johansson, I., Lundqvist, E. and Ingelman-Sundberg, M. (1993) 'Molecular basis for rational megaprescribing in ultrarapid hydroxylators of debrisoquine', *Lancet* 341: 63.

Bertilsson, L., Eichelbaum, M., Mellström, B., Säwe, J., Schulz, H. U. and Sjöqvist, F. (1980) 'Nortriptyline and antipyrine clearance in relation to debrisoquine hydroxylation in man', *Life Sciences* 27: 1673–7.

Bertilsson, L., Henthorn, T. K., Sanz, E., Tybring, G., Säwe, J. and Villén, T. (1989b) 'Importance of genetic factors in the regulation of diazepam metabolism: relationship to S-mephenytoin, but not debrisoquine hydroxylation phenotype', *Clin. Pharmacol. Ther.* 45: 348–55.

Bertilsson, L. and Kalow, W. (1993) 'Why are diazepam metabolism and polymorphic S-mephenytoin hydroxylation associated with each other in white and Korean populations, but not in Chinese populations?', *Clin. Pharmacol. Ther.* 53: 608–10.

Bertilsson, L., Lou, Y. Q., Du, Y. L., Liu, Y., Kuang, T. Y., Liao, X. M., Wang, K. Y., Reviriego, J., Iselius, L. and Sjöqvist, F. (1992) 'Pronounced differences between native Chinese and Swedish populations in the polymorphic hydroxylations of debrisoquine and S-mephenytoin', *Clin. Pharmacol. Ther.* 51: 388– 97.

Beutler, E. (1990) 'The genetics of glucose-6-phosphate dehydrogenase deficiency', *Seminars in Hematology* 27: 137–64.

Beutler, E. (1992) 'The molecular biology of G6PD variants and other red cell enzyme defects', *Annu. Rev. Med.* 43: 47–59.

Beutler, E. (1993) 'Study of glucose-6-phosphate dehydrogenase: history and molecular biology', *Am. J. Hematol.* 42: 53–8.

Blum, M., Demierre, A., Grant, D. M., Heim, M. and Meyer, U. A. (1991) 'Molecular mechanism of slow acetylation of drugs and carcinogens in humans', *Proc. Nat. Acad. Sci. USA* 88: 5237–41.

Bonicke, R. and Reif, W. (1953) 'Enzymatische inaktivierung von Isonicotinsaure-hydrazid im menschlichen und tierischen Organismus', *Arch. Exper. Path. u. Pharmakol.* 220: 321–33.

Bosron, W. F. and Li, T. K. (1986) 'Genetic polymorphism of human liver alcohol and aldehyde dehydrogenases, and their relationship to alcohol metabolism and alcoholism', *Hepatology* 6: 502–10.

Böttiger, Y., Tybring, G., Götharson, E. and Bertilsson, L. (1997) 'Inhibition of the sulfoxidation of omeprazole by ketoconazole in poor and extensive metabolizers of S-mephenytoin', *Clin. Pharmacol. Ther.* 62: 384–91.

Brewer, G. J. (1986) 'Pharmacogenetic interaction of glucose-6-phosphate dehydrogenase deficiency with acetylation and hydroxylation', in A. Yoshida and E. Beutler (eds) *Glucose-6-phosphate Dehydrogenase*, Orlando: Academic Press, pp. 13–23.

Broly, F., Gaedigk, A., Heim, M., Eichelbaum, M., Morike, K. and Meyer, U. A. (1991) 'Debrisoquine/sparteine hydroxylation genotype and phenotype: analysis of common mutations and alleles of CYP2D6 in a European population', *DNA Cell Biol.* 10: 545–58.

Brøsen, K., Sindrup, S. H., Skjelbo, E. *et al.* (1993) 'Role of genetic polymorphism in psychopharmacology – an update, in L. F. Gram, G. P. Balant, H. Y. Meltzer *et al.* (eds) *Clinical Pharmacology in Psychiatry*, Berlin and Heidelberg: Springer-Verlag, pp. 199–211.

Burnell, J. C. and Bosron, W. F. (1989) 'Genetic polymorphism of human liver alcohol dehydrogenase and kinetic properties of the isoenzymes', in K. E. Crow and R. D. Batt (eds) *Human Metabolism of Alcohol, Vol. 2*, Boca Raton: CRC Press, pp. 65–75.

Carro-Ciampi, G., Gray, S. and Kalow, W. (1983) 'Paraoxonase phenotype distribution in Canadian Indian and Inuit populations', *Can. J. Physiol. Pharmacol.* 61: 336–40.

Carson, P. E., Flanagan, C. L., Iokes, C. E. and Alving, A. S. (1956) 'Enzymatic deficiency in primaquine-sensitive erythrocytes', *Science* 124: 484–5.

Cavalli-Sforza, L. L., Menozzi, P. and Piazza, A. (1994) *The History and Geography of Human Genes*, Princton: Princeton University Press.

Cavalli-Sforza, L. L., Piazza, A., Menozzi, P. and Mountain, J. (1988) 'Reconstruction of human evolution: bringing together genetic, archaeological, and linguistic data', *Proc. Nat. Acad. Sci. USA* 85: 6002–6.

Chang, M., Dahl, M. L., Tybring, G., Götharson, E. and Bertilsson, L. (1995) 'Use of omeprazole as a probe drug for CYP2C19 phenotype in Swedish Caucasians

– comparison with S-mephenytoin hydroxylation phenotype and CYP2C19 genotype', *Pharmacogenetics* **5**: 358–63.

Comas-Diaz, L. and Jacobsen, F. M. (1991) 'Ethnocultural transference and coutertransference in the therapeutic dyad', *Amer. J. Orthopsychiat.* **61**: 392–402.

Crabbe, J. C. and Harris, R. A. (eds) (1991) *The Genetic Basis of Alcohol and Drug Actions*, New York: Plenum Press.

Czeizel, A., Benkmann, H. G. and Goedde, H. W. (eds) (1991) *Genetics of the Hungarian Population: Ethnic Aspects, Genetic Markers, Ecogenetics and Disease Spectrum*, Budapest: Akademiai Kiado.

Dahl, M. L., Johansson, I., Bertilsson, L., Ingelman-Sundberg, M. and Sjöqvist, F. (1995) 'Ultrarapid hydroxylation of debrisoquine in a Swedish population. Analysis of the molecular genetic basis', *J. Pharmacol. Exp. Ther.* **274**: 516–20.

Dahl, M. L., Johansson, I., Porsmyr Palmertz, M. P., Ingelman-Sundberg, M. and Sjöqvist, F. (1992) 'Analysis of the CYP2D6 gene in relation to debrisoquine and desipramine hydroxylation in a Swedish population', *Clin. Pharmacol. Ther.* **51**: 12–17.

Dalén, P., Dahl, M. L., Bernal Ruiz, M. L., Nordin, J. and Bertilsson, L. (1998) '10–Hydroxylation of nortriptyline in Caucasians with 0, 1, 2, 3 and 13 functional CYP2D6 genes', *Clin. Pharmacol. Ther.* **63**: 444–52.

Daly, A. K., Brockmöller, J., Broly, F. Eichelbaum, M., Evans, W. E., Gonzales, F. J., Huang, J.-D., Idle, J. R., Ingleman-Sundberg, M., Ishizaki, T., Jacqz-Aigrain, E., Meyer, U. A., Nebert, D. W., Steen, V. M., Wolf, C. R. and Zanger, U. M. (1996) 'Nomenclature for human CYP2D6 alleles', *Pharmacogenetics* **6**: 193–201.

Deguchi, T., Mashimo, M. and Suzuki, T. (1990) 'Correlation between acetylator phenotypes and genotypes of polymorphic arylamine N-acetyltransferase in human liver', *J. Biol. Chem.* **265**: 12757–60.

De Morais, S. M. F., Wilkinson, G. R., Blaisdell, J., Meyer, U. A., Nakamura, K. and Goldstein, J. A. (1994b) 'Identification of a new genetic defect responsible for the polymorphism of (S)-mephenytoin metabolism in Japanese', *Mol. Pharmacol.* **46**: 594–8.

De Morais, S. M. F., Wilkinson, G. R., Blaisdell, J., Nakamura, K., Meyer, U. A. and Goldstein, J. A. (1994a) 'The major genetic defect responsible for the polymorphism of S-mephenytoin metabolism in humans', *J. Biol. Chem.* **269**: 15419–22.

Diepgen, T. L. and Geldmacher-von Mallinckrodt, M. (1986) 'Interethnic differences in the detoxification of organophosphates: the human serum paraoxonase polymorphism', *Arch Toxicol* **9** (Suppl): 154–8.

Dolphin, C. T., Riley, J. H., Smith, R. L., Shephard, E. A. and Phillips, I. R. (1997) 'Structural organization of the human flavin-containing monooxygenase 3 gene (FM03), the favored candidate for fish-odor syndrome, determined directly from genomic DNA', *Genomics* **46**: 260–7.

Eckerson, H. W., Oseroff, A., Lockridge, O. and La Du, B. N. (1983) 'Immunological comparison of the usual and atypical human serum cholinesterase phenotypes', *Bionchem. Genet.* **21**: 93–108.

Edenberg, H. J., Brown, C. J., Hur, M. W., Kotagiri, S., Li, M., Zhang, L. and Zhi, X. (1996) 'Regulation of the seven human alcohol dehydrogenase genes', in H. Weiner, R. Lindahl, D. W. Crabb and T. G. Flynn (eds) *Enzymology and Molecular Biology of Carbonyl Metabolism 6*, New York: Plenum Press, pp. 339–45.

Eichelbaum, M., Baur, M. P., Dengler, H. J., Osikowska-Evers, B. O., Tieves, G., Zekorn, C. and Rittner, C. (1987) 'Chromosomal assignment of human cytochrome P450 (debrisoquine/sparteine type) to chromosome 22', *Br. J. Clin. Pharmacol.* **23**: 455–8.

Eichelbaum, M., Bertilsson, L., Säwe, J. and Zekorn, C. (1982) 'Polymorphic oxidation of sparteine and debrisoquine. Related pharmacogenetic entities', *Clin. Pharmacol. Ther.* **31**: 184–6.

Eichelbaum, M. and Gross, A. S. (1992) 'The genetic polymorphism of debrisoquine/sparteine metabolism – clinical aspects', in W. Kalow (ed.) *Pharmacogenetics of Drug Metabolism*, New York: Pergamon Press, pp. 625–48.

Eichelbaum, M., Spannbrucker, N., Steinke, B. and Dengler, H. J. (1979) 'Defective N-oxidation of sparteine in man: a new pharmacogenetic defect', *Eur. J. Clin. Pharmacol.* **16**: 183–7.

Etler, D. A. (1992) 'Recent developments in the study of human biology in China: a review', *Hum. Biol.* **64**: 567–85.

Evans, D. A. P. (1992) 'N-Acetyltransferase', in W. Kalow (ed.) *Pharmacogenetics of Drug Metabolism Int Encycl Pharmacol Therap Sect. 137,* New York: Pergamon Press, pp. 95–178.

Ferguson, R. A. and Goldberg, D. M. (1997) 'Genetic markers of alcohol abuse', *Clin. Chim. Acta.* **257**: 199–250.

Fernandez-Salguero, P., Hoffman, S. M., Cholerton, S., Mohrenweiser, H., Raunio, H., Rautio, A., Pelkonen, O., Huang, J. D., Evans, W. E., Idle, J. R. *et al.* (1995) 'A genetic polymorphism in coumarin 7–hydroxylation: sequence of the human CYP2A genes and identification of variant CYP2A6 alleles', *Am. J. Hum. Genet.* **57**: 651–60.

Freis, E. D. (1986) 'Antihypertensive agents', in W. Kalow, H. W. Goedde and D. P. Agarwal (eds) *Ethnic Differences in Reactions to Drugs and Xenobiotics,* New York: Alan R. Liss, pp. 313–22.

Fuhr, U., Klittich, K. and Staib, A. H. (1993) 'Inhibitory effect of grapefruit juice and the active component naringenin on CYP1A2 dependent metabolism of caffeine in man', *Br. J. Clin. Pharmac* **35**: 431–6.

Furuta, T., Ohashi, K., Kamata, T., Takashima, M., Kosuge, K., Kawasaki, T., Hanai, H., Kubota, T., Ishizaki, T. and Kaneko, E. (1998) 'Effect of genetic differences in omeprazole metabolism on cure rates for *Helicobacter pylori* infection and peptic ulcer', *Ann. Int. Med.* **129**: 1027–30.

Gaedigk, A., Blum, M., Gaedigk, R., Eichelbaum, M. and Meyer, U. A. (1991) 'Deletion of the entire cytochrome P450 CYP2D6 gene as a cause of impaired drug metabolism in poor metabolizers of the debrisoquine/sparteine polymorphism', *Am. J. Hum. Genet.* **48**: 943–50.

Gaffney, D. and Campbell, R. A. (1994) 'A PCR based method to determine the Kalow allele of the cholinesterase gene: the Elk allele frequency and its significance in the normal population', *J. Med. Genet.* **31**: 248–50.

Goedde, H. W. and Agarwal, D. P. (1986) 'Aldehyde oxidation: ethnic variation in metabolism and response', in W. Kalow, H. W. Goedde and D. P. Agarwal (eds) *Ethnic Differences in Reactions to Drugs and Xenobiotics*, New York: Alan R. Liss, pp. 113–138.

Goedde, H. W. and Agarwal, D. P. (eds) (1987) *Genetics and Alcoholism.* New York: Alan R Liss.

Goedde, H. W. and Agarwal, D. P. (1992) 'Pharmacogenetics of aldehydo dehydrogenase', in W. Kalow (ed.) *Pharmacogenetics of Drug Metabolism Int Encycl Pharmacol Therap Sect 137*, New York: Pergamon Press, pp. 281–311.

Goldstein, J. A., Faletto, M. B., Romkes-Sparks, M., Sullivan, T., Kitareewan, S., Raucy, J. L., Lasker, J. M. and Ghanayem, B. I. (1994) 'Evidence that CYP2C19 is the major (S)-mehenytoin 4'-hydroxylase in humans', *Biochemistry* 33: 1743–52.

Gonzalez, F. J. (1992) 'Human cytochrome P450: problems and prospects', *Trends Pharmacol. Sci.* 13: 346–52.

Gorelick, D. A. (1997) 'Enhancing cocaine metabolism with butyrylcholinesterase as a treatment strategy', *Drug Alcohol Depend.* 48: 159–65.

Graf, T., Broly, F., Hoffman, F., Probst, M., Meyer, U. A. and Howald, H. (1992) 'Prediction of phenotype for acetylation and for debrisoquine hydroxylation by DNA-tests in healthy human volunteers', *Eur. J. Clin. Pharmacol.* 43: 399–403.

Grant, D. M. (1993) 'Molecular genetics of the N-acetyltransferases', *Pharmacogenetics* 3: 45–50.

Grant, D. M., Blum, M., Beer, M. and Meyer, U. A. (1991) 'Monomorphic and polymorphic human arylamine N-acetyltransferases: a comparison of liver isozymes and expressed products of two cloned genes', *Mol. Pharm.* 39: 184–91.

Grant, D. M., Hughes, N. C., Janezic, S. A., Goodfellow, G. H., Chen, H. J., Gaedigk, A., Yu, V. L. and Grewal, R. (1997) 'Human acetyltransferase polymorphisms', *Mutation Research* 376: 61–70.

Grant, D. M., Morike, K., Eichelbaum, M. and Meyer, U. A. (1990) 'Acetylation pharmacogenetics. The slow acetylator phenotype is caused by decreased or absent arylamine N-acetyltransferase in human liver', *J. Clin. Invest.* 85: 968– 72.

Griffith, M. W. (1977) 'The influences of race on the psychotherapeutic relationship', *Psychiatry* 40: 27–40.

Hahn, R. A. (1992) 'The state of federal health statistics on racial and ethnic groups', *JAMA* 267: 268–71.

Harada, S., Agarwal, D. P. and Goedde, H. W. (1978) 'Isozyme variations in acetaldehyde dehydrogenase (EC1.2.1.3.) in human tissues', *Hum Genet* 44: 181–5.

Hasumura, Y. and Takeuchi, J. (1991) 'Alcoholic liver disease in Japanese patients: a comparison with caucasians', *J. Gastroenterol. Hepat.* 6: 520–7.

Hayes, R. B., Bi, W., Rothman, N., Broly, F., Caporaso, N., Feng, P., You, X., Yin, S., Woosley, R. L. and Meyer, U. A. (1993) 'N-acetylation phenotype and genotype and risk of bladder cancer in benzidine-exposed workers', *Carcinogenesis* 4: 675–8.

Heim, H. M. and Meyer, U. A. (1990) 'Genotyping of poor metabolisers of debrisoquine by allele-specific PCR amplification', *Lancet* 336: 529–32.

Heim, H. M. and Meyer, U. A. (1992) 'Evolution of a high polymorphic human cytochrome P450 gene cluster: CYP2D6', *Genomics* 14: 49–58.

Hempel, J., Kaiser, R. and Jörnvall, H (1985) 'Mitochondrial aldehyde dehydrogenase from human liver: primary structure, differences in relation to the cytosolic enzyme and functional correlations', *Eur. J. Biochem.* 153: 13–28.

Herrlin, K., Massele, A. Y., Jande, M., Alm, C., Tybring, G.. Aden, Abdi.,Y., Wennerholm. A., Johansson, I., Dahl, M. L., Bertilsson, L. and Gustafsson, L. L. (1998) 'Bantu Tanzanians have a decreased capacity to metabolize omeprazole and mephenytoin in relation to their CYP2C19 genotype', *Clin. Pharmacol. Ther.* 64: 391–401.

Hickman, D. and Sim, E. (1991) 'N-acetyltransferase polymorphism: comparison of phenotype and genotype in humans', *Biochem. Pharmacol.* 42: 1007–14.

Higuchi, S. (1994) 'Polymorphisms of ethanol metabolizing enzyme genes and alcoholism', *Alcohol & Alcoholism* Suppl 2: 29–34.

Higuchi, S., Parrish, K. M., Dufour, M. C., Towle, L. H. and Harford, T. C. (1992) 'The relationship between three subtypes of the flushing response and DSM-III alcohol abuse in Japanese', *J. Studies on Alcohol* 53: 553–60.

Hirono, A. and Beutler, E. (1988) 'Molecular cloning and nucleotide sequence of cDNA for human glucose-6-phosphate dehydrogenase variant A(-)', *Proc. Natl. Acad. Sci. USA* 85: 3951–4.

Hoffman, R. S., Henry, G. C., Howland, M. A., Weisman, R. S., Weil, L. and Goldfrank, L. R. (1992) 'Association between life-threatening cocaine toxicity and plasma cholinesterase activity', *Ann. Emerg. Med.* 21: 247–53.

Holloway, M. and Yam, P. (1992) 'Reflecting differences: health care begins to address needs of women and minorities', *Scientific American* 13–18.

Horai, Y., Nakano, M., Ishizaki, T., Ishikawa, K., Zhou, H. H., Zhou, B. I., Liao, C. L. and Zhang, L. M. (1989) 'Metoprolol and mephenytoin oxidation polymorphisms in Far Eastern Oriental subjects: Japanese versus mainland Chinese', *Clin. Pharmacol. Ther.* 46: 198–207.

Hughes, H. B., Biehl, J. P., Jones, A. P. and Schmidt, L. H. (1954) 'Metabolism of isoniazid in man as related to the occurrence of peripheral neuritis', *Am. Rev. Tuberculosis* 70: 266–73.

Hughes, N., Janezic, S. A., McQueen, K. L., Jewett, M. A. S., Castranio, T., Bell, D. A. and Grant, D. M. (1998) 'Identification and characterization of variant alleles of human acetyltransferase NAT1 with defective function using p-aminosalicylate as an in-vivo and in-vitro probe', *Pharmacogenetics* 8: 55–66.

Hurley, T. D., Bosron, W. F., Stone, C. L. and Amzel, L. M. (1994) 'Structures of three human beta alcohol dehydrogenase variants. Correlations with their functional differences', *J. Mol. Biol.* 239: 415–29.

Hurley, T. D., Ehrig, T., Edenberg, H. J. and Bosron, W. F. (1990) 'Characterization of human alcohol dehydrogenases containing substitutions at amino acids 47 and 51', in H. Weiner, B. Wermuth and D. W. Crabb (eds) *Enzymology and Molecular Biology of Carbonyl Metabolism 3,* New York: Plenum Press, pp, 271–5.

Ilett, K. F., Chriswell, G. M., Spargo, R. M., Platt, E. and Minchin, R. F. (1993) 'Acetylation phenotype and genotype in aboriginal leprosy patients from the north-west region of Western Australia', *Pharmacogenetics* 5: 264–9.

Inaba, T., Jurima, M., Mahon, W. A. and Kalow, W. (1985) 'In vitro inhibition studies of two isozymes of human liver cytochrome P-450. Mephenytoin p-hydroxylase and sparteine monooxygenase', *Drug Metab. Dispos.* 13: 443–8.

Ingelman-Sundberg, M., Oscarsson, M. and McLellan, R. A. (1999) 'Polymorphic human cytochrome P450 enzymes: an opportunity for individualized drug treatment', *Trends in Pharmacol. Sci.* 20: 324–49.

Ishizaki, T., Sohn, D. R., Kobayashi, K., Chiba, K., Lee, K. H., Shin, S. G., Andersson, T, Regårdh, C. G., Lou, Y. C., Zhang, Y., Dahl, M. L. and Bertilsson, L. (1994) 'Interethnic differences in omeprazole metabolism in the two S-mephenytoin hydroxylation phenotypes studied in Caucasians and Orientals', *Ther. Drug Monit.* 16: 214–5.

Jeanes, C. W. L., Schaefer, O. and Eidus, L. (1972) 'Inactivation of isoniazid by Canadian Eskimos and Indians', *Can. Med. Assoc. J.* 106: 331–5.

Jensen, F. S., Nielsen, L. R. and Schwartz, M. (1996) 'Detection of the plasma cholinesterase K variant by PCR using an amplification-created restriction site', *Hum. Hered.* 46: 26–31.

Jensen, F. S., Schwarz, M. and Viby-Mogensen, J. (1995) 'Identification of human plasma cholinesterase variants using molecular biological techniques', *Acta Anaesthesiol. Scand.* **39**: 142–9.

Johansson, I., Lundqvist, E., Bertilsson, L., Dahl, M. L., Sjöqvist, F. and Ingelman-Sundberg, M. (1993) 'Inherited amplification of an active gene in the cytochrome P450 CYP2D-locus as a cause of ultrarapid metabolism of debrisoquine', *Proc. Natl. Acad. Sci. USA* **90**: 11825–9.

Johansson, I., Oscarsson, M., Yue, Q. Y., Bertilsson, L., Sjöqvist, F. and Ingelman-Sundberg, M. (1994) 'Genetic analysis of the Chinese CYP2D locus. Characterization of variant CYP2D6 genes present in subjects with diminished capacity for debrisoquine hydroxylation', *Mol. Pharmacol.* **46**: 452–9.

Johansson, I., Yue, Q. Y., Dahl, M. L., Heim, M., Säwe, J., Bertilsson, L., Meyer, U. A., Sjöqvist, F. and Ingelman-Sundberg, M. (1991) 'Genetic analysis of the interethnic difference between Chinese and Caucasians in the polymorphic metabolism of debrisoquine and codeine', *Eur. J. Clin. Pharmacol.* **40**: 553–6.

Johnson, J. A. (1997) 'Influence of race or ethnicity on pharmacokinetics of drugs', *J. Pharmaceut. Sci.* **86**: 1328–33.

Jordan, T. J., Lewit, E. M. and Reichman, L. B. (1991) 'Isoniazid preventive therapy for tuberculosis: decision analysis considering ethnicity and gender', *Am. Rev. Respir. Dis.* **144**: 1357–60.

Jornvall, H. and Hoog, J. O. (1995) 'Nomenclature of alcohol dehydrogenases', *Alcohol and Alcoholism* **30**: 153–61.

Jurima, M., Inaba, T., Kadar, D. and Kalow, W. (1985) 'Genetic polymorphism of mephenytoin *p* (4')-hydroxylation: difference between Orientals and Caucasians', *Br. J. Clin. Pharmacol.* **19**: 483–7.

Kalow, W. (1962) *Pharmacogenetics. Heredity and the Response to Drugs*, Philadelphia: W. B. Saunders Company.

Kalow, W. (1982a) 'Ethnic differences in drug metabolism', *Clin. Pharmacokinet.* **7**: 373–400.

Kalow, W. (1982b) 'The metabolism of xenobiotics in different populations', *Can. J. Physiol. Pharmacol.* **60**: 1–12.

Kalow, W. (1984a) 'Pharmacoanthropology: drug metabolism', *Federation Proceedings* **43**: 2326–31.

Kalow, W. (1984b) 'Pharmacoanthropology: outline, problems and the nature of case histories', *Federation Proceedings* **43**: 2314–8.

Kalow, W. (1988) 'Entwicklungen der pharmakogenetik – ein ruckblick zum 75', *Geburtstag von Hans Herken. Klin Wochenschr* **66**: 229–35.

Kalow, W. (1991) 'Interethnic variation of drug metabolism', *Trends Pharmacol. Sci.* **12**: 102–7.

Kalow, W. (1992a) 'Pharmacoanthropology and the genetics of drug metabolism', in W. Kalow (ed.) *Pharmacogenetics of Drug Metabolism Internatl Encycl Pharmacol Therap Sect 137*, New York: Pergamon Press, pp. 865–77.

Kalow, W. (ed.) (1992b) *Pharmacogenetics of Drug Metabolism, Int Encycl Pharmacol Therap Sect 137*, New York: Pergamon Press.

Kalow, W. (1993) 'Pharmacogenetics: its biologic roots and the medical challenge', *Clin. Pharmacol. Ther.* **54**: 235–41.

Kalow, W. and Bertilsson, L. (1994) 'Interethnic factors affecting drug response', in B. Testa and U. A. Meyer (eds) *Adv. in Drug Research, vol 25*, London: Academic Press, pp. 1–53.

Kalow, W. and Genest, K. (1957) 'A method for the detection of atypical forms of human serum cholinesterase. Determination of dibucaine numbers', *Can. J. Biochem. Physiol.* **35**: 339–46.

Kalow, W., Goedde, H. W. and Agarwal, D. P. (eds) (1986) *Ethnic Differences in Reactions to Drugs and Xenobiotics*, New York: Alan R. Liss.

Kalow, W. and Gunn, D. R. (1957) 'The relation between dose of succinylcholine and duration of apnea in man', *J. Pharmac. Exp. Therap.* **120**: 203–14.

Kalow, W., Ozdemir, V., Tang, B. K., Tothfalusi, L. and Endrenyi, L. (1999) 'The science of pharmacological variability: an essay', *Clin. Pharmacol. Ther.* **66**: 445–7.

Kalow, W. and Tang, B. K. (1993) 'The use of caffeine for enzyme assays: a critical apraisal', *Clin. Pharmacol. Ther.* **53**: 503–14.

Kalow, W., Tang, B. K. and Endrenyi, L. (1998) 'Hypothesis: comparisons of inter- and intra-individual variations can substitute for twin studies in drug research', *Pharmacogenetics* **8**: 283–9.

Kalow, W. and Tyndale, R. (1992) 'Debrisoquine/sparteine monooxygenase and other P-450s in brain', in W. Kalow (ed.) *Pharmacogenetics of Drug Metabolism. In Encycl. Pharmacol Therap. Sect. 137*, New York: Pergamon Press, pp. 649–56.

Kaneko, A., Lum, J. K., Yaviong, J., Takahashi, N., Ishizaki, T., Bertilsson, L., Kobayakawa, T. and Björkman, A. (1999) 'High and variable frequencies of *CYP2C19* mutations: medical consequences of poor drug metabolism in Vanuatu and other Pacific islands', *Pharmacogenetics* **9**: 581–90.

Kaplan, M., Renbaum, P., Levy-Lahad, E., Hammerman, C., Lahad, A. and Beutler, E. (1997) 'Gilbert syndrome and glucose-6-phosphate dehydrogenase deficiency: a dose-dependent genetic interaction crucial to neonatal hyperbilirubinemia', *Proc. Nat. Acad. Sci. USA* **94**: 12128–32.

Kassam, J. P., Tang, B. K., Kadar, D. and Kalow, W. (1989) 'In vitro studies of human liver alcohol dehydrogenase variants using a variety of substrates', *Drug Metab. Dispos.* **17**: 567–72.

Kattamis, C. (1986) 'Favism: epidemiological and clinical aspects', in A.Yoshida and E. Beutler (eds) *Glucose-6-phosphate Dehydrogenase*, Orlando: Academic Press, pp. 25–43.

Katz, M. (1979) 'Transcultural psychopharmacology in depression: east and west', *Psychopharmacology Bulletin* **15**: 24–6.

Kay, A. C., Kuhl, W., Prchal, J. and Beutler, E. (1992) 'The origin of glucose-6-phosphate-dehydrogenase (G6PD) polymorphisms in African-Americans', *Am. J. Hum. Genet.* **50**: 394–8.

Kedishvili, N. Y., Stone, C. L., Popov, K. M. and Chernoff, E. A. G. (1996) 'Role of alcohol dehydrogenases in steroid and retinoid metabolism', in H. Weiner, R. Lindahl, D. W. Crabb and T. G. Flynn (eds) *Enzymology and Molecular Biology of Carbonyl Metabolism 6* , New York: Plenum Press, pp. 321–9.

Koymans, L., Vermeulen, N. P., Van Acker, S. A., te Koppele, J. M., Heykants, J. J., Lavrijsen, K., Meuldermans, W.. and Donne-Op den Kelder, G. M. (1992) 'A predictive model for substrates of cytochrome P450–debrisoquine (2D6)', *Chem. Res. Toxicol.* **5**: 211–9.

Krisch, K. (1968) 'Enzymatische Hydrolyse von Diathyl-p-nitrophenylphosphat durch menschliches Serum', *Chem. Klin. Biochem.* **6**: 41–5.

Kudzma, E. C. (1992) 'Drug response: all bodies are not created equal', *Am. J. Nursing* **92**: 48–50.

Küpfer, A. and Preisig, R. (1984) 'Pharmacogenetics of mephenytoin: a new drug hydroxylation polymorphism in man', *Eur. J. Clin. Pharmacol.* **26**: 753–9.

La Du, B. N. (1992) 'Human serum paraoxonase/arylesterase', in W. Kalow (ed.) *Pharmacogenetics of Drug Metabolism Int Encycl Pharmacol Therap Sect 137*, New York: Pergamon Press, pp. 321–9.

La Du, B.N. (1995) 'Butyrylcholinesterase variants and the new methods of molecular biology', *Acta Anaesthesiol. Scand.* **39**: 139–41.

La Du, B. N. and Adkins, S. (1986) 'Analysis of the serum paraoxonase/arylesterase polymorphism in some Sudanese families', in W. Kalow, H. W. Goedde and D. P. Agarwal (eds) *Ethnic Differences in Reactions to Drugs and Xenobiotics*, New York: Alan R. Liss, pp. 87–98.

Lefley, H. P. (1990) 'Culture and chronic mental illness', *Hosp. Commun. Psychiatry* **41**: 277–86.

Leviev, I., Negro, F. and James, R. W. (1997) 'Two alleles of the human paraoxonase gene produce different amounts of mRNA. An explanation for differences in serum concentrations of paraoxonase associated with the (Leu-Met54) polymorphism', *Arterioscler. Thromb. Vasc. Biol.* **17**: 2935–9.

Lin, K. M. and Finder, E. (1983) 'Neuroleptic dosage for Asians', *Am. J. Psychiatry* **140**: 490–1.

Lin, K. M., Poland, R. E., Lau, J. K. and Rubin, R. T. (1988) 'Haloperidol and prolactin concentrations in Asians and Caucasians', *J. Clin. Psychopharmacol.* **8**: 195–201.

Lin, K. M., Poland, R. E. and Nakasaki, G. (1993) *Psychopharmacology and Psychobiology of Ethnicity*, Progress in Psychiatry No. 39, Washington, London: American Psychiatric Press.

Lin, K. M., Poland, R. E., Smith, M. W., Strickland, T. L. and Mendoza, R. (1991) 'Pharmacokinetic and other related factors affecting psychotropic responses in Asians', *Psychopharmacol. Bull.* **27**: 427–39.

Lin, H. J., Probst-Hensch, N. M., Hughes, N. C., Sakamoto, G. T., Louie, A. D., Kau, I. H., Lin, B. K., Lee, D. B., Lin, J., Frankl, H.D., Lee, E. R., Hardy, S., Grant, D. M. and Haile, R. W. (1998) 'Variants of N-acetyltransferase NAT1 and a case-control study of colorectal adenomas', *Pharmacogenetics* **8**: 269– 81.

Llerena, A., Alm, C., Dahl, M. L., Ekqvist, B. and Bertilsson, L. (1992) 'Haloperidol disposition is dependent of debrisoquine hydroxylation phenotype', *Ther. Drug Monit.* **14**: 92–7.

Llerena, A., Edman, G., Cobaleda, J., Benitez, J., Schalling, D. and Bertilsson, L. (1993) 'Relationship between personality and debrisoquine hydroxylation capacity – suggestion of an endogenous neuroactive substrate or product of the cytochrome P4502D6', *Acta Psych. Scand.* **87**: 23–8.

Lockridge, O. (1992) 'Genetic variants of human serum butyrylcholinesterase influence the metabolism of the muscle relaxant succinylcholine', in W. Kalow (ed.) *Pharmacogenetics of Drug Metabolism Int Encycl Pharmacol Therap Sect 137*, New York: Pergamon Press, pp. 15–50.

Lou, Y. C. (1990) 'Differences in drug metabolism polymorphisms between Orientals and Caucasians', *Drug. Metab. Rev.* **22**: 451–72.

Lou, Y. C., Liu, Y., Bertilsson, L. and Sjöqvist, F. (1987) 'Low frequency of slow debrisoquine hydroxylation in a native Chinese population', *Lancet* **II**: 852–3.

Luzzatto, L. (1986) 'Glucose-6-phosphate dehydrogenase and other genetic factors interacting with drugs', in W. Kalow, H. W. Goedde and D. Agarwal (eds) *Ethnic Differences in Reactions to Drugs and Xenobiotics*, New York: Alan R. Liss, pp. 385–99.

Luzzatto, L. and Mehta, A. (1989) 'Glucose-6-phosphate dehydrogenase deficiency', in C. R. Scriver, A. L. Beaudet, W. S. Sly and D. Vall (eds) *The Metabolic Basis of Inherited Disease*, New York: McGraw-Hill Information Services Company, pp. 2237–65.

Mackness, B., Durrington, P. N. and Mackness, M. I. (1998) 'Human serum paraoxonase', *Gen. Pharmacol.* 31: 329–36.

Mackness, B., Mackness, M. I., Arrol, S., Turkie, W. and Durrington, P. N. (1997) 'Effect of the molecular polymorphisms of human paraoxonase (PON1) on the rate of hydrolysis of paraoxon', *Br. J. Pharmacol.* 122: 265–8.

McLellan, R. A., Oscasson, M., Seidegård, J. E., Evans, D. A. P. and Ingelman-Sundberg, M. (1997) 'Frequent occurrence of *CYP2D6* gene duplication in Saudi Arabians', *Pharmacogenetics* 7: 187–91.

Maezawa, Y., Yamauchi, M., Toda, G., Suzuki, H. and Sakurai, S. (1995) 'Alcohol-metabolizing enzyme polymorphisms and alcoholism in Japan', *Alcohol Clin. Esp. Res.* 19: 951–4.

Mahgoub, A., Idle, J. R., Dring, D. G., Lancaster, R. and Smith, R.L. (1977) 'Polymorphic hydroxylation of debrisoquine in man', *Lancet* 2: 584–6.

Malo, D. and Skamene, E. (1994) 'Genetic control of host resistance to infection', *Trends in Genetics* 10: 365–71.

Masimirembwa, C. M., Beke, M., Hasler, J. A., Tang, B. K. and Kalow, W. (1995) 'Low CYP1A2 activity in rural Shona children of Zimbabwe', *Clin. Pharmacol. Ther.* 57: 25–31.

Masimirembwa, C., Hasler, J., Bertilsson, L., Johansson, I., Ekberg, O. and Ingelman-Sundberg, M. (1996a) 'Phenotype and genotype analysis of debrisoquine hydroxylase (CYP2D6) in a black Zimbabwean population. Reduced enzyme activity and evaluation of metabolic correlation of CYP2D6 probe drugs', *Eur. J. Clin. Pharmacol.* 51: 117–22.

Masimirembwa, C., Persson, I., Bertilsson, L., Hasler, J. and Ingelman-Sundberg, M. (1996b) 'A novel mutant variant of the CYP2D6 gene (CYP2D6*17) 'common in a black African population: association with diminished debrisoquine hydroxylase activity', *Br. J. Clin. Pharmacol.* 42: 713–9.

Masson, P., Legrand, P., Bartels, C. F., Froment, M. T., Schopfer, L. M. and Lockridge, O. (1997) 'Role of aspartate 70 and tryptophan 82 in binding of succinyldithiocholine to human butyrylcholinesterase', *Biochemistry* 36: 2266–77.

Mattes, C. E., Lynch, T. J., Singh, A., Bradley, R. M., Kellaris, P. A., Brady, R.O. and Dretchen, K. L. (1997) 'Therapeutic use of butyrylcholinesterase for cocaine intoxication', *Toxicol. Applied Pharmacol* 145: 372–80.

Mellström, B., Bertilsson, L., Säwe, J., Schulz, H. U. and Sjöqvist, F. (1981) 'E- and Z-hydroxylation of nortriptyline in man – relationship to polymorphic hydroxylation of debrisoquine', *Clin. Pharmacol. Ther.* 30: 189–93.

Mihara, K., Suzuki, A., Kondo, T., Yasui, N., Furukori, H., Nagashima, U., Otani, K., Kaneko, S. and Inoue, Y. (1999) 'Effects of the *CYP2D6*10* allele on the steady-state plasma concentrations of haloperidol and reduced haloperidol in Japanese patients with schizophrenia', *Clin. Pharmacol. Ther.* 65: 291–4.

Morita, S., Shimoda, K., Someya, T., Yoshimura, Y., Kamijima, K. and Kato, N. (2000) 'Steady-state plasma levels of nortriptyline and its hydroxylated metabolites in Japanese patients: impact of *CYP2D6* genotype on the hydroxylation of nortriptyline', *J. Clin. Psychopharmacol.* 20: 141–9.

Motulsky, A. G. (1996) 'Nutritional ecogenetics: homocysteine-related arteriosclerotic vascular disease, neural tube defects, and folic acid', *Am. J. Hum. Genet.* **58**: 17–20.

Nakamura, K., Goto, F., Ray, W. A., McAllister, C. B., Jacqz, E., Wilkinson, G. R. and Branch, R. A. (1985) 'Interethnic differences in genetic polymorphism of debrisoquine and mephenytoin hydroxylation between Japanese and Caucasian populations', *Clin. Pharmacol.* **38**: 402–8.

Nei, M. (1987) *Molecular Evolutionary Genetics,* New York: Columbia University Press.

Nei, M. and Saitou, N. (1986) 'Genetic relationship of human populations and ethnic differences in reaction to drugs and food', in W. Kalow, H. W. Goedde and D. P. Agarwal (eds) *Ethnic Differences in Reactions to Drugs and Xenobiotics,* New York: Alan R. Liss, pp. 21–37.

Nielsen, K. K., Brøsen, K., Hausen, M. G. J. and Gram, L. F. (1994) 'Single-dose limetics of clomipramine relationship to the sparteine and S-mephenytoin oxidation polymorphisms', *Clin. Pharmacol. Ther.* **55**: 518–27.

Niznik, H. B., Tyndale, R. F., Sallee, R. F., Gonzalez, F. J., Hardwick, J. P., Inaba, T. and Kalow, W. (1990) 'The dopamine transporter and cytochrome P450IID1 (debrisoquine 4–hydroxylase) in brain: resolution and identification of two distinct [^{3}H] GBR-12935 binding proteins', *Arch. Biochem. Biophys.* **276**: 424–32.

Nyberg, S., Farde, L., Halldin, C., Dahl, M. L. and Bertilsson, L. (1995) 'D2 dopamine receptor occupancy during low-dose treatment with haloperidol decanoate', *Am. J. Psychiatry* **152**: 173–8.

O'Dowd, B. F., Rothhammer, F. and Israel, Y. (1990) 'Genotyping of mitochondrial aldehyde dehydrogenase locus of native American Indians', *Alcoholism Clinical and Experimental Research* **14**: 531–3.

Okey, A. B. (1992) 'Enzyme induction in the cytochrome P-450 system', in W. Kalow (ed.) *Pharmacogenetics of Drug Metabolism Int Encycl Pharmacol Therap Sect 137,* New York: Pergamon Press, pp. 549–608.

Persidis, A. (1998) 'The business of pharmacogenomics', *Nat. Biotechnol.* **16**: 209–10.

Pianezza, M. L., Sellers, E. M. and Tyndale, R. F. (1998) 'Nicotine metabolism defect reduces smoking', *Nature* **393**: 750.

Playfer, J. R., Eze, L. C., Bullen, M. F. and Evans, D. P. (1976) 'Genetic polymorphism and interethnic variability of plasma paroxonase activity', *J. Med. Genet.* **13**: 337–42.

Potkin, S. E., Shen, Y., Pardes, H., Phelps, B. H., Zhou, D., Shu, L., Korpi, E. and Wyatt, R. J. (1984) 'Haloperidol concentrations elevated in Chinese patients', *Psychiatry Res.* **12**: 167–72.

Primo-Parmo, S. L., Bartels, C. F., Wiersema, B., van der Spek, A. F., Innis, J. W. and La Du, B. N. (1996b) 'Characterization of 12 silent alleles of the human butyrylcholinesterase (BCHE) gene', *Am. J. Hum. Genet.* **58**: 52–64.

Primo-Parmo, S., Sorenson, R. C., Teiber, J. and La Du, B. N. (1996a) 'The human serum paraoxonase/arylesterase gene (PON1) is one member of a multigene family', *Genomics* **33**: 1–10.

Reich, T., Edenberg, H. J., Goate, A., Williams, J. T., Rice, J. P., Van Eerdewegh, P., Foroud, T., Hesselbrock, V., Schuckit, M. A., Bucholz, K., Porjesz, B., Li, T. K., Conneally, P. M., Nurnberger, J. I. Jr., Tischfield. J. A., Crowe, R. R., Cloninger, C. R., Wu, W., Shears, S., Carr, K., Crose, C., Willig, C. and Begleiter, H. (1998)

'Genome-wide search for genes affecting the risk for alcohol dependence', *Am. J. Med. Genet.* 81: 207–15.

Roh, H. K., Chung, J. Y., Oh, D. Y., Park, C. S., Svensson, J. O., Dahl, M. L. and Bertilsson, L. (2001) 'Plasma concentrations of haloperidol and its reduced metabolite and related to the *CYP2D6* genotype at low, but not high doses of haloperidol in Korean schizophrenic patients', *Br. J. Clin. Pharmacol.* (in press).

Roh, H. K., Dahl, M. L., Johansson, I., Ingelman-Sundberg, M., Cha, Y. N. and Bertilsson, L. (1996a) 'Debrisoquine and S-mephenytoin hydroxylation phenotypes and genotype in a Korean population', *Pharmacogenetics* 6: 441–7.

Roh, H. K., Dahl, M. L., Tybring, G., Yamada, H., Cha, Y. N. and Bertilsson, L. (1996b) 'CYP2C19 genotype and phenotype determined by omeprazole in a Korean population' *Pharmacogenetics* 6: 547–51.

Rosenberg, L. E. (1984) 'Inborn errors of nutriet metabolism Garrod's lessons and legacies', in A. Velazquex and H. Bourges (eds) *Genetic Factors in Nutrition*, Orlando: Academic Press, pp. 61.

Roy, A. C., Saha, N., Tay, J. S. H. and Ratnam, S. S. (1991) 'Serum paraoxonase polymorphism in three populations of southeast Asia', *Hum. Hered.* 41: 265–9.

Rubinstein, H. M.., Dietz, A. A. and Lubrano, T. (1978) 'E$^k_1$, another quantitative variant at cholinesterase locus l', *J. Med. Genet.* 15: 27–9.

Rudorfer, M. V., Lane, E. A., Chang, W. H., Zhang, M. D. and Potter, W. Z. (1984) 'Desipramine pharmacokinetics in Chinese and Caucasian volunteers', *Br. J. Clin. Pharmacol.* 17: 433–40.

Sachse, C., Brockmöller, J., Bauer, S. and Roots, I. (1997) 'Cytochrome P450 2D6 variants in a Caucasian population: allele frequencies and phenotypic consequences', *Am. J. Hum. Genet.* 60: 284–95.

Sagar, M., Tybring, G., Dahl, M. L., Bertilsson, L. and Seensalu, R. (2000) 'Effects of omeprazole on intragastric pH and gastrin are dependent on the *CYP2C19* polymorphism', *Gastroenterology* 119: 670–76.

Sanghera, D. K., Aston, C. E., Saha, N. and Kamboh, M. I. (1998) 'DNA polymorphisms in two paraoxonase genes (PON1 and PON2) are associated with the risk of coronary heart disease', *Am. J. Hum. Genet.* 62: 36–44.

Sanz, E. J., Villén, T., Alm, C. and Bertilsson, L. (1989) 'S-mephenytoin hydroxylation phenotype in a Swedish population – determined after coadministration with debrisoquine', *Clin. Pharmacol. Ther.* 45: 495–9.

Schwartz, H. J. and Johnson, D. (1996) 'In vitro competitive inhibition of plasma cholinesterase by cocaine: normal and variant genotypes', *J. Toxicol. Clin. Toxicol.* 34: 77–81.

Schönbaum, E. and Lomax, P. (1993) *Thermoregulation Pathology, Pharmacology, and Therapy*, New York: Pergamon Press.

Shen, Y. C., Fan, J. H., Edenberg, H. J., Li, T. K., Cui, Y. H., Wang, Y. F., Tian, C. H., Zhou, C. F., Zhou, R. L., Wang, J., Zhao, Z. L. and Xia, G. Y. (1997) 'Polymorphism of ADH and ALDH genes among four ethnic groups in China and effects upon the risk for alcoholism', *Alcohol Clin. Esp. Res.* 21: 1272–7.

Shibuta, K., Abe, M. and Suzuki, T. (1994) 'A new detection method for the K variant of butyrylcholinesterase based on PCR primer introduced restriction analysis (PCR-PIRA)', *J. Med. Genet.* 31: 576–9.

Shimoda, K., Jerling, M., Böttiger, Y., Yasuda, S., Morita, S. and Bertilsson, L. (1999) 'Pronounced differences in disposition of clomipramine between Japanese and Swedish patients', *J. Clin. Psychopharmacol.* 19: 393–400.

Singh, S., Fritze, G., Fang, B., Harada, S., Paik, Y. K., Eckey, R., Agarwal, D. P. and Goedde, H. W. (1989) 'Inheritance of mitochondrial aldehyde dehydrogenase: genotyping in Chinese, Japanese and South Korean families reveals dominance of the mutant allele', *Hum. Genet.* **83**: 119–21.

Skjelbo, E., Brøsen, K., Hallas, J. and Gram, L. F. (1991) 'The mephenytoin oxidation polymorphism is partially responsible for the N-demethylation of imipramine', *Clin. Pharmacol. Ther.* **49**: 18–23.

Skoda, R. C., Gonzalez, F. J., Demierre, A. and Meyer, U. A. (1988) 'Two mutant alleles of the human cytochrome P450 db1 gene (P450 II D1) associated with genetically deficient metabolism of debrisoquine and other drugs', *Proc. Natl. Acad. Sci. USA* **85**: 5240–3.

Smolen, A,, Eckerson, H. W. and La Du, B. N. (1982) 'Purification of arylesterases A and B from human serum', *Am. J. Hum. Genet.* **34**: 63A.

Sohn, D. R., Kobayashi, K., Chiba, K., Lee, K. H., Shin, S. G. and Ishizaki, T. (1992a) 'Disposition kinetics and metabolism of omeprazole in extensive and poor metabolizers of S-mephenytoin 4′-hydroxylation recruited from an Oriental population', *J. Pharmacol. Exp. Ther.* **262**: 1195–202.

Sohn, D. R., Kusaka, M., Ishizaki, T., Shin, S. G., Jang, I. J., Shin, J. G. and Chiba, K. (1992b) 'Incidence of S-mephenytoin hydroxylation deficiency in a Korean population and the interphenotypic differences in diazepam pharmacokinetics', *Clin. Pharmacol. Ther.* **52**: 160–9.

Sohn, D. R., Shin, S. G., Park, C. W., Kusaka, M., Chiba, K. and Ishizaki, T. (1991) 'Metoprolol oxidation polymorphism in a Korean population: comparison with native Japanese and Chinese populations', *Br. J. Clin. Pharmacol.* **32**: 504–7.

Spielberg, S. P. (1996) 'N-acetyltransferases: pharmacogenetics and clinical consequences of polymorphic drug metabolism', *J. Pharmacokin. Biopharmaceut.* **24**: 509–19.

Strasser, F., Huyng, M. N. and Plapp, B. V. (1996) 'Activity of liver alcohol dehydrogenases of steroids', in H. Weiner, R. Lindahl, D. W. Crabb and T. G. Flynn (eds) *Enzymology and Molecular Biology of Carbonyl Metabolism 6*, New York: Plenum Press, pp. 313–20.

Suddendorf, R. F. (1989) 'Research on alcohol metabolism among Asians and its implications for understanding causes of alcoholism', *Public Health Reports* **104**: 615–20.

Sudo, K., Maekawa, M., Akizuki, S., Magara, T., Ogasawara, H. and Tanaka, T. (1997) 'Human butyrylcholinesterase L3301 mutation belongs to a fluoride-resistant gene, by expression in human fetal kidney cells', *Biochem. Biophys. Res. Commun.* **240**: 372–5.

Suzuki, A., Otani, K., Mihara, K., Yasui, N., Kaneko, S., Inoue, Y. and Hayashi, K. (1997) 'Effects of the CYP2D6 genotype on the steady-state plasma concentrations of haloperidol and reduced haloperidol in Japanese schizophrenic patients', *Pharmacogenetics* **7**: 415–8.

Tanaka, F., Shiratori,Y,. Yokosuka, O., Imazeki, F., Tsukada, Y. and Omata, M. (1996) 'High incidence of ADH2*1/ALDH2*1 genes among Japanese alcohol dependents and patients with alcoholic liver disease', *Hepatology* **23**: 234–9.

Tanigawara, Y., Aoyama, N., Kita, T., Shirakawa, K., Komada, F., Kasuga, M. and Okumura, K. (1999) 'CYP2C19 genotype-related efficacy of omeprazole for the treatment of infection caused by *Helicobacter pylori*', *Clin. Pharmacol. Ther.* **66**: 528–34.

Thomasson, H. R., Edenberg, H. J., Crabb, D. W., Mai, X. L., Jerome, R. E., Li, T. K., Wang, S. P., Lin, Y. T., Lu, R. B. and Yin, S. J. (1991) 'Alcohol and aldehyde dehydrogenase genotypes and alcoholism in Chinese men', *Am. J. Hum. Genet.* 48: 677–81.

Träskman, L., Åsberg, M., Bertilsson, L., Cronholm, B., Mellström, B., Neckers, L. M., Sjöqvist, F., Thorén, P. and Tybring, G. (1979) 'Plasma levels of chlorimipramine and its demethyl metabolite during treatment of depression', *Clin. Pharmacol. Ther.* 26: 600–10.

Tucker, G. T., Silas, J. H., Iyun, A. O., Lennard, M. S. and Smith, A. J. (1977) 'Polymorphic hydroxylation of debrisoquine in man', Lancet 2: 718.

Usanga, E. A. and Luzzatto, L. (1985) 'Adaptation of plasmodium falciparum to glucose 6-phosphate dehydrogenase-deficient host red cells by production of parasite-encoded enzyme', *Nature* 313: 793–5.

Vasiliou, V. (1997) 'Appendix B, aldehyde dehydrogenase genes', in H. Weiner, R. Lindahl, D. W. Crabb and T. G. Flynn (eds) *Enzymology and Molecular Biology of Carbonyl Metabolism 6*, New York, Plenum Press, pp. 595–600.

Vatsis, K. P., Martell, K. J. and Weber, W. W. (1991) 'Diverse point mutations in the human gene for polymorphic N-acetyltransferase', *Proc. Natl. Acad. Sci. USA* 88: 6333–7.

Vatsis, K. P., Weber, W. W., Bell, D. A., Dupret, J. M., Price Evans. D. A., Grant. D. M., Hein, D. W., Lin, H. J., Meyer, U. A., Relling, M. V., Sim, E., Suzuki, T. and Yamazoe, Y. (1995) 'Nomenclature for N-acetyltransferases', *Pharmacogenetics* 5: 1–17.

Velazquez, A. and Bourges, H. (1984) *Genetic Factors in Nutrition*, New York: Academic Press.

Vesell, E. S. (1992) 'Pharmacogenetic perspectives gained from twin and family studies', in W. Kalow (ed.) *Pharmacogenetics of Drug Metabolism Int Encycl Pharmacol Therap Sect 137*, New York: Pergamon Press, pp. 843–63

von Wartburg, J. P., Bethune, J. L. and Vallee, B. L. (1964) 'Human liver alcohol dehydrogenase. Kinetic and physcochemical properties', *Biochemistry* 3: 1775–82.

Vulliamy, T., Mason, P. and Luzzatto, L (1992) 'The molecular basis of glucose-6-phosphate dehydrogenase deficiency', *Trends in Genetics* 8: 138–43.

Walcher, D. N. and Kretchmer, N. (1993) *Food, Nutrition and Evolution. Food as an Environmental Factor in the Genesis of Human Variability,* New York: Masson Publishing USA.

Wang, S. L., Huang, J. D., Lai, M. D., Liu, B. H. and Lai, M. L. (1993) 'Molecular basis of genetic variation in debrisoquine hydroxylation in Chinese subjects: polymorhism in RFLP and DNA sequence of CYP2D6', *Clin. Pharmacol. Ther.* 53: 410–8.

Ward, S. A., Helby, N. A., Skjelbo, E., Brøsen, K., Gram, L. F. and Breckenridge, A. M. (1991) 'The activation of the biguanide antimalarial proguanil co-segregates with the mephenytoin oxidation polymorphism – a panel study', *Br. J. Clin. Pharmacol.* 31: 689–92.

Ward, S. A., Walle, T., Walle, U. K., Wilkinson, GR. and Branch, R. A. (1989) 'Propranolol's metabolism is determined by both mephenytoin and debrisoquine hydroxylase activities', *Clin. Pharmacol. Ther.* 45: 72–9.

Weber, W. W. (1987) *The Acetylator Genes and Drug Response,* New York: Oxford University Press.

Wedlund, P. J., Aslanian, W. S., McAllister, C. B., Wilkinson, G. R. and Branch, R. A. (1984) 'Mephenytoin hydroxylation deficiency in Caucasians: frequency of a new oxidative drug metabolism polymorphism', *Clin. Pharmacol. Ther.* **36:** 773–80.

Weiner, H., Lindahl, R., Crabb, D. W. and Flynn, T. G. (1997) *Enzymology and Molecular Biology of Carbonyl Metabolism 6,* New York: Plenum Press.

Wennerholm, A., Johansson, I., Massele, A. Y., Jande, M., Alm, C., Aden Abdi, Y., Dahl, M. L., Ingelman-Sundberg, M., Bertilsson, L. and Gustafsson, L. L. (1999) 'Decreased capacity for debrisoquine metabolism among black Tanzanians: analyses of the *CYP2D6* genotype and phenotype' *Pharmacogenetics* **9:** 707–14.

Whitfield, J. B. (1997) 'Meta-analysis of the effects of alcohol dehydrogenase genotype on alcohol dependence and alcoholic liver disease', *Alcohol & Alcoholism* **32:** 613–9.

Whittaker, M. (1986) 'Cholinesterase', *Monographs in Human Genetics. Vol 11,* Basel: Karger.

Wilkinson, G. R., Guengerich, F. P. and Branch, R. A.. (1992) 'Genetic polymorphism of S-mephenytoin hydroxylation', in W. Kalow (ed.) *Pharmacogenetics of Drug Metabolism,* New York: Pergamon Press, pp. 657–85.

Winkleby, M. A., Ragland, D. R., Syme, S. L. and Fisher, J. M. (1988) 'Heightened risk of hypertension among black males: the masking effects of covariables', *Am. J. Epidem.* **128:** 1075–83.

Wood, A. J. and Zhou, H. H. (1991) 'Ethnic differences in drug disposition and responsiveness', *Clin. Pharmacokinet.* **20:** 350–73.

Woolhouse, N. M., Eichelbaum. M., Oates, N. S., Idle, J. R. and Smith, R. L. (1985) 'Dissociation of coregulatory control of debrisoquine/phenformin and sparteine oxidation in Ghanians', *Clin. Pharmacol. Ther.* **37:** 512–21.

Wrighton, S. A., Stevens, J. C., Becker, G. W. and VandenBranden, M. (1993) 'Isolation and characterization of human liver cytochrome P4502C19: correlation between 2C19 and S-mephenytoin 4′-hydroxylation', *Arch. Biochem. Biophys.* **306:** 240–5.

Yoshida, A. and Beutler, E. (1986) *Glucose-6-phosphate Dehydrogenase,* Orlando: Academic Press.

Yue, Q. Y., Bertilsson, L., Dahl-Puustinen, M. L., Säwe, J., Sjöqvist, F., Johansson, I. and Ingelman-Sundberg, M. (1989a) 'Disassociation between debrisoquine hydroxylation phenotype and genotype among Chinese', *Lancet* **II:** 870.

Yue, Q. Y., Svensson, J. O., Alm, C. Sjöqvist, F. and Säwe, J. (1989b) 'Inter-individual and interethnic differences in the demethylation and glucuronidation of codeine', *Br. J. Clin. Pharm.* **28:** 629–37.

Yue, Q. and Säwe, J. (1992) 'Interindividual and interethnic differences in codeine metabolism', in W. Kalow (ed) *Pharmacogenetics of Drug Metabolism. Int Encycl Pharmacol Therap Sect 137,* New York: Pergamon Press, pp. 721–7.

Yue, Q. Y., Zhong, Z. H., Tybring, G., Dalén, P., Dahl, M. L., Bertilsson, L. and Sjöqvist, F. (1998) 'Pharmacokinetics of nortriptyline and its 10–hydroxy meta-bolite in Chinese subjects of different CYP2D6 genotypes', *Clin. Pharmacol. Ther.* **64:** 384–90.

Zhang, Y., Reviriego, J., Lou, Y. Q., Sjöqvist, F. and Bertilsson, L. (1990) 'Diazepam metabolism in native Chinese poor and extensive hydroxylators of S-mephenytoin: interethnic differences in comparison with white subjects', *Clin. Pharmacol. Ther.* **48:** 496–502.

Chapter 3

Development and ageing as sources of variability in drug metabolism

A. Rane

Background

The elimination processes may be envisaged as a chemical defense of the body in the absence of which extensive toxicity to drugs and other chemicals would ensue. Just as with other physiological processes, metabolism of drugs varies throughout maturation and ageing. The variability in drug metabolism is two-dimensional. First, there is a variation along the age axis. Second, and perpendicular to the age axis, there is a variation at each stage of development and ageing. The former kind of variation has been extensively explored and described (O'Mahony and Woodhouse, 1994; Woodhouse and Wynne, 1992; Rane, 1995), whereas only little information about the latter dimension of variability is available.

Data interpretation

Practical and ethical constraints set a limit to the type of pharmacokinetic studies that can be performed and that give the best information about drug metabolic capacity in infants, children, and adults. Most commonly, plasma half-life $(t_{1/2})$ is described in the literature. However, the $t_{1/2}$ may not reflect only the drug-clearing capacity.

The drug metabolism capacity is preferably estimated by the clearance term (Cl) which is the volume of blood or plasma that is irreversibly cleared from the drug in unit time. Drug clearance is measured on the basis of the plasma concentration profile, i.e. the area under the plasma concentration versus time curve (AUC), after an oral (o), or an intravenous (i.v.) dose. If the dose is administered orally, a bioavailability factor (F) has to be introduced. F is the fraction of the oral dose that reaches the systemic circulation without being bound/metabolised in the gut wall and liver after absorption. Accordingly,

$$Cl_{iv} = D_{iv}/AUC_{iv} \qquad (1)$$
$$Cl_o = F \times D_o/AUC_o \qquad (2)$$

Presystemic binding and/or metabolism equals $1-F$ and is collectively called "first pass elimination", or presystemic elimination (E). It follows that

$$F=1-E \tag{3}$$

A low value of F indicates high presystemic elimination and/or incomplete absorption of the drug.

A physiological approach to drug clearance (Rowland *et al.*, 1973; Wilkinson and Shand, 1975) has established that extraction over the metabolising organ, in most cases the liver, E_H, is a function not only of the drug-metabolising enzyme activity (Cl_i=total intrinsic hepatic clearance) but also of the hepatic blood flow (Q), according to the following equations:

$$Cl_H=Q \times E_H \tag{4}$$
$$Cl_H=Q \, [Cl_i/Q+Cl_i] \tag{5}$$

The Cl_i is defined as the maximum capacity to remove drug from the blood in the absence of flow limitations. From this equation it is obvious that changes in liver blood flow will preferentially affect clearance of drugs with high values of Cl_i, which may be observed as changes in plasma half-life $(t_{1/2})$. In contrast, changes in enzymatic activity will particularly affect the clearance of drugs with low values of Cl_i. Such changes affect the AUC after both oral and intravenous administration, such that the AUC is decreased when the enzyme activity increases.

The hepatic clearance is also dependent on drug binding in blood, and this is accounted for by modification of equation (5):

$$Cl_H=Q \, [f_u \times Cl'_i : Q+f_u \times Cl'_i] \tag{6}$$

In equation (6), f_u denotes the unbound fraction in blood and Cl'_i is the intrinsic hepatic clearance of unbound drug. This equation shows that drug binding in blood has little importance for E and Cl_H if Cl'_i is high. In contrast, it may influence the Cl_H if the value of Cl'_i is low (Wilkinson and Shand, 1975).

As a consequence of these pharmacokinetic considerations, caution must be exercised in the interpretation of differences in the $t_{1/2}$ and/or AUC of drugs that are eliminated by metabolism; do they reflect differences in metabolic drug clearance or in blood flow of the drug metabolising organ, notably the liver? This obviously depends on the magnitude of Cl_i and only a few drugs have been classified according to this system. In the discussion of drug kinetics in different age groups it is thus essential to differentiate between "low clearance" and "high clearance" drugs.

By definition, the oral clearance of a drug (Cl_o) that is completely absorbed and metabolised only by the liver is equivalent to the intrinsic hepatic clearance of the drug. Unfortunately, there are few clinical situations that will permit measurement of Cl_o of such drugs. Therefore, the $t_{1/2}$ must be used as an estimate of the hepatic drug-metabolising activity when this is appropriate. It must be kept in mind that $t_{1/2}$ of a drug is also related to volume of distribution (V_d) according to

$$t_{1/2} = 0.693 \times V_d / Cl_H \tag{7}$$

In the absence of large variation in V_d, $t_{1/2}$ will reflect the hepatic enzyme activity for "low extraction" drugs, and hepatic blood flow for "high extraction" drugs, or both (for drugs with intermediate values of Cl_i).

For drugs without non-metabolic elimination pathways the drug-metabolising capacity is also reflected by the steady-state concentration (C_{ss}) according to equation (8).

$$C_{ss} = F \times D / Cl_H \times \tau \tag{8}$$

in which τ denotes the dosing interval.

In summary, it is obvious that the clinical situation and ethical constraints will yield few possibilities to study drug-metabolising capacity beyond determinations of C_{ss} and $t_{1/2}$ in children or adults. These parameters may, however, reflect drug-metabolic capacity in as much as the fraction metabolised and the clearance characteristics are known.

Clinical data

Relatively little interest has been devoted to studies of the variability in drug metabolism, particularly at the extremes of age. Relatively few drugs with known "extraction ratio" characteristics have been studied in infants and children, or in elderly subjects. Thus, there are limited possibilities to compare the variability in drug-metabolic disposition in infants, children, middle-aged subjects, and the elderly. Because of differences between laboratories in methodology and experimental approach, the best information is obtained when studies were performed in the same research group. Tables 3.1 and 3.2 list some studies that included one or several of the following age groups: newborns (0–1 month), infants (1 month–2 years), children (2–17 years), "middle-aged" adults (18–69 years), and elderly individuals (more than 70 years of age).

The frequency distribution of drug-metabolising ability is most often unimodal with widely separated extremes. For CYP3A, which is an important human liver enzyme with numerous endogenous and exogenous substrates including drugs, this variation may be five to twenty-fold (Wilkinson, 1996). The major causes of variation include genetic, physiological, and environmental factors. Obviously, genetic factors are constant

Table 3.1 Kinetics of some oxidised drugs in children and adults comparing the variability in half-life and clearance

Drug	Plasma or serum half-life (h)			Reference
	Newborns	Infants/ Children	Adults	
Acyclovir	105±42[a]		260±81	Blum et al., 1982
Amylobarbitone	17.4–59.5 (39)		11.6–27.2 (16)	Krauer et al, 1973
Carbamazepine	8.2–28.1	10.3–20.7 13.7–18.9	16.4–26.6	Rane et al., 1975 Eichelbaum et al., 1975 Bertilsson et al., 1980 Rane et al., 1976
Diazepam	25–100		15–25	Morselli et al., 1973
Phenobarbitone	21–100		52–120	Garretson and Dayton, 1970 Jalling, 1976 Butler et al., 1954 Lous, 1954
Phenylbutazone	21–34		12–30	Gladtke, 1968
Phenytoin	6.6–34.0		11–29	Rane et al., 1974 Lund et al., 1974
Theophylline	14.4–57.7	1.4–7.9	3.5–8.0	Aranda et al., 1976
Tolbutamide	10–40		4.4–9.0	Nitowsky et al., 1966

Notes

The numbers give average values with or without standard deviation or ranges and means (within parentheses).

[a] Clearance ml/min/1.73 m^2.

throughout life, whereas age as well as factors related to environmental influence will vary.

The variability in disposition of several drugs expressed as fold variation in half-life, or standard deviation (SD)/mean ratio for half-life or clearance is shown in Figures 3.1 and 3.2. It is obvious that the variation is larger at the young ages than in adults. There are no reasons at present to believe that environmental factors would cause the greater variation in half-life in the young age groups. Age itself appears to contribute to the variation as in the young age group. The degree of maturation of drug-metabolising enzymes may vary widely between subjects. It is plausible that endocrine factors play a role. Such factors may include transplacentally transferred maternal steroids, onset of certain endocrine processes in early life, etc. Other physiological determinants may also be important for the metabolic clearance by CYP enzymes.

In the elderly, clearance of many drugs may be as low as half of that in young cohorts. Age may affect the CYP3A catalysed clearance of drugs. Thus, elderly subjects may have as much as 30–50% less activity than young individuals (Wilkinson, 1996).

Many drugs must be used with caution in elderly patients because of low clearance and/or long half-lives. This enhances the risk of adverse drug

Table 3.2 Kinetics, and variation in kinetic parameters of some oxidised drugs in middle-aged adults and elderly individuals

Drug	Parameter	Age groups		Reference
		Adults	Elderly	
Amlodipine	Half-life (h)	42±8	58±11	Abernethy, 1994
	Clearance (l/h)	25.4±6.8	18.8±5.1	Abernethy, 1994
Antipyrine	Half-life (h)	6.6–14.5	8.4–25.9	Greenblatt et al., 1982
	Clearance (ml/min/kg)	0.55–1.46	0.22–0.94	Greenblatt et al., 1982
Desmethyldiazepam	Half-life (h)	51±6.2	151±60	Klotz et al., 1979
	Clearance (ml/min)	11.3±3.1	4.3±1.5	Klotz et al., 1979
Desmethyldiazepam	Half-life (h)	29.2–99.0	57.8–223.5	Allen et al., 1980
	Intrinsic clearance (ml/min/kg)	5.8–18.4	2.9–13.2	Allen et al., 1980
Nitrazepam	Half-life (h)	25.5±3.3	37.8±13.8	Jochemsen et al., 1983a
	Intrinsic clearance (ml/min)	489±100	456±103	Jochemsen et al., 1983a
Brotizolam	Half-life (h)	3.1–6.3	5.6–18.4	Jochemsen et al., 1983b
	Unbound clearance (ml/min/kg)	965–2026	313–725	Jochemsen et al., 1983b
Clobazam	Half-life (h)	11–23	29–77	Greenblatt et al., 1981a
	Unbound clearance (ml/min/kg)	4.0–8.6	1.6–5.1	Greenblatt et al., 1981a
Nitrazepam	Half-life (h)	28.9±7.4	40.4±16.2	Kangas et al., 1979
Desalkylflurazepam	Half-life (h)	37–118	71–289	Greenblatt et al., 1981b

Note
Values are given as range or mean ± standard deviation.

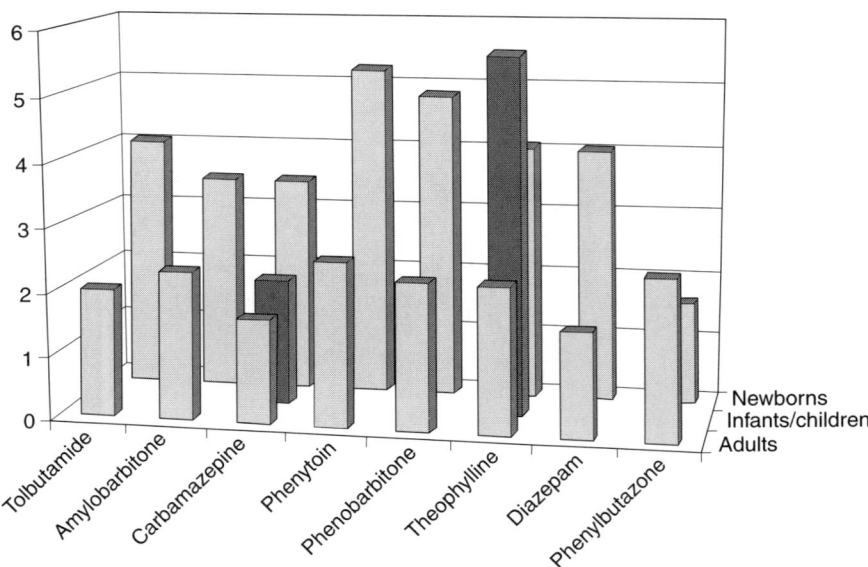

Figure 3.1 Pharmacokinetic variability of some drugs that are predominantly metabolised. Variation in half-life (fold-variation) in groups of newborns, infants/children, and adults. For literature reference, see Table 3.1.

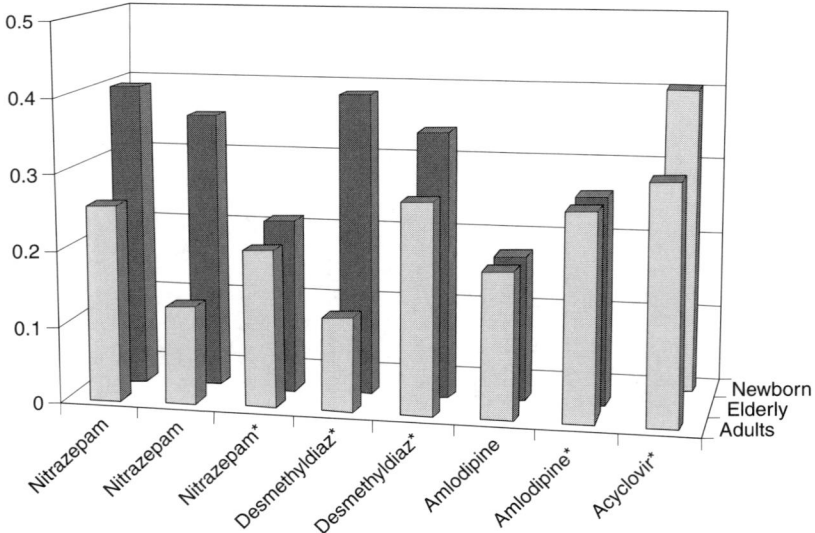

Figure 3.2 Pharmacokinetic variability of some drugs that are predominantly metabolised. Variability in half-life, clearance, or intrinsic clearance expressed as standard deviation (SD)/mean value ratios. Adults are compared with elderly individuals and, for acyclovir, newborns. No asterisk denotes half-life; an asterisk denotes clearance or intrinsic clearance. For literature reference and actual values, see Tables 3.1 and 3.2.

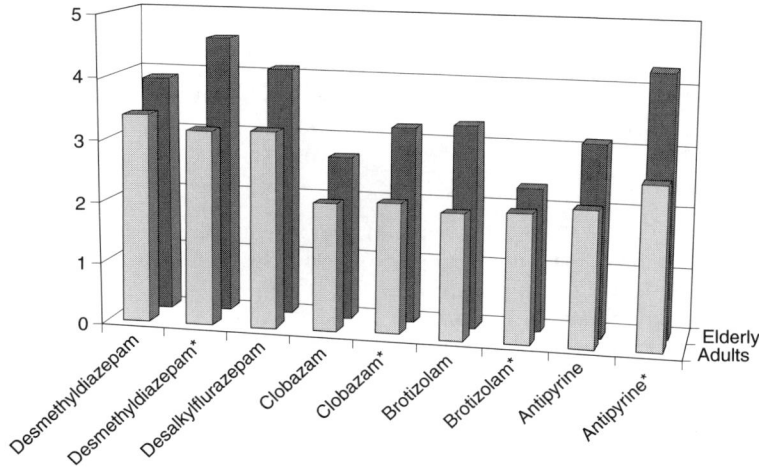

Figure 3.3 Pharmacokinetic variability of some drugs that are predominantly metabolised. Variation in half-life or clearance (fold-variation) in adults and elderly individuals. No asterisk denotes half-life; an asterisk denotes clearance or intrinsic clearance. For literature reference and actual values, see Table 3.2.

reactions. Drugs belonging to this group of agents include benzodiazepines (e.g. diazepam), hypoglycemic drugs (e.g. chlorpropamide), antidepressants (e.g. amitriptyline), etc.

A larger variability in disposition kinetics seems to exist more in the elderly than in middle-aged adult individuals (Table 3.2, Figures 3.2, 3.3). The data are based on half-lives or clearance and expressed as SD/mean ratios (Figure 3.2) or fold variation (Figures 3.1 and 3.3). This poses an additional safety problem if standard doses to all patients are used. It is thus obvious that information on age-dependent differences in variability should be highlighted in the documentation of drugs before use on a larger scale.

Other aspects of variability are worthy of discussion and investigation. There is no doubt that pharmacokinetic parameters will vary less when studied in only one of the sexes. Sex differences in drug disposition have been described in humans, although they are not as pronounced as in rats. Several drug substrates of CYP3A have been shown to be cleared at higher rates in women than in men (Watkins *et al.*, 1993; Hunt *et al.*, 1992; Watkins *et al.*, 1989; Hulst *et al.*, 1994) whereas the reverse has been described for CYP1A2 (Relling *et al.*, 1992). The literature appears to lack information on variability in men and women separately.

In conclusion, little attention has been paid to the variation in drug metabolism in different age periods of life. Available data indicate that endocrine/physiological factors are the major determinants of this difference in variation. Further studies are needed, as variation in metabolism is a major cause of concern in dose optimisation.

Acknowledgements

Part of this work was supported by grants from the Swedish Medical Research Council (04496) and Biomedical Research at European Commission, Brussels (BMH1–CT94–1622).

References

Abernethy, D. R. (1994) 'An overview of the pharmacokinetics and pharmaco-dynamics of amlodipine in elderly persons with systemic hypertension', *Am. J. Cardiol.* **73**: 10A–17.

Allen, M. D., Greenblatt, D. J., Harmatz, J. S. and Shader, R. I. (1980) 'Desmethyl-diazepam kinetics in the elderly after oral prazepam', *Clin. Pharmacol. Ther.* **28**: 196–202.

Aranda, J. V., Sitar, D. S., Parsons, D. V., Loughnan, P. M. and Neims, A. H. (1976) 'Pharmacokinetic aspects of theophylline in premature newborns', *N. Engl. J. Med.* **295**: 413–6.

Bertilsson, L., Höjer, B., Tybring, G., Osterloh, J. and Rane, A. (1980) 'Auto-induction of carbamazepine metabolism in children examined by a stable isotope technique', *Clin. Pharmacol. Ther.* **27**: 83–8.

Blum, M. R., Liao, S. H. T. and de Miranda, P. (1982) 'Overview of acyclovir pharmacokinetic disposition in adults and children', *Am. J. Med.* **73**: 186–92

Butler, T. C., Mahafee, C. and Wadell, W. J. (1954) 'Phenobarbital: studies on elimination, accumulation tolerance and dosage schedules', *J. Pharmacol. Exp. Ther.* **1211**: 425–35.

Eichelbaum, M., Ekbom, K., Bertilsson, L., Ringberger, V. A. and Rane, A. (1975) 'Plasma kinetics of carbamazepine and its epoxide metabolite in man after single and multiple doses. *Eur. J. Clin. Pharmacol.* **8**: 337–41.

Garretsson, L. K. and Dayton, P. G. (1970) 'Disappearance of phenobarbital and diphenylhydantoin from serum of children. *Clin. Pharmacol. Ther.* **11**: 674–9.

Gladtke, E. (1968) 'Pharmacokinetic studies on phenylbutazone in children' *Farmaco. Ed. Sci.* **23**: 897–906.

Greenblatt, D. J., Divoll, M., Abernethy, D. R., Harmatz, J. S. and Shader, R. I. (1982) 'Antipyrine kinetics in the elderly: prediction of age-related changes in benzodiazepine oxidizing capacity', *J. Pharmacol. Exp. Ther.* **220**: 120–6.

Greenblatt, D. J., Divoll, M., Puri, S. K., Ho, I., Zinny. M. A. and Shader, R. I. (1981a) 'Clobazam kinetics in the elderly', *Br. J. Clin. Pharmac.* **12**: 631–6.

Greenblatt, D. J., Divoll, M., Harmatzm, J. S., MacLaughlin, D. S. and Shader, R. I. (1981b) 'Kinetics and clinical effects of flurazepam in young and elderly noninsomniacs', *Clin. Pharmacol. Ther.* **30**: 475–86.

Hulst, L. K., Fleishaker, J. C., Peters, G. R., Harry, J. D., Wright, D. M. and Ward, P. (1994) 'Effect of age and gender on trilazad pharmacokinetics in humans', *Clin. Pharmacol. Ther.* **55**: 378–84.

Hunt, C., Westerkam, W. R. and Stave, G. M. (1992) 'Effect of age and gender on the activity of human hepatic CYP3A', *Biochem. Pharmacol.* **44**: 275–83.

Jalling, B. (1976) 'Plasma and cerebrospinal fluid concentrations of phenobarbital in infants given single doses', *Dev. Med. Child. Neurol.* **16**: 781–93.

Jochemsen, R., van Beusekom, B. R., Spoelstra, P., Janssen, A. R. and Breimer, D. D. (1983a) 'Effect of age and liver cirrhosis on the pharmacokinetics of nitra-zepam', *Br. J. Clin. Pharmac.* **15**: 295–302.

Jochemsen, R., Nandi, K. L., Corless, D., Wesselman, J. G. J. and Breimer, D. D. (1983b) 'Pharmacokinetics of brotizolam in the elderly', *Br. J. Clin. Pharmac.* **16:** 299S-307S.

Kangas, L., Iisalo, E., Kanto, J., Lehtinen, V., Pynnönen, S., Ruikka, I., Salminen, J., Sillanpää, M. and Syvälahti, E. (1979) 'Human Pharmacokinetics of nirazepam: effect of age and diseases', *Eur. J. Clin. Pharmacol.* **15:** 163-70.

Klotz, U. and Müller-Seydlitz, P. (1979) 'Altered elimination of desmethyldiazepam in the elderly', *Br. J. Clin. Pharmac.* **7:** 119-20.

Krauer, B., Draffan, G. H., Williams, F. M., Clare, R. A., Dollery, C. T. and Hawkins, D. F. (1973) 'Elimination of amobarbital in mothers and their newborn infants', *Clin. Pharmacol. Ther.* **14:** 442-7.

Lous, P. (1954) 'Blood serum and cerebrospinal fluid levels and renal clearance of phenemal in treated epileptics', *Acta. Pharmacol.* **10:** 261-80.

Lund, L. (1974) 'Anticonvulsant effect of diphenylhydantoin relative to plasma levels. A prospective three-year study in ambulant patients with generalized epileptic seizures', *Arch. Neurol.* **31:** 289-94.

Morselli, P. L., Principi, N., Tognoni, G., Reali, E., Belvedere, G., Stranden, S. M. and Sereni, F. (1973) 'Diazepam elimination in premature and full term infants and children', *J. Perinatal Med.* **1:** 133-41.

Nitowsky, H. M., Marz, L. and Berzofsky, J. A. (1966) 'Studies on oxidative drug metabolism in the full-term newborn infant', *Pediatr. Pharmacol. Ther.* **69:** 1139-49.

O'Mahony, M. S. and Woodhouse, K. W. (1994) 'Age, environmental factors and drug metabolism', *Pharmacol. Ther.* **61:** 279-87.

Rane, A. (1995) 'The major physiological factors that modulate drug metabolism in man. Implications for drug effects and toxicity', in G. M. Pacific and G. N. Fracchia (eds) *Advances in Drug Metabolism in Man*, European Commission, Directorate General XIII, Luxembourg, pp. 149-75.

Rane, A., Bertilsson, L. and Palmér, L. (1975) 'Disposition of placentally transferred carbamazepine (Tegretol®) in the Newborn', *Eur. J. Clin. Pharmacol.* **8:** 283-4.

Rane, A., Garle, M., Borgå, O. and Sjöqvist, F. (1974) 'Plasma disappearance of transplacentally transferred diphenylhydantoin in the newborn studied by mass fragmentography', *Clin. Pharmacol. Ther.* **15:** 39-45.

Rane, A., Höjer, B. and Wilson, J. T. (1976) 'Kinetics of carbamazepine and its 10,11–epoxide metabolite in children', *Clin. Pharmacol. Ther.* **19:** 276-83.

Relling, M. V., Lin, J.-S., Ayers, G. D. and Evans, W. E. (1992) 'Racial and gender differences in N-acetyltransferase, xantine oxidase, and CYP1A2 activities', *Clin. Pharmacol. Ther.* **52:** 643-58.

Rowland, M., Benet, L. Z. and Graham, G. (1973) 'Clearance concepts in pharmacokinetics', *J. Pharmacokin. Biopharm.* **1:** 123-36.

Watkins, P. B., Murray, S. A., Winkelman, L. G., Heuman, D. M., Wrighton, S. A. and Guzelian, P. S. (1989) 'Erythromycin breath test as an assay of glucocorticoid-inducible liver cytochromes P-450. Studies in rats and patients', *J. Clin. Invest.* **83:** 688-97.

Watkins, P. B., Turgeon, D. K., Jaffe, C. A., Ho, P. J. and Barkan, A. L. (1993) 'Gender pulsation frequency of growth hormone may mediate gender differences in CYP3A activity in man', *Clin. Res.* **41:** 132A.

Wilkinson, G. R. (1996) 'Cytochrome P4503A (CYP3A) metabolism: prediction of *in vivo* activity in humans', *J. Pharmacokinet. Biopharm.* **24:** 475-90.

Wilkinson, G. R. and Shand, D. G. (1975) 'A physiological approach to hepatic drug clearance. *Clin. Pharmacol. Ther.* **18**: 377–90.

Woodhouse, K. and Wynne, H. A. (1992) 'Age-related changes in hepatic function. Implications for drug therapy', *Drugs Aging* **2**: 243–55.

Chapter 4

Genetic and environmental factors causing variability in psychotropic drug response

J. Benítez, M.-L. Dahl, E. Spina and J. A. Carrillo

Large interindividual differences in drug response to psychotropic drugs is more of a rule than an exception. In fact, among patients treated with the same dose, psychotropic drug response varies widely from no effect at all to severe adverse drug reactions. Many factors contribute to this variability and, apart from the role of non-pharmacological aspects, such as psychological and social implications, it mainly results from the interaction of genetic, pathophysiological and environmental factors that lead to interindividual differences in drug pharmacokinetics and pharmacodynamics. Kinetic processess such as passive diffusion are rate-limited by the physicochemical characteristics of the drug, therefore they are not likely to vary significantly among patients unless pathophysiological factors exert an influence. In contrast, although not all the variations in psychotropic drug response involve drug metabolism, pharmacogenetic research has since the 1970s, and the discovery of the debrisoquine/sparteine hydroxylation polymorphism, expanded vigorously in the study of the interplay between environmental and genetic factors controlling the rate of drug metabolism and, hence, drug response (Sjöqvist *et al.*, 1997). Currently it is well known that the CYP-mediated reactions typically show pronounced interindividual variability, leading to large differences in steady-state plasma concentrations of drugs and, therefore, in therapeutic outcome. The variability in drug metabolism is mainly due to genetic factors which regulate the activity of CYPs. Additionally, they may be influenced by a number of factors such as concomitant drug administration, diet (coffee, alcohol, grapefruit juice, cruciferous vegetables, charcoal broiling meat), occupational exposure to environmental pollutants and smoking, among others. With a few exceptions, psychotropic drugs are lipophilic agents that undergo extensive metabolism in the liver, yielding polar metabolites that can be easily excreted in the urine (Caccia and Garattini, 1990). In general, their metabolism involves phase I oxidative reactions, catalysed by cytochrome P450 enzymes (CYPs), followed by phase II glucuronide conjugation.

In the present chapter, we review the role of genetic and environmental factors in the metabolism and therapeutic response to psychotropic drugs.

Cytochrome P450 system

Cytochrome P450 (CYP) is the collective term for a group of related enzymes or isozymes located in the membranes of the endoplasmic reticulum, mainly in the liver, but also in many extrahepatic tissues (e.g. intestinal mucosa, lung, kidney, lymphocytes, placenta, etc) (Smith *et al.*, 1998). These enzymes are responsible for the oxidative metabolism of a number of drugs and other exogenous compounds, as well as many endogenous substrates such as prostaglandins, fatty acids and steroids. The CYP superfamily is divided into families and subfamilies of enzymes that are defined on the basis of similarities in the amino acid sequence. Four of the families, CYP1 to CYP4, have been shown to be involved in the metabolism of xenobiotics, while the other families are of importance for the synthesis and metabolism of endogenous compounds (Gonzalez, 1992; Pelkonen *et al.*, 1998).

The drug-metabolising CYPs typically show a distinct, but overlapping, substrate specificity. An overview of the CYPs of major importance for the metabolism of psychotropic drugs is shown in Table 4.1. Two of these enzymes, CYP2D6 and CYP2C19, exhibit genetic polymorphism as the enzyme activity is polymorphically distributed in the population. The activity of these two enzymes is under genetic control and only to a minor extent influenced by environmental factors. On the other hand, no genetic polymorphism has been shown for the other major drug-metabolising CYPs, CYP1A2 and CYP3A4. However, it should be noted that their catalytic activities also show large inter- and sometimes intraindividual differences and a number of constitutional and environmental factors are modulating their activities in the population.

Debrisoquine/sparteine hydroxylation polymorphism (CYP2D6)

The CYP2D6 polymorphism was originally described in the 1970s when studying the metabolism of debrisoquine (Mahgoub *et al.*, 1977; Tucker *et al.*, 1977) and sparteine (Eichelbaum *et al.*, 1979). About 7% of Caucasians were shown to have a decreased capacity to metabolise these compounds, and the two reactions were later shown to cosegregate (Eichelbaum *et al.*, 1982). The capacity to hydroxylate debrisoquine is usually expressed as the ratio between the urinary recovery of debrisoquine and that of its major metabolite, the 4-hydroxydebrisoquine (debrisoquine metabolic ratio, MR) after a single oral dose of the drug. This ratio was shown to vary widely between individuals and is polymorphically distributed in Caucasian populations (Figure 4.1) (Evans *et al.*, 1980; Alvan *et al.*, 1990; Bertilsson *et al.*, 1992). About 7% of Caucasians had an MR higher than the antimode of 12.6, and were classified as poor metabolisers (PM), while the remaining subjects were extensive metabolisers (EM). The capacity to hydroxylate debrisoquine was shown to be under monogenic control and the PM phenotype inherited as an autosomal recessive trait

Table 4.1 The major human cytochrome P50 (CYP) enzymes of importance for the metabolism of psychotropic drugs as well as examples of marker drugs, inducers and inhibitors

	CYP1A2	CYP2C19	CYP2D6	CYP3A4
Substrates	amitriptyline[a]	amitriptyline[a]	amitriptyline	amitriptyline[a]
	imipramine[a]	imipramine[a]	imipramine	imipramine[a]
	clomipramine[a]	clomipramine[a]	clomipramine	clomipramine[a]
	fluvoxamine	citalopram	nortriptyline	diazepam
	mianserin	moclobemide	desipramine	midazolam
	clozapine	diazepam	fluvoxamine	triazolam
	olanzapine	desmethyldiazepam	fluoxetine	alprazolam
		carisoprodol	desmethylcitalopram	nefazodone
		hexobarbital	paroxetine	venlafaxine
		mephobarbital	mianserin	mirtazapine
			venlafaxine	clozapine
			maprotiline	sertindole
			haloperidol	
			perphenazine	
			thioridazine	
			zuclopenthixol	
			remoxipride	
			risperidone	
			olanzapine	
Marker drug(s)	caffeine	mephenytoin	debrisoquine	midazolam
	phenacetin	omeprazole	dextromethorphane	erythromycin
			sparteine	omeprazole
			metoprolol	cortisol
Potent inhibitors	fluvoxamine		quinidine	ketoconazole
Inducers	omeprazole[b]			carbamazepine
	carbamazepine			phenytoin
	phenobarbital			

Notes
[a] Demethylation pathway.
[b] This effect was reported in PMs of CYP2C19 after omeprazole 40 mg/day. A comparable induction (by 28%) was obtained in EM but after 120 mg/day.

(Evans *et al.*, 1980). The CYP2D6 phenotype can be similarly determined by administration of an oral dose of sparteine, dextromethorphan or metoprolol as probe drugs, followed by determination of the parent compound and its urinary metabolites (Table 4.1).

Following the phenotypic characterisation of the debrisoquine/sparteine hydroxylation polymorphism, efforts were made to clarify the molecular genetic background. The absence of the CYP2D6 protein in the liver of PMs was shown using antibodies raised against the rat P450db1, the rat

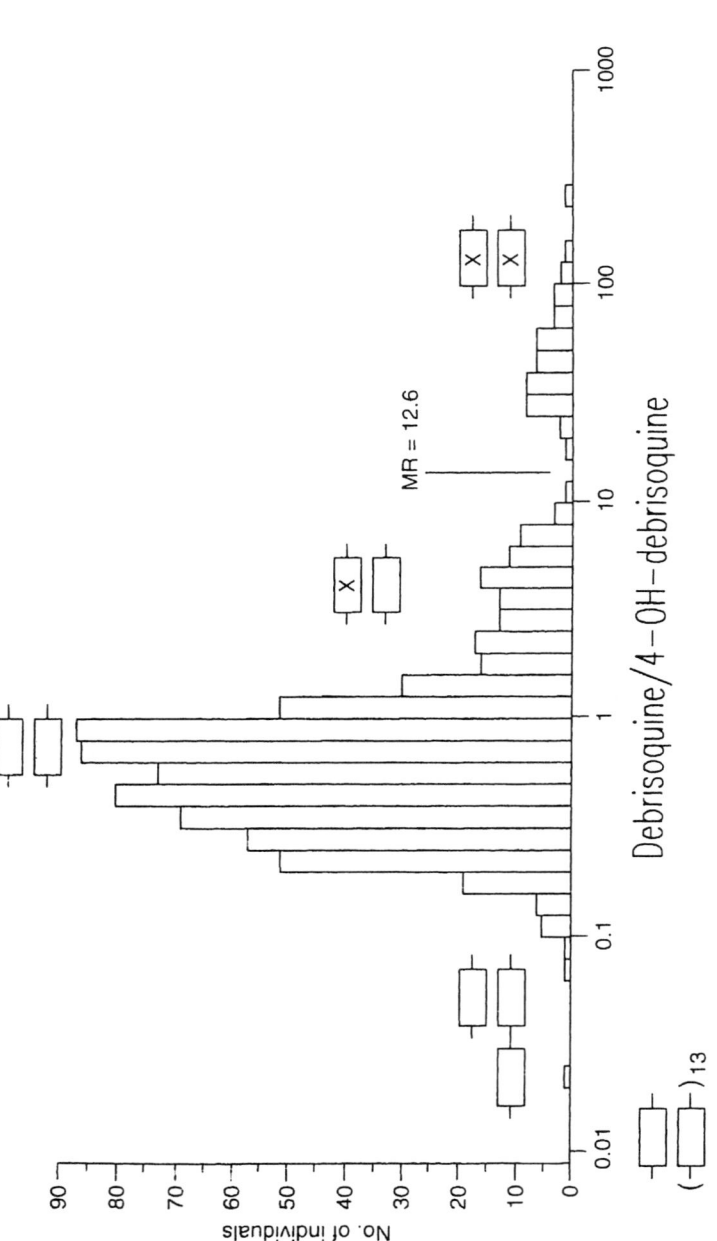

Figure 4.1 Schematic presentation of the relationship between the debrisoquine metabolic ratio (MR) and the major cytochrome P450 CYP2D6 genotypes causing altered CYP2D6 activity in healthy volunteers. The debrisoquine MR distribution is from a Swedish population.

homologue with high specific activity for 4-hydroxylation of debrisoquine (Gonzalez et al., 1987; Zanger et al., 1988). The three major defect allelic variants of CYP2D6 associated with the PM phenotype were subsequently identified (Gough et al., 1990; Heim and Meyer, 1990; Kagimoto et al., 1990; Gaedigk et al., 1991). The most common defect allele causing a deficient enzyme is CYP2D6*4, which has a frequency of about 21% in European populations. This gene has seven mutations compared with the wild-type (wt) gene, the detrimental one being the G1934→A mutation in the intron 3-exon 4 junction, causing a splicing defect (Kagimoto et al., 1990). CYP2D6*3 has an allele frequency of about 2%, and has a base deletion causing a frame shift. In the third, CYP2D6*5, the entire functional gene is deleted (Gaedigk et al., 1991). This haplotype has a frequency of about 5% across a number of different ethnic populations. In addition to these three alleles, a number of rare defect CYP2D6 alleles associated with the PM phenotype have been identified (Griese et al., 1998). Analysis of CYP2D6*3, *4 and *5 allows the prediction of the phenotype (EM versus PM) with 90–95% accuracy in European white populations (Heim and Meyer, 1990; Broly et al., 1991; Dahl et al., 1992). A better prediction would require the analysis of all the rare defect alleles.

The CYP2D6 activity varies largely within the EM phenotype, as shown by the span of MRs from 0.01 to over 10 (Figure 4.1). Individuals heterozygous for the defect alleles have a higher median MR compared with homozygous EM, indicating a gene dose effect (Broly et al., 1991; Dahl et al., 1992). In addition, several functional variants of the CYP2D locus causing decreased or increased enzyme activity contribute to this variability. The CYP2D6*9 allele was initially thought to be associated with the PM phenotype (Tyndale et al., 1991), but subsequently shown to cause the expression of an enzyme with decreased catalytic activity (Broly and Meyer, 1993). The CYP2D6*10 and CYP2D6*17 alleles are associated with decreased, but not absent, enzyme activity in Oriental and Black African populations, respectively (see hereafter).

Alleles causing increased CYP2D6 activity include duplication or multi-duplication of a functional CYP2D6*2 gene. This phenomenon was originally described in two Swedish families with extremely high CYP2D6 activity (debrisoquine MR of 0.01 to 0.1). In one of the families, the CYP2D6*2 gene was present in one extra copy, and in the other one in thirteen copies (Johansson et al., 1993). Duplicated and multiduplicated CYP2D6*2 alleles are found in 1–2% of the Swedish population (and 40% of subjects with MRs lower than 0.1), and is predictive of extremely high enzyme activity in this population (Dahl et al., 1995). Interestingly, 7% of Spaniards and as many as 29% of Ethiopians carry duplicated/multi-duplicated CYP2D6*2 genes (Agundez et al., 1995; Aklillu et al., 1996).

Numerous studies in Caucasian populations have shown very similar frequency distribution curves for the debrisoquine and sparteine MRs, and with a fairly constant incidence of the PM phenotype. Oriental populations, however, show a much lower incidence of PM (less than 1%) (Nakamura et al., 1985; Sohn et al., 1991; Bertilsson et al., 1992). Secondly, the distribution of the MRs is shifted to the right towards higher MR values in Oriental EMs compared with Caucasian EMs, indicating a lower average CYP2D6 activity in the Oriental population (Bertilsson et al., 1992). The differences in CYP2D6 activity between Oriental and Caucasian EMs are due to a high frequency (about 50%) among Orientals of an allele designated CYP2D6*10. This allele has a mutation in exon 1 causing an amino acid exchange and yielding an unstable enzyme with low catalytic activity (Johansson et al., 1994). On the other hand, the low incidence of PMs in Orientals is inherent in the low frequency of CYP2D6*4 (less than 1%). In Black African populations, the distribution of the MRs among EMs is also shifted towards higher values compared with Caucasian EMs (Masimirembwa et al., 1996). In a Zimbabwean population, this decreased CYP2D6 activity is related to the presence of yet another allelic variant of CYP2D6, CYP2D6*17, causing decreased, but not absent, enzyme activity (Masimirembwa et al., 1996).

S-mephenytoin hydroxylation polymorphism (CYP2C19)

The hydroxylation of the S-enantiomer of the anticonvulsant mephenytoin, catalysed by CYP2C19 (Wrighton et al., 1993; Goldstein et al., 1994) is also polymorphically distributed. About 3% of Caucasians, but as many as 15–25% of Orientals are classified as PM of mephenytoin (Jurima et al., 1985; Bertilsson et al., 1992; Sohn et al., 1992). In Black Africans (Tanzanians, Zimbabweans), PM frequencies of 4 to 7% have been reported (Masimirembwa et al., 1995; Persson et al., 1996; Herrlin et al., 1998). The PM phenotype is also in this case inherited as an autosomal recessive trait. The hydroxylation of omeprazole cosegregates with the 4-hydroxylation of S-mephenytoin thus, omeprazole has been validated as an alternative probe drug for CYP2C19 (Chang et al., 1995b).

The major defect CYP2C19 allele responsible for the PM phenotype in both Caucasian, Oriental and Black African populations is CYP2C19*2 (de Morais et al., 1994b; Persson et al., 1996). The second defect allele CYP2C19*3 has been found identified in Oriental populations and, taken together, these two alleles account for almost 100% of the PM alleles in Orientals (de Morais et al., 1994a; Roh et al., 1996). Two additional rare defect alleles have recently been described (Fergusson et al., 1998; Ibeanu et al., 1998). A gene dose effect has been shown for CYP2C19, as the heterozygous EM subjects show higher median S/R-mephenytoin ratios (and omeprazole/hydroxyomeprazole ratios) compared with homozygous EM (Chang et al., 1995a; Roh et al., 1996).

Table 4.2 List of factors, other than drugs, which are known to affect the CYP1A2 metabolic activity in humans

Factors	Effect on CYP1A2 activity
Coffee	Increase
Cruciferous vegetables	Increase
Ethanol	Decrease
Grapefruit juice	Decrease
Grilled meat	Increase
Liver disease	Decrease
Gender?	
Males	Increase
Females	Decrease
Menstrual cycle?	Decrease (luteal phase)
Pregnancy	Decrease
Smoking	Increase

Note: ?, not fully elucidated.

CYP1A2

The role of CYP1A2 in the metabolism of drugs is increasingly acknowledged and, as shown in Table 4.1, CYP1A2 is involved in the metabolism of several clinically important psychotropic drugs. Although CYP1A2 is not polymorphically distributed, this enzyme is inducible by smoking and shows a large variability in humans (Kalow and Tang, 1993; Carrillo and Benítez, 1994). Table 4.2 lists several constitutional and environmental factors which are known to influence the CYP1A2 metabolic activity in humans and hence, cause variability in psychotropic drug response (Carrillo and Benítez, 2000). Therefore, the availability of a reliable probe drug providing a measure of CYP1A2 activity is of considerable interest. In fact, CYP1A2 is the main enzyme catalysing the N-3-demethylation of caffeine (1,3,7–trimethylxanthine) to paraxanthine (1,7-dimethylxanthine) (Butler et al., 1989). The N-7-demethylation of paraxanthine to 1-methylxanthine is also catalysed by this enzyme (Kalow and Tang, 1993). Thus, CYP1A2 is the most important enzyme accounting for the biotransformation of caffeine and this compound has become a model drug of choice for the quantitative measurement of CYP1A2 in vivo (Kalow and Tang, 1993; Carrillo et al., 2000).

CYP3A4

CYPs belonging to the CYP3A gene subfamily account for up to 30% of the total cytochrome P450 present in adult human liver and for the majority of cytochrome P450 in human small bowel (Shimada et al., 1994). Therefore, CYP3A4 is quantitatively the major CYP in the liver, and is also expressed in intestinal mucosa. This enzyme is also involved in the metabolism of a number of psychotropic drugs (Table 4.1). Several approaches with drugs, including erythromycin, midazolam, cortisol, nifedipine, dapsone and lignocaine (Watkins et al., 1992; Watkins, 1994; Stein et al., 1996; Carrillo et al., 1998b) have been utilised to investigate the regulation mechanisms of CYP3A isoforms. Large variations in the oral bioavailability of CYP3A substrates are frequently observed and mainly related to differences in hepatic and intestinal "first-pass metabolism" (Watkins, 1994; Paine et al., 1996; Thummel et al., 1996), but the factors controlling such a variability have so far not been elucidated. This enzyme is also inducible by, for example, antiepileptics and inhibited by a number of compounds including ketoconazole, erythromycin, and grapefruit juice (Bailey et al., 1998; Pelkonen et al., 1998).

Antidepressants

Since the early 1950s, when imipramine was first introduced, tricyclic antidepressants (TCAs) have been the cornerstone of antidepressant pharmacotherapy for over 25 years and, despite the considerable advances in the treatments available for mood disorders over the past generation, TCAs still remain an important option for the pharmacotherapy of depression (Goodnick, 1994; Burke and Preskorn, 1999; Rudorfer and Potter, 1999). Several chemically unrelated agents have been developed and introduced in the past decade, to supplement the earlier antidepressants. At present, the selective serotonin reuptake inhibitors (SSRIs) are considered by many physicians, to be the first-line pharmacotherapy for the management of depressive disorders. In addition, other apparently selective agents namely, maprotiline, mianserin, mirtazapine, moclobemide, nefazodone, trazodone, venlafaxine, reboxetine and tianeptine are now available as antidepressants (Caccia, 1998; Burke and Preskorn, 1999; Dahl and Sjöqvist, 2000; Moller, 2000). Our current knowledge of the isoenzymes involved in the various oxidation pathways and their relevance for potential drug interactions varies from a considerable amount for most of the TCAs, SSRIs and nefazodone, to minimal for reboxetine and tianeptine (Caccia, 1998).

Tricyclic antidepressants

TCAs have been for many years the standard drug treatment for depressive illness. A major problem in the clinical use of these compounds is the large interindividual variability in their metabolism leading to pronounced differences in plasma concentrations and hence, in drug response. In fact, these agents have a relatively narrow therapeutic index and several studies support the existence of a relationship between plasma concentrations and clinical effects of TCAs (Perry et al., 1987; Orsulak, 1989). Optimal plasma concentrations for antidepressant activity have been suggested and, in addition, cardiovascular and CNS toxicity usually occur at concentrations well above the upper concentration limit (Preskorn *et al.*, 1988; Preskorn and Jerkovich, 1990).

TCAs are extensively metabolised in the liver by microsomal enzymes. In general their biotransformation includes an initial oxidative reaction (N-demethylation and/or ring hydroxylation), catalysed by cytochrome P450 isoenzymes, followed by conjugation with glucuronic acid (Rudorfer and Potter, 1999). The tertiary amines amitriptyline, imipramine and clomipramine are demethylated to the active metabolites nortriptyline, desipramine and desmethylclomipramine, respectively. Amitriptyline and nortriptyline are subsequently hydroxylated, mainly by 10-hydroxylation, while imipramine and desipramine are hydroxylated at position 2. The hydroxymetabolites are rapidly glucuronidated and excreted in the urine. The hydroxymetabolites of TCAs possess pharmacological activity and may contribute to the antidepressant effects of the parent drug (Goodnick, 1994; Bertilsson and Dahl, 1996; Rudorfer and Potter, 1999).

The possible role of genetic factors in the disposition of tricyclics had been hypothesised already at the end of the 1960s, when early pharmacokinetic studies revealed pronounced variability in steady-state plasma concentrations of these compounds among patients receiving the same oral dose (Hammer and Sjöqvist, 1967). This was proposed to be mainly due to differences in the activity of the hydroxylating enzymes. Subsequent twin and family studies clearly established that genetic factors were the major determinants of this variability, but the exact nature of the genetic control could not be detected (Alexanderson *et al.*, 1969; Åsberg *et al.*, 1971). In particular, in a classical study (Alexanderson *et al.*, 1969), an identical dose of nortriptyline to several twin pairs, led to very similar steady-state plasma concentrations in monozygotic twins, whereas significant intrapair differences were observed in about half of the dizygotic twins. Furthermore, cross-over studies showed that the steady-state plasma concentrations of nortriptyline and desipramine were interrelated, so that patients who developed high or low concentrations of nortriptyline also developed similarly high or low concentrations of desipramine, suggesting that both drugs are metabolised by the same enzyme (Hammer *et al.*, 1969; Alexanderson, 1972). Moreover, the kinetics of amitriptyline and clomipramine strongly correlated within an individual, indicating that the demethylation occurred through the same enzyme (Mellström *et al.*, 1979).

The discovery of the polymorphic debrisoquine oxidation aroused a renewed interest in the pharmacogenetics of tricyclic compounds. In recent years, *in vivo* and *in vitro* studies have indicated that the hydroxylation reactions of tricyclic antidepressants are catalysed by CYP2D6, whereas N-demethylation reactions seem to be catalysed by CYP1A2, CYP2C19 and CYP3A4 (Bertilsson and Dahl, 1996; Bertilsson *et al.*, 1997). With regard to the hydroxylation reactions, pharmacokinetic studies in panels of healthy, drug-free EMs and PMs have in fact suggested that the 10-hydroxylation of amitriptyline (Balant-Gorgia et al., 1982) and nortriptyline (Mellström et al., 1981), the 2-hydroxylation of imipramine (Brøsen et al., 1986b) and desipramine (Spina et al., 1987b), and the hydroxylation of clomipramine (Balant-Gorgia et al., 1986) are associated with the debrisoquine/sparteine oxidation (CYP2D6) phenotype (Table 4.1). Significant interphenotypic differences in the kinetics of secondary amines nortriptyline and desipramine have been observed: PMs reach higher peak plasma concentrations, have longer plasma half-lives, lower total and metabolic clearances and excrete less hydroxymetabolites than do EMs (Mellström et al., 1981; Spina et al., 1987b). Furthermore, a population and family study in Swedish subjects clearly established that the 2-hydroxylation of desipramine cosegregates with the polymorphic debrisoquine oxidation (Dahl et al., 1992). Recently, the pharmacokinetics of nortriptyline and its active major metabolite 10-hydroxynortriptyline were shown to be highly dependent on the CYP2D6 genotype both in Swedish and Chinese healthy volunteers (Dalen et al., 1998; Yue et al., 1998). The single dose study in Swedish subjects included, in addition to PM subjects (no functional CYP2D6 gene), heterozygous EMs (one functional gene), homozygous EMs (two functional genes) and ultrarapid hydroxylators with 3, 4 or 13 functional CYP2D6 genes (Dalen et al., 1998). In the study in Chinese subjects, the CYP2D6*10 allele was shown to be associated with significantly higher plasma levels of nortriptyline compared with the CYP2D6*1 allele (Yue et al., 1998). As additional evidence, in vitro biochemical studies showed a positive correlation between the rate of hydroxylation of nortriptyline or desipramine and that of debrisoquine in human liver microsomes from different individuals. It clearly indicated the involvement of the same CYP in these oxidative reactions (von Bahr et al., 1983; Spina et al., 1984). Such interphenotypic differences in the kinetics of secondary amines may be reduced by the effect of some functional characteristics of CYP2D6, i.e. saturation or inhibition, which are more evident in EMs (Brøsen and Gram, 1989). The CYP2D6 activity is of high affinity and low capacity character, resulting in saturability at low concentrations of the substrate. This may lead to dose-dependent kinetics in EMs as reported for imipramine and desipramine (Brøsen et al., 1986a; Nelson and Jatlow, 1987; Brøsen and Gram, 1988). Moreover, the activity of CYP2D6 in EMs may be decreased by concomitant administration of either other substrates or inhibitors of the polymorphic enzyme, as described further in this chapter.

The demethylation reactions of TCA are rather complex. The clearance by demethylation of both imipramine and amitriptyline was found not to be associated with CYP2D6 polymorphism (Mellström et al., 1983; Brøsen et al., 1986c). However, when only non-smokers were studied, a significant correlation was found between amitriptyline demethylation clearance and urinary debrisoquine MRs (Mellström *et al.*, 1986). This suggested that the demethylation reactions might be catalysed by two enzymes, one inducible by smoking and the other under the same genetic control as the hydroxylation of debrisoquine. *In vivo* and *in vitro* studies have recently indicated that other enzymes, such as the smoking-inducible CYP1A2 (Lemoine *et al.*, 1993), the polymorphic CYP2C19 (Skjelbo *et al.*, 1991; 1993; Chiba *et al.*, 1994) and CYP3A4 (Lemoine *et al.*, 1993; Ohmori *et al.*, 1993), are probably involved in the demethylation of tertiary TCAs. The role of these isoenzymes in the demethylation of TCA has been confirmed by kinetic studies with inhibitors of CYP1A2, such as fluvoxamine (Spina *et al.*, 1993; Xu *et al.*, 1996), and of CYP3A4, such as ketoconazole (Spina *et al.*, 1997a) and troleandomycin (Wang *et al.*, 1997).

The potential clinical implications of polymorphic CYP2D6 activity in relation to treatment with tricyclics are quite obvious if we consider that hydroxylation is the rate-limiting step in the elimination of tricyclics and that their therapeutic and toxic effects are concentration dependent. Depressed patients of the PM phenotype may achieve high plasma concentrations when treated with conventional doses and may develop severe side-effects. Conversely, patients with an extremely high rate of metabolism may not reach optimal plasma levels with subsequent therapeutic failure. In previous studies, indirect indices of CYP2D6 activity, such as the debrisoquine or sparteine metabolic ratio, as well as the desipramine hydroxylation index, were found to be good predictors of steady-state plasma concentrations of desipramine and nortriptyline in depressed patients (Bertilsson and Åberg-Wistedt, 1983; Nordin et al., 1985; Brøsen *et al.*, 1986b; Spina *et al.*, 1987a). The CYP2D6 genotype is also of value to predict pharmacokinetics of nortriptyline accurately (Dahl *et al.*, 1996; Dalen *et al.*, 1998; Yue *et al.*, 1998). Therefore, knowledge of the oxidation phenotype might help in identifying the two patient groups that, being at the extreme of this variation, pose clinical problems, i.e. the PM and the rapid EM. While low doses are probably needed in PM, ultrarapid metabolisers with duplicated or multiduplicated CYP2D6 genes may require increased doses (Bertilsson *et al.*, 1985, 1993b). In principle, a simple phenotyping or genotyping test before treatment with a tricyclic compound may be of value in selecting the starting dose to enhance therapeutic efficacy and to prevent toxicity. However, despite theoretical consideration, the potential usefulness of such an approach for the everyday clinical practice in psychiatry has been limited so far to a few reports in patients with extremely high or low rates of drug oxidation (Bertilsson *et al.*, 1981, 1985; Balant-Gorgia *et al.*, 1989; Bluhm *et al.*, 1993). However, in a large retrospective study of patients taking imipramine, no association was found between the debrisoquine oxidation capacity and the frequency or severity of side-effects (Meyer *et al.*, 1988). In a recent prospective study in depressed patients starting treatment with oral desipramine, plasma

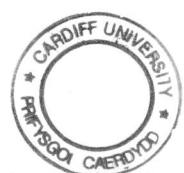

desipramine levels were significantly correlated with CYP2D6, assessed by
the dextromethorphan test before treatment (Figure 4.2) (Spina *et al.*,
1997b). The two patients with the PM phenotype showed the highest
plasma concentrations of desipramine and complained of severe adverse
effects, requiring dosage reduction. No significant correlation was found
between plasma levels of either desipramine or desipramine plus 2-hydroxy-
desipramine and antidepressant effect. These findings indicate that the
dextromethorphan metabolic ratio, as other indices of CYP2D6 activity, is
a relatively good predictor of steady-state plasma levels of desipramine in
depressed patients and may identify subjects at risk for severe concen-
tration-dependent adverse effects, but does not seem to predict the degree
of clinical improvement.

The metabolism of TCAs may be modified by environmental factors, in
particular by concomitant administration of other compounds interfering
with hepatic CYPs system. These agents may be substrates for the different
isoenzymes involved in the metabolism of TCAs or inhibitors and inducers
of their activity.

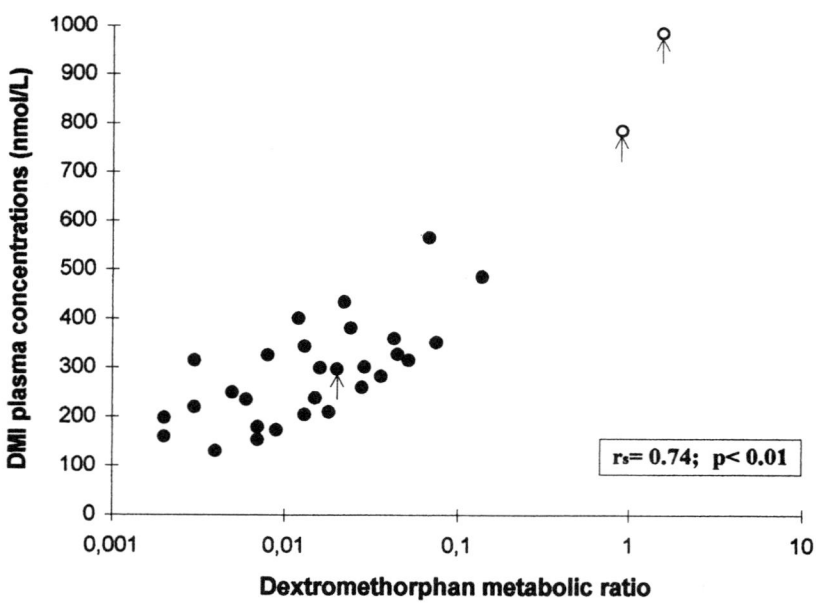

Figure 4.2 Relationship between dextromethorphan metabolic ratio and steady-state
plasma desipramine (DMI) concentrations in thirty-one depressed patients
during treatment with DMI, 100 mg daily for three weeks. The two patients
with a poor CYP2D6 metaboliser phenotype are indicated by open symbols.
Arrows indicate three patients in whom DMI dosage had to be reduced to
50 mg daily after 5–10 days because of severe adverse effects.

As previously anticipated, the genetically determined CYP2D6 activity may be influenced by concomitant treatment with potent inhibitors of this isoenzyme or other substrates with higher affinity. As a consequence, patients treated with TCA are at risk of clinically significant pharmacokinetic interactions, whose potential is greater in EM, in case of coadministration of these compounds. Dosage reductions might therefore be necessary to avoid the hazardous toxicity encountered at high plasma tricyclic concentrations. There are several examples of medications which may impair the CYP2D6-mediated elimination of TCAs.

Quinidine is the most powerful inhibitor of CYP2D6 and markedly inhibits the hydroxylation of TCAs (Brøsen and Gram, 1988; Steiner *et al.*, 1988; Ayesh *et al.*, 1991). The inhibitory effect is dramatic in EMs, while it is not observed in PMs which show a genetically determined lack of functional CYP2D6 in the liver (Steiner *et al.*, 1988).

Many neuroleptics, such as perphenazine, thioridazine, zuclopenthixol and haloperidol are metabolised, at least in part, by CYP2D6 (Bertilsson and Dahl, 1996). These agents are not only substrates, but also potent inhibitors of CYP2D6 and may competitively inhibit the metabolism of TCAs, thereby potentially raising plasma tricyclic concentrations into the toxic range (Gram and Overo, 1972; Nelson and Jatlow, 1980; Loga *et al.*, 1981). Plasma levels of TCAs may increase by up to 100% in patients receiving antipsychotic medication. Although comorbidity is very frequent in psychiatric patients, this pharmacokinetic interaction seriously questions the rationale for combining TCAs and neuroleptics. A particularly dangerous interaction may occur when thioridazine is given in combination with a TCA, since both compounds are known to produce cardiac toxicity (Heiman, 1977; Hirschowitz *et al.*, 1983).

SSRIs may interfere with the elimination of TCAs, as they inhibit, to a varying degree, the activity of different CYPs. In particular, with regard to the effect of the five marketed SSRIs on the functional activity of CYP2D6, *in vitro* studies in human liver microsomes (Brøsen and Skjelbo, 1991; Crewe *et al.*, 1992; Skjelbo and Brøsen, 1992; Otton *et al.*, 1993) and *in vivo* studies using dextromethorphan as probe drug (Ereshefsky, 1996a) have indicated that fluoxetine and paroxetine are potent inhibitors of CYP2D6, while fluvoxamine, sertraline and citalopram minimally affect this isoform. Similar results were obtained in formal pharmacokinetic studies in which the effect of therapeutic doses of each SSRI on the single dose kinetics of desipramine was investigated (Bergstrom *et al.*, 1992; Brøsen *et al.*, 1993a; Gram *et al.*, 1993; Spina *et al.*, 1993; Preskorn *et al.*, 1994; Alderman *et al.*, 1997). Fluoxetine and paroxetine produced a three- to five-fold decrease in the clearance of desipramine, whereas citalopram, fluvoxamine and sertraline had only a minimal, probably not clinically relevant effect. The inhibitory effect of fluoxetine and paroxetine may result in a dramatic increase in steady-state plasma concentrations after multiple dosing. In fact, addition of fluoxetine to tricyclic medication has been reported to increase plasma TCA concentrations by 100 to 300% and in some cases this effect was associated with signs of toxicity (Vaughan, 1988; Aranow *et al.*, 1989). Moreover, due to the long elimination half-lives of fluoxetine and its active metabolite norfluoxetine, plasma tricyclic concentrations may require up to three months to stabilise at a new steady-state level after addition of fluoxetine, and may remain elevated for several weeks after its discontinuation (Westermeyer, 1991). The potent inhibition of CYP2D6-mediated hydroxylation of TCAs by fluoxetine and paroxetine should be taken into account when using these agents in combination and a reduction of TCA dosage may be required. This is of obvious clinical interest, since SSRI augmentation of tricyclic therapy is believed to be a clinically useful strategy to improve response in depressed patients who are resistant to the individual therapies or to reduce the latency of antidepressant response (Nelson *et al.*, 1991).

Among SSRIs, fluvoxamine has also been reported to decrease the elimination of TCAs, but, differently from fluoxetine and paroxetine, this agent appears to affect the demethylation and not the hydroxylation reactions. In fact, the addition of fluvoxamine to an existing treatment with TCAs has been reported to produce an up to four-fold increase in plasma concentrations of amitriptyline, imipramine and clomipramine without affecting the levels of corresponding demethylated metabolites (Bertschy *et al.*, 1991; Spina *et al.*, 1992b; Härtter *et al.*, 1993; Spina *et al.*, 1993) with associated signs of TCA toxicity in some cases. Subsequent kinetic studies in healthy volunteers, indicated that fluvoxamine inhibits the demethylation of imipramine and clomipramine without affecting the hydroxylation (Spina *et al.*, 1993; Härtter *et al.*, 1995). As fluvoxamine is a potent *in vitro* inhibitor of CYP1A2 activity (Brosen *et al.*, 1993b), such findings confirm the major role played by CYP1A2 in the demethylation of TCAs. Concurrent inhibition by fluvoxamine of CYP2C19 and CYP3A4 may also contribute to pharmacokinetic interaction with TCAs by affecting demethylation via these enzymes.

The histamine H2-receptor antagonist cimetidine, a nonspecific inhibitor of the hepatic CYP system, has been reported to decrease the elimination of TCAs and increase their plasma concentrations to potentially toxic levels (Amsterdam *et al.*, 1984).

The anti-epileptic agents phenobarbital, phenytoin, carbamazepine and primidone are potent inducers of the hepatic drug metabolising system and have been reported to reduce plasma concentrations of several TCAs (Burrows and Davies, 1971; Ballinger *et al.*, 1974; Braithwaite *et al.*, 1975; Leinonen *et al.*, 1991). This may be explained in terms of induction of CYP1A2 and/or CYP3A4 by these agents. However, the induction of the 2–hydroxylation of desipramine, which is catalysed by CYP2D6, by carbamazepine and phenobarbital is unlikely to be mediated by this enzyme which is not inducible (Spina *et al.*, 1995; 1996). This suggests that other low-affinity CYPs, contributing to the reaction, may be induced. Since inadequate plasma levels of TCAs may result in therapeutic failure, it is likely that larger daily doses of TCAs may be required in patients treated chronically with enzyme-inducing anti-epileptic drugs for full clinical efficacy to be achieved (Brøsen and Kragh-Sorensen, 1993).

Chronic alcohol consumption has been reported to decrease plasma concentrations of TCAs, suggesting induction of their metabolism (Ciraulo *et al.*, 1988).

SSRIs

Over the past decade, the SSRIs have supplemented TCAs as antidepressants of first choice due to their greater safety and tolerability profile (Caccia, 1998). Unlike TCAs, SSRIs have a wide therapeutic index and no clear-cut correlation between plasma levels and clinical response has been demonstrated. As a consequence, genetically or environmentally induced differences in their elimination are less likely to be of great clinical concern. However, the possible clinical implications of variability in the metabolism of SSRIs may have been underestimated so far (Richelson, 1997; Caccia, 1998; Greenblatt *et al.*, 1999; Dahl and Sjöqvist, 2000).

Fluoxetine is N-demethylated to the active metabolite norfluoxetine and both fluoxetine and norfluoxetine are racemates. The N-demethylation of both fluoxetine enantiomers is probably metabolised by the same CYP enzyme(s), as a significant correlation between the rates at which human liver microsomes catalyze the reactions has been reported (Stevens and Wrighton, 1993).

Both fluoxetine and norfluoxetine are very potent inhibitors of CYP2D6-mediated oxidative reactions in human liver microsomes (Brøsen and Skjelbo, 1991; Crewe *et al.*, 1992; Skjelbo and Brøsen, 1992; Otton *et al.*, 1993) the S-enantiomers being more potent than the corresponding R-enantiomers (Stevens and Wrighton, 1993). N-demethylation of fluoxetine was found to correlate with CYP2D6 levels in human liver microsomes, but was inhibited only 20% by quinidine and 27% by antisera to CYP2D6, and occurred in human microsomes lacking the CYP2D6 enzyme, suggesting that other isozymes may be responsible for the fluoxetine demethylation *in vitro* (Stevens and Wrighton, 1993). On the other hand, in a recent *in vivo* study, significant differences in the disposition of racemic fluoxetine and norfluoxetine were observed between PM and EM, suggesting that the polymorphic CYP2D6 plays an important role in the demethylation of fluoxetine to norfluoxetine (Hamelin *et al.*, 1996). A recent single dose study in PM and EM of sparteine showed that CYP2D6 catalyses the metabolism of both R- and S-fluoxetine and most likely the further metabolism of S-norfluoxetine, but not of R-norfluoxetine (Fjordside *et al.*, 1999).

Fluvoxamine undergoes extensive oxidative reactions in the liver and eleven different metabolites have been identified in the urine. Significantly lower plasma fluvoxamine concentrations have been reported in smokers as compared with non-smokers, suggesting a possible role of CYP1A2 in the metabolism of fluvoxamine, since this isoform is induced by cigarette smoke (van Harten et al., 1992; Spigset et al., 1995). The role of CYP1A2 was further supported by another study in healthy volunteers (Carrillo et al., 1996). The same authors have also shown evidence for the contribution of CYP2D6 in the metabolism of fluvoxamine as PM subjects had higher plasma concentrations of fluvoxamine than EM after a single oral dose of the drug (Carrillo et al., 1996; Spigset et al., 1997). No data are available concerning the specific metabolic pathways of fluvoxamine catalysed by CYP2D6, CYP1A2, or other CYPs.

Paroxetine is oxidised to inactive metabolites which are then conjugated and inactivated. The median area under the plasma concentration-time curve (AUC) was seven times higher in PM than in EM after a single oral dose of paroxetine (Sindrup et al., 1992b). However, CYP2D6 is a high-affinity saturable enzyme and non-linear kinetics were seen in EMs, but not in PMs, after repeated and increased dosing. Thus, in the same subjects, the difference in median AUC was only two-fold between EM and PM at steady state (Sindrup et al., 1992b). A twenty-five-fold variation in the steady state plasma levels of paroxetine at a dose level of 30 mg/day was seen between PM and fast EM subjects (Sindrup et al., 1992a). Within the EM group there was a significant correlation between the steady state levels and the sparteine MR. The pharmacokinetic data in EM were best described by a model assuming elimination by at least two distinct processes, one a high-affinity saturable process (CYP2D6) and one low-affinity linear process (Sindrup et al., 1992a). In agreement with the in vivo studies, it has been shown that quinidine, a potent inhibitor of CYP2D6, only blocked about two thirds of paroxetine metabolism in human liver microsomes (Bloomer et al., 1992). The residual one third probably reflects paroxetine oxidation by other low affinity CYPs.

Sertraline is N-demethylated to the inactive metabolite desmethyl-sertraline. The metabolism of sertraline appears not to be dependent on genetically determined CYP2D6 activity, as no significant differences between EMs and PMs were found for sertraline and desmethylsertraline pharmacokinetics (Hamelin et al., 1996). Moreover, the in vitro conversion of sertraline to desmethylsetraline was found to correlate better with CYP3A4 activity than with CYP2D6 activity, suggesting an involvement of CYP3A4 in sertraline demethylation (Pollock, 1994).

With regard to citalopram, both CYP2D6 and CYP2C19 oxidation polymorphisms appear to contribute to the metabolism of this SSRI, based on a study comparing steady-state plasma concentrations of citalopram and its metabolites in EMs and PMs for both sparteine (CYP2D6) and mephenytoin (CYP2C19) polymorphisms (Sindrup *et al.*, 1993). The primary metabolic pathway of citalopram, demethylation to desmethylcitalopram, cosegregates with the CYP2C19 activity, while the further metabolism of desmethylcitalopram to didesmethylcitalopram is dependent on the polymorphic CYP2D6 activity. *In vitro* studies have indicated the involvement not only of CYP2C19, but also CYP3A4 in the N-demethylation of citalopram (Kobayashi *et al.*, 1997; Rochat *et al.*, 1997).

Several agents have been reported to inhibit CYP isoenzymes responsible for the metabolism of SSRIs, thereby increasing their plasma concentrations to potentially toxic levels. Treatment with antipsychotics may influence the elimination of some SSRIs. A two- to ten-fold increase in plasma fluvoxamine concentrations was reported in patients treated with antipsychotics of the butyrophenone class (Härtter and Hiemke, 1992). In another study, plasma concentrations of citalopram were elevated by 36% during coadministration of phenothiazines (Oyehaugh *et al.*, 1984). Coadministration of desipramine, which is a substrate of CYP2D6, was found to increase plasma levels of fluoxetine and paroxetine, but not sertraline (Preskorn *et al.*, 1994; Alderman *et al.*, 1997). In studies in healthy volunteers, cimetidine, a nonspecific inhibitor of hepatic microsomal enzymes, increased the plasma concentrations of paroxetine, citalopram and sertraline by 50, 43 and 24%, respectively (Bannister *et al.*, 1989).

Enzyme-inducing anti-epileptic drugs may stimulate the oxidative metabolism of concurrently prescribed SSRIs. In particular, phenobarbital was reported to cause a 25% decrease in plasma concentrations of paroxetine (Greb *et al.*, 1989; Andersen *et al.*, 1991).

As described briefly above, the SSRIs differ with respect to their inhibitory effects on the drug-metabolising CYPs. Fluoxetine and paroxetine are potent inhibitors of CYP2D6, fluvoxamine is a potent inhibitor of CYP1A2 and a moderate inhibitor of CYP2C19 and CYP3A4, while citalopram and sertraline are weak inhibitors of these isoenzymes. Although a detailed evaluation of this topic is beyond the scope of this article, the potential pharmacokinetic drug interactions between SSRIs and other drugs metabolised by these enzymes should be acknowledged (Lane, 1996).

Other antidepressants

Maprotiline

The metabolism of the tetracyclic antidepressant maprotiline appears to co-segregate with the CYP2D6 polymorphic debrisoquine hydroxylation. The mean C_{max} of maprotiline in six PMs of debrisoquine was 2.7-fold greater than that in six EMs and the mean AUC (0, 48 h) was 3.5 times higher. It has been suggested that such differences in the pharmacokinetics of maprotiline between EMs and PMs may lead to differences in pharmacodynamics, especially with respect to the side-effect profile (Firkusny and Gleiter, 1994). However, it has been suggested that isozymes other than CYP2D6 or CYP1A2 are involved in the metabolism of the drug (Vormfelde et al., 1997).

Mianserin

Mianserin and its major metabolite desmethylmianserin appear to be metabolised by the polymorphic CYP2D6. PMs of debrisoquine were found to reach significantly higher concentrations of mianserin and desmethylmianserin than EMs after a single oral dose of the drug (Dahl et al., 1994b). In addition, the two extremely rapid EMs participating in the study had the lowest mianserin concentrations and no detectable desmethylmianserin in serum. The CYP2D6-dependent metabolism showed marked stereoselectivity for the major and more potent S(+)-enantiomer of mianserin. A study in depressed Japanese patients suggested that the CYP2D6 genotype plays a major role in controlling the steady state plasma concentrations of the S(+)-enantiomer of mianserin (Mihara et al., 1997b).

Mirtazapine

In vitro studies with microsomes from human liver and cells expressing different CYPs have revealed that racemic mirtazapine is predominantly metabolised by CYP2D6 and (Dahl et al., 1997). To determine the effect of the CYP2D6 polymorphism on mirtazepine kinetics in vivo, a single oral dose of mirtazepine was given to seven EMs and seven PMs of mirtazapine. No significant differences in the pharmacokinetic parameters of mirtazapine and its desmethyl metabolite were found between EM and PM subjects using a non-enantioselective method, indicating that the disposition of mirtazapine is not to a major extent dependent of CYP2D6 activity (Dahl et al., 1997). However, analysis of the enantiomers of mirtazapine showed CYP2D6-related differences in the plasma levels of the minor mirtazapine enantiomer (Delbressine et al., 1997). The clinical implications of this CYP2D6-dependent metabolism are however likely to be minor.

Moclobemide

A panel study in healthy volunteers has indicated that the selective and reversible monoamine oxidase A inhibitor moclobemide is a substrate of CYP2C19 (Gram et al., 1995). The clinical significance of this association is unclear.

Nefazodone

Nefazodone, a $5HT_{2A}$ antagonist and serotonin reuptake inhibitor, is extensively metabolised in the liver to hydroxynefazodone, to p-hydroxy-nefazodone, to a triazoledione metabolite and via cleavage of the molecule to m-chlorophenyl-piperazine (mCCP), which is further hydroxylated. *In vitro* and *in vivo* data indicate that nefazodone and hydroxynefazodone are potent inhibitors of CYP3A4 (Schmider *et al.*, 1996) and it has been postulated that the major isoenzyme involved in the metabolism of nefazodone is most likely CYP3A4. However, no data clearly demonstrating the role of CYP3A4 in the metabolism of nefazodone have been found in the literature. In a recent study in EMs and PMs of dextro-methorphan, no significant differences in pharmacokinetic parameters of nefazodone or hydroxynefazodone were noted between the two phenotypes, indicating that CYP2D6 is probably not involved in the primary metabolism of nefazodone (Barbhaiya *et al.*, 1996). However, plasma concentrations of mCCP were higher in PM than in EM subjects, suggesting that the metabolism of mCCP is mediated by CYP2D6. *In vitro* studies in human liver microsomes and cells expressing single CYP enzymes have confirmed that CYP2D6 catalyses the metabolism of mCCP to its main metabolite p-hydroxy-mCCP (Rotzinger *et al.*, 1998).

Trazodone

The antidepressant trazodone undergoes oxidative cleavage, yielding m-chlorophenylpiperazine (mCPP), which is also a metabolic product of nefazodone. CYP2D6 has been suggested to be involved in the metabolism of both trazodone and mCCP (Yasui *et al.*, 1995). However, in a recent investigation, CYP2D6 genotype was found not to predict steady-state plasma concentrations of trazodone or mCPP in depressed Japanese patients (Mihara *et al.*, 1997a). Other enzymes, i.e. CYP1A2 and CYP3A4, are probably also involved in the metabolism of these compounds, as their plasma concentrations are significantly lower in smokers than in non-smokers and during coadministration of carbamazepine, an inducer of CYP3A4 (Ishida *et al.*, 1995; Otani *et al.*, 1996).

Venlafaxine

Venlafaxine, a serotonin and noradrenaline reuptake inhibitor, is biotrans-formed in humans to a major active metabolite O-desmethylvenlafaxine, and in parallel to N-desmethylvenlafaxine. *In vitro* studies in human liver microsomes indicate that the O-demethylation of venlafaxine is catalysed by CYP2D6, while CYP3A4 is probably involved in the N-demethylation pathway (Otton *et al.*, 1996). Since venlafaxine and O-desmethylvenlafaxine have similar pharmacological properties, the clinical implications of polymorphic venlafaxine metabolism are uncertain.

Reboxetine

Based on *in vitro* studies, the metabolism of the (S,S)- and (R,R)-reboxetine enantiomers in humans seems to be principally mediated via CYP3A (Wienkers *et al.*, 1999). In addition, both compounds were found to be competitive inhibitors of CYP2D6 and CYP3A4 (K(i)=2.5 and 11 µM, respectively) (Wienkers *et al.*, 1999). On the contrary, in a recent investigation in ten healthy volunteers and, using dextromethorphan as a model CYP2D6 substrate (Avenoso *et al.*, 1999), there were no changes in the urinary dextromethorphan/dextrorphan ratio in the reboxetine phase when compared with the control session. It suggests that reboxetine is unlikely to cause clinically significant interactions with substrates of CYP2D6 (Avenoso *et al.*, 1999).

In conclusion, intensive research has demonstrated that most antidepressants are metabolised, at least in part, by the polymorphic CYP2D6. This explains the pronounced interindividual variability in plasma concentrations of these agents and the interactions observed when these drugs are used in combination with other substrates or inhibitors of the enzyme. The clinical significance of this association is most pronounced for TCAs, as they have a small therapeutic index and their effects are concentration dependent. Patients with a decreased capacity to eliminate these drugs, either due to a genetic or environmentally induced deficiency in CYP2D6 may develop severe adverse effects with conventional doses. Conversely, ultrarapid metabolisers with duplicated or multiduplicated CYP2D6 genes may require higher than normal doses for optimal treatment. The clinical implications of polymorphic metabolism of the newer antidepressants remain to be demonstrated.

Antipsychotic drugs

Schizophrenia is a chronic and debilitating disorder whose pharmacological management is often less than optimal. For several decades, drug treatment for this disorder consisted of classical antipsychotics such as haloperidol and phenotiazine-derivatives. However, the limitations in the clinical use of these drugs arise from the high incidence of extrapyramidal side-effects and lack of effect on negative symptoms. Therefore, it has driven the development of newer agents, often referred to as atypical antipsychotics that include clozapine, risperidone, olanzapine, sertindole, quetiapine, and ziprasidone among others. They have an enhanced 5-hydroxytryptamine/dopaminergic receptors (5-HT2/D2) affinity ratio and undergo extensive biotransformation. All antipsychotic drugs are subject to extensive metabolism in the liver, and many of them have pharmacologically active metabolites. However, as with antidepressants, the dosage requirement and therapeutic response vary widely between patients treated with the same dose, indicating interindividual differences in the elimination kinetics and in the steady state plasma levels achieved during treatment (Dahl, 1986). It should be noted that the polymorphic CYP2D6 is involved in the metabolism of most antipsychotics so far investigated (Dahl and Bertilsson, 1993; Fang and Gorrod, 1999; Bertilsson *et al.*, 1993a), but the role of other enzymes such as the smoking-inducible CYP1A2 and CYP3A4 is increasingly acknowledged in psychopharmacology.

Classical antipsychotics

Perphenazine

Perphenazine was the first antipsychotic drug studied in relation to the polymorphism of debrisoquine (CYP2D6). In a panel study in healthy volunteers, the mean peak serum concentration of perphenazine was three to four times higher in PMs than in EMs, indicating the involvement of CYP2D6 in the first pass extraction of the drug (Figure 4.3) (Dahl-Puustinen *et al.*, 1989). A similar difference between the phenotypes was seen in the systemic elimination of perphenazine. The study showed that the elimination of perphenazine after oral administration is to a great extent dependent on the activity of CYP2D6, which also has an effect on the oral bioavailability of the drug (Dahl-Puustinen, *et al.*, 1989). In addition, a three-fold difference in oral clearance of perphenazine between PM and homozygous EM genotypes was seen in patients on long-term therapy with the antipsychotic (Jerling, *et al.*, 1996).

Further *in vivo* evidence about the involvement of CYP2D6 in the metabolism of the drug was obtained after adding paroxetine, a potent inhibitor of the polymorphic CYP2D6 (Jeppesen *et al.*, 1996), to eight EMs for CYP2D6. Perphenazine peak plasma concentrations increased from two-fold to thirteen-fold. This was associated with a significant increase in central nervous system side-effects of perphenazine, including oversedation, extrapyramidal symptoms, and impairment of psychomotor performance and memory in the volunteers (Özdemir, *et al.*, 1997).

Zuclopenthixol

Zuclopenthixol has a chemical structure very similar to that of perphenazine and in a similar manner, the plasma elimination half-life was significantly longer in six PMs compared with six EMs of debrisoquine after a single oral dose of the antipsychotic zuclopenthixol (Dahl *et al.*, 1991). The apparent oral clearance was significantly lower in PMs than in EMs. However,

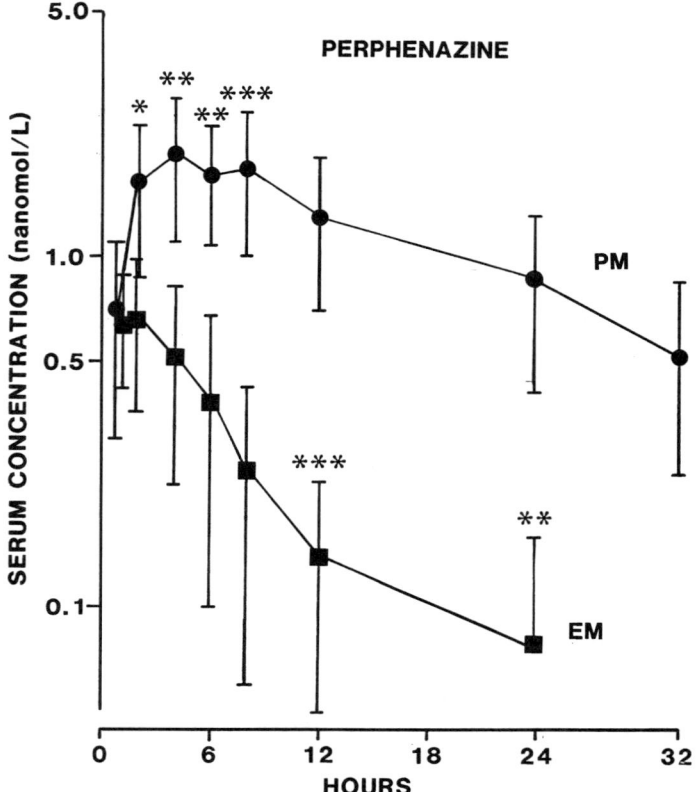

Figure 4.3 Serum concentrations of perphenazine (mean±SD) in six poor metabolisers (PM) and six extensive metabolisers (EM) of debrisoquine after a single oral dose of 6 mg perphenazine. Significant differences in serum concentrations between EM and PM are indicated: *p<0.05; **p<0.01; ***p<0.001 (modified from Dahl-Puustinen *et al.*, 1989).

CYP2D6 seems to be more important for the elimination of perphenazine than of zuclopenthixol due to the more extensive impact of CYP2D6 on the first pass metabolism of perphenazine (Dahl and Bertilsson, 1993). Accordingly, the difference in the oral clearances of zuclopenthixol between PM and homozygous EM was two-fold for zuclopenthixol compared with three-fold for perphenazine (Jerling *et al.*, 1996).

Haloperidol

Haloperidol has for many years been one of the most commonly used drugs in psychiatry. It is metabolised by reduction of the ketone group to form reduced haloperidol, as well as by N-dealkylation and aromatic hydroxylation. Interconversion of haloperidol and reduced haloperidol is known to occur, as haloperidol is found in plasma after the administration of reduced haloperidol and vice versa (Chakraborty *et al.*, 1989).

PMs of debrisoquine eliminated haloperidol significantly more slowly than did EMs, with mean plasma elimination half-lives of 29.4 and 16.3 h and mean CL values of 1.2 and 2.5 l/h/kg, respectively (Llerena *et al.*, 1992a). The plasma levels of reduced haloperidol were also higher in PMs than in EMs (Llerena *et al.*, 1992b).

In eight patients with schizophrenia treated with haloperidol decanoate, the dopamine D2 receptor occupancy was determined by positron emission tomography 1 and 4 weeks after intramuscular injection of the drug (Nyberg *et al.*, 1995b). One of the patients was genotypically a PM of debrisoquine; of the group, he had the highest plasma concentration of haloperidol and also the highest D2 receptor occupancy. Thus, there also appears to be a relationship between the CYP2D6 genotype and D2 receptor occupancy by haloperidol.

Further evidence for the role of CYP2D6 in the metabolism of haloperidol, has been provided in a clinical study showing a pharmacokinetic interaction between the CYP2D6 inhibitor fluoxetine (Otton *et al.*, 1993; Jeppesen *et al.*, 1996) and haloperidol in 13 schizophrenic patients with prominent negative symptoms (Avenoso *et al.*, 1997). However, the specific enzymes mediating the metabolism of haloperidol have not been definitively established, and haloperidol concentrations in serum were markedly elevated by fluvoxamine, a potent inhibitor of the CYP1A2 and CYP2C19 metabolic activities, in three schizophrenic patients (Daniel *et al.*, 1994). Additionally, smoking may induce the metabolism of haloperidol, which results in lower plasma haloperidol concentrations in smokers than in nonsmokers, particularly at low doses of haloperidol (Shimoda *et al.*, 1999). This finding provided further indirect evidence about the involvement of CYP1A2 in the metabolism of haloperidol. Since elevated plasma concentrations of haloperidol and reduced haloperidol were found during itraconazole administration, the CYP3A4 is also probably involved in the metabolism of the antipsychotic (Yasui *et al.*, 1999).

Thioridazine

Thioridazine is extensively biotransformed into two active metabolites, the thioridazine 2-sulfoxide (THD 2-SO or mesoridazine) and thioridazine 2-sulfone (THD 2-SO$_2$ or sulforidazine) and a non-antipsychotic metabolite, the thioridazine 5-sulfoxide (THD 5-SO), which is cardiotoxic (Dahl, 1982; Hale and Poklis, 1996). However, the specific enzymes mediating the metabolism of thioridazine have not been fully established. It is known that the polymorphic CYP2D6 is involved in the formation of mesoridazine from thioridazine (von Bahr *et al.*, 1991; Eap *et al.*, 1996) and also probably partially in the formation of thioridazine 5-sulfoxide, but not in the formation of sulforidazine from mesoridazine (Eap *et al.*, 1996). Additionally, the polymorphic CYP2C19 is not involved in the formation of the aforementioned compounds, but it seems to contribute, along with CYP1A2, to further degradation of thioridazine and its metabolites into yet unidentified compounds (Eap *et al.*, 1996; Carrillo *et al.*, 1999).

In a study carried out in schizophrenic patients, the addition of a low dose of fluvoxamine (25 mg twice a day) led to a pharmacokinetic interaction with thioridazine (Carrillo *et al.*, 1999). After addition of fluvoxamine, the mean concentrations of thioridazine increased by 225%, those of mesoridazine by 220%, and those of sulforidazine by 250%. On the other hand, the metabolism of fluvoxamine, a compound that exhibits a non-linear kinetics (Härtter *et al.*, 1998; Spigset *et al.*, 1998), is mainly determined by CYP2D6 (Carrillo *et al.*, 1996; Spigset *et al.*, 1997), an enzyme strongly inhibited by thioridazine (Yasui *et al.*, 1995). Thus, a reciprocal inhibition is expected so high levels of thioridazine could also contribute to a slow elimination of fluvoxamine. Therefore, it could explain the fact that despite fluvoxamine discontinuation for two weeks, three patients still showed elevated concentrations of thioridazine and its metabolites in the aforementioned study (Carrillo *et al.*, 1999). This study indicated the involvement of CYP1A2 and/or CYP2C19 in the mechanism of the interaction between thioridazine and fluvoxamine. Therefore, clinicians should be aware of the potential for a pharmacokinetic interaction between thioridazine and fluvoxamine and unless otherwise indicated, this drug association should be avoided in clinical practice.

Atypical antipsychotics

Clozapine

Clozapine was the first marketed antipsychotic agent labeled as atypical. While the metabolism of most of investigated classical antipsychotic drugs cosegregate with the polymorphic debrisoquine hydroxylation (Bertilsson *et al.*, 1993a), no such relationship was found for clozapine (Dahl *et al.*, 1994a; Arranz *et al.*, 1995). In contrast, a pharmacokinetic interaction was observed in patients between the potent CYP1A2 inhibitor fluvoxamine (Brøsen *et al.*, 1993b), and clozapine (Jerling *et al.*, 1994). In order to obtain further evidence about the role of CYP1A2 in the metabolism of clozapine, a study involving 14 healthy volunteers was carried out (Bertilsson *et al.*, 1994). A high correlation between a clearance measure of clozapine and an index of CYP1A2 ($r_s=0.84$) was found. An *in vitro* study also confirmed the involvement of CYP1A2 and CYP3A4 in the demethylation and CYP3A4 in the N-oxidation of clozapine (Eiermann *et al.*, 1997).

It has already been mentioned that a number of factors may influence the CYP1A2 metabolic activity and hence, drug response (Carrillo and Benítez, 2000). Smoking induces CYP1A2 (Kalow and Tang, 1993; Carrillo and Benítez, 1994) and plasma concentrations of clozapine have been found to be lower in smokers than in nonsmokers (Haring *et al.*, 1989; 1990). In fact, a grand mal seizure following smoking cessation has been described in a patient who was treated with clozapine, probably due to increased plasma concentrations after giving up smoking (McCarthy, 1994).

Caffeine is a compound that frequently occurs in psychiatric patients, and a clinically defined risk of toxicity when coadministering caffeine and clozapine has been reported (Vainer and Chouinard, 1994). This was interpreted as a pharmacodynamic interaction at the receptor level, but it could be due to an interaction at the CYP1A2 enzyme level (Carrillo *et al.*, 1995).

A pharmacokinetic interaction between clozapine and dietary caffeine was found in a recent clinical study involving seven schizophrenic patients (six males and one female) receiving monotherapy with clozapine at 271 ± 102 mg/day (3.73 ± 1.4 mg/kg) (Carrillo *et al.*, 1998a). Plasma clozapine concentrations significantly decreased by 50% after a caffeine-free diet for 5 days; the largest percentage decrease (-80%) was registered in the patient with heaviest smoking behavior (40 cigarettes/day), who also had the lowest plasma clozapine levels over time.

Since both clozapine and caffeine are CYP1A2 substrates, drastic changes in the consumption of caffeine and/or smoking could influence the pharmacokinetics of clozapine, and monitoring of clozapine and metabolite levels may be warranted in such situations (Carillo and Benítez, 1996; Carrillo *et al.*, 1998a).

The elimination of clozapine may be affected by concurrent administration of compounds interfering with the isoenzymes involved in its metabolism. In particular, a five- to ten-fold elevation of plasma clozapine concentrations was described after addition of fluvoxamine (Hiemke *et al.*, 1994; Jerling *et al.*, 1994), while anticonvulsant agents with enzyme-inducing properties, such as carbamazepine and phenobarbital, were reported to decrease plasma levels of clozapine (Jerling *et al.*, 1994; Facciola *et al.*, 1998).

Olanzapine

Olanzapine is an atypical antipsychotic drug that shares many pharmacological properties with clozapine (Stockton and Rasmussen, 1996). The N-glucuronidation pathway seems to be the most important one for olanzapine metabolism (Ereshefsky, 1996b; Kassahun *et al.*, 1997), but *in vitro* (Ring *et al.*, 1996a, 1996b) and *in vivo* (Fulton and Goa, 1997; Kassahun *et al.*, 1997) investigations have demonstrated that the smoking-inducible CYP1A2 along with the polymorphic CYP2D6 isozymes are also involved in its metabolism. In an investigation in eight schizophrenic patients (four males and four females), olanzapine therapy for 15 days caused a significant reduction (by 40%) in the overall 0–24 h caffeine urinary metabolite index of CYP1A2 activity from baseline (Carrillo *et al.*, 1998c). It was intriguing to find in this study, two smoking patients registering the highest CYP1A2 indices, who were unresponsive to olanzapine. Furthermore, one of them also failed to show any response to previous treatment with clozapine (Carrillo *et al.*, 1998c). Hence, these data support the hypothesis of a clinically important role of CYP1A2 and related factors in causing variability in drug response to olanzapine. Conversely, in a study conducted in healthy volunteers (Macias *et al.*, 1998) olanzapine did not affect the pharmacokinetics of theophylline, a substrate of CYP1A2 (Sarkar *et al.*, 1992; Rasmussen and Brøsen, 1997).

Risperidone

Risperidone is an antagonist of postsynaptic serotonin-2 and dopamine D2 receptors (Nyberg *et al.*, 1993; Farde *et al.*, 1995). The pharmacokinetics of risperidone, and the prolactin response were studied in twelve dextromethorphan-phenotyped healthy males after administration of 1 mg risperidone intravenously, intramuscularly, and orally (Huang *et al.*, 1993). The formation of the equipotent major and also active metabolite, 9-hydroxyrisperidone exhibited CYP2D6-related polymorphism. The plasma area under the concentration-time curve from time zero to infinity (AUC 0–∞) ratio of 9-hydroxyrisperidone to risperidone averaged three (intravenous and intramuscular) and six (oral administration) in the extensive metabolisers and 0.2 in the poor metabolisers. Risperidone half-life was about 3 hours in EMs and 22 hours in PMs (Huang *et al.*, 1993). A positron emission tomography (PET) study confirmed that the plasma concentrations of risperidone were higher and the elimination half-life longer in two PM than in three EM subjects. However, no differences were found in the plasma concentrations of the active moiety (sum of risperidone and of 9-hydroxyrisperidone), suggesting that the 9-hydroxy metabolite contributes to the *in vivo* effects of risperidone (Nyberg *et al.*, 1995a). Further confirmation for the role of CYP2D6, came from a recent study in which steady-state plasma concentrations of risperidone and its major metabolite were measured in thirty-seven schizophrenic patients stabilised on risperidone. The risperidone/9-hydroxyrisperidone ratio in plasma was strongly associated with CYP2D6 genotype: the highest ratios were observed in PM, heterozygous EM had significantly higher ratios than homozygous

EM, while ultrarapid metabolisers had some of the lowest ratios (Scordo *et al.*, 1999).

Other antipsychotics

Sertindole

Sertindole is extensively metabolised by CYP3A and also CYP2D6. The major identified metabolites are dehydrosertindole, resulting from imidazoline ring oxidation and subsequent dehydration and norsertindole, which can be formed directly from sertindole or from dehydrosertindole (Sakamoto *et al.*, 1995). Sertindole appeared to be cardiotoxic. In fact, it produces prolongation of the QT interval even at therapeutic doses in humans and since a few cases of sudden death have been reported, its safety has been debated widely, leading to market withdrawal of the product (Lewis *et al.*, 2000).

Zotepine

Zotepine is a dibenzothiepine derivative antipsychotic drug developed in Japan. Two major metabolites of the drug, desmethylzotepine-S-oxide and 7-hydroxy-desmethylzotepine-O-sulphate, had previously been identified in humans, but the pharmacological activities of these metabolites are unknown (Noda *et al.*, 1979). It has been suggested that neither smoking nor CYP2C19 status affects the metabolism of zotepine and the elevation in plasma concentrations of zotepine after coadministration of diazepam may be a result of competitive inhibition of zotepine metabolism by diazepam via isoenzymes other than CYP2C19, e.g. CYP3A4 (Kondo *et al.*, 1996). In fact it has recently been suggested that both the N-demethylation and S-oxidation of zotepine are mediated mainly by CYP3A4, and that CYP1A2 and 2D6 play an important role in the 2- and 3-hydroxylation of zotepine, respectively (Shiraga *et al.*, 1999).

Quetiapine

The dibenzothiazepine quetiapine, also offers an alternative to conventional antipsychotics for the treatment of schizophrenia, with apparently fewer side-effects (Parsa and Bastani, 1998). Preliminary observations suggest the participation of CYP3A4 in the metabolism of the drug (Misra *et al.*, 1998).

In conclusion, most of the antipsychotic drugs so far investigated are metabolised, at least in part, by CYP2D6. The activity of this enzyme is predominantly under genetic control and only to a minor extent influenced by environmental factors. Interindividual differences in the elimination kinetics and in plasma concentrations of antipsychotics resulting from genetically determined variability in the expression of CYP2D6 may thus have potentially important clinical implications. An association between the PM phenotype and acute neuroleptic-induced side-effects has been documented in a few patients (Meyer *et al.*, 1990; Spina *et al.*, 1992a). Other studies have indicated that CYP2D6 genotype might influence the occurrence and severity of antipsychotic-induced movement disorders, including tardive dyskinesia (Arthur *et al.*, 1995; Andreassen *et al.*, 1997; Armstrong *et al.*, 1997). Nevertheless, the CYP1A2 and CYP3A4 metabolic activities are increasingly acknowledged in psychopharmacology, and they are involved in the metabolism of a number of psychotropic drugs. The CYP1A2 activity has not been demonstrated to be polymorphically distributed in the population. However, it shows a wide variability in humans and since several factors such as gender, smoking and concomitant caffeine intake affect this metabolic activity, they should be taken into consideration when giving CYP1A2 substrates to psychiatric patients.

References

Agundez, J. A., Ledesma, M. C., Ladero, J. M. and Benitez, J. (1995) 'Prevalence of CYP2D6 gene duplication and its repercussion on the oxidative phenotype in a white population', *Clin. Pharmacol. Ther.* **57**: 265–69.

Aklillu, E., Persson, I., Bertilsson, L., Johansson, I., Rodrigues, F. and Ingelman-Sundberg, M. (1996) 'Frequent distribution of ultrarapid metabolizers of debrisoquine in an Ethiopian population carrying duplicated and multiduplicated functional CYP2D6 alleles', *J. Pharmacol. Exp. Ther.* **278**: 441–6.

Alderman, J., Preskorn, S. H., Greenblatt, D. J., Harrison, W., Penenberg, D., Allison, J. and Chung, M. (1997) 'Desipramine pharmacokinetics when co-administered with paroxetine or sertraline in extensive metabolizers', *J. Clin. Psychopharmacol.* **17**: 284–91.

Alexanderson, B. (1972) 'Pharmacokinetics of nortriptyline in man after single and multiple oral doses: the predictability of steady-state plasma concentrations from single-dose plasma-level data', *Eur. J. Clin. Pharmacol.* **4**: 82–91.

Alexanderson, B., Evans, D. A. and Sjöqvist, F. (1969) 'Steady-state plasma levels of nortriptyline in twins: influence of genetic factors and drug therapy', *Br. Med. J.* **4**: 764–8.

Alvan, G., Bechtel, P., Iselius, L. and Gundert-Remy, U. (1990) 'Hydroxylation polymorphisms of debrisoquine and mephenytoin in European populations', *Eur. J. Clin. Pharmacol.* **39**: 533–7.

Amsterdam, J. D., Brunswick, D. J., Potter, L. and Kaplan, M. J. (1984) 'Cimetidine-induced alterations in desipramine plasma concentrations', *Psychopharmacology* **83**: 373–5.

Andersen, B. B., Mikkelsen, M., Vesterager, A., Dam, M., Kristensen, H. B., Pedersen, B., Lund, J. and Mengel, H. (1991) 'No influence of the antidepressant paroxetine on carbamazepine, valproate and phenytoin', *Epilepsy Res.* **10**: 201–4.

Andreassen, O. A, MacEwan, T, Gulbrandsen, A. K., McCreadie, R. G. and Steen, V. M. (1997) 'Non-functional CYP2D6 alleles and risk for neuroleptic-induced movement disorders in schizophrenic patients', *Psychopharmacology (Berl.)* **131:** 174–9.

Aranow, A. B., Hudson, J. I., Pope, H. G., Jr., Grady, T. A., Laage, T. A., Bell, I. R. and Cole, J. O. (1989) 'Elevated antidepressant plasma levels after addition of fluoxetine', *Am. J. Psychiatry* **146:** 911–3.

Armstrong, M., Daly, A. K., Blennerhassett, R., Ferrier, N. and Idle, J. R. (1997) 'Antipsychotic drug-induced movement disorders in schizophrenics in relation to CYP2D6 genotype', *Br. J. Psychiatry* **170:** 23–6.

Arranz, M. J., Dawson, E., Shaikh, S., Sham, P., Sharma, T., Aitchison, K., Crocq, M. A., Gill, M., Kerwin, R. and Collier, D. A. (1995) 'Cytochrome P4502D6 genotype does not determine response to clozapine', *Br. J. Clin. Pharmacol.* **39:** 417–20.

Arthur, H., Dahl, M. L., Siwers, B. and Sjöqvist, F. (1995) 'Polymorphic drug metabolism in schizophrenic patients with tardive dyskinesia', *J. Clin. Psychopharmacol.* **15:** 211–6.

Åsberg, M., Evans, D. A. and Sjöqvist, F. (1971) 'Genetic control of nortriptyline kinetics in man: a study of relatives of propositi with high plasma concentrations', *J. Med. Genet.* **8:** 129–35.

Avenoso, A., Facciola, G., Scordo, M. G. and Spina, E. (1999) 'No effect of the new antidepressant reboxetine on CYP2D6 activity in healthy volunteers', *Ther. Drug. Monit.* **21:** 577–9.

Avenoso, A., Spina, E., Campo, G., Facciola, G., Ferlito, M., Zuccaro, P., Perucca, E. and Caputi, A. P. (1997) 'Interaction between fluoxetine and haloperidol: pharmacokinetic and clinical implications', *Pharmacol. Res.* **35:** 335–9.

Ayesh, R., Dawling, S., Hayler, A., Oates, N. S., Cholerton, S., Widdop, B., Idle, J. R. and Smith, R. L. (1991) 'Comparative effects of the diastereoisomers, quinine and quinidine in producing phenocopy debrisoquine poor metabolisers (PMs) in healthy volunteers', *Chirality* **3:** 14–18.

Bailey, D. G., Malcolm, J., Arnold, O. and Spence, J. D. (1998) 'Grapefruit juice-drug interactions', *Br. J. Clin. Pharmacol.* **46:** 101–10.

Balant-Gorgia, A. E., Balant, L. P. and Garrone, G. (1989) 'High blood concentrations of imipramine or clomipramine and therapeutic failure: a case report study using drug monitoring data', *Ther. Drug. Monit.* **11:** 415–20.

Balant-Gorgia, A. E., Balant, L. P., Genet, C., Dayer, P., Aeschlimann, J. M. and Garrone, G. (1986) 'Importance of oxidative polymorphism and levomepromazine treatment on the steady-state blood concentrations of clomipramine and its major metabolites', *Eur. J. Clin. Pharmacol.* **31:** 449–55.

Balant-Gorgia, A. E., Schulz, P., Dayer, P., Balant, L., Kubli, A., Gertsch, C. and Garrone, G. (1982) 'Role of oxidation polymorphism on blood and urine concentrations of amitriptyline and its metabolites in man', *Arch. Psychiatr. Nervenkr.* **232:** 215–22.

Ballinger, B. R., Presly, A., Reid, A. H. and Stevenson, I. H. (1974) 'The effects of hypnotics on imipramine treatment', *Psychopharmacologia* **39:** 267–74.

Bannister, S. J., Houser, V. P., Hulse, J. D., Kisicki, J. C. and Rasmussen, J. G. (1989) 'Evaluation of the potential for interactions of paroxetine with diazepam, cimetidine, warfarin, and digoxin', *Acta Psychiatr. Scand. Suppl.* **350:** 102–6.

Barbhaiya, R. H., Buch, A. B. and Greene, D. S. (1996) 'Single and multiple dose pharmacokinetics of nefazodone in subjects classified as extensive and poor metabolizers of dextromethorphan', *Br. J. Clin. Pharmacol.* **42:** 573–81.

Bergstrom, R. F., Peyton, A. L. and Lemberger, L. (1992) 'Quantification and mechanism of the fluoxetine and tricyclic antidepressant interaction', *Clin. Pharmacol. Ther.* 51: 239–48.

Bertilsson, L. and Åberg-Wistedt, A. (1983) 'The debrisoquine hydroxylation test predicts steady-state plasma levels of desipramine', *Br. J. Clin. Pharmacol.* 15: 388–90.

Bertilsson, L., Åberg-Wistedt, A., Gustafsson, L. L. and Nordin, C. (1985) 'Extremely rapid hydroxylation of debrisoquine: a case report with implication for treatment with nortriptyline and other tricyclic antidepressants', *Ther. Drug. Monit.* 7: 478–80.

Bertilsson, L., Carrillo, J. A., Dahl, M. L., Llerena, A., Alm, C., Bondesson, U., Lindstrom, L., Rodriguez de la Rubia, I., Ramos, S. and Benítez, J. (1994) 'Clozapine disposition covaries with CYP1A2 activity determined by a caffeine test', *Br. J. Clin. Pharmacol.* 38: 471–3.

Bertilsson, L. and Dahl, M. L. (1996) 'Polymorphic drug oxidation: relevance to the treatment of psychiatric disorders', *CNS Drugs* 5: 200–23.

Bertilsson, L., Dahl, M. L., Ekqvist, B. and Llerena, A. (1993a) 'Disposition of the neuroleptics perphenazine, zuclopenthixol, and haloperidol cosegregates with polymorphic debrisoquine hydroxylation', *Psychopharmacol. Ser.* 10: 230–7.

Bertilsson, L., Dahl, M. L., Sjöqvist, F., Åberg-Wistedt, A., Humble, M., Johansson, I., Lundqvist, E. and Ingelman-Sundberg, M. (1993b) 'Molecular basis for rational megaprescribing in ultrarapid hydroxylators of debrisoquine (letter)', *Lancet* 341: 63.

Bertilsson, L., Dahl, M. L. and Tybring, G. (1997) 'Pharmacogenetics of antidepressants: clinical aspects', *Acta. Psychiatr. Scand. Suppl.* 391: 14–21.

Bertilsson, L., Lou, Y. Q., Du, Y. L., Liu, Y., Kuang, T. Y., Liao, X. M., Wang, K. Y., Reviriego, J., Iselius, L. and Sjöqvist, F. (1992) 'Pronounced differences between native Chinese and Swedish populations in the polymorphic hydroxylations of debrisoquin and S-mephenytoin', *Clin. Pharmacol. Ther.* 51: 388–97.

Bertilsson, L., Mellström, B., Sjöqvist, F., Martenson, B. and Åsberg, M. (1981) 'Slow hydroxylation of nortriptyline and concomitant poor debrisoquine hydroxylation: clinical implications (letter)', *Lancet* 1: 560–1.

Bertschy, G., Vandel, S., Vandel, B., Allers, G. and Volmat, R. (1991) 'Fluvoxamine–tricyclic antidepressant interaction. An accidental finding (letter)', *Eur. J. Clin. Pharmacol.* 40: 119–20.

Bloomer, J. C., Woods, F. R., Haddock, R. E., Lennard, M. S. and Tucker, G. T. (1992) 'The role of cytochrome P4502D6 in the metabolism of paroxetine by human liver microsomes', *Br. J. Clin. Pharmacol.* 33: 521–3.

Bluhm, R. E., Wilkinson, G. R., Shelton, R. and Branch, R. A. (1993) 'Genetically determined drug-metabolizing activity and desipramine-associated cardiotoxicity: a case report', *Clin. Pharmacol. Ther.* 53: 89–95.

Braithwaite, R. A., Flanagan, R. J. and Richens, A. (1975) 'Steady-state plasma nortriptyline concentrations in epileptic patients (letter)', *Br. J. Clin. Pharmacol.* 2: 469–71.

Broly, F., Gaedigk, A., Heim, M., Eichelbaum, M., Morike, K. and Meyer, U. A. (1991) 'Debrisoquine/sparteine hydroxylation genotype and phenotype: analysis of common mutations and alleles of CYP2D6 in a European population', *DNA Cell. Biol.* 10: 545–58.

Broly, F. and Meyer, U. A. (1993) 'Debrisoquine oxidation polymorphism: phenotypic consequences of a 3-base-pair deletion in exon 5 of the CYP2D6 gene', *Pharmacogenetics* 3: 123–30.

Brøsen, K. and Gram, L. F. (1988) 'First-pass metabolism of imipramine and desipramine: impact of the sparteine oxidation phenotype', *Clin. Pharmacol. Ther.* 43: 400–6.

Brøsen, K. and Gram, L. F. (1989) 'Quinidine inhibits the 2-hydroxylation of imipramine and desipramine but not the demethylation of imipramine', *Eur. J. Clin. Pharmacol.* 37: 155–60.

Brøsen, K., Gram, L. F., Klysner, R. and Bech, P. (1986a) 'Steady-state levels of imipramine and its metabolites: significance of dose-dependent kinetics', *Eur. J. Clin. Pharmacol.* 30: 43–9.

Brøsen, K., Hansen, J. G., Nielsen, K. K., Sindrup, S. H. and Gram, L. F. (1993a) 'Inhibition by paroxetine of desipramine metabolism in extensive but not in poor metabolizers of sparteine', *Eur. J. Clin. Pharmacol.* 44: 349–55.

Brøsen, K., Klysner, R., Gram, L. F., Otton, S. V., Bech, P. and Bertilsson, L. (1986b) 'Steady-state concentrations of imipramine and its metabolites in relation to the sparteine/debrisoquine polymorphism', *Eur. J. Clin. Pharmacol.* 30: 679–84.

Brøsen, K. and Kragh-Sorensen, P. (1993) 'Concomitant intake of nortriptyline and carbamazepine', *Ther. Drug. Monit.* 15: 258–60.

Brøsen, K., Otton, S. V. and Gram, L. F. (1986c) 'Imipramine demethylation and hydroxylation: impact of the sparteine oxidation phenotype', *Clin. Pharmacol. Ther.* 40: 543–9.

Brøsen, K. and Skjelbo, E. (1991) 'Fluoxetine and norfluoxetine are potent inhibitors of P450IID6–the source of the sparteine/debrisoquine oxidation polymorphism (letter)', *Br. J. Clin. Pharmacol.* 32: 136–7.

Brøsen, K., Skjelbo, E., Rasmussen, B. B., Poulsen, H. E. and Loft, S. (1993b) 'Fluvoxamine is a potent inhibitor of cytochrome P4501A2', *Biochem. Pharmacol.* 45: 1211–4.

Burke, M. J. and Preskorn, S. H. (1999) 'Therapeutic drug monitoring of anti-depressants: cost implications and relevance to clinical practice', *Clin. Pharmacokinet.* 37: 147–65.

Burrows, G. D. and Davies, B. (1971) 'Antidepressants and barbiturates', *Br. Med. J.* 4: 113.

Butler, M. A., Iwasaki, M., Guengerich, F. P. and Kadlubar, F. F. (1989) 'Human cytochrome P-450PA (P-450IA2), the phenacetin O-deethylase, is primarily responsible for the hepatic 3-demethylation of caffeine and N-oxidation of carcinogenic arylamines', *Proc. Natl. Acad. Sci. USA* 86: 7696–700.

Caccia, S. (1998) 'Metabolism of the newer antidepressants. An overview of the pharmacological and pharmacokinetic implications', *Clin. Pharmacokinet.* 34: 281–302.

Caccia, S. and Garattini, S. (1990) 'Formation of active metabolites of psychotropic drugs. An updated review of their significance', *Clin. Pharmacokinet.* 18: 434–59.

Carrillo, J. A. and Benítez, J. (1994) 'Caffeine metabolism in a healthy Spanish population: N-acetylator phenotype and oxidation pathways', *Clin. Pharmacol. Ther.* 55: 293–304.

Carrillo, J. A. and Benítez, J. (1996) 'CYP1A2 activity, gender and smoking, as variables influencing the toxicity of caffeine', *Br. J. Clin. Pharmacol.* **41**: 605–8.

Carrillo, J. A. and Benítez, J. (2000) 'Clinically significant pharmacokinetic interactions between dietary caffeine and medications', *Clin. Pharmacokinet.* **39**: 127–53.

Carrillo, J. A., Christensen, M., Ramos, S. I., Alm, C., Dahl, M. L., Benítez, J. and Bertilsson, L. (2000) 'Evaluation of caffeine as an in vivo probe for CYP1A2 using measurements in plasma, saliva and urine', *Ther. Drug. Monit.* **22**: 409–17.

Carrillo, J. A., Dahl, M. L., Svensson, J. O., Alm, C., Rodriguez, I. and Bertilsson, L. (1996) 'Disposition of fluvoxamine in humans is determined by the polymorphic CYP2D6 and also by the CYP1A2 activity', *Clin. Pharmacol. Ther.* **60**: 183–90.

Carrillo, J. A., Herraiz, A. G., Ramos, S. I. and Benítez, J. (1998a) 'Effects of caffeine withdrawal from the diet on the metabolism of clozapine in schizophrenic patients', *J. Clin. Psychopharmacol.* **18**: 311–6.

Carrillo, J. A., Jerling, M. and Bertilsson, L. (1995) 'Comments to "interaction between caffeine and clozapine" (letter)', *J. Clin. Psychopharmacol.* **15**: 376–7.

Carrillo, J. A., Ramos, S. I., Agundez, J. A., Martinez, C. and Benítez, J. (1998b) 'Analysis of midazolam and metabolites in plasma by high-performance liquid chromatography: probe of CYP3A', *Ther. Drug. Monit.* **20**: 319–24.

Carrillo, J. A., Ramos, S. I., Herraiz, A. G., Llerena, A., Agundez, J. A., Berecz, R., Duran M. and Benítez, J. (1999) 'Pharmacokinetic interaction of fluvoxamine and thioridazine in schizophrenic patients', *J. Clin. Psychopharmacol.* **19**: 494–9.

Carrillo, J. A., Ramos, S. I., Herraiz, A. G., Lozano, L. and Benítez, J. (1998c) 'CYP1A2 activity and smoking influence the risk/benefit ratio of olanzapine in schizophrenic patients', in L. P. Balant, J. Benítez, S. G. Dahl, L. F. Gram, R. M. Pinder and W. Z. Potter (eds) *Clinical Pharmacology in Psychiatry: Finding the Right Dose of Psychotropic Drugs*, European Commision, COST B1, Brussels, pp 291–5.

Chakraborty, B. S., Hubbard, J. W., Hawes, E. M., McKay, G., Cooper, J. K., Gurnsey, T., Korchinski, E. D. and Midha, K. K. (1989) 'Interconversion between haloperidol and reduced haloperidol in healthy volunteers', *Eur. J. Clin. Pharmacol.* **37**: 45–8.

Chang, M., Dahl, M. L., Tybring, G., Gotharson, E. and Bertilsson, L. (1995a) 'Use of omeprazole as a probe drug for CYP2C19 phenotype in Swedish Caucasians: comparison with S-mephenytoin hydroxylation phenotype and CYP2C19 genotype', *Pharmacogenetics* **5**: 358–63.

Chang, M., Tybring, G., Dahl, M. L., Gotharson, E., Sagar, M., Seensalu, R. and Bertilsson, L. (1995b) 'Interphenotype differences in disposition and effect on gastrin levels of omeprazole–suitability of omeprazole as a probe for CYP2C19', *Br. J. Clin. Pharmacol.* **39**: 511–8.

Chiba, K., Saitoh, A., Koyama, E., Tani, M., Hayashi, M. and Ishizaki, T. (1994) 'The role of S-mephenytoin 4'-hydroxylase in imipramine metabolism by human liver microsomes: a two-enzyme kinetic analysis of N-demethylation and 2-hydroxylation', *Br. J. Clin. Pharmacol.* **37**: 237–42.

Ciraulo, D. A., Barnhill, J. G. and Jaffe, J. H. (1988) 'Clinical pharmacokinetics of imipramine and desipramine in alcoholics and normal volunteers', *Clin. Pharmacol. Ther.* **43**: 509–18.

Crewe, H. K., Lennard, M. S., Tucker, G. T., Woods, F. R. and Haddock, R. E. (1992) 'The effect of selective serotonin re-uptake inhibitors on cytochrome P4502D6 (CYP2D6) activity in human liver microsomes', *Br. J. Clin. Pharmacol.* **34**: 262–5.

Dahl, S. G. (1982) 'Active metabolites of neuroleptic drugs: possible contribution to therapeutic and toxic effects', *Ther. Drug. Monit.* **4**: 33–40.

Dahl, S. G. (1986) 'Plasma level monitoring of antipsychotic drugs. Clinical utility', *Clin. Pharmacokinet.* **11**: 36–61.

Dahl, M. L. and Bertilsson, L. (1993) 'Genetically variable metabolism of antidepressants and neuroleptic drugs in man', *Pharmacogenetics* **3**: 61–70.

Dahl, M. L., Bertilsson, L. and Nordin, C. (1996) 'Steady-state plasma levels of nortriptyline and its 10-hydroxy metabolite: relationship to the CYP2D6 genotype', *Psychopharmacology (Berl.)* **123**: 315–9.

Dahl, M. L., Ekqvist, B., Widen, J. and Bertilsson, L. (1991) 'Disposition of the neuroleptic zuclopenthixol cosegregates with the polymorphic hydroxylation of debrisoquine in humans', *Acta. Psychiatr. Scand.* **84**: 99–102.

Dahl, M. L., Johansson, I., Bertilsson, L., Ingelman-Sundberg, M. and Sjöqvist, F. (1995) 'Ultrarapid hydroxylation of debrisoquine in a Swedish population. Analysis of the molecular genetic basis', *J. Pharmacol. Exp. Ther.* **274**: 516–20.

Dahl, M. L., Johansson, I., Palmertz, M. P., Ingelman-Sundberg, M. and Sjöqvist, F. (1992) 'Analysis of the CYP2D6 gene in relation to debrisoquine and desipramine hydroxylation in a Swedish population', *Clin. Pharmacol. Ther.* **51**: 12–17.

Dahl, M. L., Llerena, A., Bondesson, U., Lindström, L. and Bertilsson, L. (1994a) 'Disposition of clozapine in man: lack of association with debrisoquine and S-mephenytoin hydroxylation polymorphisms', *Br. J. Clin. Pharmacol.* **37**: 71–4.

Dahl, M. L. and Sjöqvist, F. (2000) 'Pharmacogenetic methods as a complement to therapeutic monitoring of antidepressants and neuroleptics', *Ther. Drug. Monit.* **22**: 114–7.

Dahl, M. L., Tybring, G., Elwin, C. E., Alm, C., Andreasson, K., Gyllenpalm, M. and Bertilsson, L. (1994b) 'Stereoselective disposition of mianserin is related to debrisoquine hydroxylation polymorphism', *Clin. Pharmacol. Ther.* **56**: 176–83.

Dahl, M. L., Voortman, G., Alm, C., Elwin, C., Delbressine, L., Vos, R., Bogaards, J. J. P. and Bertilsson, L. (1997) 'In vitro and in vivo studies on the disposition of mirtazapine in humans', *Clin. Drug. Invest.* **13**: 37–46.

Dahl-Puustinen, M. L., Liden, A., Alm, C., Nordin, C. and Bertilsson, L. (1989) 'Disposition of perphenazine is related to polymorphic debrisoquine hydroxylation in human beings', *Clin. Pharmacol. Ther.* **46**: 78–81.

Dalen, P., Dahl, M. L., Ruiz, M. L., Nordin, J. and Bertilsson, L. (1998) '10-Hydroxylation of nortriptyline in white persons with 0, 1, 2, 3, and 13 functional CYP2D6 genes', *Clin. Pharmacol. Ther.* **63**: 444–52.

Daniel, D. G., Randolph, C., Jaskiw, G., Handel, S., Williams, T., Abi-Dargham, A., Shoaf, S., Egan, M., Elkashef, A., Liboff, S. and Linnoila, M. (1994) 'Co-administration of fluvoxamine increases serum concentrations of haloperidol', *J. Clin. Psychopharmacol.* **14**: 340–3.

de Morais, S. M., Wilkinson, G. R., Blaisdell, J., Meyer, U. A., Nakamura, K. and Goldstein, J. A. (1994a) 'Identification of a new genetic defect responsible for the polymorphism of (S)-mephenytoin metabolism in Japanese', *Mol. Pharmacol.* **46**: 594–8.

de Morais, S. M., Wilkinson, G. R., Blaisdell, J., Nakamura, K., Meyer, U. A. and Goldstein, J. A. (1994b) 'The major genetic defect responsible for the polymorphism of S-mephenytoin metabolism in humans', *J. Biol. Chem.* **269**: 15419–22.

Delbressine, L., Dahl, M. L., van den Wildenberg, H. M., Kleijn, H. J. and Bertilsson, L. (1997) 'In vivo study in humans on disposition of the enantiomers and metabolites of mirtazapine', *European Neuropsychopharmacology* **7**: S145.

Eap, C. B., Guentert, T. W., Schaublin Loidl, M., Stabl, M., Koeb, L., Powell, K. and Baumann, P. (1996) 'Plasma levels of the enantiomers of thioridazine, thioridazine 2-sulfoxide, thioridazine 2-sulfone, and thioridazine 5-sulfoxide in poor and extensive metabolizers of dextromethorphan and mephenytoin', *Clin. Pharmacol. Ther.* **59**: 322–31.

Eichelbaum, M., Bertilsson, L., Säwe, J. and Zekorn, C. (1982) 'Polymorphic oxidation of sparteine and debrisoquine: related pharmacogenetic entities', *Clin. Pharmacol. Ther.* **31**: 184–6.

Eichelbaum, M., Spannbrucker, N., Steincke, B. and Dengler, H. J. (1979) 'Defective N-oxidation of sparteine in man: a new pharmacogenetic defect', *Eur. J. Clin. Pharmacol.* **16**: 183–7.

Eiermann, B., Engel, G., Johansson, I., Zanger, U. M. and Bertilsson, L. (1997) 'The involvement of CYP1A2 and CYP3A4 in the metabolism of clozapine', *Br. J. Clin. Pharmacol.* **44**: 439–46.

Ereshefsky, L. (1996a) 'Drug-drug interactions involving antidepressants: focus on venlafaxine', *J. Clin. Psychopharmacol.* **16**: 37S-50S; discussion 50S–53S.

Ereshefsky, L. (1996b) 'Pharmacokinetics and drug interactions: update for new antipsychotics', *J. Clin. Psychiatry* **57**: 12–25.

Evans, D. A., Mahgoub, A., Sloan, T. P., Idle, J. R. and Smith, R. L. (1980) 'A family and population study of the genetic polymorphism of debrisoquine oxidation in a white British population', *J. Med. Genet.* **17**: 102–5.

Facciola, G., Avenoso, A., Spina, E. and Perucca, E. (1998) 'Inducing effect of phenobarbital on clozapine metabolism in patients with chronic schizophrenia', *Ther. Drug. Monit* **20**: 628–30.

Fang, J. and Gorrod, J. W. (1999) 'Metabolism, pharmacogenetics, and metabolic drug-drug interactions of antipsychotic drugs', *Cell. Mol. Neurobiol.* **19**: 491–510.

Farde, L., Nyberg, S., Oxenstierna, G., Nakashima, Y., Halldin, C. and Ericsson, B. (1995) 'Positron emission tomography studies on D2 and 5-HT2 receptor binding in risperidone-treated schizophrenic patients', *J. Clin. Psychopharmacol.* **15**: 19S–23S.

Ferguson, R. J., De Morais, S. M., Benhamou, S., Bouchardy, C., Blaisdell, J., Ibeanu, G., Wilkinson, G. R., Sarich, T. C., Wright, J. M., Dayer, P. and Goldstein, J. A. (1998) 'A new genetic defect in human CYP2C19: mutation of the initiation codon is responsible for poor metabolism of S-mephenytoin', *J. Pharmacol. Exp. Ther.* **284**: 356–61.

Firkusny, L. and Gleiter, C. H. (1994) 'Maprotiline metabolism appears to co-segregate with the genetically-determined CYP2D6 polymorphic hydroxylation of debrisoquine', *Br. J. Clin. Pharmacol.* **37**: 383–8.

Fjordside, L., Jeppesen, U., Eap, C. B., Powell, K., Baumann, P. and Brøsen, K. (1999) 'The stereoselective metabolism of fluoxetine in poor and extensive metabolizers of sparteine', *Pharmacogenetics* 9: 55–60.

Fulton, B. and Goa, K. L. (1997) 'Olanzapine. A review of its pharmacological properties and therapeutic efficacy in the management of schizophrenia and related psychoses', *Drugs* 53: 281–98.

Gaedigk, A., Blum, M., Gaedigk, R., Eichelbaum, M. and Meyer, U. A. (1991) 'Deletion of the entire cytochrome P450 CYP2D6 gene as a cause of impaired drug metabolism in poor metabolizers of the debrisoquine/sparteine polymorphism', *Am. J. Hum. Genet.* 48: 943–50.

Goldstein, J. A., Faletto, M. B., Romkes-Sparks, M., Sullivan, T., Kitareewan, S., Raucy, J. L., Lasker, J. M. and Ghanayem, B. I. (1994) 'Evidence that CYP2C19 is the major (S)-mephenytoin 4'-hydroxylase in humans', *Biochemistry* 33: 1743–52.

Gonzalez, F. J. (1992) 'Human cytochromes P450: problems and prospects', *Trends Pharmacol. Sci.* 13: 346–52.

Gonzalez, F. J., Matsunaga, T., Nagata, K., Meyer, U. A., Nebert, D. W., Pastewka, J., Kozak, C. A., Gillette, J., Gelboin, H. V. and Hardwick, J. P. (1987) 'Debrisoquine 4-hydroxylase: characterization of a new P450 gene subfamily, regulation, chromosomal mapping, and molecular analysis of the DA rat polymorphism', *DNA* 6: 149–61.

Goodnick, P. J. (1994) 'Pharmacokinetic optimisation of therapy with newer antidepressants', *Clin. Pharmacokinet.* 27: 307–30.

Gough, A. C., Miles, J. S., Spurr, N. K., Moss, J. E., Gaedigk, A., Eichelbaum, M. and Wolf, C. R. (1990) 'Identification of the primary gene defect at the cytochrome P450 CYP2D locus', *Nature* 347: 773–6.

Gram, L. F., Guentert, T. W., Grange, S., Vistisen, K. and Brøsen, K. (1995) 'Moclobemide, a substrate of CYP2C19 and an inhibitor of CYP2C19, CYP2D6, and CYP1A2: a panel study', *Clin. Pharmacol. Ther.* 57: 670–7.

Gram, L. F., Hansen, M. G., Sindrup, S. H., Brøsen, K., Poulsen, J. H., Aaes-Jorgensen, T. and Overo, K. F. (1993) 'Citalopram: interaction studies with levomepromazine, imipramine, and lithium', *Ther. Drug. Monit.* 15: 18–24.

Gram, L. F. and Overo, K. F. (1972) 'Drug interaction: inhibitory effect of neuroleptics on metabolism of tricyclic antidepressants in man', *Br. Med. J.* 1: 463–5.

Greb, W. H., Buscher, G., Dierdorf, H. D., Koster, F. E., Wolf, D. and Mellows, G. (1989) 'The effect of liver enzyme inhibition by cimetidine and enzyme induction by phenobarbitone on the pharmacokinetics of paroxetine', *Acta. Psychiatr. Scand. Suppl.* 350: 95–8.

Greenblatt, D. J., von Moltke, L. L., Harmatz, J. S. and Shader, R. I. (1999) 'Human cytochromes and some newer antidepressants: kinetics, metabolism, and drug interactions', *J. Clin. Psychopharmacol.* 19: 23S–35S.

Griese, E. U., Zanger, U. M., Brudermanns, U., Gaedigk, A., Mikus, G., Morike, K., Stuven, T. and Eichelbaum, M. (1998) 'Assessment of the predictive power of genotypes for the in-vivo catalytic function of CYP2D6 in a German population', *Pharmacogenetics* 8: 15–26.

Hale, P. and Poklis, A. (1996) 'Thioridazine cardiotoxicity', *J. Toxicol. Clin. Toxicol.* 34: 127–30.

Hamelin, B. A., Turgeon, J., Vallee, F., Belanger, P. M., Paquet, F. and LeBel, M. (1996) 'The disposition of fluoxetine but not sertraline is altered in poor metabolizers of debrisoquine', *Clin. Pharmacol. Ther.* **60**: 512–21.

Hammer, W., Martens, S. and Sjöqvist, F. (1969) A comparative study of the metabolism of desmethylimipramine, nortriptyline, and oxyphenylbutazone in man', *Clin. Pharmacol. Ther.* **10**: 44–9.

Hammer, W. and Sjöqvist, F. (1967) 'Plasma levels of monomethylated tricyclic antidepressants during treatment with imipramine-like compounds', *Life Sci.* **6**: 1895–903.

Haring, C., Fleischhacker, W. W., Schett, P., Humpel, C., Barnas, C. and Saria, A. (1990) 'Influence of patient-related variables on clozapine plasma levels', *Am. J. Psychiatry* **147**: 1471–5.

Haring, C., Meise, U., Humpel, C., Saria, A., Fleischhacker, W. W. and Hinterhuber, H. (1989) 'Dose-related plasma levels of clozapine: influence of smoking behaviour, sex and age', *Psychopharmacology* **99**: S38–40.

Härtter, S., Arand, M., Oesch, F. and Hiemke, C. (1995) 'Non-competitive inhibition of clomipramine N-demethylation by fluvoxamine', *Psychopharmacology (Berl.)* **117**: 149–53.

Härtter, S. and Hiemke, C. (1992) 'Determination of fluvoxamine in human plasma by HPLC-analysis including direct injection of plasma and column switching', *Pharmacopsychiatry* **25**: 103.

Härtter, S., Wetzel, H., Hammes, E. and Hiemke, C. (1993) 'Inhibition of antidepressant demethylation and hydroxylation by fluvoxamine in depressed patients', *Psychopharmacology* **110**: 302–8.

Härtter, S., Wetzel, H., Hammes, E., Torkzadeh, M. and Hiemke, C. (1998) 'Nonlinear pharmacokinetics of fluvoxamine and gender differences', *Ther. Drug. Monit.* **20**: 446–9.

Heim, M. and Meyer, U. A. (1990) 'Genotyping of poor metabolisers of debrisoquine by allele-specific PCR amplification', *Lancet* **336**: 529–32.

Heiman, E.M. (1977) 'Cardiac toxicity with thioridazine–tricyclic antidepressant combination', *J. Nerv. Ment. Dis.* **165**: 139–43.

Herrlin, K., Massele, A. Y., Jande, M., Alm, C., Tybring, G., Abdi, Y. A., Wennerholm, A., Johansson, I., Dahl, M. L., Bertilsson, L. and Gustafsson, L. L. (1998) 'Bantu Tanzanians have a decreased capacity to metabolize omeprazole and mephenytoin in relation to their CYP2C19 genotype', *Clin. Pharmacol. Ther.* **64**: 391–401.

Hiemke, C., Weigmann, H., Härtter, S., Dahmen, N., Wetzel, H. and Müller, H. (1994) 'Elevated levels of clozapine in serum after addition of fluvoxamine', *J. Clin. Psychopharmacol.* **14**: 279–81.

Hirschowitz, J., Bennett, J. A., Zemlan, F. P. and Garver, D. L. (1983) 'Thioridazine effect on desipramine plasma levels', *J. Clin. Psychopharmacol.* **3**: 376–9.

Huang, M. L., Van Peer, A., Woestenborghs, R., De Coster, R., Heykants, J., Jansen, A. A., Zylicz, Z., Visscher, H. W. and Jonkman, J. H. (1993) 'Pharmacokinetics of the novel antipsychotic agent risperidone and the prolactin response in healthy subjects', *Clin. Pharmacol. Ther.* **54**: 257–68.

Ibeanu, G. C., Blaisdell, J., Ghanayem, B. I., Beyeler, C., Benhamou, S., Bouchardy, C., Wilkinson, G. R., Dayer, P., Daly, A. K. and Goldstein, J. A. (1998) 'An additional defective allele, CYP2C19*5, contributes to the S-mephenytoin poor metabolizer phenotype in Caucasians', *Pharmacogenetics* **8**: 129–35.

Ishida, M., Otani, K., Kaneko, S., Ohkubo, T., Osanai, T., Yasui, N., Mihara, K., Higuchi, H. and Sugawara, K. (1995) 'Effects of various factors on steady state plasma concentrations of trazodone and its active metabolite m-chlorophenyl-piperazine', *Int. Clin. Psychopharmacol.* **10**: 143–6.

Jeppesen, U., Gram, L. F., Vistisen, K., Loft, S., Poulsen, H. E. and Brøsen, K. (1996) 'Dose-dependent inhibition of CYP1A2, CYP2C19 and CYP2D6 by citalopram, fluoxetine, fluvoxamine and paroxetine', *Eur. J. Clin. Pharmacol.* **51**: 73–8.

Jerling, M., Dahl, M. L., Åberg-Wistedt, A., Liljenberg, B., Landell, N. E., Bertilsson, L. and Sjöqvist, F. (1996) 'The CYP2D6 genotype predicts the oral clearance of the neuroleptic agents perphenazine and zuclopenthixol', *Clin. Pharmacol. Ther.* **59**: 423–8.

Jerling, M., Lindstrom, L., Bondesson, U. and Bertilsson, L. (1994) 'Fluvoxamine inhibition and carbamazepine induction of the metabolism of clozapine: evidence from a therapeutic drug monitoring service', *Ther. Drug. Monit.* **16**: 368–74.

Johansson, I., Lundqvist, E., Bertilsson, L., Dahl, M. L., Sjöqvist, F. and Ingelman-Sundberg, M. (1993) 'Inherited amplification of an active gene in the cytochrome P450 CYP2D locus as a cause of ultrarapid metabolism of debrisoquine', *Proc. Natl. Acad. Sci. USA* **90**: 11825–9.

Johansson, I., Oscarson, M., Yue, Q. Y., Bertilsson, L., Sjöqvist, F. and Ingelman-Sundberg M. (1994) 'Genetic analysis of the Chinese cytochrome P4502D locus: characterization of variant CYP2D6 genes present in subjects with diminished capacity for debrisoquine hydroxylation', *Mol. Pharmacol.* **46**: 452–9.

Jurima, M., Inaba, T., Kadar, D. and Kalow, W. (1985) 'Genetic polymorphism of mephenytoin p(4')-hydroxylation: difference between Orientals and Caucasians', *Br. J. Clin. Pharmacol.* **19**: 483–7.

Kagimoto, M., Heim, M., Kagimoto, K., Zeugin, T. and Meyer, U. A. (1990) 'Multiple mutations of the human cytochrome P450IID6 gene (CYP2D6) in poor metabolizers of debrisoquine. Study of the functional significance of individual mutations by expression of chimeric genes', *J. Biol. Chem.* **265**: 17209–14.

Kalow, W. and Tang, B. K. (1993) 'The use of caffeine for enzyme assays: a critical appraisal', *Clin. Pharmacol. Ther.* **53**: 503–14.

Kassahun, K., Mattiuz, E., Nyhart, E., Jr., Obermeyer, B., Gillespie, T., Murphy, A., Goodwin, R. M., Tupper, D., Callaghan, J. T. and Lemberger, L. (1997) 'Disposition and biotransformation of the antipsychotic agent olanzapine in humans', *Drug. Metab. Dispos.* **25**: 81–93.

Kobayashi, K., Chiba, K., Yagi, T., Shimada, N., Taniguchi, T., Horie, T., Tani, M., Yamamoto, T., Ishizaki, T. and Kuroiwa, Y. (1997) 'Identification of cytochrome P450 isoforms involved in citalopram N-demethylation by human liver microsomes', *J. Pharmacol. Exp. Ther.* **280**: 927–33.

Kondo, T., Tanaka, O., Otani, K., Mihara, K., Tokinaga, N., Kaneko, S., Chiba, K. and Ishizaki, T. (1996) 'Possible inhibitory effect of diazepam on the metabolism of zotepine, an antipsychotic drug', *Psychopharmacology (Berl.)* **127**: 311–4.

Lane, R. M. (1996) 'Pharmacokinetic drug interaction potential of selective serotonin reuptake inhibitors', *Int. Clin. Psychopharmacol.* **11** (suppl 5): 31–61.

Leinonen, E., Lillsunde, P., Laukkanen, V. and Ylitalo, P. (1991) 'Effects of carbamazepine on serum antidepressant concentrations in psychiatric patients', *J. Clin. Psychopharmacol.* **11**: 313–8.

Lemoine, A., Gautier, J. C., Azoulay, D., Kiffel, L., Belloc, C., Guengerich, F. P., Maurel, P., Beaune, P. and Leroux, J. P. (1993) 'Major pathway of imipramine metabolism is catalyzed by cytochromes P-450 1A2 and P-450 3A4 in human liver', *Mol. Pharmacol.* **43**: 827–32.

Lewis, R., Bagnall, A. and Leitner, M. (2000) 'Sertindole for schizophrenia', *Cochrane Database Syst. Rev.* **2**.

Llerena, A., Alm, C., Dahl, M. L., Ekqvist, B. and Bertilsson, L. (1992a) 'Haloperidol disposition is dependent on debrisoquine hydroxylation phenotype', *Ther. Drug. Monit.* **14**: 92–7.

Llerena, A., Dahl, M. L., Ekqvist, B. and Bertilsson, L. (1992b) 'Haloperidol disposition is dependent on the debrisoquine hydroxylation phenotype: increased plasma levels of the reduced metabolite in poor metabolizers', *Ther. Drug. Monit.* **14**: 261–4.

Loga, S., Curry, S. and Lader, M. (1981) 'Interaction of chlorpromazine and nortriptyline in patients with schizophrenia', *Clin. Pharmacokinet.* **6**: 454–62.

McCarthy, R. H. (1994) 'Seizures following smoking cessation in a clozapine responder', *Pharmacopsychiatry* **27**: 210–1.

Macias, W. L., Bergstrom, R. F., Cerimele, B. J., Kassahun, K., Tatum, D. E. and Callaghan, J. T. (1998) 'Lack of effect of olanzapine on the pharmacokinetics of a single aminophylline dose in healthy men', *Pharmacotherapy* **18**: 1237–48.

Mahgoub, A., Idle, J. R., Dring, L. G., Lancaster, R. and Smith, R. L. (1977) 'Polymorphic hydroxylation of debrisoquine in man', *Lancet* **2**: 584–6.

Masimirembwa, C., Bertilsson, L., Johansson, I., Hasler, J. A. and Ingelman-Sundberg, M. (1995) 'Phenotyping and genotyping of S-mephenytoin hydroxylase (cytochrome P450 2C19) in a Shona population of Zimbabwe', *Clin. Pharmacol. Ther.* **57**: 656–61.

Masimirembwa, C., Persson, I., Bertilsson, L., Hasler, J. and Ingelman-Sundberg, M. (1996) 'A novel mutant variant of the CYP2D6 gene (CYP2D6*17) common in a black African population: association with diminished debrisoquine hydroxylase activity', *Br. J. Clin. Pharmacol.* **42**: 713–9.

Mellström, B., Bertilsson, L., Lou, Y. C., Säwe, J. and Sjöqvist, F. (1983) 'Amitriptyline metabolism: relationship to polymorphic debrisoquine hydroxylation', *Clin. Pharmacol. Ther.* **34**: 516–20.

Mellström, B., Bertilsson, L., Säwe, J., Schulz, H. U. and Sjöqvist, F. (1981) 'E- and Z-10-hydroxylation of nortriptyline: relationship to polymorphic debrisoquine hydroxylation', *Clin. Pharmacol. Ther.* **30**: 189–93.

Mellström, B., Bertilsson, L., Traskman, L., Rollins, D., Åsberg, M. and Sjöqvist, F. (1979) 'Intraindividual similarity in the metabolism of amitriptyline and chlorimipramine in depressed patients', *Pharmacology* **19**: 282–7.

Mellström, B., Säwe, J., Bertilsson, L. and Sjöqvist, F. (1986) 'Amitriptyline metabolism: association with debrisoquine hydroxylation in nonsmokers', *Clin Pharmacol. Ther.* **39**: 369–71.

Meyer, J. W., Woggon, B., Baumann, P. and Meyer, U. A. (1990) 'Clinical implications of slow sulphoxidation of thioridazine in a poor metabolizer of the debrisoquine type', *Eur. J. Clin. Pharmacol.* **39**: 613–4.

Meyer, J. W., Woggon, B. and Kupfer, A. (1988) 'Importance of oxidative polymorphism on clinical efficacy and side-effects of imipramine – a retrospective study', *Pharmacopsychiatry* **21**: 365–6.

Mihara, K., Otani, K., Suzuki, A., Yasui, N., Nakano, H., Meng, X., Ohkubo, T., Nagasaki, T., Kaneko, S., Tsuchida, S., Sugawara, K. and Gonzalez, F. J. (1997a) 'Relationship between the CYP2D6 genotype and the steady-state plasma concentrations of trazodone and its active metabolite m-chlorophenylpiperazine', *Psychopharmacology (Berl.)* **133**: 95–8.

Mihara, K., Otani, K., Tybring, G., Dahl, M. L., Bertilsson L. and Kaneko, S. (1997b) 'The CYP2D6 genotype and plasma concentrations of mianserin enantiomers in relation to therapeutic response to mianserin in depressed Japanese patients', *J. Clin. Psychopharmacol.* **17**: 467–71.

Misra, L. K., Erpenbach, J. E., Hamlyn, H. and Fuller, W. C. (1998) 'Quetiapine: a new atypical antipsychotic', *S. D. J. Med.* **51**: 189–93.

Moller, H.J. (2000) 'Are all antidepressants the same?' *J. Clin. Psychiatry* **61**: 24–8.

Nakamura, K., Goto, F., Ray, W. A., McAllister, C. B., Jacqz, E., Wilkinson, G. R. and Branch, R. A. (1985) 'Interethnic differences in genetic polymorphism of debrisoquine and mephenytoin hydroxylation between Japanese and Caucasian populations', *Clin. Pharmacol. Ther.* **38**: 402–8.

Nelson, J. C. and Jatlow, P. I. (1980) 'Neuroloeptic effect on desipramine steady-state plasma concentrations', *Am. J. Psychiatry* **137**: 1232–4.

Nelson, J. C. and Jatlow, P. I. (1987) 'Nonlinear desipramine kinetics: prevalence and importance', *Clin. Pharmacol. Ther.* **41**: 666–70.

Nelson, J. C., Mazure, C. M., Bowers, M. B., Jr. and Jatlow, P. I. (1991) 'A preliminary, open study of the combination of fluoxetine and desipramine for rapid treatment of major depression', *Arch. Gen. Psychiatry* **48**: 303–7.

Noda, K., Suzuki, A., Okui, M., Noguchi, H., Nishiura, M. and Nishiura, N. (1979) 'Pharmacokinetics and metabolism of 2-chloro-11-(2-dimethylamino-ethoxy)- dibenzo[b,f]thiepine (zotepine) in rat, mouse, dog and man', *Arzneimittel-forschung* **29**: 1595–600.

Nordin, C., Siwers, B., Benítez, J. and Bertilsson, L. (1985) 'Plasma concentrations of nortriptyline and its 10-hydroxy metabolite in depressed patients–relationship to the debrisoquine hydroxylation metabolic ratio', *Br. J. Clin. Pharmacol.* **19**: 832–5.

Nyberg, S., Dahl, M. L. and Halldin, C. (1995a) 'A PET study of D2 and 5-HT2 receptor occupancy induced by risperidone in poor metabolizers of debrisoquine and risperidone', *Psychopharmacology (Berl.)* **119**: 345–8.

Nyberg, S., Farde, L., Eriksson, L., Halldin, C. and Eriksson, B. (1993) '5-HT2 and D2 dopamine receptor occupancy in the living human brain. A PET study with risperidone', *Psychopharmacology* **110**: 265–72.

Nyberg, S., Farde, L., Halldin, C., Dahl, M. L. and Bertilsson, L. (1995b) 'D2 dopamine receptor occupancy during low-dose treatment with haloperidol decanoate', *Am. J. Psychiatry* **152**: 173–8.

Ohmori, S., Takeda, S., Rikihisa, T., Kiuchi, M., Kanakubo, Y. and Kitada, M. (1993) 'Studies on cytochrome P450 responsible for oxidative metabolism of imipramine in human liver microsomes', *Biol. Pharm. Bull.* **16**: 571–5.

Orsulak, P.J. (1989) 'Therapeutic monitoring of antidepressant drugs: guidelines updated', *Ther. Drug. Monit.* **11**: 497–507.

Otani, K., Ishida, M., Kaneko, S., Mihara, K., Ohkubo, T., Osanai, T. and Sugawara, K. (1996) 'Effects of carbamazepine coadministration on plasma concentrations of trazodone and its active metabolite, m-chlorophenylpiperazine', *Ther. Drug. Monit.* **18**: 164–7.

Otton, S. V., Ball, S. E., Cheung, S. W., Inaba, T., Rudolph, R. L. and Sellers, E. M. (1996) 'Venlafaxine oxidation in vitro is catalysed by CYP2D6', *Br. J. Clin. Pharmacol.* **41**: 149–56.

Otton, S. V., Dafang, W., Joffe, R. T., Cheung, S. W. and Sellers, E. M. (1993) 'Inhibition by fluoxetine of cytochrome P450 2D6 activity', *Clin. Pharmacol. Ther.* 53: 401–9.

Oyehaugh, E., Eide, G. and Salvesen, B. (1984) 'Effect of phenothiazines on citalopram steady-state kinetics in psychiatric patients', *Nordisk Pharmacol. Acta.* 46: 37–46.

Özdemir, V., Naranjo, C. A., Herrmann, N., Reed, K., Sellers, E. M. and Kalow, W. (1997) 'Paroxetine potentiates the central nervous system side effects of perphenazine: contribution of cytochrome P4502D6 inhibition in vivo', *Clin. Pharmacol. Ther.* 62: 334–47.

Paine, M. F., Shen, D. D., Kunze, K. L., Perkins, J. D., Marsh, C. L., McVicar, J. P., Barr, D. M., Gillies, B. S. and Thummel, K. E. (1996) 'First-pass metabolism of midazolam by the human intestine', *Clin. Pharmacol. Ther.* 60: 14–24.

Parsa, M. A. and Bastani, B. (1998) 'Quetiapine (Seroquel) in the treatment of psychosis in patients with Parkinson's disease', *J. Neuropsychiatry Clin. Neurosci.* 10: 216–9.

Pelkonen, O., Mäenpää, J., Taavitsainen, P., Rautio, A. and Raunio, H. (1998) 'Inhibition and induction of human cytochrome P450 (CYP) enzymes', *Xenobiotica* 28: 1203–53.

Perry, P. J., Pfohl, B. M. and Holstad, S. G. (1987) 'The relationship between antidepressant response and tricyclic antidepressant plasma concentrations. A retrospective analysis of the literature using logistic regression analysis', *Clin. Pharmacokinet.* 13: 381–92.

Persson, I., Aklillu, E., Rodrigues, F., Bertilsson, L. and Ingelman-Sundberg, M. (1996) 'S-mephenytoin hydroxylation phenotype and CYP2C19 genotype among Ethiopians', *Pharmacogenetics* 6: 521–6.

Pollock, B. G. (1994) 'Recent developments in drug metabolism of relevance to psychiatrists', *Harv. Rev. Psychiatry* 2: 204–13.

Preskorn, S. H., Alderman, J., Chung, M., Harrison, W., Messig, M. and Harris, S. (1994) 'Pharmacokinetics of desipramine coadministered with sertraline or fluoxetine', *J. Clin. Psychopharmacol* 14: 90–8.

Preskorn, S. H., Dorey, R. C. and Jerkovich, G. S. (1988) 'Therapeutic drug monitoring of tricyclic antidepressants', *Clin. Chem.* 34: 822–8.

Preskorn, S. H. and Jerkovich, G. S. (1990) 'Central nervous system toxicity of tricyclic antidepressants: phenomenology, course, risk factors, and role of therapeutic drug monitoring', *J. Clin. Psychopharmacol* 10: 88–95.

Rasmussen, B. B. and Brøsen, K. (1997) 'Theophylline has no advantages over caffeine as a putative model drug for assessing CYP1A2 activity in humans', *Br. J. Clin. Pharmacol.* 43: 253–8.

Richelson, E. (1997) Pharmacokinetic drug interactions of new antidepressants: a review of the effects on the metabolism of other drugs', *Mayo. Clin. Proc.* 72: 835–47.

Ring, B. J., Binkley, S. N., Vandenbranden, M. and Wrighton, S. A. (1996a) 'In vitro interaction of the antipsychotic agent olanzapine with human cytochromes P450 CYP2C9, CYP2C19, CYP2D6 and CYP3A', *Br. J. Clin. Pharmacol.* 41: 181–6.

Ring, B. J., Catlow, J., Lindsay, T. J., Gillespie, T., Roskos, L. K., Cerimele, B. J., Swanson, S. P., Hamman, M. A. and Wrighton, S. A. (1996b) 'Identification of the human cytochromes P450 responsible for the in vitro formation of the major oxidative metabolites of the antipsychotic agent olanzapine', *J. Pharmacol. Exp. Ther.* **276**: 658–66.

Rochat, B., Amey, M., Gillet, M., Meyer, U. A. and Baumann, P. (1997) 'Identification of three cytochrome P450 isozymes involved in N-demethylation of citalopram enantiomers in human liver microsomes', *Pharmacogenetics* **7**: 1–10.

Roh, H. K., Dahl, M. L., Tybring, G., Yamada, H., Cha, Y. N. and Bertilsson, L. (1996) 'CYP2C19 genotype and phenotype determined by omeprazole in a Korean population', *Pharmacogenetics* **6**: 547–51.

Rotzinger, S., Fang, J., Coutts, R. T. and Baker, G. B. (1998) 'Human CYP2D6 and metabolism of m-chlorophenylpiperazine', *Biol. Psychiatry* **44**: 1185–91.

Rudorfer, M. V. and Potter, W. Z. (1999) 'Metabolism of tricyclic antidepressants', *Cell. Mol. Neurobiol.* **19**: 373–409.

Sakamoto, K., Nakamura, Y., Aikoh, S., Baba, T., Perregaard, J., Pedersen, H., Moltzen, E. K., Mulford, D. J. and Yamaguchi, T. (1995) 'Metabolism of sertindole: identification of the metabolites in the rat and dog, and species comparison of liver microsomal metabolism', *Xenobiotica* **25**: 1327–43.

Sarkar, M. A., Hunt, C., Guzelian, P. S. and Karnes, H. T. (1992) 'Characterization of human liver cytochromes P-450 involved in theophylline metabolism', *Drug Metab. Dispos.* **20**: 31–7.

Schmider, J., Greenblatt, D. J., von Moltke, L. L., Harmatz, J. S. and Shader, R. I. (1996) 'Inhibition of cytochrome P450 by nefazodone in vitro: studies of dextromethorphan O- and N-demethylation', *Br. J. Clin. Pharmacol.* **41**: 339–43.

Scordo, M. G., Spina, E., Facciola, G., Avenoso, A., Johansson, I. and Dahl, M. L. (1999) 'Cytochrome P450 2D6 genotype and steady state plasma levels of risperidone and 9-hydroxyrisperidone', *Psychopharmacology (Berl.)* **147**: 300–5.

Shimada, T., Yamazaki, H., Mimura, M., Inui, Y. and Guengerich, F. P. (1994) 'Interindividual variations in human liver cytochrome P-450 enzymes involved in the oxidation of drugs, carcinogens and toxic chemicals: studies with liver microsomes of 30 Japanese and 30 Caucasians', *J. Pharmacol. Exp. Ther.* **270**: 414–23.

Shimoda, K., Someya, T., Morita, S., Hirokane, G., Noguchi, T., Yokono, A., Shibasaki, M. and Takahashi, S. (1999) 'Lower plasma levels of haloperidol in smoking than in nonsmoking schizophrenic patients', *Ther. Drug. Monit.* **21**: 293–6.

Shiraga, T., Kaneko, H., Iwasaki, K., Tozuka, Z., Suzuki, A. and Hata, T. (1999) 'Identification of cytochrome P450 enzymes involved in the metabolism of zotepine, an antipsychotic drug, in human liver microsomes', *Xenobiotica* **29**: 217–29.

Sindrup, S. H., Brøsen, K. and Gram, L. F. (1992a) 'Pharmacokinetics of the selective serotonin reuptake inhibitor paroxetine: nonlinearity and relation to the sparteine oxidation polymorphism', *Clin. Pharmacol. Ther.* **51**: 288–95.

Sindrup, S. H., Brøsen, K., Gram, L. F., Hallas, J., Skjelbo, E., Allen, A., Allen, G. D., Cooper, S. M., Mellows, G., Tasker, T. C. G. and Zussman, B. D. (1992b) 'The relationship between paroxetine and the sparteine oxidation polymorphism', *Clin. Pharmacol. Ther.* **51**: 278–87.

Sindrup, S. H., Brøsen, K., Hansen, M. G., Aaes-Jorgensen, T., Overo, K. F. and Gram, L. F. (1993) 'Pharmacokinetics of citalopram in relation to the sparteine and the mephenytoin oxidation polymorphisms', *Ther. Drug. Monit.* **15**: 11–7.

Sjöqvist, F., Borgå, O., Dahl, M. L. and Orme, M. L. E. (1997) 'Fundamentals of clinical pharmacology', in T. M. Speight and N. H. G. Holford (eds) *Avery's Drug Treatment.* Auckland: Adis International Ltd, pp 1–73.

Skjelbo, E. and Brøsen, K. (1992) 'Inhibitors of imipramine metabolism by human liver microsomes', *Br. J. Clin. Pharmacol.* **34**: 256–61.

Skjelbo, E., Brøsen, K., Hallas, J. and Gram, L. F. (1991) 'The mephenytoin oxidation polymorphism is partially responsible for the N-demethylation of imipramine', *Clin. Pharmacol. Ther.* **49**: 18–23.

Skjelbo, E., Gram, L. F. and Brøsen, K. (1993) 'The N-demethylation of imipramine correlates with the oxidation of S-mephenytoin (S/R-ratio). A population study', *Br. J. Clin. Pharmacol.* **35**: 331–4.

Smith, G., Stubbins, M. J., Harries, L. W. and Wolf, C. R. (1998) 'Molecular genetics of the human cytochrome P450 monooxygenase superfamily', *Xenobiotica* **28**: 1129–65.

Sohn, D. R., Kusaka, M., Ishizaki, T., Shin, S.G., Jang, I. J., Shin, J. G. and Chiba, K. (1992) 'Incidence of S-mephenytoin hydroxylation deficiency in a Korean population and the interphenotypic differences in diazepam pharmacokinetics (see comments)', *Clin. Pharmacol. Ther.* **52**: 160–9.

Sohn, D. R., Shin, S. G., Park, C. W., Kusaka, M., Chiba, K. and Ishizaki, T. (1991) 'Metoprolol oxidation polymorphism in a Korean population: comparison with native Japanese and Chinese populations', *Br. J. Clin. Pharmacol.* **32**: 504–7.

Spigset, O., Carleborg, L., Hedenmalm, K. and Dahlqvist, R. (1995) 'Effect of cigarette smoking on fluvoxamine pharmacokinetics in humans', *Clin. Pharmacol. Ther.* **58**: 399–403.

Spigset, O., Granberg, K., Hagg, S., Norstrom, A. and Dahlqvist, R. (1997) 'Relationship between fluvoxamine pharmacokinetics and CYP2D6/CYP2C19 phenotype polymorphisms', *Eur. J. Clin. Pharmacol.* **52**: 129–33.

Spigset, O., Granberg, K., Hagg, S., Soderstrom, E. and Dahlqvist, R. (1998) 'Non-linear fluvoxamine disposition', *Br. J. Clin. Pharmacol.* **45**: 257–63.

Spina, E., Ancione, M., Di Rosa, A. E., Meduri, M. and Caputi, A. P. (1992a) 'Polymorphic debrisoquine oxidation and acute neuroleptic-induced adverse effects', *Eur. J. Clin. Pharmacol.* **42**: 347–8.

Spina, E., Arena, A. and Pisani, F. (1987a) 'Urinary desipramine hydroxylation index and steady-state plasma concentrations of imipramine and desipramine', *Ther. Drug. Monit.* **9**: 129–33.

Spina, E., Avenoso, A., Campo, G. M., Caputi, A. P. and Perucca, E. (1995) 'The effect of carbamazepine on the 2-hydroxylation of desipramine', *Psychopharmacology (Berl.)* **117**: 413–6.

Spina, E., Avenoso, A., Campo, G. M., Caputi, A. P. and Perucca, E. (1996) 'Phenobarbital induces the 2-hydroxylation of desipramine', *Ther. Drug Monit.* **18**: 60–4.

Spina, E., Avenoso, A., Campo, G. M., Scordo, M. G., Caputi, A. P. and Perucca, E. (1997a) 'Effect of ketoconazole on the pharmacokinetics of imipramine and desipramine in healthy subjects', *Br. J. Clin. Pharmacol.* **43**: 315–8.

Spina, E., Birgersson, C., von Bahr, C., Ericsson, O., Mellström, B., Steiner, E. and

Sjöqvist, F. (1984) 'Phenotypic consistency in hydroxylation of desmethylimipramine and debrisoquine in healthy subjects and in human liver microsomes', *Clin. Pharmacol. Ther.* **36**: 677–82.

Spina, E., Campo, G. M., Avenoso, A., Pollicino, M. A. and Caputi, A. P. (1992b) 'Interaction between fluvoxamine and imipramine/desipramine in four patients', *Ther. Drug. Monit.* **14**: 194–6.

Spina, E., Gitto, C., Avenoso, A., Campo, G. M., Caputi, A. P. and Perucca, E. (1997b) 'Relationship between plasma desipramine levels, CYP2D6 phenotype and clinical response to desipramine: a prospective study', *Eur. J. Clin. Pharmacol.* **51**: 395–8.

Spina, E., Pollicino, A. M., Avenoso, A., Campo, G. M., Perucca, E. and Caputi, A. P. (1993) 'Effect of fluvoxamine on the pharmacokinetics of imipramine and desipramine in healthy subjects', *Ther. Drug. Monit.* **15**: 243–6.

Spina, E., Steiner, E., Ericsson, O. and Sjöqvist, F. (1987b) 'Hydroxylation of desmethylimipramine: dependence on the debrisoquine hydroxylation phenotype', *Clin. Pharmacol. Ther.* **41**: 314–9.

Stein, C. M., Kinirons, M. T., Pincus, T., Wilkinson, G. R. and Wood, A. J. J. (1996) 'Comparison of the dapsone recovery ratio and the erythromycin breath test as in vivo probes of CYP3A activity in patients with rheumatoid arthritis receiving cyclosporine', *Clin. Pharmacol. Ther.* **59**: 47–51.

Steiner, E., Dumont, E., Spina, E. and Dahlqvist, R. (1988) 'Inhibition of desipramine 2-hydroxylation by quinidine and quinine', *Clin. Pharmacol. Ther.* **43**: 577–81.

Stevens, J. C. and Wrighton, S. A. (1993) 'Interaction of the enantiomers of fluoxetine and norfluoxetine with human liver cytochromes P450', *J. Pharmacol. Exp. Ther.* **266**: 964–71.

Stockton, M. E. and Rasmussen, K. (1996) 'Olanzapine, a novel atypical antipsychotic, reverses d-amphetamine- induced inhibition of midbrain dopamine cells', *Psychopharmacology (Berl.)* **124**: 50–6.

Thummel, K. E., O'Shea, D., Paine, M. F., Shen, D. D., Kunze, K. L., Perkins, J. D. and Wilkinson, G.R. (1996) 'Oral first-pass elimination of midazolam involves both gastrointestinal and hepatic CYP3A-mediated metabolism', *Clin. Pharmacol. Ther.* **59**: 491–502.

Tucker, G. T., Silas, J. H., Iyun, A. O., Lennard, M. S. and Smith, A. J. (1977) 'Polymorphic hydroxylation of debrisoquine (letter)', *Lancet* **2**: 718.

Tyndale, R., Aoyama, T., Broly, F., Matsunaga, T., Inaba, T., Kalow, W., Gelboin, H. V., Meyer, U. A. and Gonzalez, F. J. (1991) 'Identification of a new variant CYP2D6 allele lacking the codon encoding Lys-281: possible association with the poor metabolizer phenotype', *Pharmacogenetics* **1**: 26–32.

Vainer, J. L. and Chouinard, G. (1994) 'Interaction between caffeine and clozapine', *J. Clin. Psychopharmacol.* **14**: 284–5.

van Harten, J., Stevens, L. A., Raghoebar, M., Holland, R. L., Wesnes, K. and Cournot, A. (1992) 'Fluvoxamine does not interact with alcohol or potentiate alcohol-related impairment of cognitive function', *Clin. Pharmacol. Ther.* **52**: 427–35.

Vaughan, D. A. (1988) 'Interaction of fluoxetine with tricyclic antidepressants (letter)', *Am. J. Psychiatry* **145**: 1478.

von Bahr, C., Birgersson, C., Blanck, A., Goransson, M., Mellström, B. and Nilsell,

K. (1983) 'Correlation between nortriptyline and debrisoquine hydroxylation in the human liver', *Life Sci.* **33**: 631–6.

von Bahr, C., Movin, G., Nordin, C., Liden, A., Hammarlund-Udenaes, M., Hedberg, A., Ring, H. and Sjöqvist, F. (1991) 'Plasma levels of thioridazine and metabolites are influenced by the debrisoquine hydroxylation phenotype', *Clin. Pharmacol. Ther.* **49**: 234–40.

Vormfelde, S. V., Bitsch, A., Meineke, I., Gundert-Remy, U. M. and Gleiter, C. H. (1997) 'Non-response to maprotiline caused by ultra-rapid metabolism that is different from CYP2D6?' *Eur. J. Clin. Pharmacol.* **52**: 387–90.

Wang, J. S., Wang, W., Xie, H. G., Huang, S. L. and Zhou, H. H. (1997) 'Effect of troleandomycin on the pharmacokinetics of imipramine in Chinese: the role of CYP3A', *Br. J. Clin. Pharmacol.* **44**: 195–8.

Watkins, P. B. (1994) 'Noninvasive tests of CYP3A enzymes', *Pharmacogenetics* **4**: 171–84.

Watkins, P. B., Turgeon, D. K., Saenger, P., Lown, K. S., Kolars, J. C., Hamilton, T., Fishman, K., Guzelian, P. S. and Voorhees, J. J. (1992) 'Comparison of urinary 6-ß-cortisol and the erythromycin breath test as measures of hepatic P450IIIA (CYP3A) activity', *Clin. Pharmacol. Ther.* **52**: 265–73.

Westermeyer, J. (1991) 'Fluoxetine-induced tricyclic toxicity: extent and duration', *J. Clin. Pharmacol.* **31**: 388–92.

Wienkers, L. C., Allievi, C., Hauer, M. J. and Wynalda, M. A. (1999) 'Cytochrome P-450-mediated metabolism of the individual enantiomers of the antidepressant agent reboxetine in human liver microsomes', *Drug. Metab. Dispos.* **27**: 1334–40.

Wrighton, S. A., Stevens, J. C., Becker, G. W. and VandenBranden, M. (1993) 'Isolation and characterization of human liver cytochrome P450 2C19: correlation between 2C19 and S-mephenytoin 4'-hydroxylation', *Arch. Biochem. Biophys.* **306**: 240–5.

Xu, Z. H., Huang, S. L. and Zhou, H. H. (1996) 'Inhibition of imipramine N-demethylation by fluvoxamine in Chinese young men', *Chung Kuo Yao Li Hsueh Pao* **17**: 399–402.

Yasui, N., Kondo, T., Otani, K., Furukori, H., Mihara, K., Suzuki, A., Kaneko, S. and Inoue, Y. (1999) 'Effects of itraconazole on the steady-state plasma concentrations of haloperidol and its reduced metabolite in schizophrenic patients: in vivo evidence of the involvement of CYP3A4 for haloperidol metabolism', *J. Clin. Psychopharmacol.* **19**: 149–54.

Yasui, N., Otani, K., Kaneko, S., Ohkubo, T., Osanai, T., Ishida, M., Mihara, K., Kondo, T., Sugawara, K. and Fukushima, Y. (1995) 'Inhibition of trazodone metabolism by thioridazine in humans', *Ther. Drug. Monit.* **17**: 333–5.

Yue, Q. Y., Zhong, Z. H., Tybring, G., Dalen, P., Dahl, M. L., Bertilsson, L. and Sjöqvist, F. (1998) 'Pharmacokinetics of nortriptyline and its 10-hydroxy metabolite in Chinese subjects of different CYP2D6 genotypes', *Clin. Pharmacol. Ther.* **64**: 384–90.

Zanger, U. M., Vilbois, F., Hardwick, J. P. and Meyer, U. A. (1988) 'Absence of hepatic cytochrome P450bufI causes genetically deficient debrisoquine oxidation in man', *Biochemistry* **27**: 5447–54.

Chapter 5

Interindividual variability in the metabolism of cardiovascular drugs

U. Klotz and H. K. Kroemer

Introduction

Variability in drug response represents an important issue in drug development and therapy (Lin and Lu, 1997). Because of the inter-individual variability in dose/plasma concentration/response (therapeutic and/or toxic effects) relationships, patients might need different dosage regimens. Much of this variability is caused by the significant inter-individual variation in oxidative drug metabolism, resulting mostly from variability in the activity of different cytochrome P450 (CYP) enzymes in the liver and extrahepatic tissues. The sources of variability are genetic and environmental factors (including drugs and food constituents/diets), as well as age and various disease states (Vesell, 1991; Murray 1992; Tumer *et al.*, 1992; Wilkinson, 1997; Rodighiero, 1999).

Metabolism comprises several reactions, including oxidation, reduction, dealkylation, hydrolysis, hydration, condensation and conjugation. Often, the biotransformation of drugs is biphasic: first a compound undergoes a functionalisation reaction (phase I) followed by conjugation (phase II) with an endogenous agent (e.g. glucuronic acid). The class of CYP represents the most important enzymes involved in oxidative drug metabolism. The selectivity of those CYPs in terms of metabolised substrates, inducing and inhibiting agents or vulnerability towards endogenous and environmental influences is variable and overlapping. The CYP3A subfamily represents the predominant and most abundant enzymes (Shimada *et al.*, 1994) which are also expressed in the gastrointestinal tract (Krishna and Klotz, 1994; Klotz, 1998a).

The assessment of drug metabolism *in vivo* can be accomplished by direct measurement of the formation rate of the metabolites from plasma and/or urinary excretion data. However, in the past most often drug metabolism has been estimated indirectly from pharmacokinetic studies with different test compounds or probes (Kivistö and Kroemer, 1997). The most appropriate pharmacokinetic term to provide information on drug metabolism under *in vivo* conditions is the systemic clearance (CL) which measures the ability of the body to eliminate a drug (Wilkinson, 1987). The term CL represents the sum of $CL_{hepatic} + CL_{renal} + CL_{intestinal} + CL_{other\ sites}$. For orally administered drugs the phenomenon of presystemic elimination (intestinal and/or hepatic first-pass effect for so-called high clearance drugs) must be considered if the apparent oral clearance (Cl_o) is calculated.

Several different methods can be applied to identify or to measure drug-metabolising enzyme activities *in vitro* (see this book and Pacifici and Fracchia, 1995). In general, a substrate (probe drug) and cofactors are incubated with tissue samples or cell fractions (e.g. hepatocytes or human liver microsomes) under defined conditions which need to be more standardised in the future as there is considerable interlaboratory variability in the assessment of P450 activities (Boobis *et al.*, 1998). It is often assumed that such an *in vitro* evaluation can reflect – at least to some extent – the *in vivo* situation and more recently different approaches have been tried to predict the *in vivo* drug metabolism from *in vitro* data (Kroemer *et al*, 1992; Iwatsubo *et al.*, 1997; Ito *et al.*, 1998).

During the last decade it became apparent that from *in vitro* experiments and drug interaction studies in humans the major metabolic pathways and the involved CYP of several cardiovascular drugs could be assessed in qualitative and quantitative terms (see Table 5.1). Based on this information it is possible to predict whether the disposition of a drug will be affected by certain environmental or genetic factors as well as by other therapeutic agents given concomitantly (Pelkonen *et al.*, 1998).

The present chapter will describe in its first part some important factors which can affect the metabolism (pharmacokinetics) of cardiovascular drugs and thus are contributing to the intraindividual variability in drug metabolism. In the second part we will concentrate on four model drugs (lidocaine, propafenone, propranolol and verapamil) to illustrate in more detail the effect of those factors.

Determinants of drug metabolism

Genetics

The initial clinical observations of unexpected toxicity of the antihypertensive drug debrisoquine in the U.K. and that of the antiarrhythmic agent sparteine in Germany turned out to be the result of the lack of a drug metabolising enzyme which later was identified as CYP2D6 (Kroemer and Eichelbaum, 1995). From this so-called genetic polymorphism between 5 and 10% of Caucasians and about 1% of the Asian population are affected and during the last few years for several cardiovascular drugs such poor metabolisers (PM) could be identified (see Table 5.2). Similar to sparteine and debrisoquine PMs of propafenone, mexiletine or

Table 5.1 List of cardiovascular drugs whose metabolic pathways could be assigned to certain CYP enzymes

Drug	Major pathways	Mediated by CYP
Alprenolol	Aromatic hydroxylation	2D6
Amiodarone		3A4
Amlodipine		3A4
Aprindine	aromatic hydroxylation	2D6
Bufuralol	1´-hydroxylation	2D6
Bupranolol		2D6
Debrisoquine	4-hydroxylation	2D6
Encainide	O-demethylation	2D6
Felodipine	dehydrogenation	3A4
Flecainide	O-dealkylation	2D6
Metoprolol	aliphatic hydroxylation	2D6
	and O-dealkylation	2D6
Mexiletine		2D6
Nifedipine	dehydrogenation	3A4
N-propylajmaline	benzylic hydroxylation	2D6
Propafenone	aromatic hydroxylation	2D6
	N-dealkylation	1A2, 3A
	+ glucuronidation	
Propranolol	4´-hydroxylation	2D6
	N-dealkylation	2D6, 1A2
	side chain oxidation	2C19
	+ glucuronidation	
Lidocaine	dealkylation	3A4 (1A2)
Losartan		3A4, 2C9
Quinidine	3-hydroxylation, N-oxidation	3A4
Sparteine	oxidation	2D6
Timolol		2D6
Verapamil	N-demethylation	3A4, 1A2
	O-demethylation	2C9

Table 5.2 Pharmacokinetics of cardiovascular drugs in poor (PM) and extensive (EM) metabolisers of CYP2D6

Drug	Oral Cl (ml/min)		$t_{1/2}$ (h)	
	EM	PM	EM	PM
sparteine	7.2[a]	2.6[a]	2.3	6.7
propafenone	1115	264	5.5	17.2
encainide	195	4	2.3	11.3
flecainide	1041	600	6.8	11.8
mexiletine	621	315	8.9	12.6
N-propylajmaline	670	69	2.2	12.0

Notes
Modified from Fromm et al., 1997.
[a]ml/min/kg.

N-propylajmaline will have considerably higher risk of severe side-effects or drug toxicity if the dosage is not reduced properly. Since sodium channel blocking activity of encainide resides mainly in its metabolite O-desmethylencainide whose formation is catalysed by CYP2D6, EMs might have an increased risk of proarrhythmic events induced by the active metabolite. As flecainide is also eliminated by the renal route (50% of dose is excreted unchanged) PMs are likely to be at greater risk only when kidney function is additionally impaired (Fromm *et al.*, 1997).

The metabolism of several β-adrenoceptor antagonists has been shown to be catalysed at least in part by CYP2D6 (see Table 5.1). Especially bufuralol has been often used as a probe for CYP2D6 (Meyer and Zanger, 1997) and an association of PM status with side-effects has been demonstrated (Dayer *et al.*, 1982). In contrast, CYP2D6 plays only a minor role for elimination of propranolol: 4′-hydroxylation and partly N-dealkylation (+CYP1A2) are catalysed by CYP2D6 and in the side-chain oxidation of propranolol CYP2C19 (another polymorphically expressed enzyme) seems to be involved. Thus, only subjects being PMs of both CYP2D6 and CYP2C19 might have a reduced propranolol clearance (Rowland *et al.*, 1996; Ward *et al.*, 1989).

For metoprolol, however CYP2D6 phenotype dependent pharmaco-kinetics and pharmacodynamics have been observed. Aliphatic hydroxyl-ation (10% of a given dose) and partially O-demethylation (65% of a given dose) are catalysed by CYP2D6 (Lennard, 1989). Following a single oral dose of 200 mg, a 5.8-fold difference in the area under curve (AUC) between EMs and PMs was found and consequently a more pronounced and prolonged β-blockade was measurable (Lennard *et al.*, 1982; Laurent-Kenesi *et al.*, 1993).

Similar to metoprolol, interphenotypic differences in the pharmaco-kinetics and pharmacodynamics of timolol have been observed. Following a single oral dose timolol plasma concentrations were on average two- to four-fold larger in PMs if compared with EMs. As a consequence β-blockade was more pronounced in PMs (Lewis *et al.*, 1985; McGourty *et al.*, 1985).

The antihypertensive, α_1-adrenoceptor antagonist indoramin (Pierce *et al.*, 1987) and the antianginal perhexiline (Shah *et al.*, 1982) are other examples of drugs which are metabolised by CYP2D6 and which induce more side-effects in PMs. The ethnic background of a patient population has an impact not only on the frequency of PMs for CYP2D6 (see above) but will have also some influence on drug disposition and response (Wood and Zhou, 1991). Recently, racial differences between Caucasian and Chinese subjects both in the stereoselective pharmacokinetics and pharmacodynamics of propranolol have been observed (Zhou *et al.*, 1989). Following a single oral dose of 80 mg of racemic propranolol plasma concentrations of both enantiomers (AUC) were lower and CL_o higher in

Chinese than in White subjects. (Zhou and Wood, 1990). In contrast, no differences in the stereoselective steady state disposition and action of propafenone were seen between healthy male Chinese and German individuals (Li *et al.*, 1998).

Gender

Among the known variables influencing metabolic disposition of xenobiotics, gender is a factor to be considered as sex and growth hormones are also regulators of drug metabolism (Bonate, 1991). Lidocaine and propranolol represent examples of gender-related pharmacokinetics. Whereas the higher lidocaine plasma levels seen in females were attributed to a longer $t_{1/2}$ (Wing *et al.*, 1984), CL of propranolol was lower in females than in males (Walle *et al.*, 1989).

Ageing

Ageing is associated with various morphological, physiological and biochemical changes, such as decrease of liver size, hepatic blood flow and metabolic capacity (Woodhouse and Wynne, 1992; Kinirons and Crome, 1997; Le Couteur and McLean, 1998; Hämmerlein *et al.*, 1998). In addition, in the elderly, polypharmacy and multimorbidity will affect drug metabolism. Dependent on study design, data analysis and the population evaluated, controversial results were obtained for several drugs (see Table 5.3). Whereas phase II reactions seem not to be altered in the elderly it remains uncertain whether ageing will reduce phase I metabolism (Klotz, 1998b).

In most *in vitro* studies neither total levels of CYP proteins nor individual enzyme activities declined with ageing. Similarly, any age-related reduction in the *in vivo* drug metabolising ability of older individuals is likely to be small, except for the very old or the frail elderly. However, the oral bioavailability of high-clearance drugs which is dependent on liver blood flow can be significantly increased in the elderly (Wilkinson, 1997). When

Table 5.3 Influence of age on the clearance of some cardiovascular drugs

Reduced clearance	No significant change
Lidocaine	Lidocaine
Diltiazem	Digitoxin
Propranolol	Propranolol
Nifedipine	Prazosin
Verapamil	Verapamil

Note
According to reviews of LeCouteur and McLean, 1998; Woodhouse and Wynne, 1992; Hämmerlein *et al.*, 1998.

antipyrine clearance was determined in 226 patients (age range 20 to >70 years old) with "equal" slight to moderate alterations in liver histopathologic conditions, subjects over 60 years showed some significant decline (Sotaniemi et al., 1997).

Liver disease

As the liver is the major metabolic site for xenobiotics it can be anticipated that hepatic (dys)function will contribute largely to the interindividual variability of drug metabolism. Numerous studies for a large number of drugs have been performed, mainly in patients with alcoholic cirrhosis (Morgan and McLean, 1995; Wilkinson, 1997; Rodighiero, 1999). With some drugs, especially those whose metabolism is predominantly by glucuronidation, little or no alterations in disposition are associated with liver disease. In general, drugs metabolised by phase I reactions have an approximately 50% reduction in their CL. This holds true also for several cardiovascular drugs, such as digitoxin, lidocaine, propafenone, propranolol, metoprolol, labetolol, disopyramide, procainamide, quinidine, encainide, lorcainide, flecainide, mexiletine, verapamil, nifedipine, diltiazem, nicardipine, nisoldipine, nitrendipine, isradipine, amlodipine or felodipine (Rodighiero, 1999). A recent study with probes for CYP2C19 (mephenytoin) and CYP2D6 (debrisoquine) indicated that impairment in cirrhotic patients was more pronounced for mephenytoin (79%) than for debrisoquine (Adedoyin et al., 1998). In addition, based on in vitro studies with microsomes isolated from removed livers of patients with end-stage cirrhosis, it was demonstrated that CYP proteins and activities are selectively altered and that presence or absence of cholestasis affects the modified pattern (George et al., 1995).

For high clearance drugs if given orally a profound increase in bioavailability can be observed since intra- and extrahepatic vascular shunting seen in chronic liver disease will diminish the extent of any first-pass metabolism. In addition, total hepatic blood flow may be reduced (see Table 5.4). Several studies using liver biopsy samples from cirrhotic patients have found variable, in general reduced microsomal levels and/or catalytic activities of various CYP-isoenzymes (Guengerich and Turvy, 1991). Unfortunately, there is no practical functional test comparable to creatinine clearance in renal disease, which can quantitatively characterise hepatic (dys)function. Therefore any prediction of the extent of metabolic impairment is extremely difficult.

Environmental factors

Among the various environmental factors smoking, ethanol consumption, diet or food (e.g. grapefruit juice) and drug intake have received most

Table 5.4 Oral bioavailability (mean±SD) of some cardiovascular drugs in healthy subjects and patients with severe liver disease

Drug	Oral bioavailability (%)	
	Control	Liver disease
Encainide	26±7	76±17
Glyceryl trinitrate	2±4	50±23
Labetalol	33±8	63±22
Metoprolol	50±11	84±10
Nifedipine	51±17	90±26
Nitrendipine	40±11	54±10
Nisoldipine	3±2	15±10
Propranolol	38±3	54±6
Verapamil	22±8	52±13
Propafenone	21±26	75±43

Note
Modified from Wilkinson, 1997.

attention (see this book). Smoking will lead to an induction of the CY1A subfamily and drugs metabolised by these enzymes (e.g. theophylline, caffeine, phenacetin) will be eliminated much faster in smokers than in nonsmokers (Miller, 1989, Dong *et al.*, 1998). Likewise, chronic ethanol intake will induce CYP2E1 and consequently substrates of CYP2E1 (e.g. chlorzoxazone, paracetamol, fluorinated volatile anesthetics and many organic solvents) show an accelerated metabolism with a more extensive formation of (reactive) metabolites which sometimes have toxicological consequences (Klotz and Ammon, 1998).

Concomitant food intake or prolonged dietary changes can also modify drug disposition (see Table 5.5). Especially drugs with a high extraction ratio whose hepatic elimination is sensitive to changes in hepatic blood flow (e.g. lidocaine, propranolol) will be affected. Thereby input rate and route of drug administration have to be considered (Walter-Sack and Klotz, 1996).

When drugs are ingested together with grapefruit juice, intestinal drug metabolism mediated by CYP3A will be inhibited and consequently the oral bioavailability of many CYP3A substrates will be profoundly increased. Among them are felodipine, nifedipine, nitrendipine, amlodipine, nimodipine, nisoldipine, verapamil and terfenadine (Walter-Sack and Klotz, 1996; Fuhr, 1998).

If patients are treated at the same time with several drugs their metabolism can be accelerated by induction or impaired by different inhibitory mechanisms. As numerous drug interactions on the level of metabolism have been reported in the literature (Lin and Lu, 1997; Guengerich, 1997; Klotz and Kivistö, 1999) it is beyond the scope of this article to deal with them in more detail.

Table 5.5 Influence of diet on the disposition of some cardiovascular drugs

Dietary conditions	Drug studied	Effect on drug disposition
Concomitant food intake	metoprolol, labetalol, lidocaine	increased F
	labetalol (i.v.)	decrease in AUC
	hydralazine (fast release preparation)	increased F (no effect with sustained release preparations)
	perindoprilat	decreased F
High-protein meal	propranolol (infusion)	decreased C_{ss}
	lidocaine (infusion)	increased CL
Prolonged high protein intake	propranolol	increased oral CL

Notes
Modified from Walter-Sack and Klotz, 1996.
AUC, area under the concentration time curve; C_{SS}, steady state plasma concentration; CL, clearance; F, oral bioavailability; i.v., intravenous.

In conclusion, all the above-mentioned factors will have some more or less pronounced effect on the metabolism of drugs including cardiovascular agents. Thus, it is conceivable that those factors contribute significantly to the interindividual variability in drug response.

Lidocaine

The high clearance drug lidocaine is rapidly and extensively metabolised in the liver. Its clearance is dependent on hepatic blood flow. The major primary metabolite monoethylglycinexylidide (MEGX) is formed by CYP3A4 and the metabolic rate of MEGX in microsomes of fourteen human livers varied from about 120 to 850 nmoles/mg protein an hour (Bargetzi *et al.*, 1989). Based on the above pathway, the so-called MEGX test has been developed to assess liver function (Oellerich *et al.*, 1987). The test has been widely used to measure pre- and post-transplant liver function and as a prognostic indicator of different surgical procedures or for survival in cirrhosis (Oellerich *et al.*, 1989, 1990; Arrigoni *et al.*, 1994; Reichel *et al.*, 1995). More recently lidocaine was used as a suitable probe for measuring individual CYP3A4 activity (Kivistö and Kroemer, 1997).

In healthy volunteers, a mean CL value of about 10 ml/min/kg can be assumed and different disease states can affect hepatic elimination of lidocaine (see Table 5.6). In patients with heart failure the variable CL (range about 2.5–11 ml/min/kg) was dependent on the cardiac output (Thomson *et al.*, 1973). Patients with myocardial infarction receiving constant infusions of lidocaine were subdivided into two groups with ($n=7$) and without ($n=6$) cardiac failure. Steady state concentrations of

Table 5.6 Clearance values (ml/min/kg) of lidocaine in different patient populations

Healthy volunteers	Heart failure	Liver cirrhosis	Reference
10 (n=10)	6.3 (n=8)	6.0 (n=8)	Thomson et al.,1973
16.3 (n=16) (11.0–20.4)	–	7.8 (n=12) (5.4–10.2)	Oellerich et al.,1990
26.9±7.2 (n=16)[a]	–	11.7±6.5 (n=27)[a]	Colli et al.,1988
	chronic hepatitis 19.4±2.0 (n=12)[b]	7.3±0.4 (n=53)[b]	Huet and Villeneuve, 1983

Notes
[a]Mean±S.E.
[b]Mean±S.D.

lidocaine at termination of infusion were 46% higher in the patients with cardiac failure than in those without cardiac failure (Prescott *et al.*, 1976).

Following infusions of lidocaine for 24 h in two groups of patients (*n*=19 and 32) with unstable angina, acute myocardial infarction, and malignant ventricular arrhythmias a time-dependent decline in CL was observed: after 4 h infusion CL ranged from about 5 to 20 ml/min/kg and after 24 h from about 2 to 15 ml/min/kg. Likewise, steady-state serum levels varied about four-fold between the different patients (Wong and Hurwitz, 1985).

In patients with liver cirrhosis there is an about 50% reduction in CL of lidocaine, whereas patients with chronic hepatitis have apparently a normal CL (see Table 5.6). The impairment of the metabolism of lidocaine in severe liver disease can be also visualised by the MEGX test, as the plasma concentrations of the metabolite measured 15 min after an intravenous test dose of lidocaine are much lower in those patients (Oellerich *et al.*, 1990; Reichel *et al.*, 1995; Gremse *et al.*, 1990; Pritchard-Davies *et al.*, 1994). Likewise, dependent on the severity of the liver disease a gradual decrease of MEGX measured fifteen min after the injection of 1 mg/kg of lidocaine can be observed (Sotaniemi *et al.*, 1995). As expected for a high clearance drug the pronounced hepatic first-pass effect results in a low (about 20–25%) oral bioavailability which, however will increase to about 70 to 75% in patients with cirrhosis (Huet and Villeneuve, 1983; Pomier-Layrargues *et al.*, 1988).

When lidocaine disposition was compared in nine healthy males and females, CL averaged 12.5 and 14.3 ml/min/kg respectively (ns). However, oral bioavailability was significantly (*p* <0.01) higher in females (39%) than in males (24%) and smoking appeared to have no influence (Wing *et al.*, 1984).

Since hepatic blood flow declines with age (Sherlock *et al.*, 1950), one would expect a reduction in CL of the high clearance drug lidocaine. Surprisingly, systemic CL (50 mg i.v.) was nearly identical in young volunteers

(20–34 years old) and elderly patients (83–87 years): 5.3 (range 1.9–10.4) versus 5.0 (range 2.7–10.8) ml/min/kg, respectively. However, as oral CL (250 mg p.o.) was lower ($p < 0.02$) in the elderly (18.8 ml/min/kg) than in the young (43.4 ml/min/kg), bioavailability was increased ($p < 0.05$) from 12.8% (young group) to 26.6% in the elderly patients (Cusack et al., 1985). When MEGX concentrations following a single i.v. dose of 1 mg/kg were measured after 15, 30 and 60 min, either lower concentrations were noted in elderly subjects (Orlando and Palatini, 1997) or no correlation with increasing age was observed (Pritchard-Davies et al., 1994). Hepatic blood flow may also depend on posture. However, before and after 7 days of total recumbency CL of lidocaine (4.6 ± 0.7 versus 4.7 ± 0.7 ml/min/kg) was not different in eight subjects tested (Kates et al., 1980).

Thus, it appears that cardiac output and liver function are the most important determinants for the hepatic elimination of lidocaine.

Propafenone

Elimination of the racemic propafenone is primarily by hepatic metabolism. Following single and multiple oral or intravenous dosing nonlinear (dose-dependent) pharmacokinetics of propafenone and its metabolites were found (Hollmann et al., 1983; Conolly et al., 1984; Vozeh et al., 1990). After oral administration bioavailability (F) is variable and low (3–30%) because of an extensive first-pass effect. Part of the variability can be explained by the nonlinear nature of the pharmacokinetics: for 150 mg F ranged from 2.2 to 10.3%, for 300 mg from 3 to 27% (Hollmann et al., 1983) and for 300 to 450 mg from 5 to 31% (Vozeh et al., 1990). 5-Hydroxylation and N-dealkylation constitute the major pathways and both metabolites have antiarrhythmic activities comparable to those of propafenone (Thompson et al., 1988). Based on in vitro studies with liver microsomes of four human kidney donors CYP2D6 was identified to catalyse the formation of 5–hydroxypropafenone and V_{max} values for this reaction ranged from 1.3 to 23.9 pmol 5-OH-propafenone formed per µg protein an hour (Kroemer et al., 1989). Therefore it is not surprising that humans with a deficiency of CYP2D6, known as PM phenotype, have much lower 5-hydroxypropafenone plasma levels if compared with the EM phenotype (Siddoway et al., 1987).

In similar in vitro experiments it was elucidated that N-dealkylation is mediated by CYP1A2 and CYP3A. With seven human livers a wide interindividual variability in intrinsic clearance (V_{max}/K_m) was observed (from 0.01 to 0.1 ml/h/mg protein). Also in vivo (fourteen patients dosed with 150 mg propafenone t.i.d.) steady state plasma concentrations of N-desalkylpropafenone varied widely from 4 to 293 ng/ml (Botsch et al., 1993).

Based on the metabolic pattern of propafenone and the enzymes involved, genetic constitution can explain a large part of the interindividual variability in the disposition of propafenone (see Tables 5.2 and 5.7). Patients with a PM phenotype will have much higher propafenone levels than EM whereas 5-hydroxypropafenone plasma concentrations can not be detected in PM (Lee *et al.*, 1990). For the correct phenotype assignment normally a test dose of either debrisoquine, sparteine or dextromethorphan is applied. However, phenotyping can be also performed during propafenone therapy by analysing the urinary excretion of intact glucuronides of propafenone (Botsch *et al.*, 1994).

In healthy EM, systemic CL of racemic propafenone ranged between 600 and 1,500 ml/min (Vozeh *et al.*, 1990) and apparent oral CL varied widely from 250 to 5,000 ml/min as did metabolic clearance to 5–hydroxy-propafenone with 120 to 1,950 ml/min (Funck-Brentano *et al.*, 1989). In contrast in PM, oral CL of propafenone is much lower (see also Table 5.2) ranging from 100 to 300 ml/min (Funck-Brentano *et al.*, 1989, 1990).

It should be remembered that propafenone is a racemate. Thus, its disposition should be evaluated in a stereoselective manner. During oral treatment with racemic propafenone oral CL of its two enantiomers is different and dependent on the phenotype. In any case, oral CL of (R)-propafenone is always significantly larger than that of (S)-propafenone (Kroemer *et al.*, 1989, 1994) and apparently there is no difference in the stereoselective disposition of propafenone between Caucasians and Chinese subjects (Li *et al.*, 1998). However, it should be noted that both enantiomers exhibit nonlinear pharmacokinetics which is evident from a much higher oral clearance following a single dose if compared with steady state conditions (see Table 5.8).

Table 5.7 Trough steady state plasma concentrations of propafenone and its two major metabolites in five poor (PM) and nine extensive (EM) metabolisers of CYP2D6 following different dosage

Concentration mean (±SD) μmoles/l	150 mg tid		225 mg tid		300 mg tid	
	EM	PM	EM	PM	EM	PM
Propafenone	0.56 (0.54)	3.18[a] (0.76)	1.20 (1.14)	4.75[a] (0.79)	2.53 (2.46)	5.46[b] (0.66)
5-OH-propafenone	0.27 (0.15)	nd	0.35 (0.15)	nd	0.50 (0.19)	nd
N-desalkyl-propafenone	0.07 (0.26)	0.26[b] (0.09)	0.15 (0.16)	0.36[b] (0.11)	0.34 (0.22)	0.45 (0.14)

Notes
Modified from Lee *et al.*, 1990.
nd, not detected; [a]$p<0.01$; [b]$p<0.05$; (PM versus EM).

When both enantiomers of propafenone were given separately and their disposition compared with that following racemic administration, a mutual enantiomer–enantiomer interaction could be verified. Thus, when the racemate was given, the elimination of (S)-propafenone was impaired and that of the (R)-form accelerated compared with single enantiomer administration (Kroemer *et al.*, 1994; Li *et al.*, 1998). *In vitro* experiments indicated that competitive inhibition could partly account for this surprising observation (Kroemer *et al.*, 1991).

Substantial changes in the pharmacokinetics of propafenone are seen in patients with liver failure resulting from alcoholic liver cirrhosis or gastrointestinal disorders. An up to five-fold increase in oral bioavailability and an about 40% reduction of oral CL (down to 500 ml/min) was seen in severe cases and kinetic changes correlated significantly with some laboratory test parameters, such as serum albumin and prothrombin time (Lee *et al.*, 1987).

In addition to oxidation some part of propafenone and its metabolites are subject to glucuronidation and the glucuronides are excreted via the kidneys (Botsch *et al.*, 1994). Thus, renal function might have some indirect effect of the disposition of propafenone. Following a single i.v.-dose of propafenone pharmacokinetics of the parent compound was unchanged in five patients with renal insufficiency (mean $CL_{creatinine}$ 40 ml/min) if compared with five healthy volunteers (Burgess *et al.*, 1989). During oral treatment with propafenone for ventricular arrhythmias four patients (62 ± 6 years old) with chronic renal failure had almost identical dose-corrected steady-state levels of racemic propafenone if compared to five age-matched (59 ± 5 years old) control patients ($CL_{creatinine}$: 74–116 ml/min). However, the plasma levels for the glucuronides of (S)- and (R)-propafenone were significantly ($p < 0.05$) higher in patients with chronic renal failure. If the control group was compared with seven young (29 ± 5 years old) healthy male volunteers it appeared that both glucuronides were elevated in the older patients (Fromm *et al.*, 1995).

In conclusion, the major cause for the interindividual variability in the

Table 5.8 Oral clearance (ml/min) of (S)- and (R)-propafenone following single or multiple dosing (150 mg p.o. every six or eight h) with racemic drug

EM (mean ± SD)		PM		Reference
S	R	S	R	
5814 ± 3894 (*n*=4)	11161 ± 6378	375 ± 108 (*n*=4)	535 ± 231	Gross *et al.*, 1989[a]
424 ± 126 (*n*=5)	735 ± 226	53/164 (*n*=2)	113/243	Kroemer *et al.*, 1989[b]
920 ± 300 (*n*=7)	1460 ± 480	–	–	Kroemer *et al.*, 1994[b]
1226 ± 751 (*n*=8)	1678 ± 625	–	–	Li *et al.*, 1998[b]

Notes
[a] Single dose; [b] steady state conditions.

metabolism of propafenone is the CYP2D6 phenotype. In addition, actual liver function and the dose-dependent kinetics will contribute significantly to the variability in propafenone's metabolism.

Propranolol

The hepatic metabolism of propranolol results in a large number of metabolites; at least six have been recovered from urine and less than 1% of a dose is excreted unchanged in the urine. The racemic propranolol is metabolised through three distinct pathways: ring oxidation to 4'-hydroxy-propranolol with subsequent O-glucuronidation and O-sulfatation, side-chain oxidation to α-naphthoxylactic acid and direct O-glucuronidation at the side-chain (Walle et al., 1985). 4'-Hydroxylation and partly N-dealkylation (+CYP1A2) are catalysed by CYP2D6 and in the side-chain oxidation of propranolol CYP2C19 seems to be involved (Ward et al., 1989; Walle et al., 1986). However, glucuronidation of propranolol is another important pathway (Walle et al., 1979). Nevertheless oral CL of propranolol is higher in the EM phenotype of CYP2D6 (219±53 l/h) if compared with PM (75±13 l/h). The difference is even more impressive if the fractional clearance to 4'-hydroxypropranolol is calculated: 34±10 versus 2.9±1.0 l/h. Both clearances are about four-fold higher in EM and PM when rifampicin is coadministered (Shaheen et al., 1989).

Some of these metabolic pathways are stereoselective (Ward et al., 1989; Walle et al., 1984). (R)-propranolol is cleared more rapidly than (S)-propranolol and consequently concentrations of the latter are usually 30 to 60% higher than those of the former (Silber et al., 1982; Lalonde et al., 1988). There are also stereoselective differences in the plasma protein binding of propranolol enantiomers and as CL of propranolol is of the restrictive type (Wilkinson, 1987) variability in this binding will contribute to differences in hepatic elimination (Walle et al., 1983).

The high hepatic extraction ratio is dose-dependent and during chronic therapy averages about 0.7. As in the case of lidocaine, CL of propranolol is variable (600–1,000 ml/min) and limited by hepatic blood flow. Oral bioavailability is rather low (30–40%) because of an extensive first-pass effect (Shand and Ragno, 1972; Walle et al., 1985) and F seems to be dependent on the input rate which can also influence the S/R-concentration ratio (Bleske et al., 1995).

Stereoselective disposition of propranolol was similar in White male healthy subjects and in Chinese males following a single oral dose of 80 mg (see Table 5.9). However, both enantiomers were cleared more rapidly in Chinese subjects (60 and 37 ml/min/kg for (R)- and (S)-propranolol) than in Caucasians (36 and 23 ml/min/kg, respectively), whereas elimination half-life (3.5 to 4 h) did not differ significantly between the two groups or between the two enantiomers (Zhou and Wood, 1990).

Table 5.9 Oral clearance (mean±SD) of propranolol enantiomers in healthy subjects

CL_O, ml/min/kg		n (age in years)	Oral dose, mg	Reference
R	S			
34.0±17.2	23.9±12.5	12 (29)	3×80 mg for 6 days	Hunt et al., 1990
36.3± 8.7 (SEM)	22.7±3.8	9 (28±9)	80 mg	Zhou and Wood, 1990
30.3± 9.6 (179±46)[a]	22.8±6.7 (175±40)[a]	10 (23–33)	3×80 mg for 6 days	Lalonde et al., 1990
26.2±14.3 (170±84)[a]	19.0±9.5 (168±76)[a]	10 (55–75)	3×80 mg for 6 days	Lalonde et al., 1990

Note
[a]Values refer to unbound propranolol.

Besides genetics and ethnic origin, gender represents another determinant contributing to variability in the metabolism of propranolol. In a large population study, females had about 80% higher serum levels than males (Walle et al., 1985). Whereas following a single i.v. dose of 0.1 mg/kg males and females had a very similar systemic CL (17.7±2.0 versus 15.1±0.8 ml/min/kg), total oral CL of propranolol (single dose of 80 mg p.o.) was significantly ($p < 0.02$) lower in 13 females (40±6 ml/min/kg; ±SEM) if compared with 15 males (66±8 ml/min/kg). Also the fractional clearances to the propranolol glucuronide and to α-naphthoxylactic acid were higher in males than in females (Walle et al., 1989).

Similar to rifampicin, smoking can induce the metabolism of propranolol. Oral CL of propranolol was significantly ($p < 0.02$) higher in six cigarette smokers (94±14 ml/min/kg; ±SEM) if compared to seven nonsmokers (53±6 ml/min/kg). Ring oxidation appeared to be only slightly affected whereas both side-chain oxidation and glucuronidation were increased by 110 and 55%, respectively. This would suggest that the enzymes involved in the latter two reactions are inducible by aromatic hydrocarbons (Walle et al., 1987).

As the liver is the major site for the metabolism of propranolol hepatic (dys)function will markedly affect its disposition. Already in 1975, Branch et al. reported that following an i.v. bolus of 40 mg (+)-propranolol, a decrease in its CL was seen with increasing severity of liver disease. This could be due to loss of enzyme activity, altered liver blood flow including vascular shunting and altered drug binding in blood. Several studies (for review see Morgan and McLean, 1995; Rodighiero, 1999) indicated that in cirrhotic patients reduction observed in estimated liver flow is rather low (15%) and that intrinsic clearance of propranolol always fell to a much greater extent (70 to 80%). Following a single i.v. dose, systemic CL was reduced by 30 to 60% (Branch et al., 1976a, b; Pessayre et al., 1978;

Wood *et al.*, 1978). During steady state conditions (80 mg p.o. t.i.d. for two days) apparent oral CL of total and unbound propranolol averaged 2.43 and 28.0 l/min in nine normal subjects and 1.27 and 13.9 l/min in seven patients with cirrhosis. The differences were less marked following a labelled i.v. bolus: systemic CL of total and unbound propranolol were 0.86 and 9.7 l/h in the controls and 0.58 and 6.3 l/h in the cirrhotics. The kinetic changes resulted in an increase of the bioavailability of propranolol from normally 38 to 54% in the cirrhotic patients (Wood *et al.*, 1978).

When the blood is shunted around the liver, e.g. by a portacaval (PC) shunt for recurrent variceal bleeding, relative oral bioavailability of propranolol (80 mg p.o.) expressed as AUC was much higher (1098 ± 84 ng/ml/h) in three cirrhotic patients with PC shunt than in six cirrhotics (357 ± 38 ng/ml/h) or in six healthy subjects (321 ± 25 ng/ml/h). In addition, bioavailability was affected by time of day of administration (Semenowicz-Siuda *et al.*, 1984).

In seven patients with clinical and laboratory evidence of liver disease indicating diagnostic liver biopsy, liver blood flow, P450 content and oral CL of propranolol were measured. Whereas hepatic perfusion appeared quite normal and of low variation (range 1.426 to 2.049 ml/min), P450 content (range 1.7 to 17.1 nmol/g) oral CL of propranolol (range 1.0 to 10.4 l/min) showed a much larger interindividual variability. Between the latter two parameters a significant ($r=0.833$; $p<0.05$) relationship was found, indicating that liver enzyme activity plays a dominant role in the elimination of propranolol (Pirttiaho *et al.*, 1980).

Since in a group of nine elderly subjects (mean age 77 years) higher plasma levels of racemic propranolol (single oral dose of 40 mg) were observed than in nine young (27 years) individuals (Castleden *et al.*, 1975) a more extensive study was performed by the same group (Castleden and George, 1979). In a single i.v. (0.15 mg/kg) versus p.o. (40 mg) cross-over study in seven young (mean age 29 years) and eight older (78 years) subjects, systemic CL was significantly ($p<0.02$) lower in the elderly (7.8 ± 1.3 ml/min/kg) compared with young subjects (13.2 ± 1.4 ml/min/kg). Plasma concentration following the oral dose were about two-fold higher in the elderly as first-pass extraction of $45 \pm 8\%$ was significantly ($p<0.05$) less than in the young ($70 \pm 5\%$). Likewise during multiple oral dosing (40 mg four times a day for 2 days) steady state plasma concentrations of racemic propranolol were two- to three-fold higher in the elderly during the measured dosing interval of 6 hours. This suggests that intrinsic clearance of propranolol is affected by ageing (Castleden and George, 1979).

A similar, about 2.5-fold increase in the AUC of racemic propranolol (80 mg tid for 2 days) was seen in old (mean ages 66 and 68 years, respectively) smokers and nonsmokers if compared with matched young (20–30 years) controls. Surprisingly, smoking did not affect the AUC of propranolol in both populations (Hitzenberger *et al.*, 1982). Conversely, an age-related decrease in oral CL of propranolol was only seen in smokers, but no apparent change was seen in nonsmokers (Vestal *et al.*, 1979). Similarly, in another study, no significant decrease in oral CL was seen in a small number of young and old subjects (Rigby *et al.*, 1985).

As the disposition of propranolol is stereoselective and (S)-propranolol is about 100 times more active as a β-adrenergic receptor blocker than (R)-propranolol (Barrett and Cullum, 1968), these pharmacological properties have to be considered in age studies as done more recently by Lalonde *et al.* (1990). As can be seen from Table 5.9, there was no age effect on oral CL of both enantiomers for either total propranolol or unbound propranolol. Based on the existing studies it remains unclear whether old age is associated with a significant change in the metabolism of propranolol.

In conclusion, the stereoselective disposition of propranolol is affected to same extent by genetics, ethnic origin, gender and smoking habits. Plasma protein binding and especially liver function determine disposition and bioavailability of propranolol.

Verapamil

The metabolic pattern of verapamil in human is very complex and so far twelve different metabolites have been identified in urine (Eichelbaum *et al.*, 1979). The major pathways include N-demethylation to norverapamil by CYP3A4 and to D-703 by CYP3A4 and CYP1A2 as well as O-demethylation to D-703 and D-702 by CYP2C9 (Kroemer *et al.*, 1993; Busse *et al.*, 1995).

Based on *in vitro* experiments with microsomes from ten human livers, the calculated intrinsic clearances (V_{max}/K_m) for the formation of the enan-

Table 5.10 Mean clearance values for the enantiomers of verapamil

Subjects (n)		Systemic CL, ml/min.		Oral CL, l/min.		Reference
		S	R	S	R	
Healthy subjects		1411	797	7.5	1.7	Hoon et al., 1986
Young males	(12)	–	–	9.1	1.8	Karim and Piergies, 1995
Young subjects	(11)	–	–	9.5	0.8	Bhatti et al., 1995
Young males	(6)	–	–	9.2	1.9	Mikus et al., 1990
Young males	(15)	1700	1017	4.1	1.0	Abernethy et al., 1993
Elderly males	(15)	1283	750	2.7	0.7	Abernethy et al., 1993
Young subjects[a]	(8)	930	841	–	–	Schwartz et al., 1993
Elderly subjects[a]	(8)	610	691	–	–	Schwartz et al., 1993
Young males	(8)	1177	695	8.6	1.7	Fromm et al., 1996
Elderly males	(8)	1119	599	8.9	1.6	Fromm et al., 1998

Note
[a] Enantiomers were infused (15 min) separately.

tiomers of norverapamil, D-702, D-703 and D-617 showed coefficients of variation between 61 and 89% (median 76%). In parallel *in vivo* studies in four healthy male volunteers metabolic clearance rates of the four metabolites followed the same sequence (D-617>norverapamil>D-703>D-702) as *in vitro*. Under both conditions metabolism was preferential for S-verapamil (Kroemer *et al.*, 1992). The calcium channel blocker verapamil is administered as a racemate and its stereoselective disposition has to be considered since the cardiovascular effects are attributable mainly to the S-enantiomer (Echizen *et al.*, 1985; Hoon *et al.*, 1986). This active moiety is subject to preferential hepatic first-pass metabolism leading to an R/S ratio of plasma concentrations of about 5 after oral administration of verapamil (Vogelsang *et al.*, 1984).

Verapamil represents a high clearance drug and because of an extensive presystemic metabolism by the gut wall and the liver oral bioavailability is low: under steady state conditions about 15% for S-verapamil and approximately 35 to 40% for the R-enantiomer (Fromm *et al.*, 1996, 1998). The oral CL of verapamil exhibits considerable inter- and intra-individual variation, ranging between 26 and 85% and 12 and 48%, respectively (Eichelbaum and Somogyi, 1984). Because of the stereoselective and to some extent saturable first-pass metabolism of verapamil the bioavailability of both enantiomers is also dependent on the oral input-rate, e.g. differences in F and R/S ratios could be observed between immediate versus controlled-release formulations (Harder *et al.*, 1991; Bhatti *et al.*, 1995; Karim and Piergies, 1995). In addition, the time of administration represents another variable as some circadian variation in the pharmacokinetics of verapamil has been observed (Eldon *et al.*, 1989; Jespersen *et al.*, 1989).

As verapamil has a low (about 20%) oral availability despite complete absorption, extraction by the liver must be high. This could be verified by indirect estimations (comparison of AUC following i.v. and p.o. administration and calculation of hepatic blood flow Q_H), as well as by direct measurements in eight patients with organic heart disease undergoing diagnostic catheterisation. The calculated hepatic extraction ratio E of racemic propranolol ranged from 0.83 to 0.89 (Woodcook *et al.*, 1981a, b). Therefore it was not surprising that hepatic elimination of racemic verapamil was reduced by about 50% in patients with cirrhosis (decrease in E and Q_H), e.g. systemic plasma clearance fell from a mean of 1.258 ml/min in six normal subjects to 616 ml/min in seven patients with liver cirrhosis. In the same individuals, oral clearance was reduced from 6.4 l/min to 1.3 l/min and consequently bioavailability increased ($p < 0.001$) from 22% (controls) to 52% in cirrhotics (Somogyi *et al.*, 1981). Surgical meso-caval shunting can lead to almost complete bioavailability (Eichelbaum *et al.*, 1980).

Concerning the effect of age on the clearance of verapamil, contradictory results have been reported. In some studies an age-related reduction of about 50% of oral CL could be seen (Abernethy *et al.*, 1993; Gupta *et al.*, 1995; Sasaki *et al.*, 1993) whereas in other studies no significant difference was observed between young and elderly populations (Abernethy *et al.*, 1986; Ahmed *et al.*, 1991; Fromm *et al.*, 1998). Schwarz *et al.* (1993, 1994) detected no significant reductions in systemic CL of R-verapamil in healthy, older subjects, but systemic CL of S-verapamil was decreased in the older people. The observed discrepancies (see also Table 5.10) might be due to differences in populations investigated, verapamil preparations used, study design and data analysis.

In summary, the complex extra-/hepatic metabolism of verapamil is stereoselective and sensitive to changes in hepatic perfusion. Liver function represents the key determinant affecting the disposition of verapamil.

Conclusions

With different substrates (e.g. lidocaine, propafenone, propranolol, verapamil) metabolised by various enzyme subfamilies (e.g. CYP3A, CYP2D6, CYP2C9, CYP1A2) a large (about ten-fold) variation in drug metabolism was observed in *in vitro* experiments with human liver microsomes. In general, interindividual variability of systemic and/or oral drug clearance was lower *in vivo* (about three-fold) if genetic polymorphisms are excluded. The major cause of variability represents the hepatic function which shows major impairments in cirrhosis and sometimes might be slightly reduced in elderly populations. For substrates of CYP2D6 (e.g. propafenone) the genetic background contributes profoundly (up to a factor of 10) to the interindividual variability. Some cardiovascular drugs (e.g. lidocaine for CYP3A4 or sparteine/debrisoquine/propafenone for CYP2D6) can be used as probes to estimate the drug metabolising activities of an individual subject. The different confounding factors described here for lidocaine, propafenone, propranolol and verapamil should be taken into account to estimate their impact on the interindividual variability in the metabolism and disposition of any cardiovascular drugs on the premise that their pharmacokinetic properties are known.

Acknowledgements

This work was supported by the Robert Bosch Foundation Stuttgart and a grant of the EU (BMH 1–CT 94–1622). The secretarial help of Mrs. G. Wilder and H. Köhler is highly appreciated.

References

Abernethy, D. R., Schwartz, J. B., Todd, E. L., Luchi, R. and Snow, E. (1986) 'Verapamil pharmacodynamics and disposition in young and elderly hypertensive patients. Altered electrocardiographic and hypotensive responses', *Ann. Intern. Med.* **105**: 329–36.

Abernethy, D. R., Wainer, I. W., Longstreth, J. A. and Andrawis, N. S. (1993) 'Stereoselective verapamil disposition and dynamics in aging during racemic verapamil administration', *J. Pharmacol. Exp. Ther.* **266**: 904–11.

Adedoyin, A., Arns, P. A., Richards, W. O., Wilkinson, G. R. and Branch, R. A. (1998) 'Selective effect of liver disease on the activities of specific metabolizing enzymes: investigations of cytochrome P4502C19 and 2D6', *Clin. Pharmacol. Ther.* **64**: 8–17.

Ahmed, J. H., Meredith, P. A., and Elliott, H. L. (1991) 'The influence of age on the pharmacokinetics of verapamil', *Pharmacol. Res.* **24**: 227–33.

Arrigoni, A., Gindro, T., Aimo, G., Cappello, N., Meloni, A., Benedetti, P., Molino, G.P., Verme, G. and Rizetto, M. (1994) Monoethylglycinexylidide test: a prognostic indicator of survival in cirrhosis', *Hepatology* **20**: 383–7.

Bargetzi, M. J., Aoyama, T., Gonzalez, F. J. and Meyer, U. A. (1989) 'Lidocaine metabolism in human liver microsomes by cytochrome P450IIIA4', *Clin. Pharmacol. Ther.* **46**: 521–7.

Barrett, A. M. and Cullum, V. A. (1968) 'The biological properties of the optical isomers of propranolol and their effects on cardiac arrhythmias', *Br. J. Pharmacol.* **34**: 43–55.

Bhatti, M. M., Lewanczuk, R. Z., Pasutto, F. M. and Foster, R. T. (1995) 'Pharmacokinetics of verapamil and norverapamil enantiomers after administration of immediate and controlled-release formulations to humans: evidence suggesting input-rate determined stereoselectivity', *J. Clin. Pharmacol.* **35**: 1076–82.

Bleske, B. E., Welage, L. S., Rose, S., Amidon, G. L. and Shea, M. J. (1995) 'The effect of dosage release formulations on the pharmacokinetics of propranolol stereoisomers in humans', *J. Clin. Pharmacol.* **35**: 374–8.

Bonate, P. L. (1991) 'Gender-related differences in xenobiotic metabolism', *J. Clin. Pharmacol.* **31**: 684–90.

Boobis, A. R., McKillop, D., Robinson, D. T., Adams, D. A. and McCormick, D. J. (1998) 'Interlaboratory comparison of the assessment of P450 activities in human hepatic microsomal samples', *Xenobiot* **28**: 493–506.

Botsch, S., Gautier, J.-C., Beaune, P., Eichelbaum, M. and Kroemer, H. K. (1993) 'Identification and characterization of the cytochrome P450 enzymes involved in D-dealkylation of propafenone: molecular base for interaction potential and variable disposition of active metabolites', *Mol. Pharmacol.* **43**: 120–6.

Botsch, S., Heinkele, G., Meese, C. O., Eichelbaum, M. and Kroemer, H. K. (1994) 'Rapid determination of CYP2D6 phenotype during propafenone therapy by analysing urinary excretion of propafenone glucuronides', *Eur. J. Clin. Pharmacol.* **46**: 133–5.

Branch, R. A., James, J. and Read, A. E. (1975) 'The pharmacokinetics of (+)-propranolol in normal subjects and patients with chronic liver disease', *Br. J. Clin. Pharmacol.* **2**: 183P–4P.

Branch, R. A., James, J. and Read, A. F. (1976a) 'A study of factors influencing drug disposition in chronic liver disease using the model drug (+)-propranolol', *Br. J. Clin. Pharmacol.* **3**: 242–9.

Branch, R. A. and Shand, D. G. (1976b) 'Propranolol disposition in chronic liver disease. A physiological approach', *Clin. Pharmacokinet.* **1**: 264–79.

Burgess, E., Duff, H. and Wilkes, P. (1989) 'Propafenone disposition in renal insufficiency and renal failure', *J. Clin. Pharmacol.* 29: 112–13.

Busse, D., Cosme, J., Beaune, P., Kroemer, H. K. and Eichelbaum, M. (1995) 'Cytochromes of the P4502C subfamily are the major enzymes involved in the O-demethylation of verapamil in humans', *Naunyn Schmiedebergs Arch. Pharmacol.* 353: 116–21.

Castleden, C. M. and George, C. F. (1979) 'The effect of aging on the hepatic clearance of propranolol', *Br. J. Clin. Pharmacol.* 7: 49–54.

Castleden, C. M., Kaye, C. M. and Parsons, R. L. (1975) 'The effect of age on plasma levels of propranolol and practolol in man', *Br. J. Clin. Pharmacol.* 2: 303–6.

Colli, A., Buccino, G., Cocciolo, M., Parravicini, R. and Scaltrini, G. (1988) 'Disposition of a flow-limited drug (lidocaine) and a metabolic capacity-limited drug (theophylline) in liver cirrhosis', *Clin. Pharmacol. Ther.* 44: 642–9.

Conolly, S., Lebsack, C., Winkle, R. A., Harrison, D. C. and Kates, R. E. (1984) 'Propafenone disposition kinetics in cardiac arrhythmia', *Clin. Pharmacol. Ther.* 36: 163–8.

Cusack, B., O'Malley, K., Lavan, J., Noel, J. and Kelly, J. G. (1985) 'Protein binding and disposition of lignocaine in the elderly', *Eur. J. Clin. Pharmacol.* 29: 323–9.

Dayer, P., Kubli, A., Küpfer, F., Courvoisier, F., Balant, L. and Fabre, J. (1982) 'Defective hydroxylation of bufuralol associated with side-effects of the drug in poor metabolizers', *Br. J. Clin. Pharmacol.* 13: 750–2.

Dong, S. X., Ping, Z. Z., Xiao, W. Z., Shu, C. C., Bartoli, A., Gatti. G., D'Urso, S., Perucca, E. (1998) 'Effect of active and passive cigarette smoking on CYP1A2-mediated phenacetin disposition in Chinese subjects', *Ther. Drug Monit.* 20: 371–5.

Echizen, H., Vogelsang, B. and Eichelbaum, M. (1985) 'Effects of d, l-verapamil on atrioventricular conduction in relation to its stereoselective first-pass metabolism', *Clin. Pharmacol. Ther.* 38: 71–6.

Eichelbaum, M., Albrecht, M., Kliems, K., Schäfer, K. and Somogyi, A. (1980) 'Influence of meso-caval shunt surgery on verapamil kinetics, bioavailability and response', *Br. J. Clin. Pharmacol.* 10: 527–9.

Eichelbaum, M., Ende, M., Remberg, G., Schomerus, M. and Dengler, H.J. (1979) 'The metabolism of DL-(^{14}C)verapamil in man', *Drug Metab. Disp.* 7: 145–8.

Eichelbaum, M. and Somogyi, A. (1984) 'Inter- and intra-subject variations in the first-pass elimination of highly cleared drugs during chronic dosing', *Eur. J. Clin. Pharmacol.* 26: 47–53.

Eldon, M. A., Battle, M. M., Voigtman, R. E. and Colburn, W. A. (1989) 'Differences in oral verapamil absorption as a function of time of day', *J. Clin. Pharmacol.* 29: 989–93.

Fromm, M. F., Botsch, S., Heinkele, G., Evers, J. and Kroemer, H. K. (1995) 'Influence of renal function on the steady-state pharmacokinetics of the antiarrhythmic propafenone and its phase I and phase II metabolites', *Eur. J. Clin. Pharmacol.* 48: 279–83.

Fromm, M. F., Busse, D., Kroemer, H. K. and Eichelbaum, M. (1996) 'Differential induction of prehepatic and hepatic metabolism of verapamil by rifampin', *Hepatology* 24: 796–801.

Fromm, M. F., Dilger, K., Busse, D., Kroemer, H. K., Eichelbaum, M. and Klotz, U. (1998) 'Gut wall metabolism of verapamil in older people: effects of rifampicin-mediated enzyme induction', *Br. J. Clin. Pharmacol.* **45**: 247–55.

Fromm, M. F., Kroemer, H. K. and Eichelbaum, M. (1997) 'Impact of P450 genetic polymorphism on the first-pass extraction of cardiovascular and neuroactive drugs', *Adv. Drug Delivery Rev.* **27**: 171–99.

Fuhr, U. (1998) 'Drug interactions with grapefruit juice. Extent, probable mechanism and clinical relevance', *Drug Safety* **18**: 251–72.

Funck-Brentano, C., Kroemer, H. K., Lee; J. T. and Roden, D. M. (1990) 'Propafenone', *N. Engl. J. Med.* **322**: 518–25.

Funck-Brentano, C., Kroemer, H. K., Pavlou, H., Woosley, R. L. and Roden, D. M. (1989) 'Genetically determined interaction between propafenone and low dose quinidine: role of active metabolites in modulating net drug effect', *Br. J. Clin. Pharmacol.* **27**: 435–44.

George, J., Murry, M., Byth, K. and Farrell, G. F. (1995) 'Differential alterations of cytochrome P450 proteins in livers from patients with severe chronic liver disease', *Hepatology* **21**: 120–8.

Gremse, D. A., A-Kader, H. H., Schroeder, T. J. and Balistreri, W. F. (1990) 'Assessment of lidocaine metabolite formation as a quantitative liver function test in children', *Hepatology* **12**: 565–9.

Gross, A. S., Trenk, D., Kroemer, H. K., Meese, C. O., Jähnchen, E. and Eichelbaum, M. (1997) 'Stereoselective propafenone disposition in poor and extensive metabolisers of sparteine', *Eur. J. Clin. Pharmacol.* **36** (Suppl.): A200.

Guengerich, F. P. (1997) 'Role of cytochrome P450 enzymes in drug-drug interactions', *Adv. Pharmacol.* **43**: 7–35.

Guengerich, F. P. and Turvy, C. G. (1991) 'Comparison of levels of several human microsomal cytochrome P450 enzymes and epoxide hydrolase in normal and disease status using immunochemical analysis of surgical liver samples', *J. Pharmacol. Exp. Ther.* **256**: 1189–94.

Gupta, S. K., Atkinson, L., Tu, T. and Longstreth, J. A. (1995) 'Age and gender related changes in stereoselective pharmacokinetics and pharmacodynamics of verapamil and norverapamil', *Br. J. Clin. Pharmacol.* **40**: 325–31.

Hämmerlein, A., Derendorf, H. and Lowenthal, D. T. (1998) 'Pharmacokinetic and pharmacodynamic changes in the elderly. Clinical implications', *Clin. Pharmacokinet.* **35**: 49–64.

Harder, S., Thürmann, P., Siewert, M., Blume, H., Huber, Th. and Rietbrock, N. (1991) 'Pharmacodynamic profile of verapamil in relation to absolute bioavailability: investigations with a conventional and a controlled-release formulation', *J. Cardiovasc. Pharmacol.* **17**: 207–12.

Hitzenberger, G., Fitscha, P., Beveridge, T., Nüesch, E. and Pacha, W. (1982) 'Effects of age and smoking on the pharmacokinetics of pindolol and propranolol', *Br. J. Clin. Pharmacol.* **13**: 217S-22S.

Hollmann, M., Brode, E., Hotz, E., Kaumeier, S., and Kehrhahn, O.H. (1983) 'Investigations on the pharmacokinetics of propafenone in man', *Arzneim.-forsch.* **33**: 763–70.

Hoon, T. J., Baumann, J. L., Rodvold, K. A., Gallestegui, J. and Hariman, R. J. (1986) 'The pharmacodynamic and pharmacokinetic differences of the D- and

L-isomers of verapamil: implications in the treatment of paroxysmal supra-ventricular tachycardia', *Amer. Heart J.* **112**: 396–403.

Huet, P.-M. and Villeneuve, J.-P. (1983) 'Determinants of drug disposition in patients with cirrhosis', *Hepatology* **3**: 913–8.

Hunt, B. A., Bottorff, M. B., Herring, V. L., Self, T. H., Lalonde, R. L. (1990) 'Effects of calcium channel blockers on the pharmacokinetics of propranolol stereoisomers', *Clin. Pharmacol. Ther.* **47**: 584–91.

Ito, K., Iwatsubo, T., Kanamitsu, S., Nakajima, Y. and Sugiyama, Y. (1998) 'Quantitative prediction of in vivo drug clearance and drug interactions from in vitro data on metabolism, together with binding and transport', *Annu. Rev. Pharmacol. Toxicol.* **38**: 461–99.

Iwatsubo, T., Hirota, N., Ooie, T., Suzuki, H., Shimada, N., Chiba, K., Ishizaki, T., Green, C. E., Tyson, C. A. and Sugiyama, Y. (1977) 'Prediction of *in vivo* drug metabolism in the human liver from *in vitro* metabolism data', *Pharmacol. Ther.* **73**: 147–71.

Jespersen, C. M., Fredericksen, M., Hansen, J. F., Klitgaard, N. A. and Sorum, C. (1989) 'Circadian variation in the pharmacokinetics of verapamil', *Eur. J. Clin. Pharmacol.* **37**: 613–5.

Karim, A. and Piergies, A. (1995) 'Verapamil stereoisomerism: enantiomeric ratios in plasma dependent on peak concentrations, oral input rate, or both', *Clin. Pharmacol. Ther.* **58**: 174–84.

Kates, R. E., Harapat, S. R., Keefe, D. L. D., Goldwater, D. and Harrison, D. C. (1980) 'Influence of prolonged recumbancy on drug disposition', *Clin. Pharmacol. Ther.* **28**: 624–8.

Kinirons, M. T. and Crome, P. (1997) 'Clinical pharmacokinetic considerations in the elderly. An update', *Clin. Pharmacokinet.* **33**: 302–12.

Kivistö, K. T. and Kroemer, H. K. (1997) 'Use of probe drugs as predictors of drug metabolism in humans', *J. Clin. Pharmacol.* **37**: 40S-8S.

Klotz, U. (1998a) 'Drug metabolism in the intestinal wall', in H. E. Blum, J. Ch. Bode, Ch. Bode and R. B. Sartor (eds.) *Gut and the Liver*, Dordrecht: Kluwer Academic Publ. pp. 163–76.

Klotz, U. (1998b) 'Effect of age on pharmacokinetics and pharmacodynamics in man', *Internat. J. Clin. Pharmacol. Ther.* **36**: 581–5.

Klotz, U. and Ammon, E. (1998) 'Clinical and toxicological consequences on the inductive potential of ethanol', *Eur. J. Clin. Pharmacol.* **54**: 7–12.

Klotz, U. and Kivistö, K. T. (1999) 'Enzyme inhibition and induction – PK/PD impact', in G. T. Tucker (ed.) *Variability in Human Drug Response*, Amsterdam: Excerpta Medica, pp. 29–37.

Krishna, D. R. and Klotz, U. (1994) 'Extrahepatic metabolism of drugs in humans', *Clin. Pharmacokinet.* **26**: 144–60.

Kroemer, H. K., Echizen, H., Heidemann, H. and Eichelbaum, M. (1992) 'Predictability of the *in vivo* metabolism of verapamil from *in vitro* data: contribution of individual metabolic pathways and stereoselective aspects', *J. Pharmacol. Exp. Ther.* **260**: 1052–7.

Kroemer, H. K. and Eichelbaum, M. (1995) '"It's the genes, stupid". Molecular bases and clinical consequences of genetic cytochrome P450 2D6 polymorphism', *Life Sci.* **56**: 2285–98.

Kroemer, H. K., Fischer, E., Meese, C. O. and Eichelbaum, M. (1991) 'Enantiomer/ enantiomer interaction of (S)- and (R)-propafenone for cytochrome P450IID6–catalyzed 5–hydroxylation: *in vitro* evaluation of the mechanism', *Mol. Pharmacol.* 40: 135–42.

Kroemer, H. K., Fromm, M. F., Bühl, K., Terefe, H., Blaschke, G. and Eichelbaum, M. (1994) 'An enantiomer-enantiomer interaction of (S)- and (R)-propafenone modifies the effects of racemic drug therapy', *Circulation* 89: 2396–400.

Kroemer, H. K., Funck-Brentano, C., Silberstein, D. J., Wood, A. J. J., Eichelbaum, M., Woosley, R. L. and Roden, D. M. (1989) 'Stereoselective disposition and pharmacologic activity of propafenone enantiomers', Circulation 79: 1068–76.

Kroemer, H. K., Gautier, J.-C., Beaune, P., Henderson, C., Wolf, R. and Eichelbaum, M. (1993) 'Identification of P450 enzymes involved in metabolism of verapamil in humans', *Naunyn Schmiedebergs Arch. Pharmacol.* 348: 332–7.

Kroemer, H. K., Mikus, G., Kronbach, T., Meyer, U. A. and Eichelbaum, M. (1989) 'In vitro characterization of the human cytochrome P450 involved in polymorphic oxidation of propafenone', *Clin. Pharmacol. Ther.* 45: 28–33.

Lalonde, R. L., Bottorff, M. B., Straka, R. J., Tenero, D. M., Pieper, J. A. and Wainer, I. W. (1988) 'Nonlinear accumulation of propranolol enantiomers', *Br. J. Clin. Pharmacol.* 26: 100–2.

Lalonde, R. L., Tenero, D. M., Burlew, B. S., Herrings, V. L. and Bottorff, M. B. (1990) 'Effects of age on the protein binding and disposition of propranolol stereoisomers', *Clin. Pharmacol. Ther.* 47: 447–55.

Laurent-Kenesi, M. A., Funck-Brentano, C., Poirier, J. M., Decolin, D. and Jaillon, P. (1993) 'Influence of CYP2D6–dependent metabolism on the steady-state pharmacokinetics and pharmacodynamics of metoprolol and nicardipine, alone and in combination', *Br. J. Clin. Pharmacol.* 36: 531–8.

Le Couteur, D. G. and McLean, A. J. (1998) 'The aging liver. Drug clearance and an oxygen diffusion barrier hypothesis', *Clin. Pharmacokinet.* 34: 359–73.

Lee, J. T., Kroemer, H. K., Silberstein, D. J., Funck-Brentano, C., Lineberry, M. D., Wood, A. J. J., Roden, D. M. and Woosley, R. M. (1990) 'The role of genetically determined polymorphic drug metabolism in the beta-blockade produced by propafenone', *N. Engl. J. Med.* 322: 1764–8.

Lee, J. T., Yee, Y.-G., Dorian, P. and Kates, R. E. (1987) 'Influence of hepatic dysfunction on the pharmacokinetics of propafenone', *J. Clin. Pharmacol.* 27: 384–9.

Lennard, M. S. (1989) 'The polymorphic oxidation of beta-adrenoceptor antagonists', *Pharmacol. Ther.* 41: 461–77.

Lennard, M. S., Silas, J. H., Freestone, S., Ramsay, L. E., Tucker, G. T. and Woods, H. F. (1982) 'Oxidation phenotype – a major determinant of metoprolol metabolism and response', *N. Engl. J. Med.* 307: 1558–60.

Lewis, R. V., Lennard, M. S., Jackson, P. R., Tucker, G. T., Ramsey, L. E. and Woods, H. F. (1985) 'Timolol and atenolol: relationships between oxidation phenotype, pharmacokinetics and pharmacodynamics', *Br. J. Clin. Pharmacol.* 19: 329–33.

Li, G., Gong, P.-L., Qiu, J., Zeng, F.-D. and Klotz, U. (1998) 'Stereoselective steady state disposition and action of propafenone in Chinese subjects', *Br. J. Clin. Pharmacol.* 46: 441–5.

Lin, J.H. and Lu, Y.H. (1997) 'Role of pharmacokinetics and metabolism in drug discovery and development', *Pharmacol. Rev.* **49**: 403–49.

McGourty, J. C., Silas, J. H., Fleming, J. J., McBurney, A. and Ward, J. W. (1985) 'Pharmacokinetics and beta-blocking effects of timolol in poor and extensive metabolizers of debrisoquine', *Clin. Pharmacol. Ther.* **38**: 409–13.

Meyer, U. A. and Zanger, U. M. (1997) 'Molecular mechanisms of genetic polymorphisms of drug metabolism', *Ann. Rev. Pharmacol. Toxicol.* **37**: 269–96.

Mikus, G., Eichelbaum, M., Fischer, C., Gumulka, S., Klotz, U. and Kroemer, H. K. (1990) 'Interaction of verapamil and cimetidine: stereochemical aspects of drug metabolism, drug disposition and drug action', *J. Pharmacol. Exp. Ther.* **253**: 1042–8.

Miller, L. G. (1989) 'Recent developments in the study of the effects of cigarette smoking on clinical pharmacokinetics and clinical pharmacodynamics', *Clin. Pharmacokinet.* **17**: 90–108.

Morgan, D. J. and McLean, A. J. (1995) 'Clinical pharmacokinetic and pharmacodynamic considerations in patients with liver disease. An update', *Clin. Pharmacokinet.* **29**: 370–91.

Murray, M. (1992) 'P450 enzymes. Inhibition mechanisms, genetic regulation and effects of liver disease', *Clin. Pharmacokinet.* **23**: 132–46.

Oellerich, M., Burdelski, M., Lautz, H.-U., Schulz, M., Schmidt, F.-W. and Herrmann, H. (1990) 'Lidocaine metabolite formation as a measure of liver function in patients with cirrhosis', *Ther. Drug Monit.* **12**: 219–26.

Oellerich, M., Burdelski, M., Ringe, B., Lamesch, P., Gubernatis, G., Bunzendahl, H., Pichlmayer, R. and Herrmann, H. (1989) 'Lignocaine metabolite formation as a measure of pre-transplant liver function', *Lancet* **1**: 640–2.

Oellerich, M., Raude, E., Burdelski, M., Schulz, M., Schmidt, F. W., Ringe, B., Lamesch, P., Pichlmayr, R., Raith, H., Scheruhn, M., Wrenger, M. and Witteking, Ch. (1987) 'Monoethylglycinexylidide formation kinetics: a novel approach to assessment of liver function', *J. Clin. Chem. Clin. Biochem.* **25**: 845–53.

Orlando, R.. and Palatini, P. (1997) 'The effect of age on plasma MEGX concentrations', *Br. J. Clin. Pharmacol.* **44**: 206–8.

Pacifici, G. M. and Fracchia, G. N. (eds) (1995) *Advances in Drug Metabolism in Man*, European Commission (EUR 15439 – ISBN 92–827–3982–1), Luxembourg/Brussels.

Pelkonen, O., Maenpaa, J., Taavitsainen, P., Rautio, A. and Raunio, H. (1998) 'Inhibition and induction of human cytochrome P450 (CYP) enzymes', *Xenobiot.* **28**: 1203–54.

Pessayre, D., Lebrec, D., Descatoire, D., Peignouxe, M. and Benhamou, J. P. (1978) 'The mechanism for reduced drug clearance in patients with cirrhosis', *Gastroenterology* **74**: 566–71.

Pierce, D. M., Abrams, S. M. and Franklin, R. A. (1987) 'Pharmacokinetics and systemic availability of the antihypertensive agent indoramin and its metabolite 6–hydroxyindoramin in healthy subjects', *Eur. J. Clin. Pharmacol.* **32**: 619–23.

Pirttiaho, H. I., Sotaniemi, E. A., Pelkonen, R. O., Pitkänen, U., Anttila, M. and Sundqvist, H. (1980) 'Roles of hepatic blood flow and enzyme activity in the kinetics of propranolol and sotalol', *Br. J. Clin. Pharmacol.* **9**: 399–405.

Pomier-Layrargues, G., Huet, P.-M., Infante-Rivard, C., Villeneuve, J.-P., Marleau, D., Duguay, L., Tanguay, S. and Lavoie, P. (1988) 'Prognostic value of indocyanine green and lidocaine kinetics for survival and chronic hepatic encephalopathy in cirrhotic patients following elective end-to-side portacaval shunt', *Hepatology* 8: 1506–10.

Prescott, L. F., Adjepon-Yomoah, K. K. and Talbot, R. G. (1976) 'Impaired ligno-caine metabolism in patients with myocardial infarction and cardiac failure', *Br. Med. J.* 1: 939–41.

Pritchard-Davies, R., Gross, A. S. and Shenfield, G. M. (1994) 'The effect of liver disease and food on plasma MEGX concentrations', *Br. J. Clin. Pharmacol.* 37: 298–301.

Reichel, C., Wienkoop, G., Nacke, A. and Spengler, U. (1995) 'Monoethyl-glycinxilidin (MEGX)-Test. Ein Test zur Einschätzung der Prognose vor und nach Lebertransplantation', *Dtsch. Med. Wschr.* 120: 179–83.

Rigby, J.W., Scott, A. K., Hawksworth, G. M. and Petrie, J. C. (1985) 'A comparison of the pharmacokinetics of atenolol, metoprolol, oxprenolol and propranolol in elderly hypertensive and young healthy subjects', *Br. J. Clin. Pharmacol.* 20: 327–31.

Rodighiero, V. (1999) 'Effects of liver disease on pharmacokinetics. An update', *Clin. Pharmacokinet.* 37: 399–431.

Rowland, K., Ellis, S. W., Lennard, M. S. and Tucker, G. T. (1996) 'Variable contribution of CYP2D6 to the N-dealkylation of S- (-) propranolol by human liver microsomes', *Br. J. Clin. Pharmacol.* 42: 390–3.

Sasaki, M., Tateishi, T. and Ebihara, A. (1993) 'The effects of age and gender on the stereoselective pharmacokinetics of verapamil', *Clin. Pharmacol. Ther.* 54: 278–85.

Schwarz, J. B., Capili, H. and Wainer, I. W. (1994) 'Verapamil stereoisomers during racemic verapamil administration: effects of aging and comparisons to admini-stration of individual stereoisomers', *Clin. Pharmacol. Ther.* 56: 368–76.

Schwartz, J. B., Troconiz, I. F., Verotta, D., Liu, S. and Capili, H. (1993) 'Aging effects on stereoselective pharmacokinetics and pharmacodynamics of verapamil', *J. Pharmacol. Exp. Ther.* 265: 690–8.

Semenowicz-Siuda, K., Markiewicz, A. and Korczynska-Wardecka, J. (1984) 'Circadian bioavailability and some effects of propranolol in healthy subjects and in liver cirrhosis', *Internat. J. Clin. Pharmacol. Ther. Toxicol.* 22: 653–8.

Shah, R. R., Oates, N. S., Idle, J. R., Smith, R. L. and Lockhart, J. D. (1982) 'Impaired oxidation of debrisoquine in patients with perhexiline neuropathy', *Br. Med. J. Clin. Res.* 284: 295–9.

Shaheen, O., Biollaz, J., Koshakji, R. P., Wilkinson, G. R. and Wood, A. J. J. (1989) 'Influence of debrisoquin phenotype on the inducibility of propranolol meta-bolism', *Clin. Pharmacol. Ther.* 45: 439–43.

Shand, D. G. and Ragno, R. E. (1972) 'The disposition of propranolol. I. Elimination during oral absorption in man', *Pharmacology* 7: 159–68.

Sherlock, S., Bearn, A. G., Billing, B. H. and Patterson, J. C. S. (1950) 'Splanchnic blood flow in man by the bromosulphalein method: the relation of peripheral plasma bromosulphalein level to the calculated flow', *J. Lab. Clin. Med.* 35: 923–32.

Shimada, T., Yamazaki, H., Mimura, M., Inui, Y. and Guengerich, F.P. (1994) 'Interindividual variations in human liver cytochrome P-450 enzymes involved in oxidation of drugs, carcinogens and toxic chemicals: studies with liver microsomes of 30 Japanese and 30 Caucasians', *J. Pharmacol. Ther.* **270**: 414–22.

Siddoway, L. A., Thompson, K. A., McAllister, C. B., Wang; T., Wilkinson, G. R., Roden, D. M. and Woosley, R. L. (1987) 'Polymorphism of propafenone metabolism and disposition in man: clinical and pharmacokinetic consequences', *Circulation* **75**: 785–91.

Silber, B., Holford, N. H. G. and Riegelman, S. (1982) 'Stereoselective disposition and glucuronidation of propranolol in humans', *J. Pharm. Sci.* **71**: 699–704.

Somogyi, A., Albrecht, M., Kliems, G., Schäfer, K. and Eichelbaum, M. (1981) 'Pharmacokinetics, bioavailability and ECG response of verapamil in patients with liver cirrhosis', *Br. J. Clin. Pharmacol.* **12**: 51–60.

Sotaniemi, E. A., Arranto, A. J., Pelkonen, O. and Pasanen, M. (1997) 'Age and cytochrome P450–linked drug metabolism in humans: an analysis of 226 subjects with equal histopathologic conditions', *Clin. Pharmcol. Ther.* **61**: 331–9.

Sotaniemi, E. A., Rautio, A., Bäckstrom, M., Arvela, P. and Pelkonen, O. (1995) 'CYP3A4 and CYP2A6 activities marked by the metabolism of lignocaine and coumarin in patients with liver and kidney diseases and epileptic patients', *Br. J. Clin. Pharmacol.* **39**: 71–6.

Thompson, K. A., Iansmith, D. H. S., Siddoway, L. A., Woosley, R. L. and Roden, D. M. (1988) 'Potent electrophysiologic effects of the major metabolites of propafenone in canine Purkinje fibers', *J. Pharmacol. Exp. Ther.* **244**: 950–5.

Thomson, P. D., Melmon, K. L., Richardson, J. A., Cohn, K., Steinbrunn, W., Cudihee, R. and Rowland, M. (1973) 'Lidocaine pharmacokinetics in advanced heart failure, liver disease, and renal failure in humans', *Ann. Intern. Med.* **78**: 499–508.

Tumer, N, Scarpace, P. J. and Lowenthal, D. T. (1992) 'Geriatric pharmacology: basic and clinical consideration', *Annu. Rev. Pharmacol. Toxicol.* **32**: 271–303.

Vesell, E. S. (1991) 'The model drug approach in clinical pharmacology', *Clin. Pharmacol. Ther.* **50**: 239–48.

Vestal, R. E., Wood, A. J. J., Branch, R. A., Shand, D. G. and Wilkinson, G. R. (1979) 'Effect of age and cigarette smoking on propranolol disposition', *Clin. Pharmacol. Ther.* **26**: 8–15.

Vogelsang, B., Echizen, H., Schmidt, E. and Eichelbaum, M. (1984) 'Stereoselective first pass metabolism of highly cleared drugs: studies on the bioavailability of L- and D-verapamil examined with a stable isotope technique', *Br. J. Clin. Pharmacol.* **18**: 733–40.

Vozeh, S., Haefeli, W., Ha, H.-R., Vlcek, J. and Follath, F. (1990) 'Nonlinear kinetics of propafenone metabolites in healthy man', *Eur. J. Clin. Pharmacol.* **38**: 509–13.

Walle, T., Byington, R. P., Fuhrberg, C. D., McIntyre, K. M. and Vokonas, P. S. (1985) 'Biologic determinants of propranolol disposition: results from 1308 patients in the beta-blocker heart attack trial', *Clin. Pharmacol. Ther.* **38**: 509–18.

Walle, T., Fagan, T. C., Conradi, E. C., Walle, U. K. and Gaffney, T. E. (1979) 'Presystemic and systemic glucuronidation of propranolol', *Clin. Pharmacol.* **26**: 167–72.

Walle, U. K., Oehlenschlager, W. F. and Walle, T. (1986) 'Oxidative metabolism of propranolol is catalyzed by two different P-450 activities', *Pharmacologist* **28**: 216.

Walle, U. K., Walle, T., Bai, S. and Olanoff, S. (1983) 'Stereoselective binding of propranolol to human plasma, alpha-1–acid glycoprotein, and albumin', *Clin. Pharmacol. Ther.* **34**: 718–23.

Walle, T., Walle, K., Cowart, D. and Conradi, E. C. (1989) 'Pathway-selective sex differences in the metabolic clearance of propranolol in human subjects', *Clin. Pharmacol. Ther.* **46**: 257–63.

Walle, T., Walle, U. K., Cowart, T. D., Conradi, E. C. and Gaffney, T. E. (1987) 'Selective induction of propranolol metabolism by smoking: additional effects on renal clearance of metabolites', *J. Pharmacol. Exp. Ther.* **241**: 928–33.

Walle, T., Walle, U. K. and Olanoff, L. S. (1985) 'Quantitative account of propranolol metabolism in urine of normal man', *Drug Metab. Dispos.* **13**: 204–9.

Walle, T., Walle, U. K., Wilson, M. J., Fagan, T. C. and Gaffney, T. E. (1984) 'Stereoselective ring oxidation of propranolol in man', *Br. J. Clin. Pharmacol.* **18**: 741–7.

Walter-Sack, I. and Klotz, U. (1996) 'Influence of diet and nutritional status on drug metabolism', *Clin. Pharmacokinet.* **31**: 47–64.

Ward, S. A., Walle, T., Walle, U. K., Wilkinson, G. R. and Branch, R. A. (1989) 'Propranolol's metabolism is determined by both mephenytoin and debrisoquine hydroxylase activities', *Clin. Pharmacol. Ther.* **45**: 72–9.

Wilkinson, G. R. (1987) 'Clearance approaches in pharmacology', *Pharmacol. Rev.* **39**: 1–47.

Wilkinson, G. R. (1997) 'The effects of diet, aging and disease-states on pre-systemic elimination and oral bioavailability in humans', *Adv. Drug Delivery Rev.* **27**: 129–59.

Wing, L. M. H., Miners, J. O., Birkett, J., Foenander, T., Lillywhite, K. and Wanwimolrok, S. (1984) 'Lidocaine disposition – sex differences and effects of cimetidine', *Clin. Pharmacol. Ther.* **35**: 695–701.

Wong, Y. S. and Hurwitz, A. (1985) 'Simple method for maintaining serum lidocaine levels in the therapeutic range', *Arch. Intern. Med.* **145**: 1588–91.

Wood, A. J. J., Kornhauser, D. M., Wilkinson, G. R., Shand, D. G. and Branch, R. A. (1978) 'The influence of cirrhosis on steady-state blood concentrations of unbound propranolol after oral administration', *Clin. Pharmacokinet.* **3**: 478–87.

Wood, A. J. J. and Zhou, H.-H. (1991) 'Ethnic differences in drug disposition and responsiveness', *Clin. Pharmacokinet.* **20**: 350–73.

Woodcock, B. G., Rietbrock, I., Vöhringer, H. F. and Rietbrock, N. (1981a) 'Verapamil disposition in liver disease and intensive-care patients: kinetics, clearance and apparent blood flow relationships', *Clin. Pharmacol. Ther.* **29**: 27–34.

Woodcock, B. G., Schulz, W., Kober, G. and Rietbrock, N. (1981b) 'Direct determination of hepatic extraction of verapamil in cardiac patients', *Clin. Pharmacol. Ther.* **30**: 52–6.

Woodhouse, K. and Wynne, H. A. (1992) 'Age-related changes in hepatic function. Implications for drug therapy', *Drugs Aging* **2**: 243–55.

Zhou, H.-H., Kozhakji, R. P., Silberstein, D. J., Wilkinson, G. R. and Wood, A. J. J. (1989) 'Racial differences in drug response. Altered sensitivity to and clearance of propranolol in men of Chinese descent as compared with American whites', *N. Engl. J. Med.* **320**: 565–70.

Zhou, H.-H. and Wood, A. J. J. (1990) 'Differences in stereoselective disposition of propranolol do not explain sensitivity differences between white and Chinese subjects: correlation between the clearance of (−) and (+)-propranolol', *Clin. Pharmacol. Ther.* **47**: 719–23.

Chapter 6

Interindividual variability in the metabolism of anti-epileptic drugs and its clinical implications

G. Gatti, M. Furlanut and E. Perucca

It is difficult to think of a disease which has benefited more than epilepsy from advances in clinical pharmacological knowledge. The contribution of clinical pharmacology to an improved treatment of epilepsy originated in the late 1960s with the demonstration that the pharmacokinetics of anti-epileptic drugs (AEDs) show a large variability, and that this plays a major role in determining interindividual differences in drug response (Perucca and Richens, 1981). This, in turn, led to the development of therapeutic drug monitoring as an aid for the individualisation of dosage and to a greater understanding of the role of genetic, developmental and environmental factors affecting the kinetics of anti-epileptic drugs. This information has been applied on a vast scale to rationalise treatment schedules and to improve the quality of care for people with epilepsy (Eadie, 1998; Jannuzzi *et al.*, 2000).

Among factors affecting the variability in the kinetics of anti-epileptic drugs, differences in rate of drug metabolism are by far the most important (Perucca and Richens, 1995; Perucca, 1999; Tanaka, 1999). Changes in biotransformation rate under the influence of age, disease and drug interactions are commonplace in patients with epilepsy, and their characterisation has major implications for the implementation of a correct dosing schedule. The present chapter will provide a concise overview of the role of drug metabolism in the disposition of individual anticonvulsants, and its implications for a rational use of these drugs in clinical practice.

Phenytoin

The advent of phenytoin in 1938 provided a major breakthrough in epilepsy treatment, because it led to the demonstration that seizure protection can be achieved effectively without inducing sedation. Because of its effectiveness against partial and generalised tonic-clonic seizures, phenytoin was prescribed widely and it soon became clear that it also had the potential of causing troublesome side-effects such as dizziness, incoordination and cognitive impairment. Both therapeutic and toxic effects were clearly dependent on dosage, and it was surprising that in many individuals small changes in dosage caused disproportionately large changes in clinical response.

Extensive work carried out by clinical pharmacologists in the early 1970s led to the demonstration that a peculiar metabolic pattern is responsible for the unusual dose–response relationship. Unlike most other drugs, phenytoin shows saturable metabolism within the therapeutic dose range, resulting in a non-linear relationship between steady-state serum concentration and dosage (Perucca *et al.*, 1978a). When the enzyme system responsible for phenytoin metabolism becomes progressively saturated, small increments in dosage produce a disproportionate rise in serum drug concentration with the attendant risk of toxicity (Richens and Dunlop, 1975). Since the dosage at which enzyme saturation occurs varies from one subject to another (Figure 6.1), this metabolic pattern is also responsible for the wide variation in serum drug concentrations among patients receiving the same daily dosage (Figure 6.2). Under saturation conditions, elimination is not log-linear and a true half-life can not be calculated for phenytoin; however, estimates based on the decay of radioactivity after a

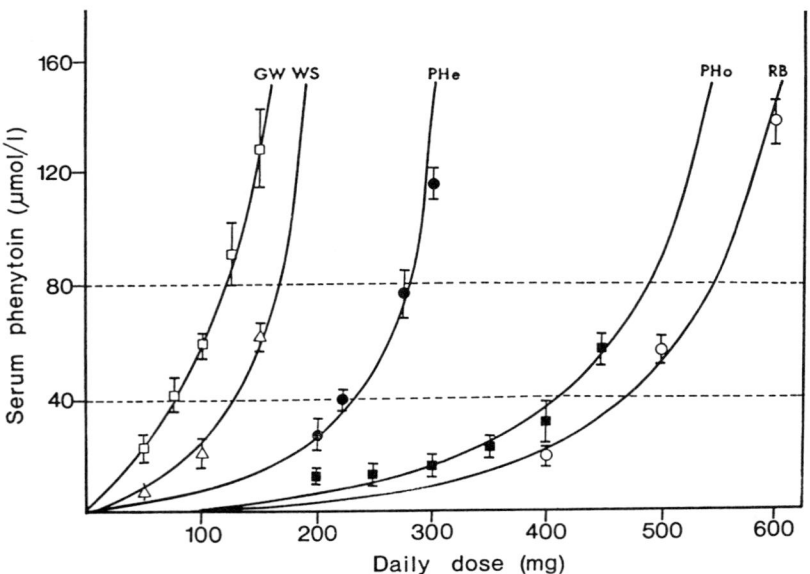

Figure 6.1 Relationship between steady-state serum phenytoin concentration and dosage in five patients with epilepsy. Each value is the mean±SD of three to eight separate determinations at each dose. Horizontal lines indicate the commonly quoted range of optimal concentrations. Modified from Richens and Dunlop, 1975, with permission.

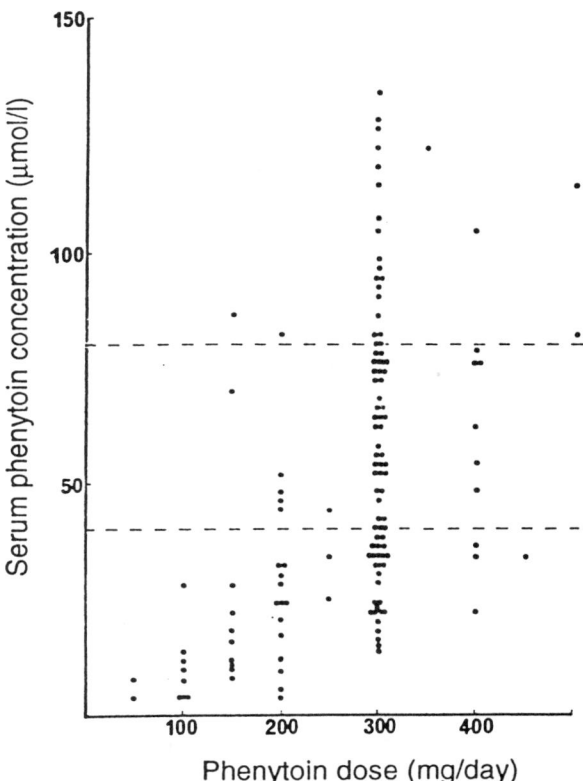

Figure 6.2 Variability in serum phenytoin concentration in 137 patients with epilepsy stabilised on chronic treatment. Horizontal lines indicate the commonly quoted range of optimal concentrations. Reproduced from Perucca and Richens, 1983, with permission.

tracer dose of carbon-labelled drug in chronically treated patients show half-lives in the range of 8 to 140 h, the longest values being observed in patients with high steady-state serum concentrations (>80 μmol/l) (Richens, 1979).

The rate of phenytoin metabolism is also subject to considerable variation under the influence of pathophysiological factors and drug interactions (Table 6.1). In particular, metabolism is faster during childhood (Battino *et al.*, 1995), pregnancy (Perucca, 1987) and, possibly, female gender (Benetello *et al.*, 1987). Administration of folic acid may stimulate phenytoin metabolism (Furlanut *et al.*, 1978), whereas a slower clearance rate is observed in patients comedicated with a number of drugs, including felbamate, sulthiame, fluoxetine, viloxazine, phenylbutazone, isoniazid, chloramphenicol, disulfiram, omeprazole, some sulphonamides, miconazole,

Table 6.1 A list of factors affecting the metabolism of the major AEDs

Drug	Main conditions associated with enhanced (↑) or reduced (↓) metabolic rate	Examples of exogenous compounds causing enhanced (↑) or reduced (↓) metabolic rate
Phenytoin	(↑) childhood[a] (↑) pregnancy (↓) CYP2C19 poor metaboliser status (↓) elderly	(↑) folic acid (↓) allopurinol, amiodarone, amitriptyline, azapropazone, bishydroxycoumarin, chloramphenicol, cimetidine, dicoumarol, diltiazem, disulfiram, erythromycin, felbamate, fluconazole, fluoxetine, fluvoxamine, isoniazid, miconazole, omeprazole, phencoupromon, phenylbutazone, propoxyphene, sertraline, some sulphonamides, sulphinpyrazone, sulthiame, tamoxifen, ticlopidine, viloxazine
Carbamazepine	(↑) childhood (↑) pregnancy (↓) elderly	(↑) carbamazepine (autoinduction), felbamate, phenobarbital, phenytoin, primidone (↓) cimetidine, danazol, diltiazem, erythromycin, fluconazole, grapefruit juice, isoniazid, ketoconazole, metronidazol, nefazodone, progabide[b], propoxyphene, remacemide, sertraline, troleandomycin, valnoctamide[b], valproic acid[b], valpromide[b], verapamil, viloxazine
Oxcarbazepine	(↑) childhood (MHD metabolism)	(↑) phenobarbital, phenytoin (inducers of MHD metabolism)
Valproic acid	(↑) childhood[a] (↓) elderly	(↑) carbamazepine, phenytoin, phenobarbital, primidone, rifampicin, cigarette smoking (↓) chlorpromazine, cimetidine, clobazam, erythromycin, felbamate, fluoxetine, isoniazid
Phenobarbital	(↑) childhood[a] (↓) perinatal asphyxia (↓) hepatic cirrhosis	(↑) rifampicin, folic acid (↓) chloramphenicol, dextropropoxyphene, dicoumarol, felbamate, influenza vaccine, isoniazid, phenytoin, quinine, valproic acid
Primidone[c]	(↑) childhood (↓) pregnancy	(↑) carbamazepine, phenobarbital, phenytoin (↓) chloramphenicol, methsuximide, isoniazid, nicotinamide
Ethosuximide	(↑) childhood	(↑) carbamazepine, phenytoin, phenobarbital, primidone, rifampicin (↓) isoniazid (?), valproic acid

Table 6.1 (continued)

Drug	Main conditions associated with enhanced (↑) or reduced (↓) metabolic rate	Examples of exogenous compounds causing enhanced (↑) or reduced (↓) metabolic rate
Lamotrigine	(↑) childhood (↑) pregnancy (↓) elderly (↓) Gilbert's syndrome (↓) hepatic cirrhosis	(↑) carbamazepine, phenytoin, phenobarbital, primidone, oxcarbazepine (↓) valproic acid, sertraline
Topiramate	(↑) childhood	(↑) carbamazepine, phenobarbital (?), phenytoin
Tiagabine	(↑) childhood (↓) severe liver disease	(↑) carbamazepine, phenobarbital, phenytoin, primidone
Felbamate	(↑) childhood	(↑) carbamazepine, phenytoin, phenobarbital (↓) valproic acid
Zonisamide	(↑) childhood	(↑) carbamazepine, phenobarbital, phenytoin, primidone (↓) ketoconazole[d], miconazole[d], cyclosporin A[d]

Notes
[a]Premature newborns may exhibit decreased metabolic capacity.
[b]Inhibitors of epoxide hydrolase and carbamazepine-10,11-epoxide metabolism.
[c]For factors affecting the biotransformation of metabolically derived phenobarbital, see phenobarbital.
[d]Predictions based on *in vitro* data.

fluconazole, azapropazone, propoxyphene, cimetidine, amiodarone, diltiazem and ticlopidine (Anderson and Graves, 1994; Anderson, 1998; Donahue *et al.*, 1999; Klaassen, 1998; Pisani *et al.*, 1990). Genetically determined impairment of phenytoin metabolism has been also described (Kutt *et al.*, 1964).

Like carbamazepine and barbiturates, phenytoin is a potent inducer of oxidative drug metabolism, with special reference to reactions mediated by cytochrome P450 (CYP) (Perucca and Richens, 1995). The P450 isoenzymes responsible for phenytoin metabolism are being elucidated (Table 6.2). The main metabolic pathway, which involves parahydroxylation, appears to be catalysed by cytochromes CYP2C9, CYP2C18 and CYP2C19 (Levy and Bajpai, 1995; Bajpai *et al.*, 1996; Mamiya *et al.*, 1998). Parahydroxylation gives rise to two enantiomers, (R)- and (S)-p-5-hydroxyphenyl-5-phenyl-hydantoin (pHPPH), and metabolism is stereoselective. Evidence has been provided that CYP2C9 favors the formation of (S)-pHPPH, while the formation of (R)-pHPPH is catalysed preferentially by CYP2C18 and CYP2C19 (Bajpai *et al.*, 1996, Mamiya *et al.*, 1998) and cosegregates with

Table 6.2 AED metabolites and, in brackets, enzymes involved in their formation

Drug	Reaction	Metabolites (enzymes)
Phenytoin	p-hydroxylation[a,b]	**(S)-pHPPH,** (R)-pHPPH (**CYP2C18, CYP2C19, CYP2C9**)
	hydrolysis[a]	(R),(S)-dihydrodiol (epoxide hydrolase)
		other minor metabolites (including reactive intermediates)
Carbamazepine	epoxidation	**carbamazepine-10,11-epoxide**[c] (**CYP3A4,** CYP2C8)
	hydrolysis[d]	trans-dihydrodiol (epoxide hydrolase)
	aromatic hydroxylation	2- and 3-hydroxy-carbamazepine (CYP1A2)
	conjugation	N-glucuronide
		other minor metabolites (including reactive intermediates)
Oxcarbazepine	reduction	**monohydroxycarbazepine**[c] (**arylketone reductase**)
	conjugation [e]	MHD glucuronide (uridine diphosphoglucuronosyltransferase)
		other minor metabolites
Valproic acid	conjugation	**glucuronide (uridine diphosphoglucuronosyltransferase)**
	beta oxidation	2-en-valproic acid [c], 3-hydroxy-valproic acid, 3-oxo-valproic acid
	hydroxylation	3- , 4- and 5-hydroxy-valproic acid (CYPs)
	desaturation	4-en-valproic acid (CYPs)
		other minor metabolites
Phenobarbital	p-hydroxylation[a]	**p-hydroxy-phenobarbital (CYP2C9,** CYP2C19, CYP2E1)
	conjugation	N-glucoside
		other minor metabolites (including reactive intermediates)
Primidone	oxidation	**phenobarbital**[c,f]
	cleavage of pyrimidine ring	**phenylethylmalonamide (PEMA)**[c]
		other minor metabolites
Methylpheno barbital[b]	hydroxylation	aromatic metabolites (CYP2C19)
	demethylation	**phenobarbital**[c,f]
	conjugation	N-glucosides and glucuronides
Ethosuximide	oxidation	**2-(1-hydroxyethyl)-2-methylsuccinimide (CYP3A4,** CYP2E, CYP2B, CYP2C)
		2-ethyl-3-hydroxy-2-methylsuccinimide (as above)
		2-(2-hydroxyethyl)-2-methylsuccinimide (as above)
		other minor metabolites

Table 6.2 (continued)

Drug	Reaction	Metabolites (enzymes)
Lamotrigine	conjugation	**2-N-** and 5-N-glucuronide (uridine diphosphoglucuronosyl-transferase) other minor metabolites
Vigabatrin	–	not significantly metabolised
Gabapentin	–	not metabolised
Topiramate	hydroxylation	products hydroxylated at the isopropylidene groups
	hydrolysis	products cleaved at the isopropylidene groups other minor metabolites
Tiagabine	hydroxylation	5-oxo-tiagabine (CYP3A4) other minor metabolites
Felbamate	hydroxylation	p-hydroxy-phenyl-felbamate (CYP2E1, CYP3A4) 2-hydroxy-felbamate (CYP2E1, CYP3A4) other minor metabolites (including reactive intermediates)
Zonisamide	acetylation reduction	N-acetyl-zonisamide (N-acetyl-transferase) 2-sulphamoylacetylphenol (**CYP3A4**, CYP2C19, CYP3A5) other metabolites (see text)

Notes

[a] Reaction preceded by formation of an unstable epoxide intermediate.
[b] Metabolism is stereoselective (see text).
[c] Active metabolite.
[d] Carbamazepine-10,11–epoxide is substrate for this reaction.
[e] Monohydroxycarbazepine (MHD) is substrate for this reaction.
[f] See phenobarbital for further metabolic reactions.
Most important metabolites and enzymes are shown in bold. Most phase I metabolites are excreted as conjugates.

CYP2C19 oxidation polymorphism (Ieiri *et al.*, 1997; Mamiya *et al.*, 1997). Saturation of CYP2C9 appears to be responsible for the Michaelis–Menten kinetics of phenytoin, whereas CYP2C19 (and possibly CYP2C18) is not saturable at therapeutic drug concentrations. These observations explain the increasing fractional contribution of CYP2C19 to phenytoin metabolism with increasing dosage (Bajpai *et al.*, 1996). In patients with genetically determined deficiency of CYP2C19 activity (who may also show impaired CYP2C18 activity, due to the linked gene mutations of CYP2C19 and CYP2C18) (Mamiya *et al.*, 1998), CYP2C9 becomes the key enzyme responsible for phenytoin elimination. Ninomiya *et al.* (2000), also described a patient with genetically determined mutations in the alleles of both CYP2C9 and CYP2C19, who became intoxicated with high serum phenytoin levels (32.6 µg/ml) while receiving a small dosage (187.5 mg/day) of the drug. Evidence is also available that phenytoin oxidation may involve the formation of an arene oxide intermediate, which may play a role in mediating adverse reactions such as teratogenicity (Krauer and Dayer, 1991), hepatotoxicity (Spielberg *et al.*, 1981; Larrey and Pageaux, 1997) and aplastic anemia (Gerson *et al.*, 1983).

Because of its narrow therapeutic index and occurrence of saturation metabolism, individualising phenytoin dosage is greatly aided by monitoring serum drug concentrations. There is evidence that an optimal response is achieved often at serum concentrations between 40 and 80 µmol/l (10–20 µg/ml), but many patients do well at concentrations outside this range (Perucca and Richens, 1981; Eadie, 1998).

Fosphenytoin

Fosphenytoin, the disodium phosphate ester of 3-hydroxymethyl-5,5-diphenylhydantoin, was developed as a water soluble phenytoin prodrug with improved tolerability over existing injectable formulations of phenytoin. After intramuscular and intravenous administration, fosphenytoin is rapidly converted to phenytoin by esterases present in blood and other tissues (Perucca and Bialer, 1996). After conversion to phenytoin, the pharmacokinetics of fosphenytoin is identical to that of phenytoin.

Carbamazepine

Carbamazepine is regarded by many neurologists as the drug of choice for partial seizures (with or without secondary generalization), but it may also be useful for primary generalised tonic–clonic seizures not complicated by other seizure types.

Like phenytoin, carbamazepine is eliminated primarily by biotransformation. The main pathway involves conversion to the active metabolite carbamazepine-10,11-epoxide (CBZ-E), which is then hydrolysed to a trans-dihydrodiol (Bertilsson and Tomson, 1986). The isoenzymes responsible for conversion to the epoxide are CYP3A4 and, to a lesser extent, CYP2C8 (Kerr *et al.*, 1994), while hydration of carbamazepine-10,11-epoxide to the diol is catalysed by epoxide hydrolase (Table 6.2). Less important routes of carbamazepine biotransformation are aromatic hydroxylation, catalysed by CYP1A2, and direct conjugation with glucuronic acid (Bertilsson and Tomson, 1986; Morselli, 1995). As with phenytoin, reactive intermediates formed during oxidative metabolism have been implicated in the pathogenesis of idiosyncratic adverse drug reactions (Pirmohamed *et al.*, 1991; Larrey and Pageaux, 1997).

The metabolism of carbamazepine shows considerable inter-subject variability, resulting in a wide scatter of serum drug concentrations among patients receiving the same dosage (Figure 6.3). Both the epoxidation and the hydration steps undergo autoinduction during chronic treatment: as a result, the half-life of carbamazepine is much shorter after repeated administration (5–20 h) than after a single dose (20–55 h). During chronic treatment, the shortest half-lives are recorded in patients receiving concomitant enzyme-inducing agents such as phenytoin and barbiturates (Spina et al., 1996). Compared with adults, children metabolise carbamazepine at a faster rate and therefore require larger dosages on a body weight basis (Battino et al., 1995). In one cross-sectional pediatric study, boys have been reported to have higher clearance rates than girls (Furlanut et al., 1985). Pregnancy may also be associated with increased carbamazepine metabolism (Perucca, 1987).

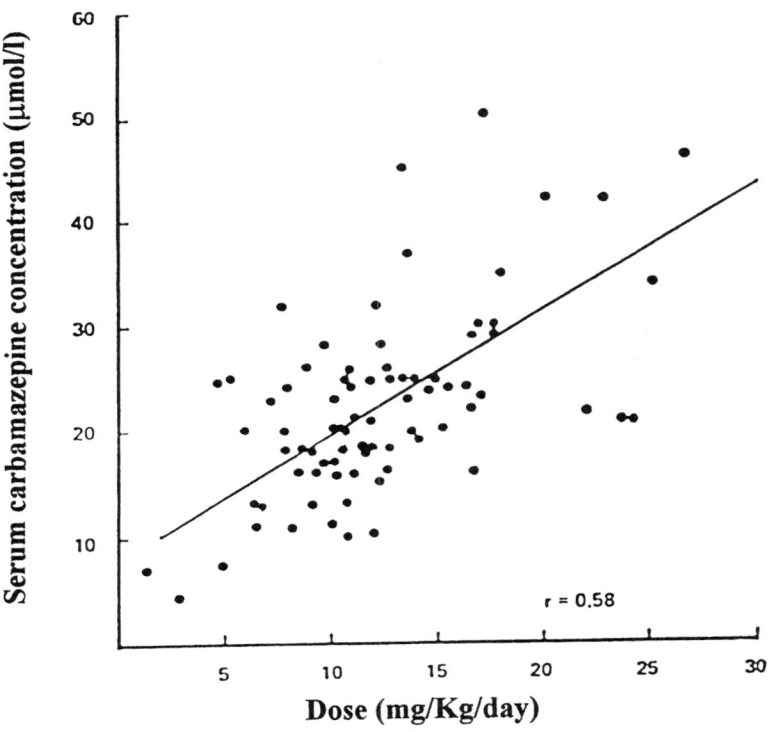

Figure 6.3 Variability in steady-state serum carbamazepine concentration as a function of the prescribed daily dosage in eighty adult patients with epilepsy. Most patients were receiving combination therapy with phenytoin or barbiturates. Reproduced from Perucca et al., 1978b, with permission.

The biotransformation of carbamazepine is highly susceptible to interactions with other drugs. As mentioned above, phenytoin, phenobarbital and primidone induce the metabolic elimination of carbamazepine and decrease its serum levels at steady-state. Conversely, carbamazepine metabolism may be inhibited by remacemide, macrolide antibiotics, isoniazid, metronidazol, certain antidepressants, verapamil, diltiazem, cimetidine, danazol, propoxyphene and, possibly, fluconazole (Spina et al., 1996; Nair and Morris, 1999) (Table 6.1). Valproic acid, valpromide, valnoctamide and progabide are inhibitors of epoxide hydrolase and may cause toxic symptoms by increasing the serum concentration of carbamazepine-10,11-epoxide (Pisani et al., 1986; Spina et al., 1996).

Since autoinduction of carbamazepine metabolism is dose-dependent, serum carbamazepine levels are non-linearly related to dose, with the change in serum drug concentration being smaller than expected from the dose increment (Perucca et al., 1980; Kudriakova et al., 1992). Most patients respond at serum drug concentrations of 17 to 47 µmol/l (4–11 µg/ml), but there are subjects who require concentrations below or above this range (Perucca and Richens, 1980; Eadie, 1998).

Oxcarbazepine

Oxcarbazepine, the 10-keto analogue of carbamazepine, has an efficacy spectrum similar to carbamazepine. Oxcarbazepine is a typical example of a drug for which factors related to metabolic disposition played an important part in the decision to proceed with development. Unlike carbamazepine which is metabolised primarily by oxidation, oxcarbazepine undergoes rapid reductive transformation to the active metabolite monohydroxycarbazepine (MHD), for which it is considered as a pro-drug (Faigle and Menge, 1990; Grant and Faulds, 1992). Conversion to MHD leads to introduction of a chiral site, and there is evidence that the enzymatic process is stereoselective and leads to preferential accumulation of S-MHD (Volosov et al., 1999). There are no major pharmacodynamic differences between the two enantiomers of the MHD metabolite (Schachter, 1999). MHD is eliminated mainly by conjugation, with a half-life of 10 to 20 h. Oxcarbazepine also differs from carbamazepine in that it does not give rise to a stable epoxide intermediate (Table 6.2). The metabolic differences between oxcarbazepine and carbamazepine lead to several pharmacokinetic advantages for the former drug, including a longer half-life, lack of autoinduction, lesser variability in pharmacokinetics and lower susceptibility to drug interactions (Baruzzi et al., 1994; Lloyd et al., 1994; Tecoma, 1999). When patients are switched from carbamazepine to oxcarbazepine, gradual loss of enzyme induction may lead to changes in the serum concentrations of concomitant antiepileptic drugs and some endogenous substrates (Isojärvi et al., 1994, 1995). The serum concentration of MHD may be reduced moderately by enzyme inducing anti-convulsants, but the extent of interaction is much lower compared with that observed with carbamazepine (Tartara *et al.* 1993). Overall, these properties facilitate the clinical use of oxcarbazepine, whose dosage can be adjusted without the need for therapeutic drug monitoring. Compared with carbamazepine, oxcarbazepine appears to be less likely to cause hypersensitivity reactions (Grant and Faulds, 1992). This may also be a consequence of metabolic differences, in view of the evidence that some idiosyncratic reactions to both drugs may be mediated by a toxic reactive metabolite (Shear *et al.*, 1988; Pirmohamed *et al.*, 1991).

Valproic acid

Valproic acid, a broad-spectrum antiepileptic drug, is also eliminated virtually entirely by metabolism. The predominant pathway is conjugation with glucuronic acid (Table 6.2), but beta, omega, omega-1 and omega-2 oxidation (and probably other minor pathways) also play a significant role (Davis *et al.*, 1994). The metabolite 2-en-valproic acid retains anticonvulsant properties, while another metabolite (4-en-valproic acid) has hepatotoxic and embryotoxic activity. The contribution of these compounds to the adverse potential of valproic acid is uncertain, but it cannot be excluded that increased conversion to toxic metabolites is the underlying mechanism for the increased susceptibility to valproate-associated hepatotoxicity in children receiving combination therapy with enzyme inducers (Kondo *et al.*, 1990).

The half-life of valproic acid is usually in the range of 8 to 16 h, the shortest values being recorded in patients taking enzyme-inducing agents. Compared with adults, children metabolise valproic acid at a faster rate and require larger dosages on a body weight basis (Zaccara *et al.*, 1988), while metabolism may be slower in the elderly (Perucca *et al.*, 1984). Valproic acid clearance may increase during pregnancy, but the reduction in serum valproic acid concentration in pregnant women is related predominantly to a decrease in its binding to plasma proteins (Perucca, 1987). Numerous drugs affect valproic acid metabolism (Table 6.1). In particular, metabolism is accelerated by carbamazepine, phenytoin and barbiturates and may be reduced by felbamate, isoniazid, fluoxetine and chlorpromazine (Perucca, 1996a).

Because of the variability in metabolic rate, patients receiving the same dosage exhibit wide differences in serum valproic acid concentration. The proposed range of optimal serum valproic acid concentrations is 350–700 µmol/l (50–100 µg/ml), but the relationship between serum concentration and clinical effect is rather poor and the monitoring of serum valproic acid levels is of limited value in clinical practice (Perucca and Richens, 1981).

Phenobarbital

Phenobarbital was introduced in therapeutic practice in 1912 and is still widely used in the management of partial and generalised seizures, except absence seizures.

The elimination of phenobarbital is partly by biotransformation and partly by renal excretion. Between 11 and 55% of an administered dose is excreted unchanged in urine, while the remainder is metabolised to p-hydroxy-phenobarbital, phenobarbital N-glucoside and other metabolites (Anderson and Levy, 1995). The oxidation pathways appear to involve cytochromes CYP2C9 (Table 6.2) and, to a lesser extent, CYP2C19 (Mamiya et al., 2000) and CYP2E1 (Hurst et al., 1997). Formation of an arene oxide intermediate has been implicated in certain hypersensitivity reactions to phenobarbital, including liver damage (Larrey and Pageaux, 1997).

The half-life of phenobarbital in adults ranges from 75 to 125 h. Elimination is slower in premature newborns, whereas children metabolise the drug at a faster rate compared with adults (Battino et al., 1995). Drugs which have been reported to inhibit phenobarbital metabolism include valproic acid (through inhibition of CYP2C9-mediated parahydroxylation), felbamate, phenytoin, propoxyphene and chloramphenicol (Table 6.1) (Pisani et al., 1990; Anderson and Graves, 1994; Hurst et al., 1997).

The optimal range of serum phenobarbital concentrations quoted in the literature is usually 40 to 170 μmol/l (10–40 μg/ml), but there is a wide variation in the levels at which therapeutic and toxic effects are observed. This is partly related to occurrence of pharmacodynamic tolerance to the sedative effect during repeated dosing (Butler et al., 1954).

Primidone

Primidone, the 2-deoxy analogue of phenobarbital, is partly excreted unchanged in urine (approximately 50% of the dose) and partly metabolised to phenylethylmalonamide (PEMA) and phenobarbital (Kauffman et al., 1977). Its half-life ranges from 4 to 22 h, the shortest values being recorded in patients on enzyme-inducing anticonvulsants (Cloyd et al., 1981). Much of the therapeutic and toxic effects of primidone are ascribed to metabolically derived phenobarbital, the contribution of the parent drug to overall pharmacological activity being unclear. Carbamazepine and phenytoin accelerate the conversion of primidone to phenobarbital (Pisani et al., 1990). Conversely, inhibition of primidone metabolism may be caused by methsuximide, isoniazid and nicotinamide (Table 6.1).

Methylphenobarbital

Methylphenobarbital is a racemic mixture of two enantiomers which exhibit marked stereoselectivity in their metabolism. While the R-enantiomer undergoes rapid CYP2C19-mediated aromatic hydroxylation (Jaqz *et al.*, 1986), the S-form is demethylated to phenobarbital, which accumulates in serum at high concentrations and is largely responsible for the pharmacological effects (Eadie and Hooper, 1995). CYP2C19 is a polymorphic enzyme and subjects with defective CYP2C19 activity are unable to hydroxylate efficiently the R-enantiomer which is then also converted to phenobarbital, whose concentrations may rise to potentially toxic levels. It is tempting to speculate that the reportedly higher frequency of adverse reactions to methylphenobarbital in Japanese can be explained by the higher prevalence of the poor CYP2C19 metaboliser phenotype in this ethnic group (Nakamura *et al.*, 1985).

Ethosuximide

Ethosuximide, the most widely used among succinimide drugs, is indicated for the management of absence seizures.

Only about 20% of an administered dose of ethosuximide is excreted unchanged in urine. The drug is extensively oxidised to a number of inactive metabolites, including the isomers of 2-(1-hydroxyethyl)-2-methyl-succinimide, 2-ethyl-3-hydroxy-2-methylsuccinimide, 2-(2-hydroxyethyl)-2-methylsuccinimide and minor metabolites (Goulet *et al.*, 1976; Bialer *et al.*, 1995). The main oxidation pathways are probably catalysed by cytochrome CYP3A4 and possibly, to a lesser extent, cytochromes CYP2E, CYP2B and/or CYP2C (Table 6.2) (Bialer *et al.*, 1995).

Ethosuximide exhibits variable pharmacokinetics, mainly as a result of interindividual differences in metabolic rate. The half-life of the drug averages 30 to 60 h in adults, while shorter values (30 to 40 h) are recorded in children (Bialer *et al.*, 1995). The metabolism of ethosuximide is inducible by concomitantly administered enzyme-inducing anticonvulsants such as carbamazepine, phenytoin and barbiturates (Table 6.1) (Giaccone *et al.*, 1996).

Ethosuximide dosage can usually be tailored on the basis of the clinical and EEG response, and monitoring of serum drug concentrations is usually unnecessary. Optimal responses are usually achieved in the range of 280 to 700 µmol/l (40–100 µg/ml), although some patients require concentrations outside this range.

Benzodiazepines

Benzodiazepines are of special value in the management of status epilepticus and they may also be used for chronic treatment in partial and generalised epilepsies, though their usefulness in long-term management is limited by side-effects and by possible loss of efficacy due to tolerance. Virtually all benzodiazepines are eliminated by biotransformation, the type of metabolic pathway and rate of elimination differing with different drugs. Half-lives are in the range of 2–3 h for midazolam, 8–25 h for lorazepam, 10–30 h for clobazam, 20–50 h for nitrazepam, 20–60 h for clonazepam and diazepam, and 30–100 h for N-desmethyldiazepam (Perucca, 1996a). Clobazam and diazepam have active metabolites with long half-lives which contribute significantly to overall pharmacological effect.

The relationship between serum benzodiazepine concentration and clinical response is rather poor and serum drug level monitoring is generally not indicated for these drugs.

Lamotrigine

Introduced into clinical practice in the early 1990s, lamotrigine is an important member of the new generation of anti-epileptic drugs. It has a broad spectrum of efficacy, and it is used primarily in the management of patients refractory to conventional agents (Goa et al., 1993).

The use of lamotrigine is complicated by considerable variability in its pharmacokinetics, largely due to the influence of drug interactions on its rate of metabolism (Goa et al., 1993; Fitton and Goa, 1995). Unlike most conventional anti-epileptic drugs, lamotrigine does not undergo oxidation but is eliminated virtually entirely by conjugation with glucuronic acid through a pathway which is stimulated by enzyme-inducing agents and inhibited by valproic acid (Tables 6.1, 6.2 and Figure 6.4). In patients receiving no concurrent treatment, its half-life is 20–30 h, but shorter values (10–20 h) are encountered in patients on phenytoin, carbamazepine or barbiturates. Oxcarbazepine also stimulates lamotrigine metabolism, though to a lesser extent compared with carbamazepine (Gatti et al., 2000; May et al., 1999). Conversely, half-life values of 50–70 h are observed in patients on valproic acid (Rambeck and Wolf, 1993). Patients receiving a combination of valproic acid and enzyme inducers have lamotrigine half-lives comparable to those recorded in patients on monotherapy. The same interactions are observed in children, who metabolise lamotrigine at a faster rate compared with adults (Figure 6.4). Pregnancy may also be associated with increased lamotrigine clearance (Tomson et al., 1997). Preliminary data suggest that lamotrigine metabolism may be inhibited by sertraline (Kaufman and Gerner, 1997).

The large variability in lamotrigine metabolic rate has important implications with respect to dosage requirements. In particular, patients comedicated with valproic acid need lower dosages compared with patients on monotherapy, whereas dose requirements are higher in patients on enzyme inducers. Patients with a slow rate of lamotrigine metabolism are at greater risk of adverse skin reactions at initiation of therapy, and lamotrigine dosage should be escalated very slowly when the drug is given

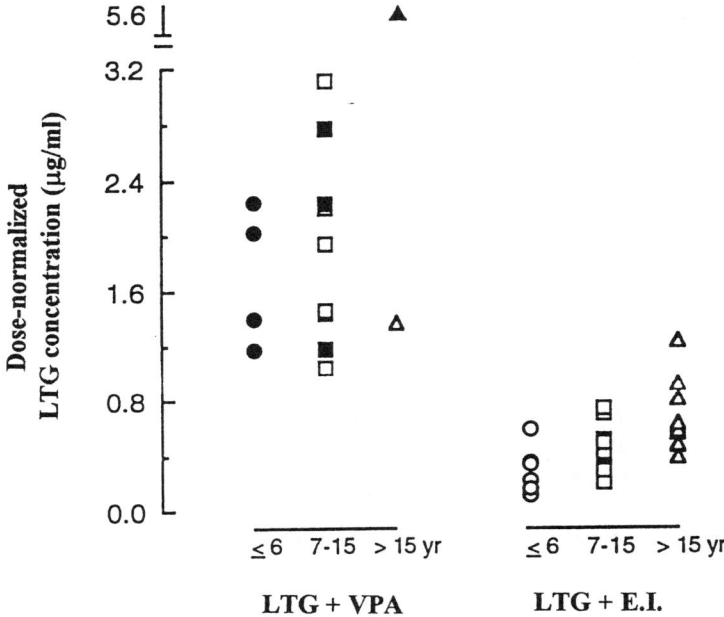

Figure 6.4 Scattergrams showing dose-normalised plasma lamotrigine (LTG) concentrations at steady-state in different age groups. Each dose-normalised concentration is the average of the values obtained in each patient by dividing the observed concentration(s) by the daily dosage (mg/kg). LTG+VPA refers to patients comedicated with sodium valproate, with (open symbols) or without (closed symbols) enzyme inducers (E.I.). LTG+E.I. refers to patients comedicated with enzyme inducers without valproate. Patients on valproate had significantly higher lamotrigine concentrations than patients in the corresponding age group receiving enzyme inducers without valproate. Among patients on enzyme inducers without valproate, lamotrigine concentrations were significantly lower in the younger age groups than in the group above 15 years. Reproduced from Bartoli *et al.*, 1997, with permission.

to subjects comedicated with valproate (Fitton and Goa, 1995). A therapeutic range of serum lamotrigine concentrations has not been clearly identified, and routine monitoring of serum levels is not recommended with this drug (Bartoli *et al.*, 1997).

Vigabatrin

Vigabatrin, an irreversible enzyme-activated suicide inhibitor of GABA transaminase (Grant and Heel, 1991), is used primarily in the management of refractory partial seizures (with or without secondary generalisation) and in the treatment of infantile spasms. Vigabatrin differs from most other anti-epileptic drugs in that it is extensively excreted unchanged in urine and it is not metabolised to any important extent (Rey *et al.*, 1992). Because of this, it shows relatively small kinetic variability. Its half-life is about 7 h, but duration of effect is prolonged due to its irreversible mode of action. There are currently no indications for the routine monitoring of serum vigabatrin levels other than as a check for compliance (Perucca, 2000).

Gabapentin

Gabapentin is a recently developed drug which is used mainly in the treatment of refractory partial seizures, with or without secondary generalization. Like vigabatrin, gabapentin is excreted in urine in unchanged form and its half-life is 5 to 7 h (Goa and Sorkin, 1993). Due to saturable absorption, serum gabapentin levels show considerable variability, but the clinical value of serum drug level monitoring has not been demonstrated. Possibly, monitoring serum gabapentin levels may be used in patients receiving large dosages, to determine whether a further dose increment can produce an increase in serum concentration despite saturable gastro-intestinal absorption (Perucca, 2000).

Topiramate

Together with tiagabine, topiramate is one of the latest additions to the therapeutic armamentarium against epilepsy. Topiramate seems to have a broad spectrum of efficacy, and it is used primarily in the treatment of refractory seizures.

The contribution of metabolism to topiramate elimination varies depending on type of comedication (Perucca and Bialer, 1996). In patients not receiving enzyme inducers, between 50 and 70% of an administered dose is excreted unchanged in urine and metabolic pathways involving hydroxylation and hydrolysis at the two isopropylidene groups (Table 6.1) account for less than 40% of drug clearance. However, in patients comedicated with phenytoin, carbamazepine and, presumably, barbiturates, metabolism becomes the main determinant of drug clearance and the fraction of the dose which is excreted unchanged in urine falls to 30% (Perucca, 1997).

The half-life of topiramate is about 20 to 30 h, but shorter values (about 12 h) are recorded in patients taking enzyme-inducing anticonvulsants. Topiramate is eliminated at a faster rate in children than in adults. For any given mg/kg dosage, serum topiramate concentrations are approximately 30% lower in children than in adults (Perucca, 1997; 1999).

A therapeutic range of serum topiramate concentrations has not yet been identified, and routine monitoring of serum drug levels is currently not indicated (Perucca, 2000).

Tiagabine

Tiagabine is an inhibitor of GABA reuptake which has been recently licensed for the add-on management of refractory partial seizures, with or without secondary generalisation (Brodie, 1997). Tiagabine is eliminated entirely by CYP3A-mediated biotransformation to inactive metabolites (Brodie, 1995; Adkins and Noble, 1998). Its half-life is about 5 to 9 h, but it is reduced to 2–3 h in patients taking enzyme-inducing anticonvulsants such as phenytoin, barbiturates or carbamazepine (Perucca, 1996b). A reduction in the rate of tiagabine metabolism would be expected with CYP3A inhibitors. Due to interindividual variation in CYP3A activity, patients receiving the same daily dosage show marked differences in tiagabine metabolism. A therapeutic range of serum tiagabine concentrations has not been identified, and individualisation of dosage should be based on clinical response (Perucca, 2000).

Felbamate

Felbamate was introduced into clinical practice in 1993 but its use has become markedly restricted due to a relatively high risk of aplastic anemia and fatal liver toxicity. Today, its main indication is the management of severe Lennox-Gastaut syndrome unresponsive to other available medications (Palmer and McTavish, 1993).

Felbamate is eliminated partly by renal excretion (about 50% of the dose) and partly by oxidative CYP2E1- and CYP3A4-mediated metabolism (Glue et al., 1997), with a half-life of 15 to 23 h. The shortest half-lives are recorded in patients comedicated with enzyme inducers. It has been suggested that formation of reactive metabolites may be involved in the idiosyncratic toxicity of felbamate, and studies designed to evaluate this possibility are in progress (Bialer et al., 1999). Although a therapeutic range of felbamate concentration of 50 to 110 mg/l in fasting morning samples has been proposed in a retrospective analysis (Troupin et al., 1997), further studies are required to confirm the potential usefulness of monitoring the serum levels of this drug.

Zonisamide

Zonisamide is a recently developed anti-epileptic drug which has been reported to have broad spectrum efficacy. It is currently licensed in Japan and South Korea (Seino et al., 1995).

Zonisamide undergoes extensive biotransformation. Metabolic pathways identified in animals include glucuronide conjugation, acetylation, hydroxylation of the benzene ring, cleavage of the N–O bond of the isoxazole ring, and hydroxylation followed by oxidation of the methylene carbon of the sulfamoyl group, finally resulting in loss of the sulfamoyl group (Seino *et al.*, 1995). Metabolites identified in humans include N-acetyl-zonisamide and a glucuronide conjugate of a metabolite with an open isoxazole ring (Perucca and Bialer, 1996). A cytochrome CYP3A is probably involved in cleavage of the isoxazole ring. *In vitro* data suggest CYP3A4 is the main isozyme responsible for zonisamide metabolism in humans, with CYP2C19 and CYP3A5 having a smaller role (Nakasa *et al.*, 1998). The half-life of zonisamide is around 60 h, but shorter values (around 30 h) are described in patients comedicated with enzyme inducing anticonvulsants (Peters and Sorkin, 1993; Perucca and Bialer, 1996). Because of variability in metabolic rate, there are considerable differences in plasma zonisamide concentrations among patients receiving the same dosage. Compared with adults, children metabolise zonisamide at a faster rate (Leppik, 1999).

The correlation between plasma or blood zonisamide concentration and therapeutic response is rather variable (Perucca and Bialer, 1996). Although zonisamide levels are sometimes monitored in clinical practice, they should be interpreted flexibly in the light of clinical response (Perucca and Bialer, 1996; Perucca, 2000).

Conclusions

Anti-epileptic drugs provide excellent examples of how differences in rate of metabolism may influence therapeutic response and mode of drug use. Complex metabolic patterns which have been identified with anti-epileptic drugs include enzyme saturation (phenytoin), dose-dependent autoinduction (carbamazepine), stereoselective activation and inactivation (phenytoin, methylphenobarbital), genetic metabolic polymorphisms (phenytoin, methylphenobarbital), formation of toxic reactive metabolites (phenytoin, carbamazepine, and other drugs) and susceptibility to heteroinduction (carbamazepine, valproic acid, lamotrigine, and other drugs) and enzyme inhibition (phenytoin, carbamazepine, phenobarbital, lamotrigine, and other drugs). These factors play an essential role in determining inter-individual differences in pharmacokinetics and drug response. For a number of drugs, monitoring drug concentrations provides a useful tool which allows control for this variability and facilitates tailoring of dosage to individual needs. In no case, however, measurement of serum drug concentrations is a substitute for rational prescribing based on clinical pharmacological knowledge and careful monitoring of clinical response. Table 6.1 and 6.2 summarise main AEDs metabolites, enzymes involved in their formation, drug interactions and other factors affecting the metabolism of the major AEDs.

References

Adkins, J. C. and Noble, S. (1998) 'Tiagabine. A review of its pharmacodynamic and pharmacokinetic properties and therapeutic potential in the management of epilepsy', *Drugs* 55: 437–60.

Anderson, G. D. (1998) 'A mechanistic approach to antiepileptic drug interactions', *Ann. Pharmacother.* 32: 554–63.

Anderson, G. D. and Graves, N. M. (1994) 'Drug interactions with antiepileptic agents. Prevention and management', *CNS Drugs* 2: 268–79.

Anderson, G. D. and Levy, R. H. (1995) 'Phenobarbital. Chemistry and biotransformation', in R. H. Levy, R. H. Mattson and B. S. Meldrum (eds) *Antiepileptic Drugs*, New York: Raven Press, pp. 371–7.

Bajpai, M., Roskos, L. K., Shen, D. D. and Levy, R. H. (1996) 'Roles of cytochrome P4502C9 and cytochrome P4502C19 in the stereoselective metabolism of phenytoin to its major metabolite', *Drug. Metab. Disp.* 24: 1401–3.

Bartoli, A., Guerrini, R., Belmonte, A., Alessandrì, M. G., Gatti, G. and Perucca, E. (1997) 'The influence of dosage, age and comedication on steady-state plasma lamotrigine concentrations in epileptic children: a prospective study with preliminary assessment of correlations with clinical response', *Ther. Drug Monit.* 19: 100–7.

Baruzzi, A., Albani, F. and Riva, R. (1994) 'Oxcarbazepine: pharmacokinetic interactions and their clinical significance', *Epilepsia* 35 (Suppl. 3): 14–19.

Battino, D., Estienne, M. and Avanzini, G. (1995) 'Clinical pharmacokinetics of antiepileptic drugs in paediatric patients. Parts I and II', *Clin. Pharmacokinet.* 29: 257–86 and 341–69.

Benetello, P., Furlanut, M., Pasqui, R., Carmillo, L., Perlotto, N. and Testa, G. (1987) 'Absence of effect of cigarette smoking on serum concentrations of some anticonvulsants in epileptic patients', *Clin. Pharmacokinet.* 12: 302–4.

Bertilsson, L. and Tomson, T. (1986) 'Clinical pharmacokinetics and pharmacological effects of carbamazepine and carbamazepine-10,11–epoxide, an update', *Clin. Pharmacokinet.* 11: 177–98.

Bialer, M., Johannessen, S. I., Kupferberg, H. J., Levy, R. H., Loiseau, P. and Perucca, E. (1999) 'Progress report on new antiepileptic drugs. A summary of the fourth Eilat Conference', *Epilepsy Res.* 34: 1–41.

Bialer, M., Xiaodong, S. and Perucca, E. (1995) 'Ethosuximide. Absorption, distribution, and excretion', in R. H. Levy, R. H. Mattson and B. S. Meldrum (eds) *Antiepileptic Drugs,* New York: Raven Press, pp. 659–65.

Brodie, M. J. (1995) 'Tiagabine pharmacology profile', *Epilepsia* 36 (Suppl. 6): 7–9.

Brodie, M. J. (1997) 'Tiagabine in the management of epilepsy', *Epilepsia* 38 (Suppl. 2): 23–7.

Butler, T. C., Mahaffee, C. and Waddell, W. J. (1954) 'Phenobarbital: studies of elimination, accumulation, tolerance, and dosage schedules', *J. Pharmacol. Exp. Ther.* 111: 425–35.

Cloyd, J., Miller, K. and Leppik, I. E. (1981) 'Primidone kinetics: effects of concurrent drugs and duration of therapy', *Clin. Pharmacol. Ther.* 29: 402–7.

Davis, R., Peters, D. H. and McTavish, D. (1994) 'Valproic acid. A reappraisal of its pharmacological properties and clinical efficacy in epilepsy', *Drugs* 47: 332–72.

Donahue, S., Flockart, D. A., Abernethy, D. R. (1999) 'Ticlopidine inhibits pheny-toin clearance', *Clin. Pharmacol. Ther.* **66**: 563–8.

Eadie, M. J. (1998) 'Therapeutic drug monitoring – antiepileptic drugs', *Brit. J. Clin. Pharmacol.* **46**: 185–94.

Eadie, M. J. and Hooper, W. D. (1995) 'Other barbiturates. Methylphenobarbital and metharbital', in R. H. Levy, R. H. Mattson and B. S. Meldrum (eds) *Antiepileptic Drugs*, New York: Raven Press, pp. 421–37.

Faigle, J. W. and Menge, G. P. (1990) 'Pharmacokinetic and metabolic features of oxcarbazepine and their clinical significance: comparison with carbamazepine', *Int. Clin. Psychopharmacol.* **5**: 73–82.

Fitton, A. and Goa, K. L. (1995) 'Lamotrigine. An update of its pharmacology and therapeutic use in epilepsy', *Drugs* **50**: 691–713.

Furlanut, M., Benetello, P., Avogaro, A. and Dainese, R. (1978) 'Effects of folic acid on phenytoin kinetics in healthy subjects', *Clin. Pharmacol. Ther.* **24**: 294–7.

Furlanut, M., Montanari, G., Bonin, P. and Casara, G. L. (1985). 'Carbamazepine and carbamazepine-10,11–epoxide serum concentrations in epileptic children', *J. Pediat.* **106**: 491–5.

Gatti, G., Bonomi, I., Jannuzzi, G. and Perucca, E. (2000) 'The new antiepileptic drugs: pharmacological and clinical aspects', *Current Pharmaceutical Design* **6**: 839–60.

Gerson, W. T., Fine, D. G., Spielberg, S. P. and Sensenbrenner, L. L. (1983) 'Anti-convulsant-induced aplastic anemia: increased susceptibility to toxic drug meta-bolites in vitro', *Blood* **61**: 889–93.

Giaccone, M., Bartoli, A., Gatti, G., Marchiselli, R., Pisani, F. and Perucca, E. (1996) 'Effect of enzyme inducing anticonvulsants on ethosuximide pharmaco-kinetics in epileptic patients', *Brit. J. Clin. Pharmacol.* **41**: 575–9.

Glue, P., Banfield, C. R., Perhach, J. L., Mather, G. G., Racha, J. K. and Levy, R. H. (1997) 'Pharmacokinetic interactions with felbamate. In vitro–in vivo correlation', *Clin. Pharmacokinet.* **33**: 214–24.

Goa, K. L., Ross, S. R. and Chrisp, P. (1993) 'Lamotrigine. A review of its pharmacological properties and clinical efficacy in epilepsy', *Drugs* **46**: 152–76.

Goa, K. L. and Sorkin, E. M. (1993) 'Gabapentin. A review of its pharmacological properties and clinical potential in epilepsy', *Drugs* **46**: 409–27.

Goulet, G. R., Kinkel, A. W. and Smith, T. C. (1976) 'Metabolism of ethosuximide', *Clin. Pharmacol. Ther.* **20**: 213–18.

Grant, S. M. and Faulds, D. (1992) 'Oxcarbazepine. A review of its pharmacology and therapeutic potential in epilepsy, trigeminal neuralgia and affective disorders', *Drugs* **43**: 873–88.

Grant, S. M. and Heel, R. C. (1991) 'Vigabatrin. A review of its pharmacodynamic and pharmacokinetic properties, and therapeutic potential in epilepsy and disorders of motor control', *Drugs* **41**: 889–926.

Hurst, S. I., Hargreaves J, A., Howald, W. N., Racha, J. K., Mather, G. G., Labroo, R., Carlson, S. P. and Levy, R. H. (1997) 'Enzymatic mechanism for the phenobarbital-valproate interaction', *Epilepsia* **38** (Suppl 8): 111–2.

Ieiri, I., Mamiya, K., Urae, A., Wada, Y., Kimura, M., Irie, S., Amamoto, T., Kubota, T., Yoshioka, S., Nakamura, K., Nakano, S., Tashiro, N. and Higuchi, S. (1997) 'Stereoselective 4′-hydroxylation of phenytoin: relationship to (S)-mephenytoin polymorphism in Japanese', *Brit. J. Clin. Pharmacol.* **43**: 441–5.

Isojärvi, J. I. T., Airaksinen, K. E. J., Mustonen, J. N., Pakarinen, A. J., Rautio, A., Pelkonen, O. and Myllyla, V. V. (1995) 'Thyroid and myocardial function after replacement of carbamazepine with oxcarbazepine', *Epilepsia* **36**: 810–6.

Isojärvi, J. I. T., Pakarinen, A. J., Rautio, A., Pelkonen, O. and Myllyla, V. V. (1994) 'Liver enzyme induction and serum lipid levels after replacement of carbamazepine with oxcarbazepine', *Epilepsia* **35**: 1217–20.

Jannuzzi, G., Cian, P., Gatti, G., Bartoli, A., Monaco, F. and Perucca, E. (2000) 'A multicentre randomized controlled trial on the clinical impact of therapeutic drug monitoring in patients with newly diagnosed epilepsy', *Epilepsia* **41**: 222–30.

Jaqz, E., Hall, S. D., Branch, R. A. and Wilkinson, G. R. (1986) 'Polymorphic metabolism of mephenytoin in man: pharmacokinetic interaction with a co-regulated substrate, mephobarbital', *Clin. Pharmacol. Ther.* **39**: 646–53.

Kauffman, R. E., Habersang, R. and Lansky, L. (1977) 'Kinetics of primidone excretion and metabolism in children', *Clin. Pharmacol. Ther.* **22**: 200–5.

Kaufman, K. R. and Gerner, R. (1997) 'Lamotrigine toxicity secondary to sertraline', *Epilepsia* **38** (Suppl 8): 100–1.

Kerr, B. M., Thummel, K. E. and Wurden, C. J. (1994) 'Human liver carbamazepine metabolism. Role of CYP3A4 and CYP2C8 in 10,11–epoxide formation', *Biochem. Pharmacol.* **47**: 1969–79.

Klaassen, S. L. (1998) 'Ticlopidine-induced phenytoin toxicity', *Ann. Pharmacother.* **32**: 1295–8.

Kondo, T., Otani, K., Hirano, T., Kaneko, S. and Fukushima, Y. (1990) 'The effects of phenytoin and carbamazepine on serum concentrations of mono-unsaturated metabolites of valproic acid', *Brit. J. Clin. Pharmacol.* **29**: 116–9.

Krauer, B. and Dayer, P. (1991) 'Fetal drug metabolism and its possible clinical implications', *Clin. Pharmacokinet.* **21**: 70–80.

Kudriakova, T. B., Sirota, L. A., Rozova, G. I. and Gorkov, V. A. (1992) 'Auto-induction and steady-state pharmacokinetics of carbamazepine and its major metabolites', *Brit. J. Clin. Pharmacol.* **33**: 611–5.

Kutt, H., Wolk, M., Scherman, R. and McDowell, F. (1964) 'Insufficient para-hydroxylation as a cause of phenytoin toxicity', *Neurology* **14**: 542–8.

Larrey, D. and Pageaux, G. P. (1997) 'Genetic predisposition to drug-induced hepatotoxicity', *J. Hepatol.* **26** (Suppl 2): 12–21.

Leppik, I. E. (1999) 'Zonisamide, a novel antiepileptic agent', *Today's Ther. Trends* **17**: 181–95.

Levy, R. H. and Bajpai, M. (1995) 'Phenytoin. Interaction with other drugs: mechanistic aspects', in R. H. Levy, R. H. Mattson and B. S. Meldrum (eds) *Antiepileptic Drugs,* New York: Raven Press, pp. 329–38.

Lloyd, P., Flesch, G. and Dieterle, W. (1994) 'Clinical pharmacology and pharmacokinetics of oxcarbazepine', *Epilepsia* **35** (Suppl. 3): 10–13.

May, T. W., Rambeck, B. and Jurgens, U. (1999) 'Influence of oxcarbazepine and methsuximide on lamotrigine concentrations in epileptic patients with and without valproic acid comedication: results of a retrospective study', *Ther. Drug Monit.* **21**: 175–81.

Mamiya, K., Hadama, A., Yukawa, E., Ieiri, I., Otsubo, K., Ninomiya, H., Tashiro, N., Higuchi, S. (2000) 'CYP2C19 polymorphism effect on phenobarbitone. Pharmacokinetics in Japanese patients with epilepsy: analysis by population pharmacokinetics', *Eur. J. Clin. Pharmacol.* **55**: 821–5.

Mamiya, K., Ieiri, I., Kimura, M., Wada, Y. and Higuchi, S. (1997) 'Stereoselective 4'-hydroxylation of phenytoin: relationship to CYP2C19 polymorphism', *Epilepsia* 38 (Suppl. 6): 74.

Mamiya, K., Ieiri, I., Miyahar, S., Imai, J., Higuchi, S., Ninomiya, H., Tashiro, N. and Yamada, H. (1998) 'Hydroxylation of phenytoin (PHT) and the cytochrome P450 (CYP) 2C subfamily', *Epilepsia* 39 (Suppl. 5): 82–3.

Morselli, P. L. (1995) 'Carbamazepine. Absorption, distribution and excretion', in R. H. Levy, R. H. Mattson and B. S. Meldrum (eds) *Antiepileptic Drugs*, New York: Raven Press, pp. 515–28.

Nair, D. R. and Morris, H. H. (1999) 'Potential fluconazole-induced carbamazepine toxicity', *Ann. Pharmacother.* 33: 790–2.

Nakamura, K., Goto, F. and Ray, W. A. (1985) 'Interethnic differences in genetic polymorphism of debrisoquine and mephenytoin hydroxylation between Japanese and Caucasian populations', *Clin. Pharmacol. Ther.* 38: 402–8.

Nakasa, H., Nakamura, H., Ono, S., Tsutsui, M., Kiuchi, M., Ohmori, S. and Kitada, M. (1998) 'Prediction of drug–drug interactions of zonisamide metabolism in humans from in vitro data', *Eur. J. Clin. Pharmacol.* 54: 177–83.

Ninomiya, H., Mamiya, K., Matsuo, S., Ieiri, I., Higuchi, S., Tashiro, N. (2000) 'Genetic polymorphism of the CYP2C subfamily and excessive serum phenytoin concentration with central nervous system intoxication', *Ther. Drug Monit.* 22: 230–2.

Palmer, K. J. and McTavish, D. (1993) 'Felbamate. A review of its pharmacodynamic and pharmacokinetic properties, and therapeutic efficacy in epilepsy', *Drugs* 45: 1041–65.

Perucca, E. (1987) 'Drug metabolism in pregnancy, infancy and childhood', *Pharmacol. Ther.* 34: 129–43.

Perucca, E. (1996a) 'Established drugs', in M. J. Brodie and D. M. Treiman (eds) *Modern Management of Epilepsy, Baillère's Clinical Neurology, vol 5*, London: Baillère-Tindall, pp. 693–722.

Perucca, E. (1996b) 'The new generation of antiepileptic drugs: advantages and disadvantages', *Brit. J. Clin. Pharmacol.* 42: 531–43.

Perucca, E. (1997) 'A pharmacological and clinical review of topiramate, a new antiepileptic drug', *Pharmacol. Res.* 35: 241–56.

Perucca, E. (1999) 'The clinical pharmacokinetics of new antiepileptic drugs', *Epilepsia* 40 (Suppl. 9): 7–13.

Perucca, E. (2000) 'Is there a role for the therapeutic drug monitoring of new anticonvulsants?', *Clin. Pharmacokinet.* 38: 191–204.

Perucca, E. and Bialer, M. (1996) 'The clinical pharmacokinetics of the newer antiepileptic drugs. Focus on Topiramate, zonisamide and tiagabine', *Clin. Pharmacokinet.* 31: 29–46.

Perucca, E. and Richens, A. (1980) 'Reversal by phenytoin of carbamazepine-induced water intoxication: a pharmacokinetic interaction', *J. Neurol. Neurosur. Psych.* 43: 540–5.

Perucca, E. and Richens, A. (1981) 'Antiepileptic drugs. Clinical aspects', in A. Richens and V. Marks (eds) *Therapeutic Drug Monitoring*, Edinburgh: Churchill-Livingstone, pp. 320–48.

Perucca, E. and Richens, A. (1983) 'Regulation and monitoring of drug therapy', in D. L. Williams and V. Marks (eds) *Biochemistry in Clinical Practice*, London: W. Heinemann Medical Books Ltd, pp. 379–99.

Perucca, E. and Richens., A (1995) 'Biotransformation', in R. H. Levy, R. H. Mattson and B. S. Meldrum (eds) *Antiepileptic Drugs*, New York: Raven Press, pp. 31–50.

Perucca, E., Makki, K. and Richens, A. (1978a) 'Is phenytoin metabolism dose-dependent by enzyme saturation or by feed-back inhibition?', *Clin. Pharmacol. Ther.* 26: 46–51.

Perucca, E., Garratt, A., Hebdige, S. and Richens, A. (1978b) 'Water intoxication in epileptic patients receiving carbamazepine', *J. Neurol. Neurosurg. Psych.* 41: 713–8.

Perucca, E., Bittencourt, P. and Richens, A. (1980) 'Effect of dose increments on serum carbamazepine concentration in epileptic patients', *Clin. Pharmacokinet.* 6: 576–82.

Perucca, E., Grimaldi, R., Gatti, G., Pirracchio, S., Crema, F. and Frigo, G. M. (1984) 'Pharmacokinetics of valproic acid in the elderly', *Brit. J. Clin. Pharmacol.* 17: 665–9.

Peters, D. H. and Sorkin, E. M. (1993) 'Zonisamide. A review of its pharmaco-dynamic and pharmacokinetic properties, and therapeutic potential in epilepsy', *Drugs* 45: 760–87.

Pirmohamed, M., Graham, A., Roberts, P., Smith, D., Chadwick, D., Breckenridge, A. M. and Park, B. K. (1991) 'Carbamazepine hypersensitivity: assessment of clinical and in vitro chemical cross-reactivity with phenytoin and oxcarbazepine', *Brit. J. Clin. Pharmacol.* 32: 741–9.

Pisani, F., Fazio, A., Oteri, G., Ruello, C., Gitto, C., Russo, F. and Perucca, E. (1986) 'Sodium valproate and valpromide: differential interaction with carba-mazepine in epileptic patients', *Epilepsia* 27: 548–52.

Pisani, F., Perucca, E. and Di Perri, R. (1990) 'Clinically relevant antiepileptic drug interactions', *J. Int. Med. Res.* 18: 1–15.

Rambeck, B. and Wolf, P. (1993) 'Lamotrigine clinical pharmacokinetics', *Clin. Pharmacokinet.* 25: 433–43.

Rey, E., Pons, G. and Olive, G. (1992) 'Vigabatrin clinical pharmacokinetics', *Clin. Pharmacokinet.* 23: 267–78.

Richens, A. and Dunlop, A. (1975) 'Serum phenytoin levels in management of epilepsy', *Lancet* 2: 247–8.

Richens, A. (1979) 'Clinical pharmacokinetics of phenytoin', *Clin. Pharmacokinet.* 4: 153–69.

Schachter, S. C. (1999) 'Oxcarbazepine', in M. J. Eadie and F. J. E. Vajda (eds) *Antiepileptic Drugs: Pharmacology and Therapeutics. Handbook of Experimental Pharmacology*, Berlin: Springer-Verlag, pp. 319–30,

Seino, M., Naruto, S., Ito, T. and Miyazaki, H. (1995) 'Other antiepileptic drugs. Zonisamide', in R. H. Levy, R. H. Mattson and B. S. Meldrum (eds) *Antiepileptic Drugs*, New York: Raven Press, pp. 1011–23.

Shear, N. H., Spielberg, S. P., Cannon, M. and Miller, M. (1988) 'Anticonvulsant hypersensitivity syndrome: in vitro risk assessment', *J. Clin. Invest.* 82: 1826–32.

Spielberg, S. P., Gordon, B. G., Blake, D. A., Goldstein, D. A. and Herlong, H. F. (1981) 'Predisposition to phenytoin hepatotoxicity assessed in vitro', *New Engl. J. Med.* 305: 722–7.

Spina, E., Pisani, F. and Perucca, E. (1996) 'Clinically relevant pharmacokinetic drug interactions with carbamazepine. An update', *Clin. Pharmacokinet.* 31: 198–214.

Tanaka, E. (1999) 'Clinically significant pharmacokinetic drug interactions between antiepileptic drugs', *J. Clin. Pharm. Ther.* **24**: 87–92.

Tartara, A., Galimberti, C. A., Manni, R., Morini, R., Limido, G., Gatti, G., Bartoli, A., Strada, G. and Perucca, E. (1993) 'The pharmacokinetics of oxcarbazepine and its active metabolite 10–hydroxy-carbazepine in healthy subjects and in epileptic patients treated with phenobarbitone or valproic acid', *Brit. J. Clin. Pharmacol.* **36**: 366–8.

Tecoma, E. S. (1999) 'Oxcarbazepine', *Epilepsia* **40** (Suppl. 5): 37–46.

Tomson, T., Ohman, I. and Vitols, S. (1997) 'Lamotrigine in pregnancy and lactation: a case report', *Epilepsia* **38**: 1039–41.

Troupin, A. S., Montouris, G. and Hussein, G. (1997) 'Felbamate: therapeutic range and other kinetic information', *J. Epilepsy* **10**: 26–31.

Volosov, A., Xiaodong, S., Perucca, E., Yagen, B., Sintov, A. and Bialer, M. (1999) 'Enantioselective pharmacokinetics of 10–hydroxycarbazepine after oral administration of oxcarbazepine to healthy Chinese subjects', *Clin. Pharmacol. Ther.* **66**: 547–53.

Zaccara, G., Messori, A. and Moroni, F. (1988) 'Clinical pharmacokinetics of valproic acid', *Clin. Pharmacokinet.* **15**: 367–89.

Chapter 7

Variability in the metabolism of levodopa and clinical implications

M. Furlanut, G. Wu and E. Perucca

Abbreviations

3MT, 3-methoxytyramine; 3OMD, 3-O-methyldopa; 5-HT, 5-hydroxy-tryptamine; ALDH, aldehyde dehydrogenase; ANOVA, analysis of variance; AUC, area-under-concentration-curve; COMT, catechol-O-methyltransferase; CR, controlled released preparation; CURSΣ, Columbia University Rating Scale; CV, coefficient of variation; DBH, dopamine-β-hydroxylase; DHBAC, 3,4-dihydroxybenzoic acid; DOPAC, 3,4-dihydroxyphenylacetic acid; DOPPA, 3,4-dihydroxyphenylpyruvic acid, HOPPA, 4-dihydroxyphenylpyruvic acid, HPPD, *p*-hydroxyphenylpyruvate-dioxygenase; HVA, homovanillic acid; IR, immediate released preparation; LAAD, aromatic L-amino acid decarboxylase (dopa decarboxylase); MAO, monoamino oxidase; MHBA, 3-methoxy-4-hydroxybenzylamine; SEM, standard error of mean; SD, standard deviation; TAT, tyrosine-aminotransferase; TOPA, 2,4,5-trihydroxyphenylalanine; TOPAA, 2,4,5-trihydroxyphenylacetic acid; UPDRS, the Unified Parkinson's Disease Rating Scale; VAA, vanillacetic acid; VMA, vanilmandelic acid; VPA, vanillpyruvic acid.

Introduction

Levodopa (L-3,4-dihydroxyphenylalanine) is the most effective drug available for the treatment of Parkinson's disease. It is rather unique in that the drug itself and many of its metabolites are naturally synthesised in the body. Therefore the understanding of its metabolism and the concomitant use of other drugs to modify its metabolism may improve the clinical effect. The individual variability in its metabolism may play an important role in the clinical response to this drug. This variability can be classified respectively as intraindividual and interindividual. The interindividual variability refers to the different characteristics of a patient in comparison with another, the intraindividual one mainly depends on the personal situation and external factors, both varying from time to time. On the timing scale, the interindividual variability is the variability among individuals at one time point; the intraindividual variability is the variability in an individual at different time points. Moreover, the metabolic variability of levodopa metabolism-modifying drugs adds another level of variation.

Methodologically, the interindividual variability can be assessed by calculating the coefficient of variation (CV=standard deviation/mean) with respect to the parameter of interest in a group of individuals after one measurement in each individual; the intraindividual variability can be assessed by calculating CV with respect to the parameter of interest in an individual after several measurements. Another approach involves the use of the model II (random effect) one-way analysis of variance (ANOVA). Currently, most data available in the literature are calculated according to the first approach. Hence we will use CV as an index of interindividual variability to address the interindividual variability in the metabolism of levodopa.

Levodopa metabolism

In order to understand the interindividual variability and intraindividual variability in the metabolism of levodopa, we briefly review the metabolism of levodopa in Figure 7.1 and Table 7.1. Most of the pathways are fundamentally irreversible except for the transamination pathway, e.g. 3,4-dihydroxyphenylpyruvic acid (DOPPA) can be transaminated to serve, at least in animals, as a precursor for levodopa (Hietala *et al.*, 1979; Linden, 1980) and a small amount of 3-O-methyldopa (3OMD) can be demethylated to dopa largely in erythrocytes (Tyce *et al.*, 1978; Kurama *et al.*, 1971).

When grouping the enzymes involved in the metabolism of levodopa according to the chemical reactions, we have: (a) decarboxylation, e.g. aromatic L-amino acid decarboxylase (EC 4.1.1.28, LAAD, also called dopa decarboxylase), catalyses levodopa to dopamine; (b) methylation, e.g. catechol-O-methyltransferase (EC 2.1.1.6, COMT), catalyses levodopa to 3OMD; (c) oxidation, e.g. monoamino oxidase (EC 1.4.3.4, MAO), catalyses dopamine to 3,4-dihydroxyphenylacetic acid (DOPAC); (d) transamination, e.g. tyrosine-aminotransferase (EC 2.6.1.5, TAT), catalyses levodopa to DOPPA; and (e) hydroxylation, e.g. dopamine-β-hydroxylase (EC 1.14.17.1, DBH), catalyses dopamine to norepinephrine.

When grouping the enzymes involved in the metabolism of levodopa according to their locations, we can find some enzymes ubiquitously present in various organs and tissues (LAAD is widely present in neurones, gastrointestinal cells, liver, kidney, pancreas, adrenal glands, blood and the capillary endothelium of the brain; COMT is present at high concentrations in erythrocytes, liver, and kidney; MAO is mainly present in the brain).

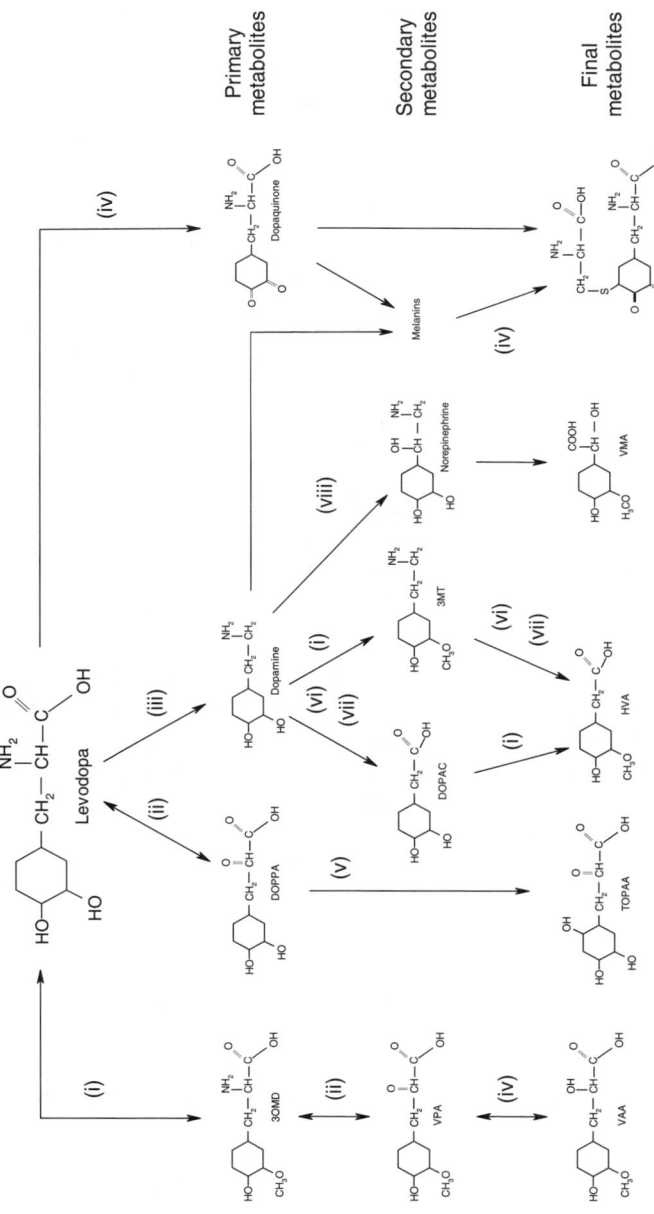

Figure 7.1 The metabolism of levodopa. (i) Catechol-*O*-methyltransferase (COMT), (ii) tyrosine-aminotransferase (TAT), (iii) L-amino aromatic acid decarboxylase (LAAD), (iv) tyrosinase or other oxidants, (v) *p*-hydroxyphenylpyruvate-dioxygenase (HPPD), (vi) monoamine oxidase (MAO), (vii) aldehyde dehydrogenase (ALDH), (viii) dopamine-β-hydroxylase (DBH). 3MT (3-methoxytyramine), 3OMD (3-*O*-methyldopa), DOPAC (3,4-dihydroxyphenylacetic acid), DOPPA (3,4-dihydroxyphenylpyruvic acid), HVA (homovanillic acid, or 3-methoxy-4-hydroxyphenylacetic acid), TOPAA (2,4,5-trihydroxyphenylacetic acid), VAA (vanillacetic acid), VMA (vanilmandelic acid or vanillinemandelic acid), VPA (vanillpyruvic acid).

Table 7.1 Enzymes involved in the metabolism of levodopa

Enzyme	Reaction	Location	Degree of stratification	Role in the metabolism of levodopa
ALDH	Oxidation	Liver	Secondary and final metabolites	
COMT	Methylation	Erythrocytes, liver, kidney	Primary and final metabolites	Metabolises about 10% of the oral dose
DBH	Hydroxylation	Brain	Secondary metabolite	Hydroxylates about 5% of dopamine
HPPD	Hydroxylation	Brain	Final metabolite	
LAAD	Decarboxylation	In all tissues	Primary metabolite	Metabolises about 65% of levodopa oral dose
MAO	Oxidation	Brain	Secondary and final metabolites	
TAT	Transamination	Liver and kidney cytosol	Primary and secondary metabolites	
Tyrosinase	Oxidation	Brain, melanocytes	Primary and final metabolites	

We can also group the enzymes involved in the metabolism of levodopa according to the stratification of metabolites of levodopa, i.e. enzymes catalysing levodopa to the primary metabolites, enzymes catalysing the primary metabolites to the secondary metabolites, and enzymes catalysing the secondary metabolites to the final metabolites.

Summarising, among numerous enzymes involved in the metabolism of levodopa, LAAD, COMT and MAO are the most important ones for the metabolism of levodopa both for interindividual variability and for clinical treatment.

Enzymes and their interindividual variability in activity

LAAD

LAAD is a multiple function enzyme and can decarboxylate numerous substrates such as 5-hydroxytryptophan, phenylalanine and tryptophan (Paterson *et al.*, 1990). LAAD has two protein isoforms as found in monkey kidney cell line (LAAD$_{480}$ and LAAD$_{442}$). The latter does not decarboxylate levodopa (O'Malley *et al.*, 1995). The interindividual variability in LAAD activity is at its lowest in the human cell line, high in the human brain and the highest in human gut (Table 7.2).

Table 7.2 Interindividual variability in enzymatic activities

Enzyme	Substrate	Tissue	K_m CV (%) (mean±SD)	V_{max} CV (%) (mean±SD)	References and Notes
HPPD	HOPPA	Control (mM)	16.7 (0.06±0.01)		Endo et al., 1983
		Hypertyrosinemia (mM)	13.0 (0.23±0.03)		
LAAD	Levodopa	Kidney cell (monkey)	9.7 (49±4.7)	14.4 (18±2.6)	O'Malley et al., 1995; (n=3); K_m=μM; V_{max}=nmol/mg/min
		Antrum (n=9)	48.5 (99±48)		Schultz 1991; K_m=μM
		Bulbum (n=8)	26.1 (161±42)		
		Jejunum (n=5)	87.8 (604±530)		
		Ileum (n=4)	120.1 (214±257)		
MAO	3MT	Amnion		13.0 (0.023±0.003)	Kawada et al., 1989; V_{max}=nmol/mg protein/min
		Chorion		27.8 (0.18±0.05)	
		Decidua		24.5 (2.69±0.66)	
MAO-A	5-HT	Brain (mouse)	18.0 (39±7)	5.6 (37.6±2.1)	Freeman et al., 1993; K_m=μM; V_{max}=pmol/mg wet tissue/min
	MHBA		22.0 (341±75)	8.3 (27.7±2.3)	
MAO-B	5-HT	Brain (mouse)	7.2 (1704±122)	2.5 (12.0±0.3)	Freeman et al., 1993; K_m=μM; V_{max}=pmol/mg wet tissue/min
	MHBA		10.2 (108±11)	2.7 (44.3±1.2)	
TAT		rat liver (U/h) (n=12)		50.0 (0.004±0.002)	Presch et al., 1997
		rat kidney (U/h) (n=12)		20.0 (0.01±0.002)	
		rat liver (unit)		21.5 (13.5±2.9)	Yang et al., 1989

Notes

If not specified, the tissue is human in origin in all the tables and figures; n=number of experiments. The data of original studies reported as mean±SEM have been converted to mean±SD in tables and figures, except Figure 7.1 and Table 7.1.

COMT

COMT is a ubiquitous enzyme occurring in micro-organisms and animals. In mammals COMT is distributed throughout various organs (Lundstrom *et al.*, 1992). Two distinct forms of COMT have been found, one mainly present in a soluble form (S-COMT) in the cytosol, and the other form is a small fraction bound to cell membranes (M-COMT) (Assicot and Bohuon, 1971; Nissinen, 1984; Jeffery and Roth, 1985; Borchardt *et al.*, 1974), both forms operating with a similar kinetic mechanism (Lotta *et al.*, 1995). The interindividual variability in COMT activity is quite large both in humans and animals (Figure 7.2). Although S-COMT and M-COMT have different kinetic properties, their interindividual variability is quite similar (Table 7.2). As COMT activity varies with age (Agathopoulos *et al.*, 1971), the interindividual variability of COMT activity changes with age too.

MAO

MAO has two isoforms, A isoform (MAO-A) and B isoform (MAO-B). MAO plays a small role in the metabolism of levodopa compared with LAAD and COMT. MAO-A is located in both neural and non-neural tissues. In brain it is present in the mitochondrial membrane of the nigro-striatal dopamine-containing neurones and of the glial cells (Waldmeier, 1987). MAO-B is located extracellularly to the dopaminergic neurones and in the serotoninergic neurones and glial cells, thus it would not interfere with the storage processes of dopamine in the dopaminergic terminals (Doudet *et al.*, 1997).

ALDH and others

Aldehyde dehydrogenase (EC 1.2.1.3, ALDH) has four isoenzymes, three existing primarily in the cytoplasm, ALHD2 in the mitochondria. ALDH2 phenotype shows two major isoenzymes with a low K_m in mitochondria and a high K_m in the cytoplasm (Harada *et al.*, 1980; Helander and Carlsson, 1990).

DBH activity in human serum is one to two orders of magnitude higher than that in any other species (Dunnette and Weinshilboum, 1983). Individuals can be classified as those with thermolabile and those with thermostable plasma DBH. The individuals with thermolabile DBH have only about 55% basal enzymatic activity compared with the individuals with stable enzyme (Dunnette and Weinshilboum, 1982).

p-Hydroxyphenylpyruvate-dioxygenase (EC 1.13.11.27, HPPD) is a crucial enzyme in plants, and is involved in the degradation of aromatic amino acids in various organisms. HPPD has recently been identified as the molecular target for new families of potent herbicides such as synthetic beta-triketones (Ellis *et al.*, 1996; Garcia *et al.*, 1997).

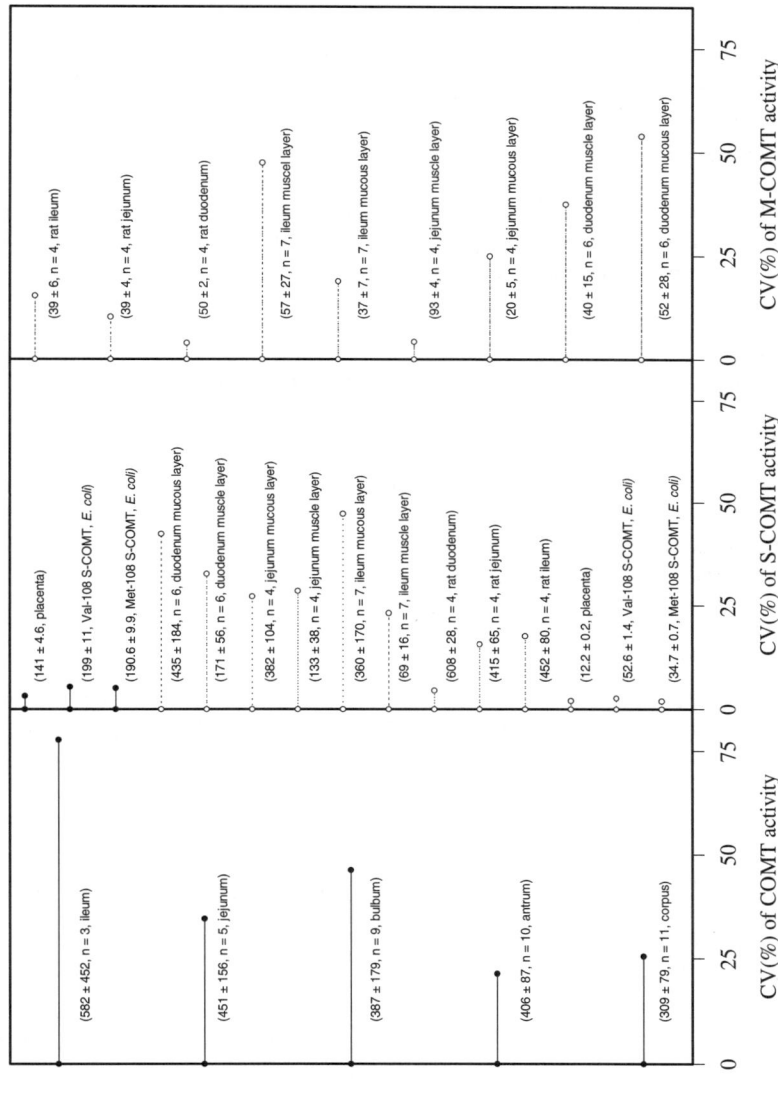

Figure 7.2 Interindividual variability in COMT activity. The solid lines with filled circles and dotted lines with unfilled circles are K_m and V_{max}. The data are obtained from humans unless specified. COMT data were calculated according to the study of Schultz (1991) and the unit of K_m is μM (levodopa as substrate). The data on S-COMT in placenta, Val-108 S-COMT and Met-108 S-COMT were calculated according to the study of Lotta *et al.*, (1995) and the units of K_m and V_{max} are μM and min⁻¹ (dopamine as substrate). The other data on S-COMT and M-COMT were calculated according to the study of Nissinen *et al.* (1988) and the unit of V_{max} is pmol/min/mg protein (DHBAC as substrate). The data in parentheses are mean±SD; *n* = the number of experiments.

CV(%) of COMT activity

(309 ± 79, n = 11, corpus)

(406 ± 87, n = 10, antrum)

(387 ± 179, n = 9, bulbum)

(451 ± 156, n = 5, jejunum)

(582 ± 452, n = 3, ileum)

CV(%) of S-COMT activity

(34.7 ± 0.7, Met-108 S-COMT, *E. coli*)

(52.6 ± 1.4, Val-108 S-COMT, *E. coli*)

(12.2 ± 0.2, placenta)

(452 ± 80, n = 4, rat ileum)

(415 ± 65, n = 4, rat jejunum)

(608 ± 28, n = 4, rat duodenum)

(69 ± 16, n = 7, ileum muscle layer)

(360 ± 170, n = 7, ileum mucous layer)

(133 ± 38, n = 4, jejunum muscle layer)

(382 ± 104, n = 4, jejunum mucous layer)

(171 ± 56, n = 6, duodenum muscle layer)

(435 ± 184, n = 6, duodenum mucous layer)

(190.6 ± 9.9, Met-108 S-COMT, *E. coli*)

(199 ± 11, Val-108 S-COMT, *E. coli*)

(141 ± 4.6, placenta)

CV(%) of M-COMT activity

(52 ± 28, n = 6, duodenum mucous layer)

(40 ± 15, n = 6, duodenum muscle layer)

(20 ± 5, n = 4, jejunum mucous layer)

(93 ± 4, n = 4, jejunum muscle layer)

(37 ± 7, n = 7, ileum mucous layer)

(57 ± 27, n = 7, ileum muscel layer)

(50 ± 2, n = 4, rat duodenum)

(39 ± 4, n = 4, rat jejunum)

(39 ± 6, n = 4, rat ileum)

Tyrosinase (EC 1.14.18.1) is a copper-containing metalloglycoprotein and temperature-sensitive for levodopa oxidation (Tripathi *et al.*, 1992).

TAT is a key enzyme involved in amino acid metabolism. TAT activity has a close correlation with glucocorticoid receptor (Ashton *et al.*, 1996; Dundjerski *et al.*, 1996).

Summarising, among COMT, LAAD and MAO, the interindividual variability is greater in the gut and lesser in the brain. This explains the reason why the levodopa disposition after oral administration displays a more extensive interindividual variability than after intravenous administration.

Levodopa, its metabolites and interindividual variability

Levodopa

Numerous factors including metabolism determine plasma levodopa concentration and half-life. The interindividual variability in each of these factors contributes to the interindividual variability in levodopa plasma concentration and half-life at varying degrees (Table 7.3).

Primary metabolites

3OMD can compete with levodopa for the amino acid transport system in the blood–brain barrier (Wade and Katzman, 1975; Pardridge, 1977; Benetello *et al.*, 1997), to cause a deterioration of the motor status in patients with Parkinson's disease (Feuerstein *et al.*, 1977; Nutt *et al.*, 1987; Wu and Furlanut, 1999), to inhibit the synaptosomal uptake of levodopa and levodopa accumulation in the corpus striatum (Reches and Fahn, 1982; Reilly *et al.*, 1980) and to be a substrate for LAAD (Ferrini and Glasser, 1964). The interindividual variability in 3OMD concentration seems to be less well investigated (Table 7.3).

DOPPA is found to be involved in animals in the oxidation and transamination of dextrodopa to levodopa by D-amino acid oxidase (EC 1.4.3.3) (Brannan *et al.*, 1996; Moses *et al.*, 1996; Karoum *et al.*, 1988). From this point of view, DOPPA might be an important intermediate between dextrodopa and levodopa, and its quantity and interindividual variability may serve as a useful index to assess the interindividual variability in the conversion of dextrodopa to levodopa.

The free dopamine is normally not detected in the cerebrospinal fluid in untreated patients with Parkinson's disease (Olanow *et al.*, 1991). The interindividual variability in dopamine plasma concentration is quite large (Table 7.3).

Dopaquinone can also be formed from L-tyrosine (Schallreuter *et al.*, 1994). Dopaquinone undergoes a rapid spontaneous auto-oxidation to

Table 7.3 Interindividual variability in levodopa and its metabolites

Substance	Parameters	CV (%) (mean±SD)	References and Notes
Levodopa	Stable patients plasma (n=15)		Contin et al., 1993; 100/25 mg (levodopa/benserazide) dose
	Absorption half-life (min)	55.8 (12.0±6.7)	
	Elimination half-life (min)	22.6 (57.2±12.9)	
	Fluctuating patients (n=25)		
	Absorption half-life (min)	62.8 (14.5±9.1)	
	Elimination half-life (min)	28.9 (50.6±14.3)	
	Half-life in monkey (min)		Hammerstad et al., 1990; 5.1 mM levodopa in 5% dextrose infusion
	Distribution in plasma (n=13)	32.7 (4.9±1.6)	
	Elimination from plasma (n=13)	39.8 (33.2±13.2)	
	Distribution in cisternal (n=9)	39.3 (8.9±3.5)	
	Elimination from cisternal (n=9)	27.2 (49.2±13.4)	
	Elimination at lumbar CSF (n=3)	26.5 (100.4±26.6)	
	Plasma C_{max} (µg/ml) (n=8)	48.1 (2.1±1.0)	Myllylä et al.; 1993; 100/25 mg (levodopa/carbidopa) dose
	Plasma t_{max} (h) (n=8)	79.8 (0.8±0.6)	
	Plasma $AUC_{0-6 h}$ (µg/ml/h) (n=8)	21.2 (3.4±0.7)	
	Plasma AUC (µg/ml/h) (n=8)	21.4 (3.6±0.8)	
	Plasma $t_{1/2}$ (h) (n=8)	13.1 (1.5±0.2)	
	Concentration in rat striatum (ng/g)	25.0 (20±5)	Männistö and Tuomainen 1991; levodopa 100 mg/kg and carbidopa 100 mg/kg i.v.
3OMD	Plasma AUC (µg/ml/h) (n=8)	53.0 (22.4±11.9)	Myllylä et al., 1993; see above for dose
	Concentration in rat striatum (ng/g)	27.3 (33±9)	Männistö and Tuomainen 1991; see above for dose
Dopamine	Plasma concentration (µg/l) (n=12)	50.0 (1±0.5)	Dutton et al., 1993; 150 to 1250 mg/day dose

Table 7.3 (continued)

Substance	Parameters	CV (%) (mean±SD)	References and Notes
DOPAC	Concentration in rat striatum (μg/g)	4.8 (2.5±0.12)	Männistö and Tuomainen 1991; see above for dose
	Excretion rate in urine	38.7 (0.58±0.22)	Mashige et al., 1994
	Plasma AUC (μg/ml/h) (n=8)	39.4 (122±48)	Myllylä et al., 1993; see above for dose
Melanin	Plasma concentration (mg/ml) (n=20)	6.2 (1.61±0.10)	Hegedus and Nayak, 1993
	Uremic plasma (mg/ml) (n=16)	14.0 (2.72±0.38)	
	Excretion rate in urine (ml/min) (n=8)	100.0 (0.48±0.48)	
Norepine-phrine	Plasma concentration (pg/ml) (n=10)	57.9 (76±44)	Kienbaum et al., 1998
	Rat plasma concentration (pg/ml)	23.7 (224±53)	Latini et al., 1998
	Fetal sheep plasma concentration (pg/ml), (n=7)	65.3 (1556±1017)	Stein et al. 1998
HVA	Concentration in rat striatum (μg/g)	5.3 (0.94±0.05)	Männistö and Tuomainen 1991; see above for dose
	Concentration in brain (ng/ml) (n=4)	26.4 (283±74.8)	Olanow et al., 1991
	Concentration in rat striatum (n=7)	24.5 (1514±370)	Brannan et al., 1992; the unit is pg/15-min dialysis
	Excretion rate in urine	40.7 (3.6±1.5)	Mashige et al., 1994
	Plasma AUC (μg/ml/h) (n=8)	39.2 (455±178)	Myllylä et al., 1993; see above for dose
VMA	Excretion rate in urine	37.7 (2.5±0.93)	Mashige et al., 1994
S-cysteinyl-dopa	Serum concentration (ng/ml)	31.6 (1.9±0.6)	Wimmer et al., 1997

leucodopachrome, which is in turn oxidised to dopachrome (Fatibello-Filho and da Cruz Vieira, 1997), then to melanins (Prota, 1988).

Secondary metabolites

DOPAC is considered an indirect marker of dopamine metabolism. The interindividual variability in brain DOPAC concentration is smaller than in urine (Table 7.3).

3-Methoxytyramine (3MT) can be viewed as an index of metabolism of dopamine after the inhibition of MAO by pargyline (Chrapusta *et al.*, 1993; Nissbrandt and Hjorth, 1992), i.e. the metabolic rate from dopamine to 3MT catalysed mainly by COMT. Table 7.3 shows the interindividual variability in 3MT.

The interindividual variability in plasma norepinephrine can be calculated from numerous studies in the literature. Table 7.3 shows some of these data. It should be noted that as the amount of norepinephrine metabolised from levodopa is extremely small, its interindividual variability has almost no relationship with levodopa metabolism.

Melanins are pigments responsible for the dark color of skin, hair, feathers, fur, insect cuticle and soil. Melanins can be found in fungi, bacteria, and pathological human urine. Among melanins, eumelanins are found in the animal kingdom and can be produced by the oxidative polymerization of 5,6-dihydroxyindoles derived enzymatically from tyrosine via dopa (Budavari, 1989) and neuromelanins arising from the oxidative metabolism of dopamine (Marsden, 1983). Unfortunately, despite an immense effort, the structure of melanins is still far from being well understood (Prota, 1988). Some data related to the interindividual variability of melanins are shown in Table 7.3.

Final metabolites

2,4,5-Trihydroxyphenylacetic acid (TOPPA) is intrinsically unstable and subject to spontaneous oxidation leading to formation of superoxide, hydrogen peroxide and a reactive quinone (Nutt and Fellman, 1984).

HVA is sometimes used in the diagnosis of neuroblastoma, especially in children (Steinmetz, 1989). A significant correlation exists between plasma and saliva HVA (Drebing *et al.*, 1989).

VMA in plasma and urine is sometimes used in clinical diagnosis of patients with cancer (Uderzo et al., 1988; Takahashi *et al.*, 1988) and hypertension (Linss and Scholze, 1990).

5-Cysteinyl-dopa can be formed in melanocytes by the action of tyrosinase, or at any other site in which superoxide and/or hydrogen peroxide flux exists (Ito and Fujita, 1982). Evidence for this reaction has been reported in humans treated with levodopa (Stewart *et al.*, 1983). The dopaquinone can undergo reactions with appropriate Lewis bases such as thiol groups and proteins (Rotman *et al.*, 1976; Wick and Fitzgerald, 1981), in which cysteine is the main source of 5-cysteinyl-dopa in human epidermal melanocytes (Benathan and Labidi, 1996). Thus 5-cysteinyl-dopa can display antioxidative activity (Benathan and Labidi, 1996). It was also suggested that plasma 5-cysteinyl-dopa may be used to diagnose melanoma for its follow-up (Peterson *et al.*, 1988) and as an index of melanogenesis (Nimmo *et al.*, 1988).

Vanillacetic acid (VAA) is almost undetectable in the urine of healthy people (Tuchman and Stocckeler, 1988).

Summarising, the interindividual variability of the metabolites of levodopa is generally smaller than that of levodopa, and the fact that the interindividual variability is larger in urine than in plasma suggests that the monitoring of metabolites of levodopa in urine has little importance in therapeutic decisions.

Genetic polymorphism in the metabolism of levodopa

The interindividual variability of the metabolism of levodopa mainly depends on genetic factors. The genetic polymorphism can explain how drugs are absorbed, metabolised and eliminated in different populations, and sub-populations, i.e. the interindividual variability depends on the population structure.

LAAD

LAAD is a multiple function enzyme, in fact the cloning of its gene can decarboxylate several substrates (Sumi *et al.*, 1990; Gudehithlu *et al.*, 1992). LAAD is not considered to be the rate limiting enzyme in the synthesis of dopamine, and its transcripts are found in almost all the brain, liver and kidney (O'Malley *et al.*, 1995). Also the detailed distribution of LAAD mRNA has been published for mouse CNS and peripheral tissues (Eaton *et al.*, 1993).

COMT

Both S-COMT and M-COMT are coded by one gene using two separate promoters (Tenhunen *et al.*, 1993). S-COMT contains 221 amino acids, whereas M-COMT has a 50- (human) and a 43- (rat) residue-long amino-terminal extension that contains the hydrophobic membrane-anchor region. The sequences of COMT from different mammalian species are very similar (Vidgren *et al.*, 1994). A common polymorphism of the human COMT gene coding includes a thermolabile low activity and a thermostable high activity, the Val-108 and Met-108 variants in gene coding could correlate with the high and low activity phenotypes of COMT (Boudikova *et al.*, 1990; Grossman *et al.*, 1992). Other high and low activity alleles are determined by the fact that the relative low activity allele is associated with a methionine residue at amino acid 158 of M-COMT, whereas a high activity variant has a valine at this site (Lachman *et al.*, 1997), as shown in human liver obtained from Caucasian females (Lachman *et al.*, 1996). Although the highest activities of COMT are found in liver and kidney (Guldberg and Marsden, 1975; Rivett *et al.*, 1983), COMT activity in erythrocytes has drawn great attention in clinical settings because of its easy assessment in vivo. Some data show, for example, that COMT activity in erythrocytes has a bimodal distribution among the Caucasian population and has a normal distribution in the Oriental population (Weinshilboum *et al.*, 1974; Weinshilboum and Raymond, 1977; Rivera-Calimlim and Reilly, 1984). De Santi *et al.* (1998) calculated the interindividual variability in COMT activity dividing the 95th percentile by the 5th percentile. They found an interindividual variability of 4.1 and 4.4 in the female and male liver, 2.6 in the human duodenum, and 5.3 in the human kidney.

MAO

MAO-A and MAO-B are encoded by two distinct genes located on the human X chromosome. A polymorphism of the gene encoding MAO-B has been identified as a single base change (A or G) in intron 13 of the X chromosome (Costa *et al.*, 1997). Several lines of evidence show that MAO-B allele 1 is likely to increase the risk of developing Parkinson's disease (Kurth *et al.*, 1993). Regarding the frequencies of alleles in different populations, MAO-B allele 1 is found in Caucasians Parkinsonian patients, but not in Japanese Parkinsonian patients (Morimoto *et al.*, 1995), and the frequency of MAO-B allele 1 is two-fold higher in Caucasians than in healthy Japanese. Another study also shows that the frequencies of MAO-B alleles 1 and 2 are 0.62 and 0.38 in Parkinsonian patients of European origin (Kurth *et al.*, 1993).

ALDH and others

Several polymorphisms exist in the gene producing ALDH enzyme. Virtually all Caucasians have two major ALDH isoenzymes, i.e. ALDH1 and ALDH2, whereas approximately 50% Japanese and other Orientals are atypical in that they have ALDH1 only (Yoshida *et al.*, 1983; Crabb *et al.*, 1989). The polymorphism in Japanese and other Orientals is due to ALDH2/2 allele (Takeshita *et al.*, 1998), and a point mutation in the human ALDH2 locus (substitution of glutamine by lysine at the position 487) leads to the enzyme inactivation (Chao *et al.*, 1994; Yoshida *et al.*,

1984). However, Neumark et al., (1998) were not able to demonstrate a similar polymorphism in the Jewish population.

The human gene for DBH was mapped on chromosome 9q34 (Perry et al., 1991), and several polymorphisms have been identified. For example, alleles of DBH*444 g/a are associated with wide differences in mean values of DBH levels in cerebrospinal fluid (Cubells et al., 1998), alleles A3/A3 and A4/A4 are associated with low and high DBH activity, whereas A3/A4 seems to keep DBH activity at a moderate level (Wei et al., 1997). Another polymorphism, DBH*304A is the common allele in African-Americans and European-Americans with allele frequencies greater than 0.80, whereas DBH*304S allele is most common in African descent and least common in East Asians and in individuals belonging to the indigenous populations of North and South America (Cubells et al., 1997).

The mutation of HPPD leads to the hereditary tyrosinemia disorder, the possible self-reactive T cell hybridomas and tolerance (Schneider and Mitchison, 1995). The structure of HPPD gene has been identified in human chromosome 12q24→qter (Awata et al., 1994; Rüetschi et al., 1997; Stenman et al., 1995). The analysis of the deduced amino acid sequence reveals a high homology with HPPD from different organisms (Ruzafa et al., 1994).

TAT gene is a liver-specific and prototypic glucocorticoid-inducible gene (Schweizer-Groyer et al., 1997). TAT has been used extensively in studies of the tissue-specific control of gene transcription, and TAT gene is located on human chromosome 16q (Scherer et al., 1989). The deficiency in hepatic TAT results in tyrosinemia type II (Richner–Hanhart syndrome), and two polymorphisms have been detected as being related to the tyrosinemia (Huhn et al., 1998; Westphal et al., 1988).

The polymorphisms in the tyrosinase gene are mainly related to the studies on oculocutaneous albinism, ocular albinism and Prader–Willi syndrome plus albinism (Lee et al., 1994). The gene is located on chromosome segment 15q11–q13 and 11q14–q21 (Colman et al., 1993; Lee et al., 1994). A common nonpathological polymorphism in Caucasians and American Blacks occurs at codon 402, the variant can be either CGA (arginine) ($p=0.85$) or CAA (glutamine) ($p=0.15$), the substitution of glutamine for arginine leading to a moderate thermoinstability in tyrosinase (Tripathi et al., 1991). However, 402CAA allele has not been found in Oriental populations. Numerous other mutations have also been identified in the tyrosinase gene related to the oculocutaneous albinism.

Summarising, besides the fact that the polymorphisms of enzymes are related to the risk of Parkinson's disease, the frequency of polymorphisms of each enzyme in a population is an important contribution to the source of interindividual variability. Unfortunately, at the present the polymorphism is usually presented as different frequencies in a population, therefore the use of the CV method is not easily applied.

Environmental factors and the metabolism of levodopa

The intraindividual variability generally depends on environmental factors (lifestyle, inhibitors, drug interactions, age, duration of disease, etc). Thus the intraindividual variability includes more random factors than the interindividual variability. However, the environmental factors also have different effects on different individuals due to the difference among individuals.

Inhibitors

Dopa decarboxylase inhibitors (LAAD inhibitors)

LAAD catalyses the conversion of levodopa to dopamine. Dopamine peripherally formed is not only unavailable for the brain but also leads to undesirable side-effects, such as nausea, vomiting and orthostatic hypotension. Thus the useful clinical inhibitors of LAAD are the peripheral ones (Pinder et al., 1976). In general, the metabolic profile of levodopa is altered by the inhibitors of LAAD in two ways: (a) an administered dose is less metabolised to HVA and DOPAC (Sandler et al., 1974; Bianchine et al., 1972); and (b) there is an absolute increase in the amount of transamination pathway end-product, i.e. VAA, and a relative increase in the amount of O-methylated product.

Carbidopa is a peripheral inhibitor usually administered in a combination of one tenth with levodopa. Normally carbidopa is undetectable in the cerebrospinal fluid of patients treated with this drug (Olanow et al., 1991). Different combinations of levodopa and carbidopa affect the metabolism of levodopa and the interindividual variability is larger in DOPAC (Figure 7.3). The interindividual variability in some carbidopa effects is shown in Table 7.4.

Benserazide is a peripheral inhibitor generally used in a combination of one fourth with levodopa. Benserazide also competes with levodopa *in vivo* for COMT (Gordonsmith et al., 1982). Different combinations of levodopa and benserazide affect the metabolism of levodopa and the interindividual variability is larger in DOPAC (Figure 7.4). The interindividual variability in several benserazide effects is shown in Table 7.4.

Inhibitors of COMT

A significant proportion of oral levodopa is metabolised to 3OMD in kidney and liver. These two organs are endowed with the highest COMT activities in the body (Axelrod et al., 1959). In the presence of LAAD inhibitors, a large proportion of levodopa is metabolised by peripheral COMT. The inhibition of COMT should therefore reduce levodopa clearance, extend the levodopa plasma concentration during a dosing

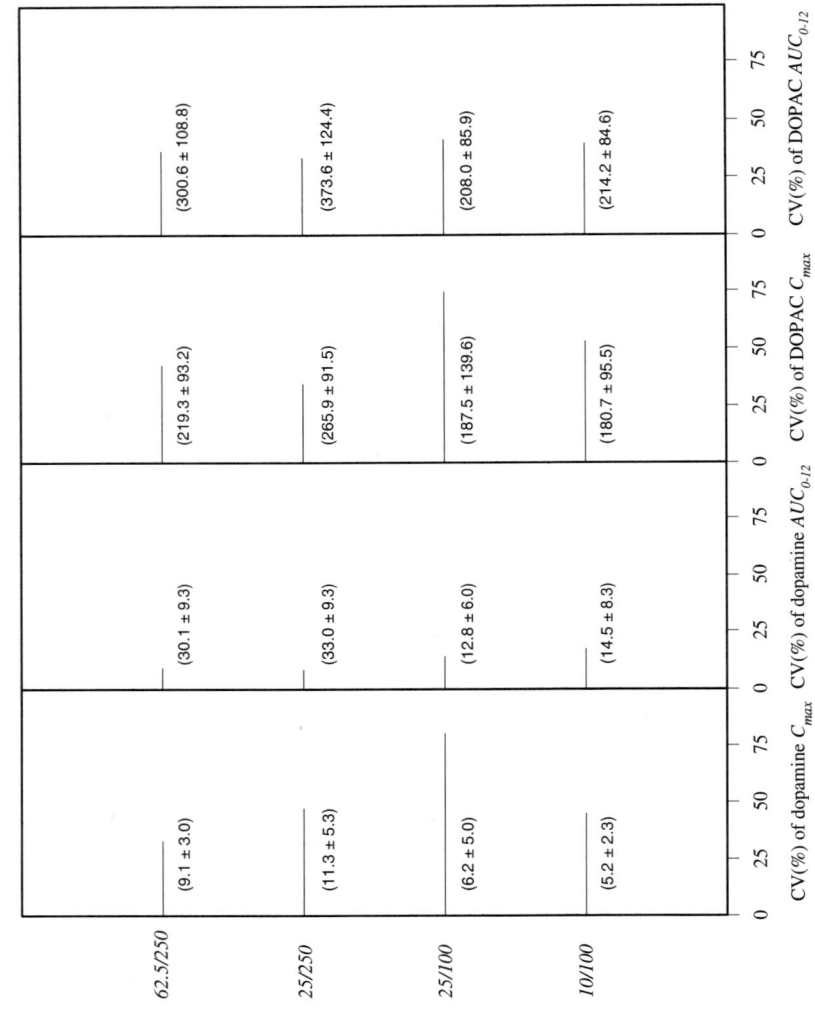

Figure 7.3 Effect of different combinations of carbidopa and levodopa on the metabolism of levodopa. CV was calculated according to the study of Kaakkola et al. (1985) in eleven healthy people. The data in parentheses are mean±SD of plasma C_{max} (ng/ml) and AUC_{0-12} (ng/ml/h).

Combination of carbidopa and levodopa (mg/mg)

62.5/250   (9.1 ± 3.0)

25/250   (11.3 ± 5.3)

25/100   (6.2 ± 5.0)

10/100   (5.2 ± 2.3)

CV(%) of dopamine C_{max}

(30.1 ± 9.3)
(33.0 ± 9.3)
(12.8 ± 6.0)
(14.5 ± 8.3)

CV(%) of dopamine AUC_{0-12}

(219.3 ± 93.2)
(265.9 ± 91.5)
(187.5 ± 139.6)
(180.7 ± 95.5)

CV(%) of DOPAC C_{max}

(300.6 ± 108.8)
(373.6 ± 124.4)
(208.0 ± 85.9)
(214.2 ± 84.6)

CV(%) of DOPAC AUC_{0-12}

Table 7.4 Interindividual variability in inhibitors of LAAD

Inhibitor	Effect	CV (%), (mean±SD)	References and Notes
Carbidopa	Decreases prolactin (%)		Kelley et al., 1996
	levodopa	3.0 (83.2±2.5)	
	levodopa/carbidopa	2.5 (80.3±2.0)	
	Uptake constant of nigrofrontal dopaminiergic pathway in Parkinsonian patients (10^{-3}) ($n=4$)	2.1 (2.89±0.06)	Otsuka et al., 1995; control=2.8±0.1 (10^{-3})
Benserazide	Reduces rat furosemide-induced diuresis (µl/min/g of kidney weight)	25.3 (8.3±2.1)	Nowicki et al., 1993; control=19.3±1.4. 25 mg/kg benserazide i.v.
	Increases levodopa accumulation in pig epithelial cells		Soares-da-Silva et al., 1998; 50 µM benserazide
	K_m (µM)	14.2 (113±16)	
	V_{max} (pmol/mg protein/6 min)	5.3 (5581±297)	
	Speeds levodopa transport rate in pig epithelial cells (pmol/mg protein/min)	11.1 (3.6±0.4)	Soares-da-Silva et al., 1997; 50 µM benserazide
	in opossum renal tubule cells (pmol/mg protein/min)	1.7 (18.1±0.3)	

interval and increase dopamine brain concentrations (Brannan *et al.*, 1992; Männistö *et al.*, 1992; Kaakkola and Wurtman, 1992). Among COMT inhibitors, nitrocatechols including nitecapone, entacapone and tolcapone have been tried in the treatment of Parkinson's disease and the latter two have entered into clinical use. The COMT in liver and kidney is sensitive to tolcapone, nitecapone, and entacapone (Bäckström *et al.*, 1989; Borgulya *et al.*, 1989; Nissinen *et al.*, 1992; Törnwall and Männistö, 1991; Törnwall *et al.*, 1994; Roth, 1992). In humans, all these three nitrocatechol COMT inhibitors inhibit the COMT activity in erythrocytes, and decrease the number of COMT-dependent metabolites of epinephrine and norepinephrine in plasma (Kaakkola *et al.*, 1994).

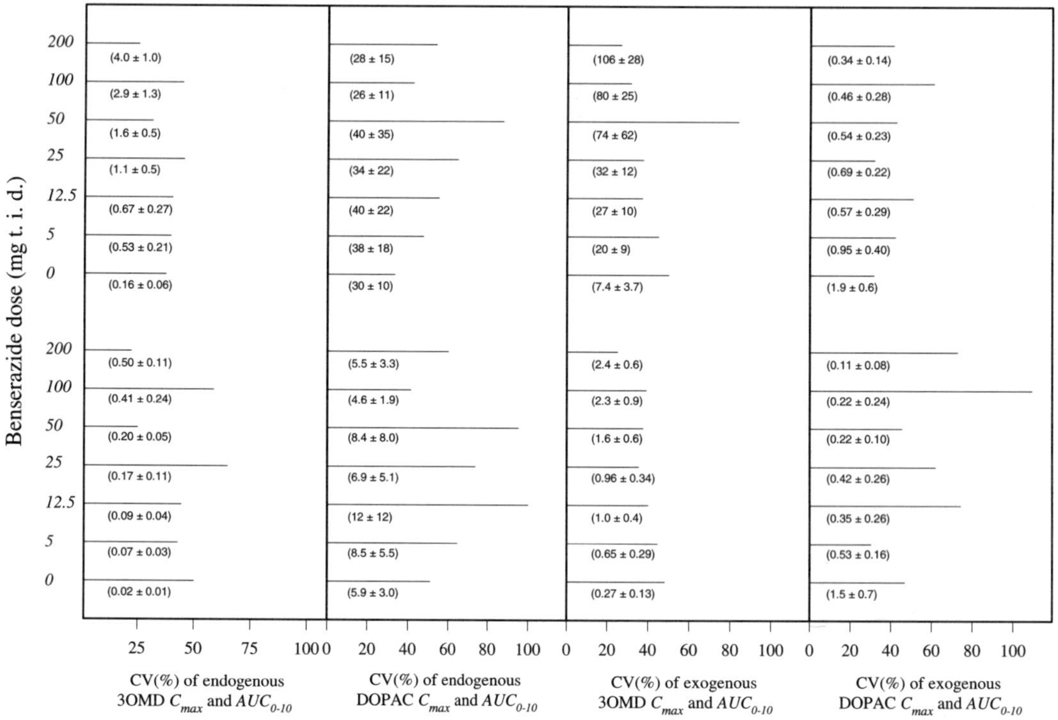

Figure 7.4 Effects of benserazide on the metabolism of endogenous and exogenous (250 mg) levodopa. CV was calculated according to the study of Dingemanse et al. (1997) in eight healthy people taking benserazide in three daily doses. The lower and upper parts present the plasma C_{max} and AUC_{0-10}. The data in parentheses are mean±SD of the plasma C_{max} and AUC_{0-10} with units of mg/l and mg/l/h for endogenous and exogenous 3OMD, and μg/l and μg/l/h for endogenous DOPAC, mg/l and mg/l/h for exogenous DOPAC. The number of healthy people in 0 mg group is sixteen.

Benserazide dose (mg t. i. d.)

	CV(%) of endogenous 3OMD C_{max} and AUC_{0-10}	CV(%) of endogenous DOPAC C_{max} and AUC_{0-10}	CV(%) of exogenous 3OMD C_{max} and AUC_{0-10}	CV(%) of exogenous DOPAC C_{max} and AUC_{0-10}
200	(4.0 ± 1.0)	(28 ± 15)	(106 ± 28)	(0.34 ± 0.14)
100	(2.9 ± 1.3)	(26 ± 11)	(80 ± 25)	(0.46 ± 0.28)
50	(1.6 ± 0.5)	(40 ± 35)	(74 ± 62)	(0.54 ± 0.23)
25	(1.1 ± 0.5)	(34 ± 22)	(32 ± 12)	(0.69 ± 0.22)
12.5	(0.67 ± 0.27)	(40 ± 22)	(27 ± 10)	(0.57 ± 0.29)
5	(0.53 ± 0.21)	(38 ± 18)	(20 ± 9)	(0.95 ± 0.40)
0	(0.16 ± 0.06)	(30 ± 10)	(7.4 ± 3.7)	(1.9 ± 0.6)
200	(0.50 ± 0.11)	(5.5 ± 3.3)	(2.4 ± 0.6)	(0.11 ± 0.08)
100	(0.41 ± 0.24)	(4.6 ± 1.9)	(2.3 ± 0.9)	(0.22 ± 0.24)
50	(0.20 ± 0.05)	(8.4 ± 8.0)	(1.6 ± 0.6)	(0.22 ± 0.10)
25	(0.17 ± 0.11)	(6.9 ± 5.1)	(0.96 ± 0.34)	(0.42 ± 0.26)
12.5	(0.09 ± 0.04)	(12 ± 12)	(1.0 ± 0.4)	(0.35 ± 0.26)
5	(0.07 ± 0.03)	(8.5 ± 5.5)	(0.65 ± 0.29)	(0.53 ± 0.16)
0	(0.02 ± 0.01)	(5.9 ± 3.0)	(0.27 ± 0.13)	(1.5 ± 0.7)

Nitecapone is a peripheral inhibitor of COMT, has natriuretic effect (Eklof *et al.*, 1997) and antioxidant properties in experimental heart transplantation (Haramaki *et al.*, 1995; Vento *et al.*, 1997). The interindividual variability in several nitecapone effects is shown in Table 7.5.

Entacapone is mainly a peripheral inhibitor of COMT. As entacapone inhibits the peripheral COMT, thus it reduces the interindividual variability in levodopa, 3OMD and HVA, but increases the interindividual variability in DOPAC (Table 7.5). The interindividual variability in the inhibition constants can be related to the interindividual variability in the metabolism of levodopa, the human lung showing a much larger interindividual variability (Table 7.5).

Tolcapone is an inhibitor of both periphery and brain in animals and humans (Dingemanse *et al.*, 1995; Yorga *et al.*, 1998; Zürcher *et al.*, 1993). It was suggested that tolcapone may allow smoother delivery of levodopa to the brain, consequently tolcapone should alleviate the 'wearing-off' effects and reduce response fluctuations to levodopa (Jorga *et al.*, 1997). The interindividual variability in the inhibition constants can be related to the interindividual variability in the metabolism of levodopa. Thus human liver shows much larger interindividual variability concerning tolcapone inhibition (Table 7.5). Different dosages have different effects on the interindividual variability of COMT inhibition in erythrocytes (Figure 7.5). Figure 7.6 shows the interindividual variability of effect of tolcapone on different combinations of levodopa and benserazide.

Inhibitors of MAO

Prevention of dopamine metabolism by MAO inhibitors further enhances dopamine accumulation. Both clorgyline and pargyline penetrate the blood–brain barrier well (Yang and Neff, 1974; Dzoljic *et al.*, 1977). Some experimental lines indicate that MAO-A inhibitor rather than MAO-B inhibitor plays a major role in the metabolism of levodopa both intra- and extraneuronally in the rat striatum (Finberg *et al.*, 1995). Suzuki *et al.* (1995) have suggested using MAO-A and -B inhibitors as neuroprotective agents to treat ischemic injury.

Selegiline (L-deprenyl) is an MAO-B inhibitor. It can also block dopamine re-uptake from the synaptic cleft, thus increasing the dopamine brain concentrations (Mahmood, 1997). One of the metabolites of selegiline, desmethylselegiline, has some MAO-B inhibitory properties, though to a lesser extent than those of selegiline (Borbe *et al.*, 1990; Heinonen *et al.*, 1997b). Experimentally, selegiline prevents neuronal cell death in various models. It was hypothesised that selegiline exerts its beneficial effects in Parkinson's disease by suppressing excitotoxic damage (Mytilineou *et al.*, 1997). The interindividual variability in several effects induced by selegiline is larger after its oral than after intravenous administration. Thus, the

Table 7.5 Interindividual variability in inhibitors of COMT

Inhibitors	Effect	CV (%) (mean±SD)	References and Notes
Nitecapone	Increases duodenal bicarbonate secretion		Knutson et al., 1993; control=149±18 μEq/cm/h
	30 mg nitecapone ($n=11$)	17.3 (277±48)	
	150 mg nitecapone ($n=11$)	8.6 (421±36)	
	Increases [^{18}F]6-flurodopa accumulation in		Laihinen et al., 1992; 100 mg nitecapone dose
	striatum (%) ($n=6$)	67.4 (20.0±13.5)	
	Increases striatum/arterial plasma ratio (%) ($n=6$)	31.4 (39.0±12.2)	
	Increases striatum/cortex 6-[18F]L-dopa ratio ($n=7$)	22.2 (2.61±0.58)	Doudet et al., 1997; 20.8±3 mg/kg nitecapone dose; control=1.86±0.19.
Entacapone	Levodopa C_{max} (μg/ml) ($n=8$)	20.9 (1.5±0.3)	Myllylä et al., 1993; see above for dose
	Levodopa $AUC_{0-6 h}$ (μg/ml/h) ($n=8$)	17.1 (4.4±0.7)	
	Levodopa AUC (μg/ml/h) ($n=8$)	18.0 (5.3±1.0)	
	Levodopa $t_{1/2}$ ($n=8$)	17.0 (2.0±0.3)	
	3OMD AUC (μg/ml/h) ($n=8$)	40.0 (17.7±7.1)	Myllylä et al., 1993, see above for dose
	DOPAC AUC (μg/ml/h) ($n=8$)	49.5 (343±170)	
	HVA AUC (μg/ml/h) ($n=8$)	23.3 (303±71)	
	IC_{50} in liver (nmol/l) ($n=5$)	8.6 (151±13)	De Santi et al., 1998; the concentrations of Entacapone and Tolcapone ranged from 62.5 to 1000 nmol/l and 125 to 4000 nmol/l, respectively
	IC_{50} in duodenum (nmol/l) ($n=3$)	8.2 (110±9)	
	IC_{50} in kidney (nmol/l) ($n=6$)	18.7 (134±25)	
	IC_{50} in lung (nmol/l) ($n=6$)	36.0 (186±67)	
	Norepinephrine (nmol/l) ($n=12$)	33.3 (2.1±0.7)	Illi et al., 1996; see Figure 7.7 for dose
Tolcapone	IC_{50} in human liver (nmol/l) ($n=5$)	24.5 (773±189)	De Santi et al., 1998, see above for dose
	IC_{50} in human duodenum (nmol/l) ($n=3$)	4.1 (812±33)	
	IC_{50} in human kidney (nmol/l) ($n=6$)	14.6 (981±241)	
	IC_{50} in human lung (nmol/l) ($n=6$)	16.3 (1389±226)	
	Increases striatum/cortex 6-[^{18}F]L-dopa ratio ($n=7$)	11.6 (2.42±0.28)	Doudet et al., 1997; 28.9±5 mg/kg tolcapone dose; control=1.86±0.19

Note
$t_{1/2}$=elimination half-life.

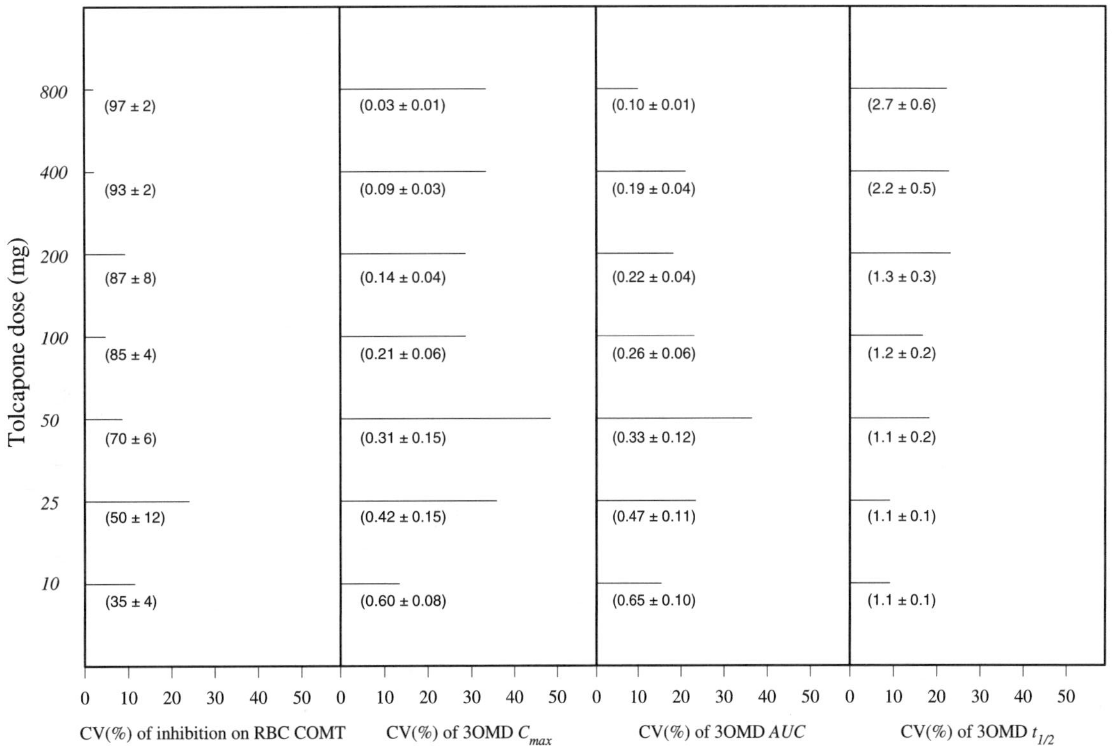

Figure 7.5 Effect of different dosages of tolcapone on the metabolism of levodopa. CV was calculated according to the study of Dingemanse et al. (1995) in six healthy people after 100/25 mg levodopa/benserazide administration. In the original study, the inhibition on RBC COMT was calculated using $(E_0 - E_{max}) \times 100/E_0$. The data in parentheses are mean±SD of the plasma C_{max}, AUC and $t_{1/2}$ with unit as ratios of parameters with tolcapone versus parameters without tolcapone. RBC=red blood cell.

Tolcapone dose (mg)	CV(%) of inhibition on RBC COMT	CV(%) of 3OMD C_{max}	CV(%) of 3OMD AUC	CV(%) of 3OMD $t_{1/2}$
800	(97 ± 2)	(0.03 ± 0.01)	(0.10 ± 0.01)	(2.7 ± 0.6)
400	(93 ± 2)	(0.09 ± 0.03)	(0.19 ± 0.04)	(2.2 ± 0.5)
200	(87 ± 8)	(0.14 ± 0.04)	(0.22 ± 0.04)	(1.3 ± 0.3)
100	(85 ± 4)	(0.21 ± 0.06)	(0.26 ± 0.06)	(1.2 ± 0.2)
50	(70 ± 6)	(0.31 ± 0.15)	(0.33 ± 0.12)	(1.1 ± 0.2)
25	(50 ± 12)	(0.42 ± 0.15)	(0.47 ± 0.11)	(1.1 ± 0.1)
10	(35 ± 4)	(0.60 ± 0.08)	(0.65 ± 0.10)	(1.1 ± 0.1)

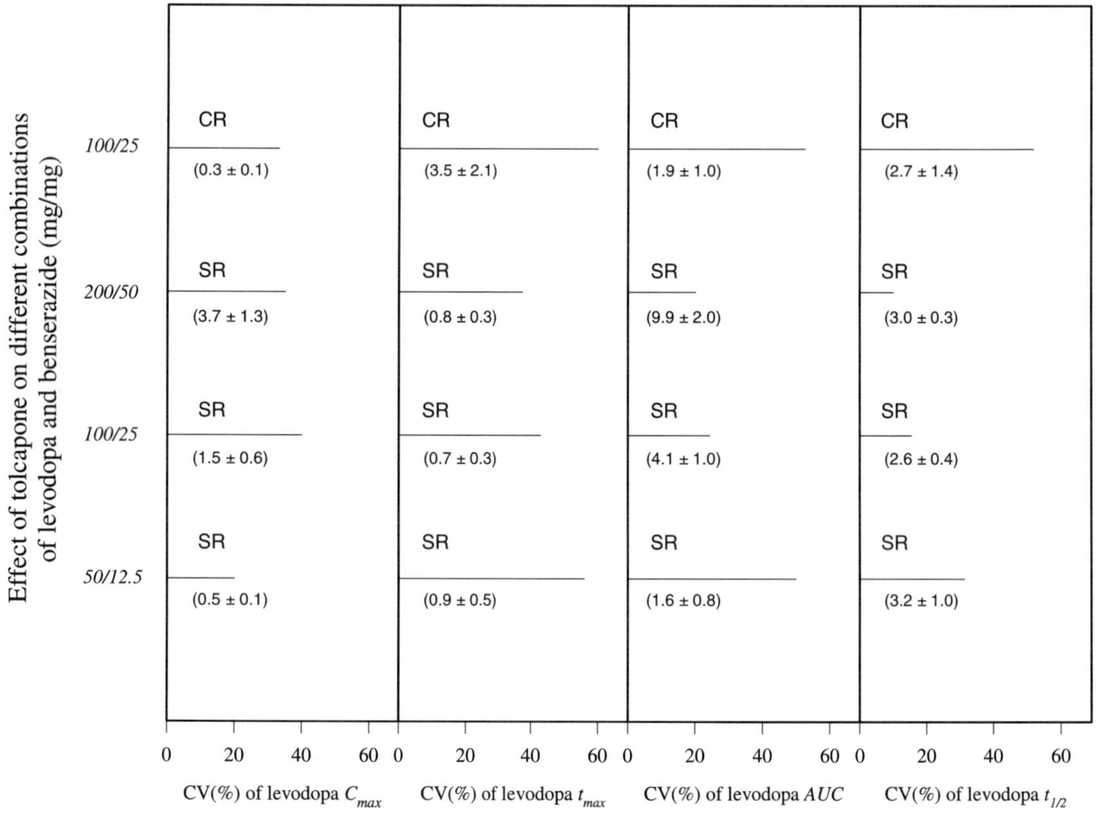

Figure 7.6
Interindividual variability of effect of tolcapone on different combinations of levodopa and benserazide in eight male healthy people with 200 mg tolcapone. CV was calculated according to the study of Jorga et al. (1997). The data in parentheses are mean±SD. CR=levodopa/benserazide controlled release preparation, SR=standard release. C_{max}, t_{max}, AUC and $t_{1/2}$ have the units of μg/ml, h, μg/ml/h and h.

Effect of tolcapone on different combinations of levodopa and benserazide (mg/mg)

levodopa/benserazide	CV(%) of levodopa C_{max}	CV(%) of levodopa t_{max}	CV(%) of levodopa AUC	CV(%) of levodopa $t_{1/2}$
100/25	CR (3.7 ± 1.3)	CR (3.5 ± 2.1)	CR (1.9 ± 1.0)	CR (2.7 ± 1.4)
200/50	SR (1.5 ± 0.6)	SR (0.8 ± 0.3)	SR (9.9 ± 2.0)	SR (3.0 ± 0.3)
100/25	SR (0.5 ± 0.1)	SR (0.7 ± 0.3)	SR (4.1 ± 1.0)	SR (2.6 ± 0.4)
50/12.5	SR (0.5 ± 0.1)	SR (0.9 ± 0.5)	SR (1.6 ± 0.8)	SR (3.2 ± 1.0)

metabolism of levodopa should have a wider interindividual variability after its oral than after its intravenous administration (Table 7.6).

Clorgyline is an inhibitor of MAO-A. Clorgyline displays a very high affinity for rat brain (Alemany *et al.*, 1995). However, Lai and Yu (1997) showed that clorgyline can enhance dopamine-induced toxicity in catecholaminergic neuroblastoma SH-SY5Y cells. The interindividual variability in several clorgyline effects is shown in Table 7.6.

Pargyline is an inhibitor on both MAO-A and B (Abdel-Fattah *et al.*, 1997), in particular on the fraction II of the serum MAO, which can be electrophoretically separated into three bands, termed as fraction I, II and III (Nakano *et al.*, 1995). The interindividual variability in several pargyline effects is shown in Table 7.6.

Co-administration of different inhibitors

Currently, it is rare to treat patients with Parkinson's disease without inhibitors of LAAD, thus the effect of two kinds of inhibitors on the interindividual variability needs to be considered.

Tolcapone and benserazide

The different combinations of these COMT and LAAD inhibitors have different effects on the interindividual variability in 3OMD C_{max}, area-under-concentration-curve (AUC) and half-life ($t_{1/2}$) with more effects on 3OMD C_{max} (Figure 7.5). Regarding clinical effect, tolcapone with levodopa-benserazide shows an interindividual variability of 99.4% CV (61.7±61.3 min, $n=10$, 200 mg tolcapone) to 81.0% CV (72.2±58.8 min, $n=10$, 400 mg tolcapone) in the duration of on-phase (Limousin *et al.*, 1995).

Entacapone and moclobemide

Co-administration of entacapone and moclobemide slightly alters the interindividual variability in clinical response as shown in Figure 7.7 (Illi *et al.*, 1996).

Tolcapone and selegiline/pargyline

The combination of these inhibitors increases the striatum/cortex 6-[18F]L-dopa ratio in monkey with an interindividual variability of 14.5% CV (2.34±0.34 versus 1.86±0.19, $n=5$, Doudet *et al.*, 1997).

Entacapone and LAAD inhibitor

Entacapone (200 and 800 mg) given concomitantly with levodopa and a dopa decarboxylase inhibitor can reduce the latency (from 70.5±30.9 to

Table 7.6 Interindividual variability in inhibitors of MAO

Inhibitors	Effect	CV (%) (mean±SD)	References and Notes
Selegiline	Inhibits platelet MAO-B (%) (n=10)	4.1 (96.4±3.9)	Heinonen et al., 1997b
	0.5 mg intravenous (n=16)	19.0 (79.6±15.1)	Heinonen et al., 1997a
	0.5 mg oral (n=16)	40.2 (23.4±9.4)	
	1 mg oral (n=16)	36.9 (40.4±14.9)	
	1.5 mg oral (n=16)	33.6 (51.5±17.3)	
	Inhibition constant IC$_{50}$ (10^{-6} M)	10.0 (1.0±0.1)	Chen et al., 1994
	Increases rat striatum dopamine release (pmol/20 min) (n=8)	11.4 (0.88±0.10)	Lamensdorf et al., 1996; 0.25 mg/kg selegiline for 21 days; control=0.34±0.04, n=13
	Prolongs rat lifespan (weeks) (n=66)	1.2 (191.9±2.3)	Knoll 1989; control=147.1±0.6.
Desmethylselegiline	Inhibits platelet MAO-B (%) (n=10)	19.9 (63.7±12.7)	Heinonen et al., 1997a
Clorgyline	Increases dopamine release (pmol/20 min) (n=7)	13.3 (0.90±0.12)	Lamensdorf et al., 1996; 0.2 mg/kg clorgyline for 21 days; control=0.34±0.04, n=13
	Inhibition constant IC$_{50}$ (10^{-10} M)	1.7 (5.8±0.1)	Chen et al., 1994
Pargyline	Decreases catechol oxidation current (% of peak height)	8.1 (143±11.6)	Milne et al., 1989
	Increases norepinephrine levels (pg/g of mice tissue)	12.4 (4122.6±509.5)	Marino et al., 1997; control=2806.7±408.9.
	Decreases accumulation of 1-methyl-4-phenylpyridinium in rat hepatocytes (%) (n=5)	17.9 (38.1±6.8)	Martel et al., 1996

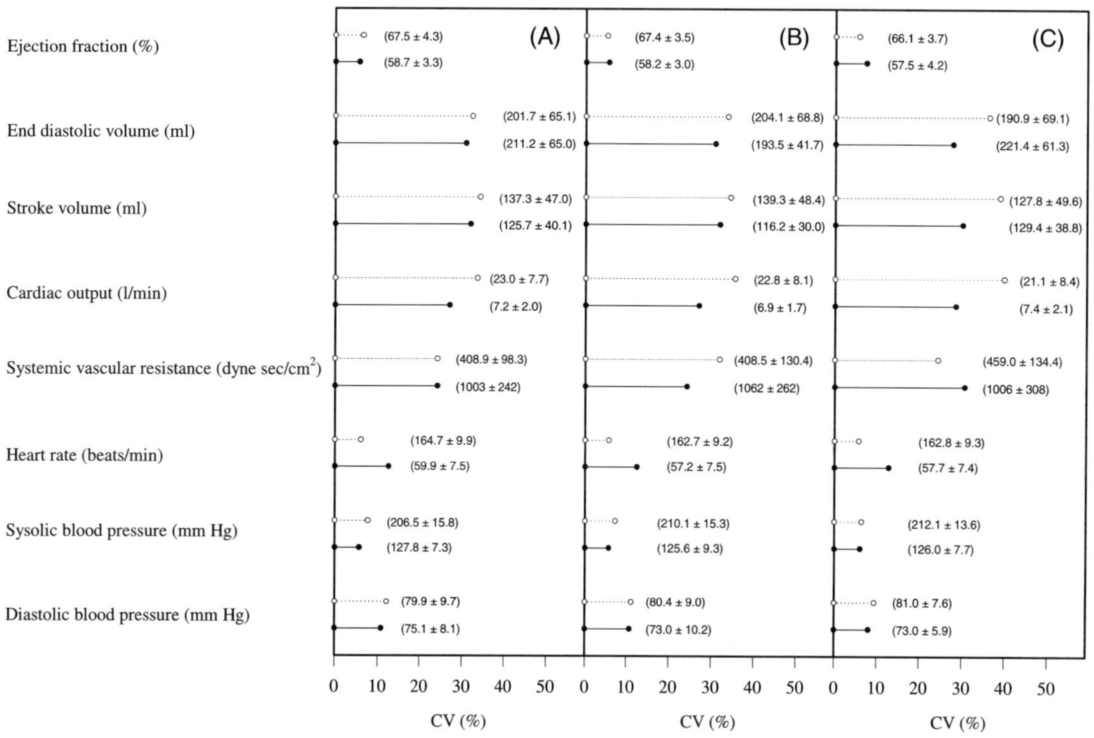

Figure 7.7 Interindividual variability in clinical response to entacapone (200 mg, A), moclobemide (150 mg, B) and both (C) in healthy male volunteers (n=12). The data in parentheses are mean±SD. Solid lines with filled circles=rest; dotted lines with unfilled circles=exercise. CV was calculated according to the study by Illi et al. (1996).

54.0 ± 17.6 min; $n=12$) and increase the duration of action (from 163.5 ± 65.4 to 168 ± 93.8 min; $n=12$) in motor fluctuating patients with Parkinson's disease with an interindividual variability ranging from 32.6 to 55.8% CV (Merello et al., 1994).

Interference of other drugs

Cyclosporine can alter the interindividual variability of K_m and V_{max} of LAAD, MAO-A, MAO-B and COMT in homogenates of rat renal tubules (Pestana et al., 1995; Pestana and Soares-da-Silva, 1994; Lee, 1993) as shown in Figure 7.8. Among these enzymes LAAD shows the maximum interindividual variability, whereas MAO-A shows the minimum.

The adenosine A_{2A} receptor antagonist, 7-(2-phenylethyl)-5-amino-2-(2-furyl)-pyrazolo-[4,3-e]-1,2,4-triazolo[1,5-c]pyrimidine, can potentiate the effects of levodopa in Parkinson's disease, as well as alter the interindividual variability as 40.2% of CV (349 ± 140 contralateral rotations, $n=7$) in levodopa group versus 44.3% of CV (758 ± 336 contralateral rotations, $n=7$) in levodopa and antagonist groups (Fenu et al., 1997).

Cabergoline with levodopa show to be effective for both advanced and de novo Parkinson patients. In addition, it alters the interindividual variability in levodopa C_{max} (11.67% of CV, 1.20 ± 0.14 µg/ml, $n=12$), t_{max} (9.6% of CV, 57.7 ± 5.54 min, $n=12$), AUC_{0-8} (15.7% of CV, 2.29 ± 0.36 µg/ml/h, $n=12$) and 3OMD AUC_{0-8} (9.2% of CV, 13.2 ± 1.2 µg/ml/h, $n=12$) (Del Dotto et al., 1997).

Co-administration of benzhexol and levodopa can lead to two or more peaks of levodopa concentrations in plasma with an interindividual variability of 32.3% CV (the second peak 2.69 ± 0.87 µg/ml, $n=10$) to 76.1% CV (the first peak 3.01 ± 2.29 µg/ml, $n=10$) (Roberts et al., 1996).

3OMD

3OMD can alter the interindividual variability of the restoration of dopamine in rat brain by levodopa after depletion of catecholamine by α-methyl-para-tyrosine (250 mg/kg), i.e. the CV (%) is 10.4 (0.96 ± 0.1 µg/g wet tissue, $n=12$), 9.1 (1.1 ± 0.1 µg/g wet tissue, $n=4$), 9.1 (1.1 ± 0.1, µg/g wet tissue, $n=11$), 10.0 (1 ± 0.1 µg/g wet tissue, $n=3$) and 9.1 (1.1 ± 0.1 µg/g wet tissue, $n=13$), 5.0 (0.2 ± 0.01 µg/g wet tissue, $n=4$), 16.7 (0.6 ± 0.1, µg/g wet tissue, $n=12$), 11.7 (0.6 ± 0.07 µg/g wet tissue, $n=4$) in control and experimental groups at 30, 60, 90, 120 min after 100 mg/kg levodopa and 200 mg/kg 3OMD i.p. (Gervas et al., 1983).

Effect of absorption pattern of levodopa on its metabolism

Although the absorption process has no direct impact on the enzymes involved in the metabolism of levodopa, the longer levodopa stays in the

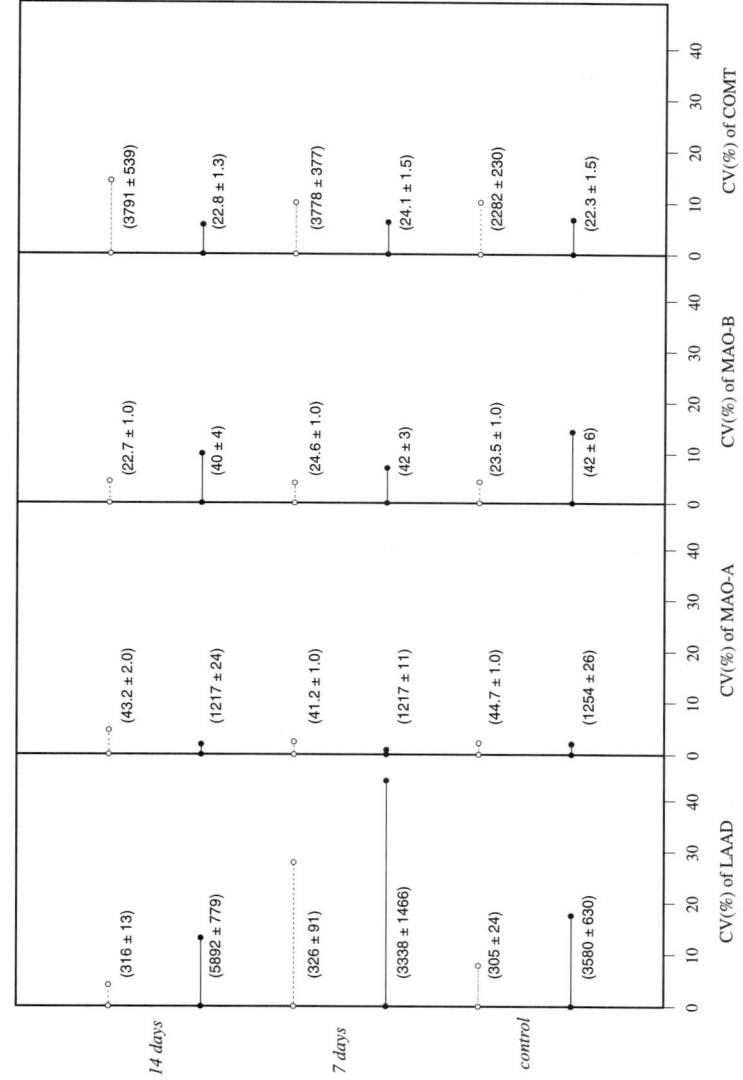

Figure 7.8 Interindividual variability in the effect of cyclosporine on K_m (μM, solid lines with filled circles) and V_{max} (pmol/mg of protein/h, dashed lines with unfilled circles) in LAAD, MAO-A, MAO-B and COMT of rat renal tubules homogenate. CV was calculated according to the study by Pestana et al. (1995) in four rats. The data in parentheses are mean±SD of K_m and V_{max}.

stomach and jejunum, the more levodopa will be biotransformed there. The duration of levodopa in the stomach and jejunum depends on the gastric emptying time and on the amount of natural amino acid present, which compete for the same transport system similar to the one across the blood–brain barrier (Wade *et al.*, 1973). Therefore the lifestyle difference among individuals and the change in personal lifestyle contribute indirectly to the interindividual and intraindividual variability in the metabolism of levodopa. In fact, the effect of food on the absorption of levodopa has been the objective of many studies. The interindividual variability regarding this aspect is beyond the subject of this chapter.

Summarising, numerous environmental factors are involved in the metabolism of levodopa, among them the inhibitors play a major role so that they may induce a remarkable effect on the individual variability of the levodopa metabolism.

Some points for debate related to interindividual variability

Dopa decarboxylase inhibitors (LAAD inhibitors)

Several lines of evidence show that LAAD inhibitors do not modify plasma levodopa half-life (Fahn, 1974; Rinne *et al.*, 1973) in the experimental group in comparison with the control one. This is naturally due to the wide interindividual variability either in both groups or in one group only. Hence LAAD inhibitors may change the interindividual variability at varying degrees.

Levodopa toxicity

Levodopa and dopamine have been reported to be cytotoxic to cells in culture (Basma *et al.*, 1995, Graham *et al.*, 1978; Parsons, 1985; Rosenberg, 1988). Mytilineou *et al.* (1993) have shown that levodopa can cause toxic effects on mesencephalic neurones in culture, thus suggesting that patients on long-term levodopa therapy might be at risk because of toxic intermediates (Steece-Collier *et al.*, 1990).

The proposed mechanism is the autoxidation into highly reactive toxic free radicals (H_2O_2, hydrogen peroxide; O_2^-, superoxide radical; and HO·, hydroxyl radical), quinones and levodopa hydroxy derivative 2,4,5-trihydroxyphenylalanine (TOPA) via an excitatory effect on glutamate receptors (Biscoe *et al.*, 1976; Aizenman *et al.*, 1990; Michel and Hefti, 1990; Olney *et al.*, 1990; Rosenberg *et al.*, 1991). A more recent study suggested that administration of levodopa reduces the growth, behavioral recovery, and tyrosine hydroxylase activity of fetal mesencephalic grafts in animals that had previously received a unilateral 6-hydroxydopamine lesion of the striatum (Felten *et al.*, 1992). One study showed that accumulation of dopamine in the extracellular fluid elicited by pargyline can be auto-oxidised, which in turn leads (possibly by an indirect mechanism) to the formation of cytotoxic OH free radicals (Obata and Yamanaka, 1995).

Biphasic effect of levodopa

Low doses of levodopa decrease motor activity in rodents whereas high doses stimulate motor activity (Stromberg, 1970; Montanaro et al., 1983; Bradbury et al., 1984). In rats dopaminergic agents usually have a biphasic effect on pain (Paalzow and Paalzow, 1983), heart rate (Paalzow and Paalzow, 1986a) and yawning (Protais et al., 1983). It was suggested that a similar biphasic dose responsiveness might contribute to the fluctuating motor response that complicates chronic levodopa therapy (Paalzow and Paalzow, 1986b). The inhibitory action of levodopa has also been observed in a clinical trial (Nutt et al., 1988), in which levodopa was given to patients by a continuous intravenous infusion at different rates, and the results suggest that levodopa causes an acute deterioration in motor function followed by an improvement. The problem of how much of this levodopa effect might be related to the interindividual variability in the metabolism of levodopa, or to dopamine receptors responsiveness, remains still unsolved.

Inhibition on LAAD by levodopa

Although levodopa is the substrate of LAAD, some studies have shown that levodopa itself can reduce the LAAD activity (Tate et al., 1971; Dairman et al., 1971; Tanaka et al., 1973). These observations have to be taken into account to correlate with the interindividual variability in the metabolism of levodopa.

Summarising, most of these data suggest that the interindividual variability in the metabolism of levodopa may play a potential role in levodopa toxicity.

Interindividual variability in clinical response

In routine clinical settings, the assessment of interindividual and intra-individual variability in clinical response to levodopa becomes problematic because of lack of control. Methodologically, the adverse effect is often assessed by the frequency of incidence of a particular symptom in a treated population. The interindividual variability being difficult to be evaluated on the basis of such data. Another difficulty in the correlation of levodopa metabolism with clinical response is that the one-to-one relationship (i.e. the higher levodopa concentration versus the higher clinical effect, the lower levodopa concentration versus the lower clinical effect) is still not yet established although several pharmacokinetic–pharmacodynamic models have been proposed.

Figure 7.7 shows the interindividual variability in clinical response respectively to entacapone or moclobemide or both and Table 7.7 shows the interindividual variability in clinical response to levodopa. Figure 7.9 shows the interindividual variability of tolcapone effects on clinical response induced by levodopa.

The interindividual variability can also appear in clinical response to different rates of levodopa infusion, for example, CV of time to onset of response after beginning levodopa administration is 25.0% (2.4±0.6 h, $n=6$), 39.1% (2.3±0.9 h, $n=10$), 46.2% (1.3±0.6 h, $n=8$) for untreated, stable, fluctuating patients at 0.8 mg/kg/h, and 27.8% (1.8±0.5 h, $n=6$), 45.5% (2.2±1.0 h, $n=10$), 50.0% (1.0±0.5 h, $n=8$) for untreated, stable, fluctuating patients at 1.6 mg/kg/h (Nutt et al., 1992), thus suggesting differences in levodopa metabolic capacity.

Summarising, the interindividual variability is smaller in clinical response than that in levodopa and levodopa metabolites, because the clinical response depends on numerous factors not only on one or two drugs.

The ways to assess individual variability

As stated in the Introduction, the assessment of individual variability can be achieved by two statistical methods: (i) the calculation of standard deviation (SD) and CV; and (ii) the calculation of model II one-way ANOVA (Sokal and Rohlfe, 1981; Rodbard, 1974; Wu et al., 1999). The former is statistically less powerful but easy and widely used, whereas the latter is more appropriate but more complicated and less used. Moreover, the assessment using the model II ANOVA is based on the statistical inference with F-test, thus one can statistically compare the interindividual variability with the intraindividual variability. By contrast, it could be not easy to compare the interindividual variability with the intraindividual variability using the first method.

Although numerous metabolites of levodopa are available, 3OMD is commonly measured in clinical settings. 3OMD variability provides an indirect assessment of the metabolism of levodopa, a measure of the inhibition of peripheral COMT, and a possible offset role for levodopa therapeutic effect.

As an example, we used the unequal sample sizes model II one-way ANOVA to calculate interindividual variability and intraindividual variability in 3OMD concentrations and AUC. It can be seen in Table 7.8 that the interindividual variability SD and CV are much wider than the intraindividual ones, even if the patients were given the same dosage of levodopa under the same conditions.

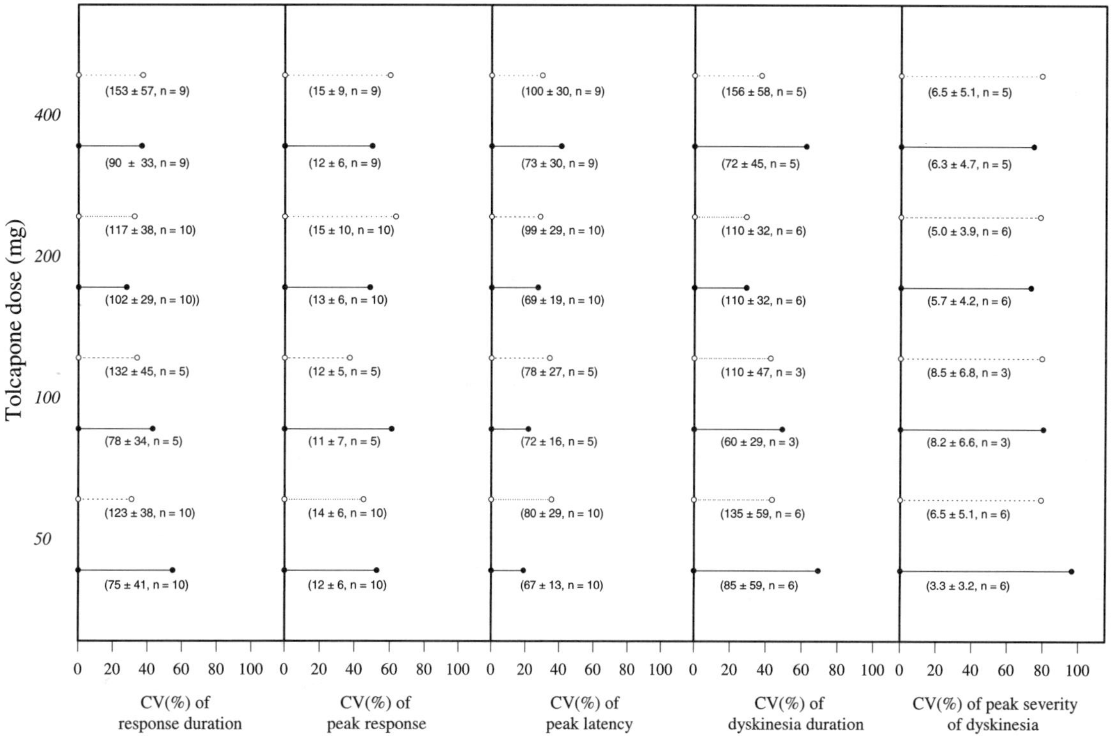

Figure 7.9 Interindividual variability in the effect of tolcapone on clinical response induced by levodopa/carbidopa association in Parkinsonian patients. CV was calculated according to the study by Roberts et al. (1994). The data in parentheses are mean±SD and number of patients. The solid lines with filled circles and dotted lines with unfilled circles are control and experimental groups.

Table 7.7 Interindividual variability in clinical response to levodopa in Parkinsian patients

Clinical response	Baseline CV (%) (mean ± SD)	Effect CV (%) (mean ± SD)	Reference and notes
Fasting tapping test (n=8)	24.7 (150±37)	56.4 (39±22)	Contin et al., 1998; 200/50 levodopa/carbidopa
Fed tapping test (n=8)	27.2 (151±41)	51.2 (41±21)	dose
CURSΣ (IR) (n=10)	25.6 (40.6±10.4)	34.9 (27.2±9.5)	Harder et al., 1995; 100/25 mg levodopa/
CURSΣ (CR) (n=10)	23.1 (39.8±9.2)	31.4 (26.1±8.2)	benserazide (IR) and 300/75 mg levodopa/
			benserazide (CR) doses
Wearing-off in oral treatment (n=9)		26.3 (1.9±0.51)	Mouradian et al., 1987; 250/25 mg
Wearing-off in i.v. treatment (n=9)		40.7 (1.4±0.57)	levodopa/carbidopa oral dose, the i.v. dose was
On–off in oral treatment (n=14)		26.7 (2.1±0.56)	optimal-dose with oral carbidopa administration
On–off in I.V. treatment (n=14)		35.8 (1.67±0.60)	
Walking with IR treatment (n=5)		60.3 (12.6±7.6)	Nutt et al., 1986; 1340±555/152±37 mg
Walking with CR-3 treatment (n=5)		47.2 (12.5±5.9)	levodopa/carbidopa (IR) and 4160±1905/
AIM with IR treatment (n=5)		105.6 (3.6±3.8)	1040±476 mg levodopa/carbidopa (CR-3) daily
AIM with CR-3 treatment (n=5)		157.1 (2.8±4.4)	
UPDRS (n=9)	41.9 (21.7±9.1)	52.6 (9.5±5.0)	Barbato et al., 1997; 200/50 mg levodopa/carbidopa
			dose

Table 7.8 3OMD plasma concentrations, AUC and their inter/intraindividual variability (SD and CV) assessed by model II ANOVA.

Concentration (ng/ml, mean±SD)	Eight patients after administration of 100 mg CR				Eleven patients after administration of 200 mg CR				
	0 h	0.5 h	1 h	2 h	0 h	0.5 h	1 h	2 h	4 h
Concentration (ng/ml, mean±SD)	2466±1432	2234±1489	2688±1520	2344±1536	3502±1556	3548±1665	3499±1624	3461±1605	3478±2087
interindividual SD (ng/ml)	147.8	1610.3	1580.4	1613.1	1614.0	1712.0	1666.0	1611.0	2358.0
interindividual CV (%)	58.1	69.2	56.3	67.0	44.9	46.9	46.3	44.6	62.1
intraindividual SD (ng/ml)	387.8	293.9	303.8	175.8	352.0	451.0	405.0	460.0	402.0
intraindividual CV (%)	15.2	12.6	10.8	7.3	10.1	12.7	11.6	13.3	11.6
AUC (ng/ml/h)		1082±759	2637±1463	4607±2952		1759±787	3521±1603	6802±3282	13881±8428
interindividual SD (ng/ml/h)		832	1535	3097		818	1661	3374	9536
interindividual CV (%)		74.1	55.9	65.5		45.2	45.9	47.6	62.7
intraindividual SD (ng/ml/h)		81	193	333		154	331	629	1156
intraindividual CV (%)		7.3	7.0	7.1		8.8	9.4	9.3	8.3

Notes
Intraindividual SD is the standard deviation within individuals and applies to the relevant concentration and AUC to a new individual from the same population.
Interindividual SD is the standard deviation between individuals if the relevant concentration and AUC are obtained from an infinite number of measurements.

Furthermore, the interindividual and intraindividual variabilities need to be considered when planning experiments (Woods *et al.*, 1989; Hills and Armitage, 1979; Evans, 1983), i.e. whether an investigation should include two parallel groups (interindividual) or a crossover design (intra-individual). The intraindividual variability is particularly important for long-term studies.

Concluding remarks

The interindividual and intraindividual variability in the metabolism of levodopa is a complicated subject, due to numerous factors. Great efforts are needed to determine the relationship between a single factor with the clinical response, and more important, to determine the relationship between multiple factors with clinical response. Finally great effort should be directed to the methodology used, such as the means to determine the interindividual variability in polymorphism.

Acknowledgements

This work was partially supported by project No. BMHCT 941622.

References

Abdel-Fattah, A. F., Matsumoto, K., Murakami, Y., Adel-Khalek Gammaz, H., Mohamed, M. F. and Watanabe, H. (1997) 'Central serotonin level-dependent changes in body temperature following administration of tryptophan to pargyline- and harmaline-pretreated rats', *Gen. Pharmacol.* **28**: 405–9.

Agathopoulos, A., Nicolopoulos, D., Matsaniotis, N. and Papadatos, C. (1971) 'Biochemical changes of catechol-O-methyltransferase during development of human liver', *Pediatrics* **47**: 125–8.

Aizenman, E., White, W. F., Loring, R. H. and Rosenberg, P. A. (1990) 'A 3,4-dihydroxyphenylalanine oxidation product is a non-N-methyl-D-aspartate glutamatergic agonist in rat cortical neurons', *Neurosci. Lett.* **116**: 168–71.

Alemany, R., Olmos, G. and Garcia-Sevilla, J. A. (1995) 'The effects of phenelzine and other monoamine oxidase inhibitor antidepressants on brain and liver I2 imidazoline-preferring receptors', *Br. J. Pharmacol.* **114**: 837–45.

Ashton, M. J., Lawrence, C., Karlsson, J. A., Stuttle, K. A., Newton, C. G., Vacher, B. Y., Webber, S. and Withnall, M. J. (1996) 'Anti-inflammatory 17beta-thioalkyl-16alpha, 17alpha-ketal and -acetal androstanes: a new class of airway selective steroids for the treatment of asthma', *J. Med. Chem.* **39**: 4888–96.

Assicot, M. and Bohuon, C. (1971) 'Presence of two distinct catechol-O-methyl-transferase activities in red blood cells', *Biochimie.* **53**: 871–4.

Awata, H., Endo, F. and Matsuda, I. (1994) 'Structure of the human 4–hydroxy-phenylpyruvic acid dioxygenase gene (HPD)', *Genomics* **23**: 534–9.

Axelrod, J., Alberts, W. and Clemente, C. (1959) 'Distribution of catechol-O-methyltransferase in the nervous system and other tissues', *J. Neurochem.* **5**: 68–71.

Bäckström, R., Honkanen, E., Pippuri, P., Kairisalo, J., Pystynen, J., Heinola, K., Nissinen, E., Lindén, I.-B., Männistö, P. T., Kaakkola, S. and Pohto, P. (1989) 'Synthesis of some novel potent and selective catechol O-methyltransferase inhibitors', *J. Med. Chem.* **32**: 841–6.

Barbato, L., Stocchi, F., Monge, A., Vacca, L., Ruggieri, S., Nordera, G. and Marsden, C. D. (1997) 'The long-duration action of levodopa may be due to a postsynaptic effect', *Clin. Neuropharmacol.* **20**: 394–401.

Basma, A. N., Morris, E. J., Nicklas, W. J. and Geller, H. M. (1995) 'L-DOPA cytotoxicity to PC12 cells in culture is via its autoxidation', *J. Neurochem.* **64**: 825–32.

Benathan, M. and Labidi, F. (1996) 'Cysteine-dependent 5-S-cysteinyldopa formation and its regulation by glutathione in normal epidermal melanocytes', *Arch. Dermatol. Res.* **288**: 697–702.

Benetello, P., Furlanut, M., Fortunato, M., Pea, F. and Baraldo, M. (1997) 'Levodopa and 3-O-methyldopa in cerebrospinal liquid after levodopa-carbidopa association', *Pharmacol. Res.* **35**: 313–5.

Bianchine, J. R., Messiha, F. S. and Hsu, T. H. (1972) 'Peripheral aromatic L-amino acids decarboxylase inhibitor in parkinsonism II: effect on metabolism of L-2-^{14}C-DOPA', *Clin. Pharmacol. Ther.* **13**: 584–94.

Biscoe, T. J., Evans, R. H., Headley, P. M., Martin, M. R. and Watkins, J. C. (1976) 'Structure-activity relations of excitatory amino acids on frog and rat spinal neurones', *Br J Pharmacol* **58**: 373–82.

Borbe, H., Niebch, G. and Nickel, B. (1990) 'Kinetic evaluation of MAO-B activity following oral administration of selegiline and desmethylselegiline in the rat', *J. Neural Transm.* **32**(Suppl.): 131–7.

Borchardt, R. T., Cheng, C. F. and Cooke, P. H. (1974) 'The purification and kinetic properties of liver microsomal-catechol-O-methyltransferase', *Life. Sci.* **14**: 1089–100.

Borgulya, J., Bruderer, H., Bernauer, K., Zürcher, G. and Da Prada, M. (1989) 'Catechol-O-methyltransferase-inhibiting pyro-catechol derivatives–synthesis and structure-activity studies', *Helv. Chim. Acta.* **72**: 952–68.

Boudikova, B., Szumlanski, C., Maidak B. and Weinshilboum, R. (1990) 'Human liver catechol-O-methyltransferase pharmacogenetics', *Clin. Pharmacol. Ther.* **48**: 381–9.

Bradbury, A. J., Costall, B. and Naylor, R. J. (1984) 'Inhibition and facilitation of motor responding of the mouse by action of dopamine agonists in the forebrain', *Neuropharmacology* **23**: 1025–31.

Brannan, T., Martinez-Tica, J. and Tahr, M. D. (1992) 'Catechol-O-methyltransferase inhibition increases striatal L-dopa and dopamine: an in vivo study in rats', *Neurology* **42**: 683–5.

Brannan, T., Prikhojan, A. and Yahr, M. D. (1996) 'Elevated striatal dopamine levels following administration of D-DOPA and its alpha-keto acid metabolite DHPPA: behavioral and physiological studies in vivo in the rat', *Brain Res* **718**: 165–8.

Budavari, S. (1989) *The Merck Index*, 11th edition (Centennial Edition) Inc. Rahway, NJ: Merck & Co., p. 991.

Chao, Y. C., Liou, S. R., Chung, Y. Y., Tang, H. S., Hsu, C. T., Li, T. K. and Yin, S. J. (1994) 'Polymorphism of alcohol and aldehyde dehydrogenase genes and alcoholic cirrhosis in Chinese patients', *Hepatology* **19**: 360–6.

Chen, K., Wu, H. F., Brimsby, J. and Shih, J. C. (1994) 'Cloning of a novel mono-amino oxidase cDNA from trout liver', *Mol. Pharmacol.* **46**: 1226–33.

Chrapusta, S. J., Karoum, F., Egan, M. F. and Wyatt, R. J. (1993) 'Haloperidol and clozapine increase intraneuronal dopamine metabolism, but not gamma-butyrolactone-resistant dopamine release', *Eur. J. Pharmacol.* **233**: 135–42.

Colman, M. A., Stevens, G., Ramsay, M., Kwon, B. and Jenkins, T. (1993) 'Exclusion of two candidate pigment loci, c and b, part of chromosome 11p, and 33 random polymorphic markers as the locus for tyrosinase-positive oculocu-taneous albinism', *Hum. Genet.* **90**: 556–60.

Contin, M., Riva, R., Martinelli, P., Albani, F. and Baruzzi, A. (1998) 'Effect of meal timing on the kinetic-dynamic profile of levodopa/carbidopa controlled is release in parkinsonian patients', *Eur. J. Clin. Pharmacol.* **54**: 303–8.

Contin, M., Riva, R., Martinelli, P., Cortelli, P., Albani, F. and Baruzzi, A. (1993) 'Pharmacodynamic modeling of oral levodopa: clinical application in Parkinson's disease', *Neurology* **43**: 367–71.

Costa, P., Checkoway, H., Levy, D., Smith-Weller, T., Franklin, G. M., Swanson, P. D. and Costa L. G. (1997) 'Association of a polymorphism in intro 13 of the monoamine oxidase B gene with Parkinson's disease', *Am. J. Med. Genet.* **74**: 154–6.

Crabb, D. W., Edenberg, H. J., Bosron, W. F. and Li, T. K. (1989) 'Genotypes for aldehyde dehydrogenase deficiency and alcohol sensitivity: the inactive ALDH$^2_2$ allele is dominant', *J. Clin. Invest.* **83**: 314–6.

Cubells, J. F., Kobayashi, K., Nagatsu, T., Kidd, K. K., Kidd, J. R., Calafell, F., Kranzler, H. R., Ichinose, H. and Gelernter, J. (1997) 'Population genetics of a functional variant of the dopamine beta-hydroxylase gene (DBH)', *Am. J. Med. Genet.* **74**: 374–9.

Cubells, J. F., van Kammen, D. P., Kelley, M. E., Anderson, G. M., O'Connor, D. T., Price, L. H., Malison, R., Rao, P. A., Kobayashi, K., Nagatsu, T. and Gelernter, J. (1998) 'Dopamine beta-hydroxylase: two polymorphisms in linkage disequilibrium at the structural gene DBH associate with biochemical phenotypic variation', *Hum. Genet.* **102**: 533–40.

Dairman, W., Christenson, J. G. and Udenfriend, S. (1971) 'Decrease in live aromatic L-amino acid decarboxylase produced by chronic administration of L-DOPA', *Proc. Natl. Acad. Sci. USA* **68**: 2117–20.

De Santi, C., Giulianotti, P. G., Pietrabissa, A., Mosca, F. and Pacifici, G. M. (1998) 'Catechol-O-methyltransferase: variation in enzyme activity and inhibition by entacapone and tolcapone', *Eur. J. Clin. Pharmacol.* **54**: 215–9.

Del Dotto, P., Colzi, A., Musatti, E., Benedetti, M. S., Periani, S., Fariello, R. and Bonuccelli U. (1997) 'Clinical and pharmacokinetic evaluation of L-dopa and cabergoline cotreatment in Parkinson's disease', *Clin. Neuropharmacol.* **20**: 455–65.

Dingemanse, J., Jorga, K., Zürcher, G., Schmitt, M., Sedek, G., Da Prada, M. and van Brummelen, P. (1995) 'Pharmacokinetic-pharmacodynamic interaction between the COMT inhibitor tolcapone and single-dose levodopa', *Br. J. Clin. Pharmacol.* **40**: 253–62.

Dingemanse, J., Kleinbloese, C. H., Zürcher, G., Wood, N. D. and Crevoisier, C. (1997) 'Pharmacodynamics of benserazide assessed by its effects on endogenous and exogenous levodopa pharmacokinetics', *Br. J. Clin. Pharmacol.* **44**: 41–8.

Doudet, D. J., Chan, G. L. Y., Holden, J. E., Pate, B. D., Morrison, K. S., Calne, D. B. and Ruth, T. J. (1997) 'Effects of monoamine oxidase and catechol-O-methyltransferase inhibition on dopamine turnover: a PET study with 6-[^{18}F]L-DOPA', *Eur. J. Pharmacol.* **334**: 31–8.

Drebing, C. J., Freedman, R., Waldo, M. and Gerhardt, G. A. (1989) 'Unconjugated methoxylated catecholamine metabolites in human saliva. Quantitation methodology and comparison with plasma levels', *Biomed. Chromatog.* **3**: 217–20.

Dundjerski, J., Butorovic, B., Kipic, J., Trajkovic, D. and Matic, G. (1996) 'Cadmium affects the activity of rat live tyrosine aminotransferase and its induction by dexamethasone', *Arch. Toxicol.* **70**: 390–5.

Dunnette, J. H. and Weinshilboum, R. M. (1982) 'Family studies of plasma dopamine-beta-hydroxylase thermal stability', *Am. J. Hum. Genet.* **34**: 84–99.

Dunnette, J. H. and Weinshilboum, R. M. (1983) 'Serum dopamine beta-hydroxylase activity in non-human primates: phylogenetic and genetic implications', *Comp. Biochem. Physiol. C–Comp. Pharmacol. Toxicol.* **75**: 85–91.

Dutton, J., Copeland, L. G., Playfer, J. R. and Roberts, N. B. (1993) 'Measuring L-dopa in plasma and urine to monitor therapy of elderly patients with Parkinson's disease treated with L-dopa and dopa decarboxylase inhibitor', *Clin. Chem.* **39**: 629–34.

Dzoljic, M. R., Bruinvels, J. and Bonta, I. L. (1977) 'Desynchronization of electrical activity in rats induced by deprenyl – an inhibitor of monamine oxidase B – and relationship with selective increase of dopamine and beta-phenylalanine', *J. Neural. Transm.–Gen. Sect.* **40**: 1–12.

Eaton, M. J., Gudehithlu, K. P., Quach, T., Silvia, C. P., Hadjiconstantinou, M. and Neff, N. H. (1993) 'Distribution of aromatic L-amino acid decarboxylase mRNA in mouse brain by in situ hybridization histology', *J. Comp. Neurol.* **337**: 640–54.

Eklof, A. C., Holtback, U., Sundelof, M., Chen, S. and Aperia, A. (1997) 'Inhibition of COMT induces dopamine-dependent natriuresis and inhibition of proximal tubular Na$^+$,K$^+$-ATPase', *Kidney Int.* **52**: 742–7.

Ellis, M. K., Whitfield, A. C., Gowans, L. A., Auton, T. R., Provan, W. M., Lock, E. A., Lee, D. L. and Smith, L. L. (1996) 'Characterization of the interaction of 2-[2–nitro-4-(trifluoromethyl)benzoyl]-4,4,6,6,-tetramethyl-cyclohexane-1,3,5–trione with rat hepatic 4-hydroxyphenylpyruvate dioxygenase', *Chem. Res. Toxicol.* **9**: 24–7.

Endo, F., Kitano, A., Uehara, I., Nagata, N., Matsuda, I., Shinka, T., Kuhara, T. and Matsumoto, I. (1983) 'Four-hydroxyphenylpyruvic acid oxidase deficiency with normal fumarylacetoacetase: a new variant form of hereditary hyper-tyrosinemia', *Pediat. Res.* **17**: 92–6.

Evans, S. J. W. (1983) 'Uses and abuses of analysis of variance', *Br. J. Clin. Pharmacol.* **15**: 629–48.

Fahn, S. (1974) "On-off" phenomenon with levodopa therapy in parkinsonism', *Neurology* **24**: 431–41.

Fatibello-Filho, O. and da Cruz Vieira, I. (1997) 'Flow injection spectrophotometric determination of L-Dopa and carbidopa in pharmaceutical formulations using a crude extract of sweet potato root (Ipomoea batatas (L.) Lam.) as enzymatic source', *Analyst* **122**: 345–50.

Felten, D. L., Felten, S. Y., Steece-Collier, K., Date, I. and Clemens, J. A. (1992) 'Age-related decline in the dopaminergic nigrostriatal system: the oxidative hypothesis and protective strategies', *Ann. Neurol.* **32** (Suppl): S133–6.

Fenu, S., Pinna, A., Ongini, E. and Morelli, M. (1997) 'Adenosine A2A receptor antagonism potentiates L-DOPA-induced turning behaviour and c-fos expression in 6-hydroxydopamine-lesioned rats', *Eur. J. Pharmacol.* **321**: 143–7.

Ferrini, R. and Glaser, A. (1964) 'In vitro decarboxylation of new phenylalanine derivatives', *Biochem. Pharmacol.* **13**: 798–800.

Feuerstein, C. L., Tanche, M., Serre, F., Gavend, M., Pellat, J. and Perret, J. (1977) 'Does 3-O-methyldopa play a role in levodopa-induced dyskinesias?' *Acta. Neurol. Scand.* **56**: 79–82.

Finberg, J. P., Wang, J., Goldstein, D. S., Kopin, I. J. and Bankiewicz, K. S. (1995) 'Influence of selective inhibition of monoamine oxidase A or B on striatal metabolism of L-DOPA in hemiparkinsonian rats', *J. Neurochem.* **65**: 1213–20.

Freeman, K. B., Bulawa, M. C., Zeng, Q. and Blank, C. L. (1993) 'Rapid and simultaneous determination of monoamino oxidase A and monoamino oxidase B activities in mouse brain homogenates by liquid chromatography with electrochemical detection', *Anal. Biochem.* **208**: 182–96.

Garcia, I., Rodgers, M., Lenne, C., Rolland, A., Sailland, A. and Matringe, M. (1997) 'Subcellular localization and purification of a p-hydroxyphenylpyruvate dioxygenase from cultured carrot cells and characterization of the corresponding cDNA', *Biochem. J.* **325**: 761–9.

Gervas, J. J., Muradás, V., Bazán, E., Aguado, E. G. and de Yébenes, J. G. (1983) 'Effects of 3-OM-dopa on monoamine metabolism in rat brain', *Neurology* **33**: 278–82.

Gordonsmith, R. H., Raworthy, M. J. and Gulliver, P. A. (1982) 'Substrate stereospecificity and selectivity of catechol-O-methyltransferase for DOPA, DOPA derivatives and α-substituted catecholamines', *Biochem. Pharmacol.* **31**: 433–7.

Graham, D. G., Tiffany, S. M., Bell, W. R. Jr. and Gutknecht, W. F. (1978) 'Autoxidation versus covalent binding of quinones as the mechanism of toxicity of dopamine, 6-hydroxydopamine, and related compounds toward C1300 neuroblastoma cells in vitro', *Mol. Pharmacol.* **14**: 644–53.

Grossman, M. H., Szumlanski, C., Littrell, J. B., Weinstein, R. and Weinshilboum, R. M. (1992) 'Electrophoretic analysis of low and high activity forms of catechol-O-methyltransferase in human erythrocytes', *Life Sci.* **50**: 473–80.

Gudehithlu, K. P., Duchemin, A. M., Silvia, C. P., Neff, N. H. and Hadjiconstantinou, M. (1992) 'Expression of cloned aromatic L-amino acid decarboxylase in *Xenopus laevis* oocytes', *Neurochem. Int.* **21**: 275–9.

Guldberg, H. C. and Marsden, C. (1975) 'Catechol-O-methyl transferase: pharmacological aspects and physiological role', *Pharmacol. Rev.* **27**: 135–206.

Hammerstad, J. P., Woodward, W. R., Gliessman, P., Boucher, B. and Nutt, J. G. (1990) 'L-Dopa pharmacokinetics in plasma and cisternal and lumbar cerebrospinal fluid of monkeys', *Ann. Neurol.* **27**: 495–9.

Harada, S., Misawa, S., Agarwal, D. P. and Goedde, H. W. (1980) 'Liver alcohol dehydrogenase and aldehyde dehydrogenase in the Japanese: isozyme variation and its possible role in alcohol intoxication', *Am. J. Hum. Genet.* **32**: 8–15.

Haramaki, N., Stewart, D. B., Aggarwal, S., Kawabata, T. and Packer, L. (1995)

'Role of ascorbate in protection by nitecapone against cardiac ischemia-reperfusion injury', *Biochem. Pharmacol.* **50**: 839–43.

Harder, S., Baas, H. and Rietbrock, S. (1995) 'Concentration-effect relationship of levodopa in patients with Parkinson's disease', *Clin. Pharmacokinet.* **29**: 243–56.

Hegedus, Z. L. and Nayak, U. (1993) 'Renal excretion of plasma soluble melanins by healthy human adults', *Arch. Int. Physiol. Biochim. Biophys.* **101**: 417–23.

Heinonen, E. H., Anttila, M. I., Karnani, H. L., Nyman, L. M., Vuorinen, J. A., Pyykkö, K. A. and Lammintausta, R. A. (1997b) 'Desmethylselegiline, a metabolite of selegiline, is an irreversible inhibitor of monoamine oxidase type B in humans', *J. Clin. Pharmacol.* **37**: 602–9.

Heinonen, E. H., Anttila, M. I., Nyman, L. M., Pyykkö, K. A., Vuorinen, J. A. and Lammintausta, R. A. (1997a) 'Inhibition of platelet monoamine oxidase type B by selegiline', *J. Clin. Pharmacol.* **37**: 597–601.

Helander, A. and Carlsson, S. (1990) 'Use of leukocyte aldehyde dehydrogenase activity to monitor inhibitory effect of disulfiram treatment', *Alcohol. Clin. Exp. Res.* **14**: 48–52.

Hietala, P., Linden, I. and Grunfors, N. (1979) 'The effects of simultaneous administration of 3,4–dihydroxyphenylpyruvic acid and L-DOPA in rat and mouse', *J. Pharm. Pharmacol.* **31**: 205–8.

Hills, M. and Armitage, P. (1979) 'The two-period cross-over clinical trial', *Br. J. Clin. Pharmacol.* **8**: 7–20.

Huhn, R., Stoermer, H., Klingele, B., Bausch, E., Fois, A., Farnetani, M., Di Rocco, M., Boue, J., Kirk, J. M., Coleman, R. and Scherer, G. (1998) 'Novel and recurrent tyrosine aminotransferase gene mutations in tyrosinemia type II', *Hum. Genet.* **102**: 305–13.

Illi, A., Sundberg, S., Ojala-Karlsson, P., Scheinin, M. and Gordin, A. (1996) 'Simultaneous inhibition of catechol-O-methyltransferase and monoamine oxidase A: effects on hemodynamics and catecholamine metabolism in healthy volunteers', *Clin. Pharmacol. Ther.* **59**: 450–7.

Ito, S. and Fujita, K. (1982) 'Conjugation of DOPA and 5–cysteinyldopa into cysteine mediated by superoxide radical', *Biochem. Pharmacol.* **31**: 2887–9.

Jeffery, D. R. and Roth, J. A. (1985) 'Purification and kinetic mechanism of human brain soluble catechol-O-methyltransferase', *J. Neurochem.* **44**: 881–5.

Jorga, K., Fotteler, B., Schmitt, M., Nielsen, T., Zürcher, G. and Aitken, J. (1997) 'The effects of COMT inhibition by tolcapone on tolerability and pharmacokinetics of different levodopa/benserazide formulations', *Eur. Neurol.* **38**: 59–67.

Kaakkola, S., Gordin, A. and Mannisto, P. T. (1994) 'General properties and clinical possibilities of new selective inhibitors of catechol O-methyltransferase', *Gen. Pharmacol.* **25**: 813–24.

Kaakkola, S., Männistö, P. T., Nissinen, E., Vuorela, A. and Mäntylä, R. (1985) 'The effect of an increased ratio of carbidopa to levodopa on the pharmacokinetics of levodopa', *Acta. Neurol. Scand.* **72**: 385–91.

Kaakkola, S. and Wurtman, R. J. (1992) 'Effects of COMT inhibitors on striatal dopamine metabolism: a microdialysis study', *Brain Res.* **11**: 241–9.

Karoum, F., Frees, W. J., Chuang, L. W., Cannon-Spoor, E., Wyatt, R. J. and Costa, E. (1988) 'D-Dopa and L-dopa similarly elevate brain dopamine and produce turning behavior in rats', *Brain Res.* **440**: 190–4.

Kawada, A., Kudo, T. and Kishimoto, Y. (1989) 'Metabolism of amniotic fluid dopamine by fetal membranes', *Asia-Oceania J. Obstet. Gynaecol.* **15**: 291–8.

Kelley, S. R., Kamal, T. J. and Molitch, M. E. (1996) 'Mechanism of verapamil calcium channel blockade-induced hyperprolactinemia', *Am. J. Physiol.* **270**: E96–100.

Kienbaum, P., Thurauf, N., Michel, M. C., Scherbaum, N., Gastpar, M. and Peters, J. (1998) 'Profound increase in epinephrine concentration in plasma and cardiovascular stimulation after mu-opioid receptor blockade in opioid-addicted patients during barbiturate-induced anesthesia for acute detoxification', *Anesthesiology* **88**: 1154–61.

Knoll, J. (1989) 'The pharmacology of selegiline ((−)deprenyl): new aspects', *Acta. Neurol. Scand.* **126** (Suppl): 83–91.

Knutson, L., Knutson, T. W. and Flemstrom, G. (1993) 'Endogenous dopamine and duodenal bicarbonate secretion in humans', *Gastroenterology* **104**: 1409–13.

Kurama, I. L., Bartholini, G., Tissot, R. and Plerscher, A. (1971) 'The metabolism of L-3–O-methyldopa, a precursor of dopa in man', *Clin. Pharmacol. Ther.* **12**: 678–82.

Kurth, J. H., Kurth, M. C., Poduslo, S. E. and Schwankhaus, J. D. (1993) 'Association of a monoamine oxidase B allele with Parkinson's disease', *Ann. Neurol.* **33**: 368–72.

Lachman, H. M., Kelsoe, J., Moreno, L., Katz, S. and Papolos, D. F. (1997) 'Lack of association of catechol-O-methyltransferase (COMT) functional polymorphism in bipolar affective disorder', *Psych. Genet.* **7**: 13–17.

Lachman, H. M., Papolos, D. F., Saito, T., Yu, Y.-M., Szumlanski, C. L. and Weinshiboum, R. W. (1996) 'Human catechol-O-methyltransferase pharmacogenetics: description of a functional polymorphism and its potential application to neuropsychiatric disorder', *Pharmacogenetics* **6**: 243–50.

Lai, C. T. and Yu, P. H. (1997) 'R(−)-deprenyl potentiates dopamine-induced cytotoxicity toward catecholaminergic neuroblastoma SH-SY5Y cells', *Toxicol. Appl. Pharmacol.* **142**: 186–91.

Laihinen, A., Rinne, J. O., Rinne, U. K., Haaparanta, M., Ruotsalainen, U., Bergman, J. and Solin, O. (1992) [18F]-6-fluorodopa PET scanning in Parkinson's disease after selective COMT inhibition with nitecapone (OR-462)', *Neurology* **42**: 199–203.

Lamensdorf, I., Youdim, M. B. and Finberg, J. P. (1996) 'Effect of long-term treatment with selective monoamine oxidase A and B inhibitors on dopamine release from rat striatum in vivo', *J. Neurochem.* **67**: 1532–9.

Latini, R., Masson, S., Jeremic, G., Luvara, G., Fiordaliso, F., Calvillo, L., Bernasconi, R., Torri, M., Rondelli, I., Razzetti, R. and Bongrani, S. (1998) 'Comparative efficacy of a DA2/alpha2 agonist and a beta-blocker in reducing adrenergic drive and cardiac fibrosis in an experimental model of left ventricular dysfunction after coronary artery occlusion', *J. Cardiovascular. Pharmacol.* **31**: 601–8.

Lee, M. R. (1993) 'Dopamine and the kidney – ten years on', *Clin. Sci.* **84**: 357–75.

Lee, S. T., Nicholls, R. D., Bundey, S., Laxova, R., Musarella, M. and Spritz, R. A. (1994) 'Mutations of the P gene in oculocutaneous albinism, ocular albinism, and Prader–Willi syndrome plus albinism', *N. Engl. J. Med.* **330**: 529–34.

Limousin, P., Pollak, P., Pfefen, J. P., Tournier-Gervason, C. L., Dubuis, R. and

Perret, J. E. (1995) 'Acute administration of levodopa-benserazide and tolcapone, a COMT inhibitor, Parkinson's disease', *Clin. Neuropharmacol.* **18**: 258–65.

Linden, I. (1980) 'Effects of 3,4–dihydroxyphenylpyruvic acid on some pharmacokinetic parameters of L-DOPA in the rat', *J. Pharm. Pharmacol.* **32**: 344–8.

Linss, G. and Scholze, J. (1990) 'Basic program for the diagnosis of arterial hypertension. Zeitschrift für die gesamte innere Medizin und ihre Grenzgebiete', **45**: 491–3.

Lotta, T., Vidgren, J., Tilgmann, C., Ulmanen, I., Melén, K., Julkunen, I. and Taskinen, J. (1995) 'Kinetics of human soluble and membrane-bound catechol O-methyltransferase: a revised mechanism and description of the thermolabile variant of the enzyme', *Biochemistry* **34**: 4202–10.

Lundstrom, K., Tilgmann, C., Peränen, J., Kalkkinen, N. and Ulmanen, I. (1992) 'Expression of enzymatically active rat liver and human placental catechol-O-methyltransferase in Escherichia coli: purification and partial characterization of the enzyme', *Biochim. Biophys. Acta.* **1129**: 149–54.

Mahmood, I. (1997) 'Clinical pharmacokinetics and pharmacodynamics of selegiline', *Clin. Pharmacokinet.* **33**: 91–102.

Männistö, P. T. and Tuomainen, P. (1991) 'Effect of high single doses of levodopa and carbidopa on brain dopamine and its metabolites: modulation by selective inhibitors of monoamine oxidase and/or catechol-O-methyltransferase in the male rat', *Naunyn–Schmiedeberg's Arch. Pharmacol.* **344**: 412–8.

Männistö, P. T., Tuomainen, P. and Tuominen, R. K. (1992) 'Different in vivo properties of three new inhibitors of catechol O-methyltransferase in the rat', *Br. J. Pharmacol.* **105**: 569–74.

Marino, F., Cosentino, M., Bombelli, R., Ferrari, M., Maestroni, G. J., Conti, A., Lecchini, S. and Frigo, G. (1997) 'Measurement of catecholamines in mouse bone marrow by means of HPLC with electrochemical detection', *Haematologica* **82**: 392–4.

Marsden, C. D. (1983) 'Neuromelanin and Parkinson's disease', *J. Neurol. Transm.* **19**(Suppl.): 121–41.

Martel, F., Martins, M. J. and Azevedo, I. (1996) 'Inward transport of 3H-MPP+ in freshly isolated rat hepatocytes: evidence for interaction with catecholamines', *Naunyn-Schmiedeberg's Arch. Pharmacol.* **354**: 305–11.

Mashige, F., Ohkubo, A., Matsushima, Y., Takano, M., Tsuchiya, E., Kanazawa, H., Nagata, Y., Takai, N., Shinozuka, N. and Sakuma, I. (1994) 'High-performance liquid chromatographic determination of catecholamine metabolites and 5–hydroxyindoleacetic acid in human urine using a mixed-mode column and an eight-channel electrode electrochemical detector', *J. Chromatog. B–Biomed. Appl.* **658**: 63–8.

Merello, M., Lees, A., Webster, R., Bovingdon, M. and Gordin, A. (1994) 'Effect of entacapone, a peripherally acting catechol-O-methyltransferase inhibitor, on the motor response to acute L-dopa administration in patients with Parkinson's disease', *J. Neurol. Neurosurg. Psych.* **57**: 186–9.

Michel, P. P. and Hefti, F. (1990) 'Toxicity of 6–hydroxydopamine and dopamine for dopaminergic neurons in culture', *J. Neurosci. Res.* **26**: 428–35.

Milne, B., Quintin, L. and Pujol, J. F. (1989) 'Fentanyl increases catecholamine oxidation current measured by in vivo voltammetry in the rat striatum', *Can. J. Anaesth.* **36**: 155–9.

Montanaro, N., Vaccheri, A., Dall'Olio, R. and Gandolfi, O. (1983) 'Time course of rat motility response to apomorphine: a simple model for studying preferential blockade of brain dopamine receptors mediating sedation', *Psychopharmacology* 81: 214–9.

Morimoto, Y., Murayama, N., Kuwano, A., Kondo, I., Yamashita, Y. and Mizuno, Y. (1995) 'Association analysis of a polymorphism of the monoamine oxidase B gene with Parkinson's disease in a Japanese population', *Am. J. Med. Genet.* 60: 570–2.

Moses, J., Siddiqui, A. and Silverman, P. B. (1996) 'Sodium benzoate differentially blocks circling induced by D- and L-dopa in the hemi-parkinsonian rat', *Neurosci. Lett.* 218: 145–8.

Mouradian, M. M., Juncos, J. L., Fabbrini, G. and Chase, T. N. (1987) 'Motor fluctuations in Parkinson's disease: pathogenetic and therapeutic studies', *Ann. Neurol.* 22: 475–9.

Myllylä, V. V., Sotaniemi, K. A., Illi, A. and Keränen, T. (1993) 'Effect of entacapone, a COMT inhibitor, on the pharmacokinetics of levodopa and on cardiovascular responses in patients with Parkinson's disease', *Eur. J. Clin. Pharmacol.* 45: 419–23.

Mytilineou, C., Han, S.-K. and Cohen, G. (1993) 'Toxic and protective effects of L-dopa on mesencephalic cell cultures', *J. Neurochem.* 61: 1470–8.

Mytilineou, C., Radcliffe, P., Leonardei, E. K., Werner, P. and Olanow, C. W. (1997) 'L-Deprenyl protects mesencephalic dopamine neurons from glutamate receptor-medicated toxicity in vitro', *J. Neurolchem.* 68: 33–9.

Nakano, H., Takamatsu, S. and Yamamoto, Y. (1995) 'Monamine oxidase (MAO)', *Jpn. J. Clin. Med.* 53: 1168–72.

Neumark, Y. D., Friedlander, Y., Thomasson, H. R. and Li, T. K. (1998) 'Association of the ADH2*2 allele with reduced ethanol consumption in Jewish men in Israel: a pilot study', *J. Stud. Alcohol.* 59: 133–9.

Nimmo, J. E., Gawkrodger, D. J., O'Docherty, C. S., Going, S. M., Percy-Robb, I. W. and Hunter, J. A. (1988) 'Plasma 5-S-cycteinyldopa as an index of melanogenesis', *Br. J. Dermatol.* 118: 487–95.

Nissbrandt, H. and Hjorth, S. (1992) 'Dopaminergic neurotransmission in somatodendritic and terminal areas of the rat brain: susceptibility to modulation by D1 and D2 receptors and to axotomy', *J. Neural. Transm.–Gen. Sec.* 90: 13–26.

Nissinen, E. (1984) 'The site of O-methylation by membrane-bound catechol-O-methyltransferase', *Biochem. Pharmacol.* 33: 3105–8.

Nissinen, E., Lindén, I.-B., Schultz, E. and Photo, P. (1992) 'Biochemical and pharmacological properties of a peripherally acting catechol-O-methyltransferase inhibitor entacapone', *Naunyn-Schmiedeberg's Arch. Pharmacol.* 346: 262–6.

Nissinen, E., Tuominen, R., Perhonien, V. and Kaakkola, S. (1988) 'Catechol-O-methyltransferase activity in human and rat small intestine', *Life Sci.* 42: 2609–14.

Nowicki, S., Levin, G. and Encro, M. A. (1993) 'Involvement of renal dopamine synthesis in the diuretic effect of furosemide in normohydrated rats', *J. Pharmacol. Exp. Ther.* 264: 1377–80.

Nutt, J. G. and Fellman, J. H. (1984) 'Pharmacokinetics of levodopa', *Clin. Neuropharmacol.* 7: 35–49.

Nutt, J. G., Gancher, S. T. and Woodward, W. R. (1988) 'Does an inhibitory action of levodopa contribute to motor fluctuations?' *Neurology* 38: 1553–7.

Nutt, J. G., Woodward, W. R. and Carter, J. H. (1986) 'Clinical and biochemical studies with controlled-release levodopa/carbidopa', *Neurology* 36: 1206–11.

Nutt, J. G., Woodward, W. R., Carter, J. H. and Gancher, S. T. (1992) 'Effect of long-term therapy on the pharmacodynamics of levodopa: relation to on-off phenomenon', *Arch. Neurol.* 49: 1123–30.

Nutt, J. G., Woodward, W. R., Gancher, S. T. and Merrick, D. (1987) '3-O-methyldopa and the response to levodopa in Parkinson's disease', *Ann. Neurol.* 21: 584–8.

O'Malley, K., Harmon, S., Moffat, M., Uhland-Smith, A. and Wong, S. (1995) 'The human aromatic L-amino acid decarboxylase gene can be alternatively spliced to generate unique protein isoforms', *J. Neurochem.* 65: 2409–16.

Obata, T. and Yamanaka, Y. (1995) 'Intracranial microdialysis of salicylic acid to detect hydroxyl radical generation by monoamine oxidase inhibitor in the rat', *Neurosci. Lett.* 188: 13–16.

Olanow, C. W., Gauger, L. L. and Cedarbaum, J. M. (1991) 'Temporal relationships between plasma and cerebrospinal fluid pharmacokinetics of levodopa and clinical effect in Parkinson's disease', *Ann. Neurol.* 29: 556–9.

Olney, J. W., Zorumski, C. F., Stewart, G. R., Price, M. T., Wang, G. and Labruyere, J. (1990) 'Excitotoxicity of L-dopa and 6–OH-dopa: implications for Parkinson's and Huntington's diseases', *Exp. Neurol.* 108: 269–72.

Otsuka, M., Ichiya, Y., Kuwabara, Y., Sasaki, M., Yoshida, T., Fukumura, T. and Masuda, K. (1995) 'Nigrofrontal dopaminergic function as assessed by 18F-dopa PET', *Nucl. Med. Comm.* 16: 1021–5.

Paalzow, G. H. M. and Paalzow, L. K. (1983) 'Opposing effects of apomorphine on pain in rats: evaluation of the dose-response curve', *Eur. J. Pharmacol.* 88: 27–35.

Paalzow, G. H. M. and Paalzow, L. K. (1986b) 'L-Dopa: how it may exacerbate parkinsonian symptoms', *TIPS* 9: 15–19.

Paalzow, L. K. and Paalzow, G. H. M. (1986a) 'Concentration-response relations for apomorphine effects on heart rate in conscious rats', *J. Pharm. Pharmacol.* 38: 28–34.

Pardridge, W. M. (1977) 'Kinetics of competitive inhibition of neutral amino acid transport across the blood-brain barrier', *J. Neurochem.* 28: 103–8.

Parsons, P. G. (1985) 'Modification of dopa toxicity in human tumour cells', *Biochem. Pharmacol.* 34: 1801–7.

Paterson, I. A., Juorio, A. V. and Boulton, A. A. (1990) '2–Phenylethylamine: a modulator of catecholamine transmission in the mammalian central nervous system?' *J. Neurochem.* 55: 1827–37.

Perry, S. E., Summar, M. L., Phillips, J. A., and Robertson, D (1991) 'Linkage analysis of the human dopamine beta-hydroxylase gene', *Genomics* 10: 493–5.

Pestana, M. and Soares-da-Silva, P. (1994) 'The renal handling of dopamine originating from L-DOPA and γ-glutamyl-L-DOPA', *Br. J. Pharmacol.* 112: 417–22.

Pestana, M., Vieira-Coelho, M. A., Pinto-do-Ó, P. C., Fernabdes, M. H. and Soares-da-Silva, P. (1995) 'Assessment of renal dopaminergic system activity during cyclosporine A administration in the rat', *Br. J. Pharmacol.* 115: 1349–58.

Peterson, L. L., Woodward, W. R., Fletcher, W. S., Palmquist, M., Tucker, M. A. and Ilias, A. (1988) 'Plasma 5-S-cysteinyldopa differentiates patients with primary and metastatic melanoma from patients with dysplastic nevus syndrome and normal subjects', *J. Am. Acad. Dermatol.* **19**: 509–15.

Pinder, R. M., Brogden, R. N., Sawyer, P. R., Speight, T. M. and Avery, G. S. (1976) 'Levodopa and decarboxylase inhibitors: a review of their clinical pharmacology and use in the treatment of parkinsonism', *Drugs* **11**: 329–77.

Presch, I., Birnbacher, R., Herkner, K. and Lubec, G. (1997) 'The effect of estradiol and ovariectomy on tyrosine hydroxylase, tyrosine aminotransferase and phenylalanine hydroxylase', *Life Sci.* **60**: 479–84.

Prota, G. (1988) 'Progress in the chemistry of melanins and related metabolites', *Med Res Rev* **8**: 525–56.

Protais, P., Dubuc, I. and Costentin, J. (1983) 'Pharmacological characteristics of dopamine receptors involved in the dual effect of dopamine agonists on yawning behaviour in rats', *Eur. J. Pharmacol.* **94**: 271–80.

Reches, A. and Fahn, S. (1982) '3-O-methyldopa blocks dopa metabolism in rat corpus striatum', *Ann. Neurol.* **12**: 267–71.

Reilly, D. K., Rivera-Calimlim, L. and Van Dyke, D. (1980) 'Catechol-O-methyltransferase activity: a determinant of levodopa response', *Clin. Pharmacol. Ther.* **28**: 278–86.

Rinne, U. K., Sonninen, V. and Siirtola, T. (1973) 'Plasma concentration of levodopa in patients with Parkinson's disease', *Eur. Neurol.* **10**: 301–10.

Rivera-Calimlim, L. and Reilly, D. K. (1984) 'Difference in erythrocyte catechol-O-methyltransferase activity between Orientals and Caucasians: difference in levodopa tolerance', *Clin. Pharmacol. Ther.* **35**: 804–9.

Rivett, A. J., Francis, A. and Roth, J. A. (1983) 'Localization of membrane-bound catechol-O-methyltransferase', *J. Neurochem.* **40**: 1494–6.

Roberts, J. W., Cora-Locatelli, G., Bravi, D., Metman, L. V., Amantea, M. A. and Chase, T. N. (1994) 'Catechol-O-methyltransferase inhibitor tolcapone prolongs levodopa/carbidopa action in parkinsonian patients', *Neurology* **44**: 2685–8.

Roberts, J., Waller, D. G., Renwick, A. G., O'Shea, N., MaCklin, B. S. and Bulling, M. (1996) 'The effects of co-administration of benzhexol on the peripheral pharmacokinetics of oral levodopa in young volunteers', *Br. J. Clin. Pharmacol.* **41**: 331–7.

Rodbard, D. (1974) 'Statistical quality control and routine data processing for radioimmunoassays and immunoradiometric assays', *Clin. Chem.* **20**: 1255–70.

Rosenberg, P. A. (1988) 'Catecholamine toxicity in cerebral cortex in dissociated cell culture', *J. Neurosci.* **8**: 2887–94.

Rosenberg, P. A., Loring, R., Xie, Y., Zaleskas, V. and Aizenman, E. (1991) '2,4,5-Trihydroxyphenylalanine in solution forms a non-N-methyl-D-aspartate glutamatergic agonist and neurotoxin', *Proc. Natl. Acad. Sci. USA.* **88**: 4865–9.

Roth, J. A. (1992) 'Membrane-bound catechol-O-methyltransferase: a reevaluation of its role in the O-methylation of the catecholamine neurotransmitters', *Rev. Physiol. Biochem. Pharmacol.* **88**: 1–29.

Rotman, A., Daly, J. W. and Creveling, C. R. (1976) 'Oxygen-dependent reaction of 6-hydroxydopamine 5,6-dihydroxytryptamine and related compounds with proteins in vitro: a model for cytotoxicity', *Mol. Pharmacol.* **12**: 837–99.

Rüetschi, U., Rymo, L. and Lindstedt, S. (1997) 'Human 4-hydroxyphenylpyruvate dioxygenase gene (HPD)', *Genomics* **44**: 292–9.

Ruzafa, C., Solano, F. and Sanchez-Amat, A. (1994) 'The protein encoded by the Shewanella colwelliana melA gene is a p-hydroxyphenylpyruvic dioxygenase', *FEMS Microbiol. Lett.* **124**: 179–84.

Sandler, M., Johnson, R. D., Ruthven, C. R. J., Reud, J. L. and Calne, D. B. (1974) 'Transamination is a major pathway of L-DOPA metabolism following peripheral decarboxylase inhibition', *Nature* **247**: 364–6.

Schallreuter, K. U., Buttner, G., Pittelkow, M. R., Wood, J. M., Swanson, N. N. and Korner, C. (1994) 'Cytotoxicity of 6-biopterin to human melanocytes', *Bioche. Biophy. Res. Com.* **204**: 43–8.

Scherer, G., Busch, E., Gaa, A. and von Deimling, O. (1989) 'Gene mapping on mouse chromosome 8 by interspecific crosses: new data on a linkage group conserved on human chromosome 16q', *Genomics* **5**: 275–82.

Schneider, S. C. and Mitchison, N. A. (1995) 'Self-reactive T cell hybridomas and tolerance. Some range of antigen dose dependence but higher numbers of self-reactive T cell hybridomas from mice in which self-tolerance has been broken by antiserum treatment', *J. Immunol.* **154**: 3796–805.

Schultz, E. (1991) 'Catechol-O-methyltransferase and aromatic L-amino acid decarboxylase activities in human gastrointestinal tissues', *Life Sci.* **49**: 721–5.

Schweizer-Groyer, G., Cadepond, F., Jibard, N., Neau, E., Segard-Maurel, I., Baulier, E. E. and Groyer, A. (1997) 'Stimulation of transcription in vitro from a liver-specific promoter by human glucocorticoid receptor (hGRalpha)', *Biochem. J.* **324**: 823–31.

Soares-da-Silva, P., Serrao, M. P., Vieira-Coelho, M. A. and Pestana, M. (1998) 'Evidence for the involvement of P-glycoprotein on the extrusion of taken up L-DOPA in cyclosporine A treated LLC-PK1 cells', *Br. J. Pharmacol.* **123**: 13–22.

Soares-da-Silva, P., Vieira-Coelho, M. A. and Serrao, M. P. (1997) 'Uptake of L 3,4-dihydroxyphenylalanine and dopamine formation in cultured renal epithelial cells', *Biochem. Pharmacol.* **54**: 1037–46.

Sokal, R. R. and Rohlfe, F. J. (1981) *Biometry: The Principles and Practice of Statistics in Biological Research*, 2nd edn, New York: W. H. Freeman and Company, pp. 205–18.

Steece-Collier, K., Collier, T. J., Sladek, C. D. and Sladek, J. R. Jr. (1990) 'Chronic levodopa impairs morphological development of grafted embryonic dopamine neurons', *Exp. Neurol.* **110**: 201–8.

Stein, P. E., White, S. E., Homan, J., Fraher, L., McGarrigle, H. H., Hanson, M. A. and Bocking, A. D. (1998) 'Fetal endocrine responses to prolonged reduced uterine blood flow are altered following bilateral sectioning of the carotid sinus and vagus nerves', *J. Endocrinol.* **157**: 149–55.

Steinmetz, J. C. (1989) 'Neonatal hypertension and cardiomegaly associated with a congenital neuroblastoma', *Pediatr. Path.* **9**: 577–82.

Stenman, G., Roijer, E., Rüetschi, U., Dellsen, A., Rymo, L. and Lindstedt, S. (1995) 'Regional assignment of the human 4-hydroxyphenylpyruvate dioxygenase gene (HPD) to 12q24→qter by fluorescence in situ hybridization', *Cytogenet Cell Genet.* **71**: 374–6.

Stewart, R. M., Miller, S. and Gunder, M. (1983) 'Urinary 5-S-cyteinylDOPA in Parkinsonism after DOPA and carbidopa', *Acta. Dermator.* **63**: 97–101.

Stromberg, U. (1970) 'Dopa effects on motility in mice: potentiation by MK 485 and dexchlorpheniramine', *Psychopharmacologia* **18**: 58–67.

Sumi, C., Ichinose, H. and Nagatsu, T. (1990) 'Characterization of recombinant human aromatic L-amino acid decarboxylase expressed in COS cells', *J. Neurochem.* **55**: 1075–8.

Suzuki, T., Akaike, N., Ueno, K., Tanaka, Y. and Himori, N. (1995) 'MAO inhibitors, clorgyline and lazabemide, prevent hydroxyl radical generation caused by brain ischemia/reperfusion in mice', *Pharmacology* **50**: 357–62.

Takahashi, Y., Kuriyama, M., Kawada, Y., Komeda, H., Horie, M. and Isogai, K. (1988) 'Multimodality treatment of adrenal ganglioncuroblastoma: a case report', *Acta. Urol. Jpn.* **34**: 2149–54.

Takeshita, T., Maruyama, S. and Morimoto, K. (1998) 'Relevance of both daily hassles and the ALDH2 genotype to problem drinking among Japanese male workers', *Alcohol. Clin. Exp. Res.* **22**: 115–20.

Tanaka, M., Oshima, T., Hayashi, C. and Kobayashi, S. (1973) 'Enhancement of the pharmacological action of 3,4–dihydroxy-L-phenylalanine (L-DOPA) and reduction of DOPA decarboxylase activity in rat liver after chronic treatment with L-DOPA', *Eur. J. Pharmacol.* **22**: 360–2.

Tate, S. S., Sweet, R., McDowell, F. H. and Meister, A. (1971) 'Decrease of the 3,4–dihydroxyphenylalanine (DOPA) decarboxylase activities in human erythrocytes and mouse tissues after administration of DOPA', *Proc. Natl. Acad. Sci. USA.* **68**: 2121–3.

Tenhunen, J., Salminen, M., Jalanko, A., Ukkonen, S. and Ulmanen, I. (1993) 'Structure of the rat catechol-O-methyltransferase gene: separate promoters are used to produce mRNA for soluble and membrane-bound forms of the enzyme', *DNA Cell. Biol.* **12**: 253–63.

Törnwall, M., Kaakkola, S., Tuomainen, P., Kask, A. and Männistö, P. T. (1994) 'Comparison of two new inhibition of catechol O-methylation on striatal dopamine metabolism: a microdialysis study in rats', *Br. J. Pharmacol.* **112**: 13–18.

Törnwall, M. and Männistö, P. (1991) 'Acute toxicity of three new selective COMT inhibitors in mice with special emphasis on interactions with drugs increasing catecholaminergic neurotransmission', *Pharmacol. Toxicol.* **69**: 64–70.

Tripathi, R. K., Giebel, L. B., Strunk, K. M. and Spritz, R. A. (1991) 'Polymorphism of the human tyrosinase gene is associated with temperature-sensitive enzymatic activity', *Gene. Expression* **1**: 103–10.

Tripathi, R. K., Hearing, V. J., Yrabe, K., Aroca, P. and Spritz, R. A. (1992) 'Mutational mapping of the catalytic activities of human tyrosinase', *J. Biol. Chem.* **267**: 23707–12.

Tuchman, M. and Stocckeler, J. S. (1988) 'Conjugated versus "free" acidic metabolites of catecholamines in random urine samples: significance for the diagnosis of neuroblastoma', *Pediatr. Res.* **23**: 576–9.

Tyce, G. M., Sharpless, N. S. and Owen, C. A. Jr. (1978) 'Demethylation in erythrocytes: a reaction involving hemoglobin', *Am. J. Physiol.* **234**: E150–7.

Uderzo, C., Rajnoldi, A. C., Schiro, R., di Lelio, A., Jankovic, M., Conter, V., Locasciulli, A. and Masera G. (1988) 'Neuroblastoma during acute lymphoblastic leukemia in remission', *Cancer* **62**: 1359–63.

Vento, A. E., Ramo, O. J., Nemlander, A. T., Nissinen, E., Holopainen, A. and Mattila, S. P. (1997) 'Nitecapone is of benefit to functional performance in experimental heart transplantation', *Res. Exp. Med.* **197**: 137–46.

Vidgren, J., Svensson, L. A. and Liljas, A. (1994) 'Crystal structure of catechol O-methyltransferase', *Nature* **368**: 354–8.

Wade, D. N., Mearrick, P. T. and Morris, J. L. (1973) 'Active transport of levodopa in the intestine', *Nature* **242**: 463–5.

Wade, L. A. and Katzman, R. (1975) '3–O-Methyldopa uptake and inhibition of L-DOPA at the blood-brain-barrier', *Life Sci.* **17**: 131–6.

Waldmeier, P. C. (1987) 'Amine oxidases and their endogenous substrates (with special reference to monoamine oxidase and the brain)', *J. Neural. Transm. – Gen. Sect.* **23**: 55–72.

Weinshilboun, R. M. and Raymond, F. A. (1977) 'Inheritance of low erythrocyte catechol-O-methyltransferase activity in man', *Am. J. Hum. Genet.* **29**: 125–35.

Weinshilboum, R. M., Raymond, F. A., Elveback, L. E. and Weidman, W. H. (1974) 'Correlation of erythrocyte catechol-O-methyltransferase activity between siblings', *Nature* **252**: 490–1.

Wej, J., Ramchand, C. N. and Hemmings, G. P. (1997) 'Possible control of dopamine beta-hydroxylase via a codominant mechanism associated with the polymorphic (GT)n repeat at its gene locus in healthy individuals', *Hum. Genet.* **99**: 52–5.

Westphal, E. M., Natt, E., Grimm, T., Odievre, M. and Scherer, G. (1988) 'The human tyrosine aminotransferase gene: characterization of restriction fragment length polymorphisms and haplotype analysis in a family with tyrosinemia type II', *Hum. Genet.* **79**: 260–4.

Wick, M. M. and Fitzgerald, G. (1981) 'Inhibition of reverse transcriptase by tyrosinase generated quinones related to levodopa and dopamine', *Chem. Biol. Interact.* **38**: 99–107.

Wimmer, I., Meyer, J. C., Seifert, B., Dummer, R., Flace, A. and Burg, G. (1997) 'Prognostic value of serum 5–S-cysteinyldopa for monitoring metastatic melanoma during immunochemotherapy', *Cancer Res.* **57**: 5073–6.

Woods, J. R., Williams, J. G. and Tavel, M. (1989) 'The two-period crossover design in medical research', *Ann. Intern. Med.* **110**: 560–6.

Wu, G., Baraldo, M. and Furlanut, M. (1999) 'Inter-patient and intra-patient variations in the baseline tapping test in patients with Parkinson's disease', *Acta. Neurol. Belgica.* **99**: 182–4.

Wu, G. and Furlanut, M. (1999) 'Pharmacodynamic modelling of levodopa, 3–O-methyldopa and their effects: an application of the Dixon equation', *Pharmacol. Res.* **39**: 203–10.

Yang, H. Y. T. and Neff, N. H. (1974) 'The monoamine oxidase of brain: selective inhibition with drugs and consequences for the metabolism of biogenic amines', *J. Pharmacol. Exp. Ther.* **189**: 733–40.

Yang, Y. L., Tan, J. X. and Xu, R. B. (1989) 'Down-regulation of glucocorticoid receptor and its relationship to the induction of rat liver tyrosine amino-transferase', *J. Steroid. Biochem.* **32**: 99–104.

Yorga, K., Fotteler, B., Heizman, P. and Zürcher, G. (1998) 'Pharmacokinetics and pharmacodynamics after oral and intravenous administration of tolcapone, a novel adjunct to Parkinson's disease therapy', *Eur. J. Clin. Pharmacol.* **54**: 443–7.

Yoshida, A., Huang, I. Y. and Ikawa, M. (1984) 'Molecular abnormality of an inactive aldehyde dehydrogenase variant commonly found in Orientals', *Proc. Natl. Acad. Sci. USA* **81**: 258–61.

Yoshida, A., Wang, G. and Dave, V. (1983) 'Determination of genotypes of human aldehyde dehydrogenase ALDH2 locus', *Am. J. Hum. Genet.* **35**: 1107–16.

Zürcher, G., Dingemanse, J. and Da Prada, M. (1993) 'Potent COMT inhibition by Ro 40–7592 in the periphery and in the brain. Preclinical and clinical findings', *Adv. Neurol.* **60**: 641–7.

Chapter 8

Interindividual variability in the disposition of anti-HIV drugs

D. J. Back, S. H. Khoo and S. E. Gibbons

Introduction

Probably the turning point in generating a belief that there were real grounds for optimism of "therapeutic success" in the treatment of HIV infection came with the introduction of protease inhibitors (PIs) in 1995. As a component of antiretroviral therapy (ART), PIs produced a dramatic decrease in mortality and morbidity in HIV infection (Palella *et al.*, 1998) most clearly demonstrated by the reduction of opportunistic infections and hospital admissions. Today, a triple-drug combination regimen containing nucleoside reverse transcriptase inhibitors (NRTIs) plus PIs or non-nucleoside reverse transcriptase inhibitors (NNRTIs) constitutes the standard of care for patients commencing therapy (see Table 8.1).

However, despite its success, combination ART still lacks sufficient potency and durability. Large prospective studies (e.g. Avanti, 1999) suggest that up to 50% of HIV-positive patients will fail to achieve adequate suppression of plasma HIV RNA (i.e. <50 copies/ml) for any of the current ART regimens. Even when this is achieved, viral rebound develops in a significant proportion of patients within 1 year of follow-up (Ledergerber *et al.*, 1999; Staszewski *et al.*, 1999; Wit *et al.*, 1999). There are also a growing number of patients who fail treatment despite exposure to most antiretroviral agents and consequently receive salvage therapy, which may include "mega-HAART" regimens (five or more drugs). Such regimens are associated with increased potential for toxicity and serious drug interactions. Treatment failure is clearly multifactorial, and may include the development of antiviral resistance, poor adherence to therapy and pharmacokinetic reasons. This review will focus on pharmacokinetic variability as an important consideration in treatment failure and current approaches to address the problem.

Pharmacokinetic variability is particularly important in relation to PIs – a group of peptidomimetic drugs (Figure 8.1) which exhibit marked potential for drug interactions leading to reduced or elevated PI plasma concentrations (Barry *et al.*, 1999; http://www.hiv-druginteractions.org).

Table 8.1 Currently licensed antiretrovirals

Protease inhibitors (PIs)	Nucleoside reverse transcriptase inhibitors (NRTIs)	Non-nucleoside reverse transcriptase inhibitors (NNRTIs)
Amprenavir	Abacavir (ABC)	Delavirdine
Indinavir	Didanosine (ddl)	Efavirenz
Nelfinavir	Lamivudine (3TC)	Nevirapine
Ritonavir	Stavudine (d4T)	
Saquinavir	Zalcitabine (ddC)	
(soft gel, hard gel)	Zidovudine (ZDV)	

Recommendation for initial treatment is:
   PI[a]+2 NRTIs
   NNRTI+2 NRTIs
   3 NRTIs[b]

Notes
[a] PI might be a combination of two PIs.
[b] Not in official guidelines, but increasingly used.

Reduced concentrations will potentially compromise efficacy while elevated concentrations will predispose to adverse events. It is in this context that therapeutic drug monitoring (TDM) in antiretroviral therapy has been considered for PIs. However, before looking in more detail at variability in PI disposition it is important to highlight the main issues around plasma concentrations of the other two main classes of antiretrovirals.

For NRTIs, establishing a relationship between plasma concentration and antiviral effect has been difficult simply because it is the intracellular triphosphate anabolite that is the active moiety (Figure 8.2). There are marked differences between the plasma half-life of the NRTIs (Table 8.2) and the intracellular half-life of the active triphosphate. Consequently, plasma concentrations of parent nucleosides and intracellular concentrations of triphosphates show only a weak correlation (Barry *et al.*, 1996; Moore *et al.*, 1999).

Data from pharmacokinetic studies of NNRTIs (see Table 8.2) (Barry *et al.*, 1999; Murphy and Montaner, 1996; Adkins and Noble, 1998) indicate that two of the drugs, efavirenz and nevirapine, have a prolonged half-life, normally achieve adequate steady-state plasma concentrations during a dosing interval and the pharmacokinetics are less variable than PIs.

Metabolism of protease inhibitors

Saquinavir was the first PI licensed for the treatment of HIV infection. The initial formulation of saquinavir was a hard gel capsule (Invirase) which exhibited low oral bioavailability, measured as 4% in healthy volunteers after a single dose and estimated to be up to 10% at steady-state in HIV-positive patients (Steimer *et al.*, 1998). In order to increase drug exposure a new soft gel formulation of saquinavir, Fortovase, was introduced with a bioavailability of approximately three times that of Invirase.

Amprenavir	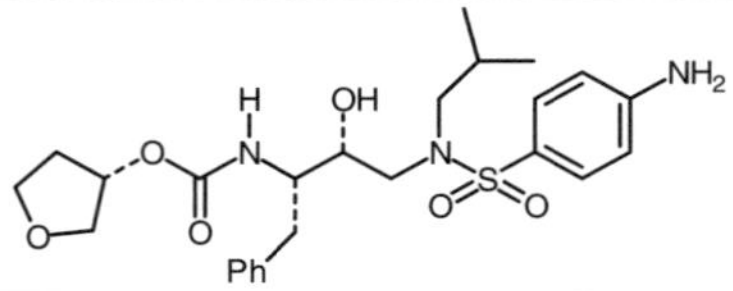
Indinavir	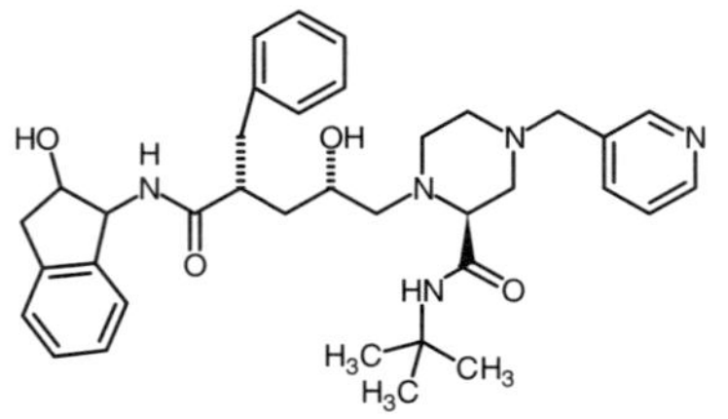
Nelfinavir	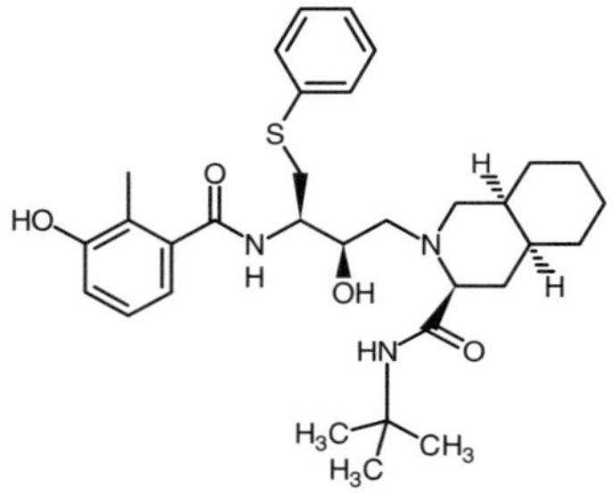
Ritonavir	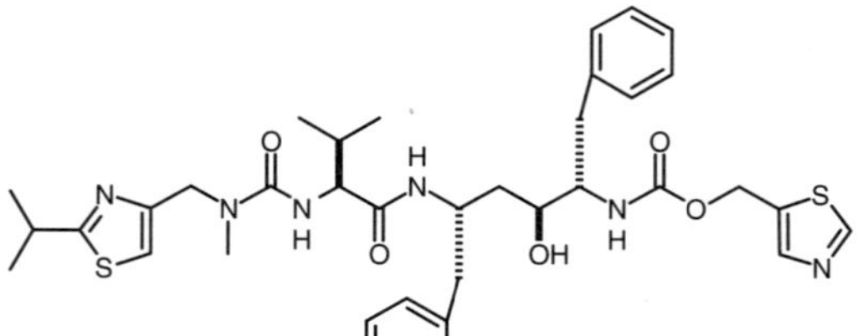
Saquinavir	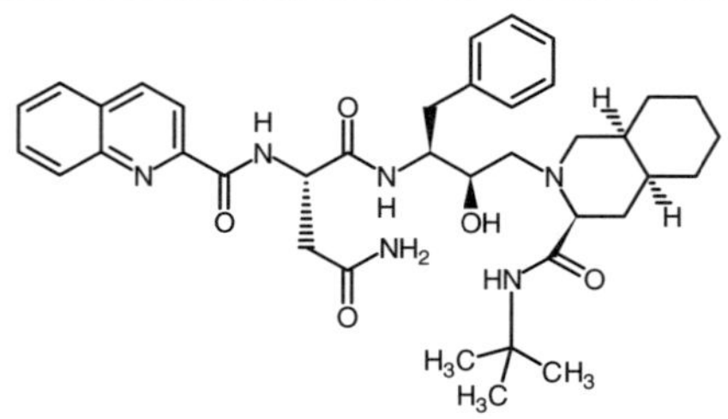

Figure 8.1 Structures of five HIV-1 protease inhibitors.

Table 8.2 Pharmacokinetic characteristics of anti-HIV drugs

Drug	Site of action	Active metabolite ?	Bioavailability	Protein binding	Plasma half-life	V_D (L/kg)	Clearance	Notes/Interactions
HIV nucleoside analogues								
Abacavir			83%	~49%	1.5 h	0.8	Renal (80%)	
Didanosine			~42%		1.5 h	1.08	Renal (50%)	
Lamivudine	Intracellular Inhibits HIV reverse transcriptase	Intracellular phosphates	80–85%	<36%	5–7 h	1.3	Renal (70%)	
Stavudine			~86%		1.3–1.4 h	0.66	Renal (40%)	
Zalcitabine			>80%	<4%	2.0 h	0.53	Renal (75%)	
Zidovudine			60–70%	34–38%	1.1 h	1.6	Hepatic	Metabolite renally excreted
HIV non-nucleoside reverse transcriptase inhibitors								
Delavirdine			not determined	~98%	6 h			Delavirdine is an inhibitor of CYP3A4
Efavirenz	Intracellular Inhibits HIV reverse transcriptase	No	not determined	>99%	45 h			Efavirenz both induces and inhibits CYP3A4
Nevirapine			~93%	~60%	25–30 h	1.21	Hepatic	Nevirapine is an inducer of CYP3A4
HIV protease inhibitors								
Amprenavir		No, apart from nelfinavir which has an active (M8) metabolite	not determined	90%	7–10 h	6.1	All PIs mainly cleared hepatically, only indinavir undergoes significant renal clearance	
Indinavir	Probably intracellular		~65%	60%	2 h	2–7		
Nelfinavir			not determined	>98%	3–5 h			
Ritonavir			not determined	98–99%	3–5 h	~0.3–0.6		
Saquinavir			12%	97%	12 h	10		

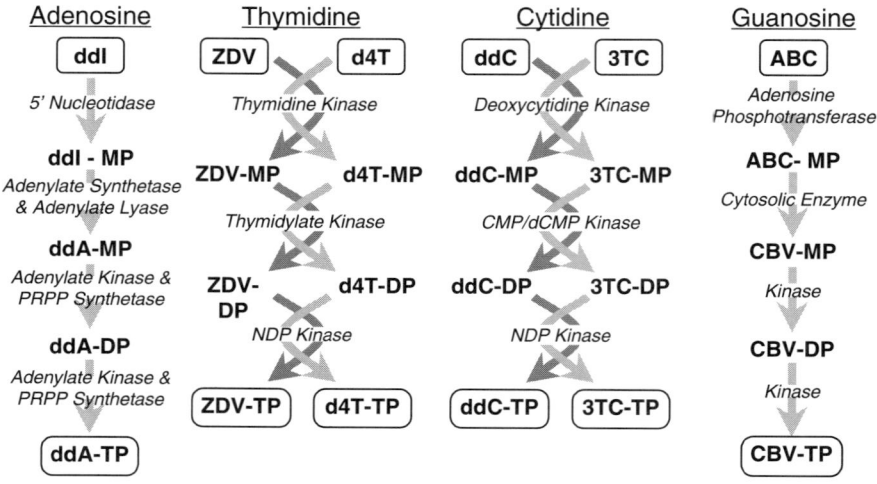

Figure 8.2 Activation pathways of nucleoside analogues.

The low oral bioavailability is due not only to extensive hepatic meta-bolism (CYP3A4), but also metabolism in the intestinal mucosa which expresses a variety of drug metabolising enzymes, with CYP3A4 being identified as the predominant cytochrome P450 isoform in human small intestinal enterocytes (Kolars *et al.*, 1991; Prueksaritanont *et al.*, 1996). In addition, the P-glycoprotein efflux pump can reduce absorption and increase gut-wall metabolism by causing drugs such as the HIV-protease inhibitors (Kim *et al.*, 1998; Profit *et al.*, 1999) to cycle through the entero-cytes, so raising their chance of pre-systemic biotransformation.

Fitzsimmons and Collins (1997) initially demonstrated the *in vitro* metabolism of saquinavir by both human intestinal and hepatic micro-somes and showed that the major metabolites of saquinavir were hydroxy-lated derivatives. They have also proposed a potential contribution for intestinal CYP3A4 in the first pass metabolism of saquinavir. More recently, Eagling *et al.* (2001) have rigorously identified saquinavir metabolites from human microsomal incubations.

CYP3A4 is also involved in the metabolism of the protease inhibitors, indinavir (Chiba *et al.*, 1997), ritonavir (Kumar *et al.*, 1996) and amprenavir (Decker *et al.*, 1998). Other isoforms (CYP2C9, CYP2D6) have also been implicated in the biotransformation of ritonavir, and ritonavir is a potent inhibitor of these CYP isoforms (Eagling *et al.*, 1998). CYPs 2C19, 2D6 and possibly CYPs 2C9 and 2E1 are also involved in the metabolism of nelfinavir (Lee *et al.*, 1997). The involvement of polymorphic CYP2C19 in the formation of a circulating metabolite of nelfinavir (M8) which possesses antiretroviral activity has also been proposed.

The data indicating PIs to be both substrates and inhibitors of P-gp are convincing (Kim *et al.*, 1998; Profit *et al.*, 1999; Lee *et al.*, 1998; Huisman *et al.*, 2000; Gutmann *et al.*, 1999). There is also evidence that saquinavir and ritonavir are substrates and inhibitors of multi-drug resistance protein (MRP1 and MRP2) (Gutmann *et al.*, 1999). In addition to the role of efflux transport proteins reducing oral absorption of a drug via effects at the enterocyte, there are hepatic effects of great importance for anti-HIV drug effects at the level of brain entry. Transporters are currently a research area of great interest and there are numerous issues to clarify in relation to HIV therapy, namely:

- Effect of drug therapies on transporter expression (up-regulation, down-regulation).
- Role of transporters in passage of drugs into CSF, semen and across the placenta.
- The feasibility of using selective transport inhibitors to increase oral bioavailability, sanctuary site penetration, etc.

Variability in plasma concentrations of protease inhibitors

PI concentrations in plasma show marked interpatient variability following standard dosing regimens. Following studies with hard-gel saquinavir which showed a greater than twenty-fold variability in trough saquinavir concentrations, it was suggested that TDM of saquinavir could have a role in improving therapeutic outcome (Barry *et al.*, 1998). This conviction has increased as plasma concentrations from patients receiving PI-containing therapies have been determined. Figure 8.3 shows trough (i.e. at the end of a dosing interval) PI concentrations from this study. There are a number of features. Clearly there is huge inter-patient variability for all the PIs. Note, for example, that a high proportion of patients receiving the original hard-gel formulation of saquinavir have trough concentrations (C_{trough}) below the calculated target minimum effective concentration (MEC). The latter is derived substantially from *in vitro* studies where the concentration of each PI to inhibit wild-type HIV is determined (IC_{50} or IC_{95} values) in the presence of 50% human serum (Molla *et al.*, 1998). The latter is important since PIs (particularly saquinavir, nelfinavir, ritonavir, amprenavir) are extensively bound to plasma proteins. Using these protein-corrected inhibitory concentration values, we and others have estimated the *in vivo* MEC for each PI (amprenavir 300–400 ng/ml; indinavir 60–100 ng/ml; nelfinavir 400–700 ng/ml; ritonavir 1500–2100 ng/ml; saquinavir 100–200 ng/ml).

Plasma concentrations following the introduction of soft-gel saquinavir are generally much higher, although some patients still present with trough concentrations below the desired value. Indinavir, ritonavir and nelfinavir show similar variability. The concentrations presented in Figure 8.3 are

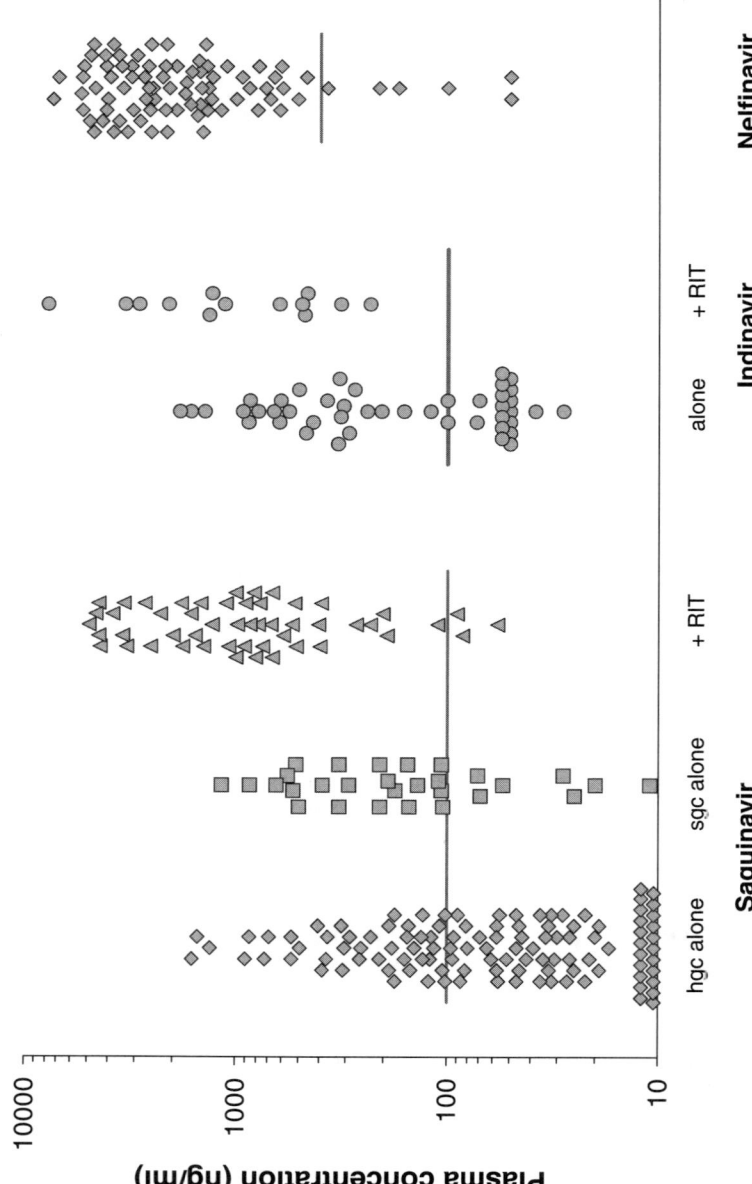

Figure 8.3 Trough plasma concentrations of saquinavir, indinavir and nelfinavir after various dosing regimens alone and in the presence of ritonavir. Data from Liverpool HIV Pharmacology Group. Hgc=hard gel capsule; sgc=soft gel capsule. The horizontal line indicates the minimum effective concentrations.

from both daily clinical practice and some carefully monitored clinical trials. They represent a cross-section of patients, some of whom will have undergone monitoring because of suspected virological failure or a potential drug interaction or a change in therapy.

In relation to the marked inter-patient variability, although it is difficult to pinpoint a single factor, we know that there are clear effects of food (on absorption), drug interactions and hepatic dysfunction. Since, as indicated, PIs are substrates for enterocytic and hepatic CYP3A4 and P-gp, drugs which inhibit CYP3A4 (e.g. other PIs; azole antifungals, such as keto-conazole or itraconazole; macrolide antibiotics, such as clarithromycin) or P-gp may result in marked elevation of PI concentrations. Conversely, the induction of CYP3A4 by drugs such as some NNRTIs, rifampicin and rifabutin may decrease PI concentrations. A patient failing a regimen will be given at least two new drugs and in salvage therapy increasingly complex combinations of drugs (as many as four to eight agents) which may include PI–PI combinations plus an NNRTI. These regimens have considerable potential for complex drug interactions and toxicity. For a complete listing of the important drug interactions in HIV therapy, see http://www.hiv-druginteractions.org.

Pre-existing liver impairment, particularly with co-existent chronic hepatitis B or C infection is not uncommon in HIV infection. Wide variability in the pharmacokinetics of nelfinavir in a small group of patients has been demonstrated (Khaliq et al., 1999) and liver dysfunction is likely to affect the disposition of all PIs. Since they are all extensively meta-bolised, determining plasma levels may assist in optimising doses, mini-mising hepatotoxocity and discriminating between drug toxicity and other causes of liver impairment.

Pharmacoenhancement

The urgent need to improve the efficacy of current antiretroviral drugs has led to the use of low-dose ritonavir as a "pharmacoenhancer" with the aim of obtaining plasma concentrations of unbound drug that are in excess of the IC_{95} of both wild-type and mutant virus (van Heeswijk et al., 1999). The benefits of using ritonavir which is one of the most potent inhibitors of CYP3A4 known (Eagling et al., 1997) include improving bioavailability through inhibition of first-pass loss (e.g. metabolism by CYP3A4 and efflux by the transporter P-gp) and reducing clearance.

The recommended dosage of indinavir is 800 mg every 8 hours. Co-administration of indinavir with (low dose) ritonavir has been shown to improve the overall pharmacokinetics of indinavir allowing for twice daily administration of reduced dosages. The steady state plasma area under the curve (AUC_{0-24h}) for indinavir in a combination of 400 mg indinavir + 400 mg ritonavir twice daily is comparable to the AUC_{0-24h} found with the conventional regimen (800 mg every 8 hours). However, the trough concentration is increased by approximately five-fold while the maximum concentration is reduced (van Heeswijk *et al.*, 1999). The higher trough concentration of indinavir is expected to enhance the potency of the drug and the lower maximum concentration to attenuate the incidence of indinavir-related urological complications which have been associated with elevated indinavir concentrations (Dieleman *et al.*, 1999). Interestingly ritonavir has been shown to significantly reduce the intersubject variability in indinavir pharmacokinetics (Hsu *et al.*, 1998).

Other data from twice daily dosing are also convincing (e.g. indinavir–ritonavir 800/100, ABT378r 400/100 mg, saquinavir–ritonavir 400/400 mg, amprenavir–ritonavir 600/100 mg), although it is probably too early to say if data from once daily dosing regimens incorporating ritonavir are anything more than promising. Eventually we will move into the once daily single agent PI (without pharmacoenhancement) and there are several drugs in the pipeline.

Therapeutic drug monitoring of antiretrovirals

One of the major problems with TDM is knowing the target concentration. Minimum target PI concentrations have largely been defined on the basis of monotherapy concentration–effect modelling or *in vitro* IC_{95} data for laboratory or clinical isolates of HIV, with allowance made for protein binding. But how are these values affected by other antiretroviral agents in a given combination? Are data derived from studies using PI monotherapy or complex four-drug regimens including dual PIs, appropriate to the general clinic population of HIV-positive patients?

In using a single target trough concentration, we assume that all patients have viral isolates with the same susceptibility. In reality many patients with resistant isolates require higher concentrations. Interindividual variability in drug absorption (for example with diet or according to disease stage) or changing patterns of adherence may confuse the picture and give TDM a poorer predictive value.

Finally there is little agreement concerning the best measure to use: AUC, C_{min} (C_{trough}), or concentrations ratios (i.e. concentration obtained at any time point related to population profile data). While AUCs represent a robust measure, there are logistical difficulties in instituting their use on a wide scale. There is currently a move to consider using C_{min}/IC_{50} values (IC_{50} being for the patient isolate) and this would certainly seem to be the way forward. In this connection the term inhibitory quotient (IQ) has been introduced where $IQ = C_{min}/IC_{50}$ and there is clearly an advantage if the IQ for a PI is in excess of 1.

The key questions such as 'does TDM improve patient outcome?' and 'is it cost-effective?' need to be addressed urgently.

References

Adkins, J. and Noble, S. (1998) 'Efavirenz', *Drugs* 56: 1055–64.

The AVANTI Steering Committee (1999) 'Analysis of HIV-1 clinical trials: statistical magic?', *Lancet* 353: 2061–64.

Barry, M. G., Khoo, S. H., Veal, G. J., Hoggard, P. G., Gibbons, S. E., Wilkins, E. G., Williams, O., Breckenridge, A. M. and Back, D. J. (1996) 'The effect of zidovudine dose on the formation of intracellular phosphorylated metabolites', *AIDS* 10: 1361–7.

Barry, M. G., Merry, C., Lloyd, J., Halifax, K., Carey, P., Mulcahy, F. and Back, D. J. (1998) 'Variability in trough plasma saquinavir concentrations in HIV patients – a case for therapeutic drug monitoring', *Br. J. Clin. Pharmacol.* 45: 501–2.

Barry, M. G., Mulcahy, F., Merry, C., Gibbons, S. and Back, D. J. (1999) 'Pharmacokinetics and potential interactions amongst anti-retroviral agents used to treat patients with HIV infection', *Clin. Pharmacokinet.* 36: 289–304.

Chiba, M., Hensleigh, M., and Lin, J. L. (1997) 'Hepatic and intestinal metabolism of indinavir, an HIV protease inhibitor, in rat and human microsomes. Major role of CYP3A', *Biochem. Pharmac.* 53: 1187–95.

Decker, C. J., Laitiner, L. M., Bridson, G. W., Raybuck, S. A., Tung, R. D. and Chaturredi, P. R. (1998) 'Metabolism of amprenavir in liver microsomes: role of CYP3A4 inhibition for drug interactions', *J. Pharm. Sci.* 87: 803–7.

Dieleman, J. P., Gyssens, I. C., van der Ende, M. E., de Marie, S. and Burger, D. M. (1999) 'Urological complaints in relation to indinavir plasma concentrations in HIV-infected patients', *AIDS* 13: 473–8.

Eagling, V. A., Back, D. J. and Barry, M. G. (1997) 'Differential inhibition of cytochrome P450 isoforms by the protease inhibitors ritonavir, saquinavir and indinavir', *Br. J. Clin. Pharmacol.* 44: 190–4.

Eagling, V. A., Tjia, J. T., and Back, D. J. (1998) 'Differential selectivity of cytochrome P450 inhibitors against probe substrates in human and rat liver microsomes', *Br. J. Clin. Pharmacol.* 45, 107–14.

Eagling, V. A., Wiltshire, H., Whitcombe, I. W. A. and Back, D. J. (2001) 'CYP3A4–mediated hepatic metabolism of the HIV-1 protease inhibitor saquinavir *in vitro*', *Xenobiotica* (in press).

Fitzsimmons, M. E. and Collins, J. M. (1997) 'Selective biotransformation of the human immunodeficiency virus protease inhibitor saquinavir by human small intestinal cytochrome P450', *Drug. Metab. Dispos.* 25: 256–67.

Gutmann, H., Fricker, G., Drewe, J., Toeroek, M. and Miller, D. S. (1999) 'Interactions of HIV protease inhibitors with ATP-dependent drug export proteins', *Mol. Pharmacol.* 56, 383–9.

Hsu, A., Granneman, G. R., Cao, G., Carothers, L., Japour, A., El-Shourbagy, T., Dennis, S., Berg, J., Erdman, K., Leonard, J. M. and Sun, E. (1998) 'Pharmacokinetic interaction between ritonavir and indinavir in healthy volunteers', *Antimicrob. Agents Chemother.* 42: 2784–91.

http://www.hiv-druginteractions.org

Huisman, M. T., Smit, J. W. and Schinkel, A. H. (2000) 'Significance of P-glycoprotein for the pharmacology and clinical use of HIV protease inhibitors', *AIDS* 14, 237–42.

Khaliq, Y., Gallicano, K., Seguin, I., Fyke, K., Carignan, G., Badley, A. and

Cameron, W. D. (1999) 'Therapeutic drug monitoring of nelfinavir in HIV patients with liver disease', paper presented at 6th Conference on Retroviruses and Opportunistic Infections, Chicago.

Kim, R. B., Fromm, M. F., Wandel, C., Leake, B., Wood, A. J. J., Roden, D. M. and Wilkinson, G. R. (1998) 'The drug transporter P-glycoprotein limits oral absorption and brain entry of HIV-1 protease inhibitors', *J. Clin. Invest.* **101**: 289–94.

Kolars, J. C., Awni, W. M., Merion, R. M., and Watkins, P. B. (1991) 'First-pass metabolism of cyclosporin by the gut', *Lancet* **338**: 1488–90.

Kumar, G. N., Rodrigues, A. D., Buko, A. M. and Denissen, J. F. (1996) 'Cytochrome P450 mediated metabolism of the HIV-1 protease inhibitor Ritonavir (ABT-538) in human liver microsomes', *J. Pharmacol. Exp. Ther.* **277**: 23–31.

Ledergerber, B., Egger, M., Opravil, M., Telenti, A., Hirschel, B., Battegay, M., Vernazza, P., Sudre, P., Flepp, M., Furrer, H., Francioli, P. and Weber, R. (1999) 'Clinical progression and virological failure on highly active anti-retroviral therapy in HIV-1 patients: a prospective cohort study', *Lancet* **353**: 863–8.

Lee, C. A., Liang, B.-H., Wu, E. Y., Grettenberger, H. M., Sandoval, T. M., Zhang, K. E. and Shetty, B. V. (1997) 'Prediction of nelfinavir mesylate (Viracept) clinical drug interactions based on its *in vitro* human P450 metabolism', paper presented at 4th Conference on Retroviruses and Opportunistic Infections, Chicago.

Lee, C. G., Gottesman, M. M., Cardarelli, C. O., Ramachandra, M., Jeang, K. T., Ambudkar, S. V., Pastan, I. and Dey, S. (1998) 'HIV-1 protease inhibitors are substrates for the MDR-1 multidrug transporter', *Biochemistry* **37**: 3594–601.

Molla, A., Vasavanonda, S., Kumar, G., Sham, H. L., Johnson, M., Grabowski, B., Denissen, J. F., Kohlbrenner, W., Plattner, J. J., Leonard, J. M., Norbeck, D. W. and Kempf, D. J. (1998) 'Human serum attenuates the activity of protease inhibitors towards wild type and mutant human immunodeficiency virus', *Virology* **250**: 255–62.

Moore, K. H., Barrett, J. E., Shaw, S., Pakes, G. E., Churchus, R., Kapoor, A., Lloyd, J., Barry, M. G. and Back, D. (1999) 'The pharmacokinetics of lamivudine phosphorylation in peripheral blood mononuclear cells from patients infected with HIV-1', *AIDS* **13**: 2239–50.

Murphy, R. L. and Montaner, J. (1996) 'Nevirapine: a review of its development, pharmacological profile and potential for clinical use', *Exp. Opin. Invest. Drugs* **5**: 1183–99.

Palella, F. J., Delaney, K. M., Moorman, A. C., Loveless, M. O., Fuhrer, J., Satten, G. A., Aschman, D. J. and Holmberg, S.D. (1998) 'Declining morbidity and mortality among patients with advanced human immunodeficiency virus infection', *N. Engl. J. Med.* **338**: 853–60.

Profit, L., Eagling, V. A. and Back, D. J. (1999) 'Modulation of P-glycoprotein function in human lymphocytes and Caco-2 cell monolayers by HIV-1 protease inhibitors', *AIDS* **13**: 1623–7.

Prueksaritanont, T., Gorham, L. M., Hochman, J. H., Tran L. O., and Vyas K. P. (1996) 'Comparative studies of drug metabolising enzymes in dog, monkey, and human small intestines, and in Caco-2 cells', *Drug Metab. Disp.* **24**: 634–642.

Staszewski, S., Miller, V., Sabin, C., Carlebach, A., Berger, A. M., Weidmann, E., Helm, E. B., Hill, A. and Phillips, A. (1999) 'Virological response to protease inhibitor therapy in an HIV clinic cohort', *AIDS* **13**: 367–73.

Steimer, J. L., Fotteler, B., Gieschke, R., Wiltshire, H., and Buss, N. (1998), Predicting the optimal dose of saquinavir via modelling of dose-exposure and exposure-effect relationships', in M. Danhof and J. L. Steimer (eds) *Measurement and Kinetics of In Vivo Drug Effects. Advances in simultaneous pharmacokinetic/pharmacodynamic modelling*, Leiden: Amsterdam Center for Drug Research, pp. 79–86.

van Heeswijk, R. P., Veldkamp, A. I., Hoetelmans, R. M., Mulder, J. W., Schreij, G., Hsu, A., Lange, J. M., Beijnen, J. H. and Meenhorst, P. L. (1999) 'The steady-state plasma concentrations of indinavir alone and in combination with a low dose of ritonavir in twice daily dosing regimens in HIV-1 infected individuals', *AIDS* **13**: F95–9

Wit, F. W., van Leeuwen, R., Weverling, G. J., Jurriaans, S., Nauta, K., Steingrover, R., Schuijtemaker, J., Eyssen, X., Fortuin, D., Weeda, M., de Wolf, F., Reiss, P., Danner, S. A. and Lange, J. M. (1999) 'Outcome and predictors of failure of highly active anti-retroviral therapy: one-year follow-up of a cohort of human immunodeficiency type-1–infected persons', *J. Infect. Dis.* **179**: 790–8.

Chapter 9

Predictive modelling of *in vivo* drug interaction from *in vitro* data

From theory to a computer-based workbench and its experimental validation

P. Bonnabry, J. Sievering, T. Leemann and P. Dayer

Introduction

The variability in the response to drugs is a major difficulty for clinicians, which can potentially induce treatment failure if concentrations are too low, or toxic events if they are too high. Both situations may lead to significant problems, depending on the pharmacological characteristics of the drug (high concentrations and small therapeutic index) and on the type of illness (lack of epilepsy control due to low concentrations).

Interactions with drugs, food and pollutants are recognised as being major determinants of environmental variability. Other important sources of uncertainty are natural (interindividual variability), genetic (polymorphisms) and to a lesser extent time-related (chronopharmacology) factors.

Interactions can occur at different levels of drug kinetics, but metabolism by the liver and by several extra-hepatic tissues is by far the most sensitive target, although absorption, binding to blood or tissue components and renal elimination may in some instances play a role. Pharmacodynamic interactions may be anticipated on the basis of known biological effects and should not be of major concern.

Enzyme selectivity

The cytochrome P450 superfamily plays a key role in drug biotransformation, elimination and interactions (Guengerich, 1997). Other drug-metabolising enzyme families, such as glucuronyltransferases, acetyltransferases, sulfotransferases, methyltransferases and glycinetransferases, play an important part in biotransformation reactions, but to date, their contribution to the development of significant drug interactions has not been studied very closely.

Multiple cytochrome P450 isozymes have been identified (Nelson *et al.*, 1996) and numerous substrates, inhibitors and inducers have been characterised (Wrighton and Stevens, 1992). Consequently, it has become more and more difficult for clinicians to manage metabolic drug interactions, because of the sheer complexity of the systems involved and the specificity of the interactions. Moreover, a large part of the basic information is obtained from *in vitro* experiments, leading to further difficulties when trying to extrapolate results to the clinical context.

To improve the understanding of cytochrome P450–dependent metabolism and drug interactions, summarising tables have been published (Guengerich, 1995; Bertz and Grannenman, 1997; Bonnabry *et al.*, 1997) or are accessible on the internet (www.dml.georgetown.edu/depts/pharmacology/davetab.html; www.hcuge.ch/Pharmacie/Listemed/Tabcasesub.PDF and .../Tabcasein.PDF). They are very useful, especially because the detailed understanding of the role of individual enzymes is an essential prerequisite for making rational predictions of *in vivo* drug metabolism and interactions. However, these tools often present major drawbacks, such as a poor updating frequency and the absence of bibliographic references.

Interpretation of *in vitro* data

At present, most basic information about drug metabolism, inhibition and induction is obtained from *in vitro* experiments. The development of several simple and cost-effective techniques (expression of specific cytochrome P450 by micro-organisms, hepatocyte tissue culture) has considerably increased this phenomenon.

Although *in vitro* experiments give very accurate and useful results, their extrapolation to the clinical situation is fraught with difficulty. For example, what should a clinician make when a 1 μM inhibition value is determined for a drug? And what is the associated risk of drug interactions for his patient?

Moreover, metabolic data obtained from recombinant micro-organisms should be considered with caution, since an apparent major biotransformation pathway may be minor *in vivo*, if the abundance of the isozyme in the metabolising organs is low.

In vitro experiments are essential, but the extrapolation of results to the *in vivo* situation is the basis of clinical impact evaluations. Although numerous *in vitro* techniques have been developed, only a few specific extrapolation techniques have been published (Rodrigues and Wong, 1997; Von Moltke *et al.*, 1998; Ito *et al.*, 1998, Nakasa *et al.*, 1998). The model proposed here was first published a few years ago (Leemann and Dayer, 1995).

In vitro–in vivo modelling of drug interactions

For reasons described above, the extrapolation of easily accessible *in vitro* data to the *in vivo* situation is an exciting challenge. Unfortunately, no single quantitative model representing all the different facets of such a complex task as predicting the risk of clinical drug interactions can possibly be sufficiently comprehensive and remain simple enough to be both widely useful and usable. Such a model should, at the same time, be very general and very specific, it should incorporate as much physiological and biological knowledge as possible, while still remaining simple. As the model becomes more and more complex, it also becomes less and less applicable, because complementary parameters are often missing.

Several studies have led to the prediction of *in vivo* drug interactions from *in vitro* data (Rodrigues and Wong, 1997; Von Moltke *et al.*, 1998; Ito *et al.*, 1998; Nakasa *et al.*, 1998). Most of them have focused on inhibitory interactions, but a few authors have also tried to predict interactions leading to enzyme induction (Kedderis, 1997). Variable strategies and models have been proposed to predict the "active" *in vivo* concentrations of inhibitors or inducers at the site of the interaction.

In place of a unique model, we have proposed a logical scheme for building extensible models to predict the impact of metabolism inhibition. These elementary building blocks are selected as required to represent key features and available data for specific situations. The strategy consists in starting from the simplest possible case and increasing the complexity only when sufficient evidence justifies it.

Simplest case model

Although the simplest model can certainly be useful for explaining many interactions, it is obviously not fully applicable to all clinical situations. Its validity is defined by the following main set of assumptions:

1   Unbound drug concentrations drive metabolism and inhibition
2   *In vivo* enzyme kinetics are identical to those characterised *in vitro*
3   Unbound inhibitor concentrations in plasma and effective concentrations at the enzyme site are identical at all times
4   Substrate biotransformation kinetics and inhibitor effect can be described by a Michaelis–Menten model
5   There is a single interaction mechanism
6   Inhibition is reversible, either competitive or non-competitive
7   Only one substance acts as an inhibitor (metabolites are not themselves inhibitors)
8   Substrate elimination kinetics are linear
9   Substrate elimination is controlled by a single enzyme
10 The substrate has a low extraction ratio

The first two assumptions are essential. Assumption 1 is central for all of pharmacology, and it is impossible to build quantitative models relating *in vitro* and *in vivo* drug metabolism data without making assumption 2.

As the systemic elimination of most compounds occurs at substrate concentrations that do not significantly saturate the enzymes catalysing their biotransformation, the effect of an inhibitor on their intrinsic clearance can be expressed as

$$Cl_{int[I]} = \frac{V_{max}}{K_m \cdot (1 + I/K_i)} = \frac{Cl_{int}}{1 + I/K_i}$$

where $CL_{int[I]}$ is the intrinsic clearance in the presence of the inhibitor, I is the effective inhibitor concentration and K_i the inhibition constant.

In the simplest form of the model, the ratio of the clearance of a drug, in the absence and in the presence of an inhibitor ($Cl_{int}/Cl_{int[I]}$) can be defined as the inhibition index (I_I). Its value is equal to 1 in the absence of an inhibiting effect and is larger than 1 when an inhibition arise. As it is usual to measure *in vivo* total concentrations in plasma, it is therefore necessary to account for plasma protein binding to integrate *in vivo* concentrations with the K_i determined *in vitro*. The *in vivo* inhibition index can thus be calculated as

$$I_I = 1 + \frac{f_u \cdot I_{pl}}{K_i}$$

where I_{pl} is the total plasma concentration, f_u the unbound fraction and K_i the inhibition constant.

This inhibition index presents interesting features: it is characteristic of a given enzyme-inhibitor pair, a specific index can be calculated for each isozyme inhibited by a substance and the kinetics of the inhibition over time can be simulated on the basis of the inhibitor's plasma kinetics.

The impact of enzyme inhibition on the pharmacokinetics of a target substrate can easily be calculated from the value of I_I:

$$Cl_{[I]} = \frac{Cl}{I_i}$$
$$t_{\frac{1}{2}[I]} = t_{\frac{1}{2}} \cdot I_I$$
$$C_{ss[I]} = C_{ss} \cdot I_I$$

Examples of more complex models

The simplest case model can be used as a first approximation, when no evidence suggests that one or several assumptions are not respected. When it becomes apparent that the use of a more complex model is necessary, the calculation model can be modified in consequence.

Intrahepatic accumulation

Intrahepatic accumulation via facilitated diffusion or active transport has been described for numerous xenobiotics (Le Blanc, 1994), especially for organic cations (anticholinergic drugs, antineoplastic drugs, neuromuscular blocking agents, local anesthetics, psychotropic amines, antihistaminics) (Meijer *et al.*, 1990) and anions (benzylpenicillin, pravastatin) (Yamazaki *et al.*, 1992; 1993).

In these cases, the inhibition index can be modeled simply as

$$I_l = 1 + \frac{\alpha \cdot f_u \cdot I_{pl}}{K_i}$$

with α being the ratio of effective inhibitor concentrations in hepatocytes to its unbound plasma concentrations. If intrahepatocyte concentration is lower than free plasma concentration, values of α are between 0 and 1.

Multiple inhibitors

In several situations, inhibiting potency of multiple inhibitors has to be modelled. Particular examples include administration of a mixture of enantiomers and substances for which both parent compound and metabolites are potential inhibitors.

When two or more substances inhibit a single isozyme by a similar mechanism, either competitive or non-competitive, the inhibition index becomes:

$$I_l = 1 + \frac{f_{u,1} \cdot I_{pl,1}}{K_{i,1}} + \frac{f_{u,2} \cdot I_{pl,2}}{K_{i,2}} + \cdots$$

where (1) and (2) subscripts refer to different inhibitors.

However, when two substances inhibit a single enzyme by different independent mechanisms, one competitive and the other non-competitive for example, the inhibition index is

$$I_l = I_{l[c]} + I_{l(nc)}$$

where the (c) and (nc) subscripts refer to the competitive and the non-competitive components, respectively.

Fraction of substrate metabolised

For many drugs more than one elimination pathway may have to be accounted for. If two elimination processes can be assumed to operate in parallel through inhibited and non-inhibited pathways, the effect of an inhibitor on a substrate's clearance can be modelled as

$$Cl_{[I]} = \frac{Cl_i}{I_i} + Cl_{ni}$$

where CL_i and CL_{ni} are the partial clearances through the inhibited and the non-inhibited pathways, respectively.

Uncertainty

Although the effect of using appropriate structural models is to reduce the degree of uncertainty, some will always remain, particularly when dealing with complex biological systems and clinical situations.

A major limitation is the absence of a general rule to predict intrahepatic concentrations of drugs from plasma concentrations. Data regarding ratios between intrahepatocyte and plasma free concentrations are very scarce, owing to the relative difficulty in measuring them and to the underestimation of the importance of this mechanism until recently. Theoretically, determination of these ratios might include the use of radiolabeled drugs, which allow an adequate estimation of intracellular concentrations and drug localisation. Some authors have suggested easier methods whereby the *in vitro* partitioning between water and liver homogenates was determined (Von Moltke *et al.*, 1994). This technique evaluates the affinity of drugs for cellular components, but the guarantee of having an appropriate estimation of enzyme exposure is not rigorously demonstrated. Published results of extrapolation data were however in accordance with known *in vivo* potential of interactions.

The role played by metabolites constitutes another source of uncertainty, since their inhibition potential, as well as their pharmacokinetic parameters are rarely determined. Their contribution to drug interactions can however be relevant, as exemplified by norfluoxetine CYP2D6 inhibition (Crewe *et al.*, 1992). In consequence, *in vitro* as well as pharmacokinetic studies should systematically include the determination of kinetic parameters for the major metabolites.

In vitro non-specific binding of drugs to microsomal proteins should be investigated more thoroughly. A study suggests significant microsomal binding of the highly plasma protein bound drugs warfarin, imipramine and propranolol (Obach, 1997). This factor, if non-negligible, can lead to a significant overestimation of *in vitro* inhibition constants (K_i) and to a subsequent underestimation of the potential for *in vivo* interactions. Unfortunately, actual knowledge of this phenomenon is very limited.

In our approach, the use of the simplest case model is often necessary, due to an absence of parameters needed to predict with more complex models (intrahepatocyte concentrations, role of metabolites). In these situations, validation of predictions by clinical studies or by comparison with *in vivo* literature data is very important.

Computer-based prediction and management of drug interactions

To manage more dynamically cytochrome P450–mediated drug inter-actions, we created an interactive digital workbench, Q-DIPS (Quantitative Drug Interactions Prediction System) (Bonnabry et al., 1999). This system is useful to collect data describing interactions between drugs and cyto-chromes P450, as well as to predict *in vivo* impact from *in vitro* data. Examples of typical questions to be answered by Q-DIPS are shown in Table 9.1.

The major steps of Q-DIPSs pharmacological development are the following:

- Systematic collection of qualitative and quantitative data describing sub-strates, inhibitors and inducers of specific cytochrome P450 isozymes
- Systematic exploration of predictive models of drug interactions
- Validation of the *in vitro/in vivo* modelling approach developed in our laboratory and described above
- Comparison of different modelling approaches
- Operational use of validated models in the context of new drug develop-ment and clinical data.

The informatic development was based on a modular approach. It allows the incorporation, at any time, of new blocks, which are automatically integrated by the program. The system actually runs with Windows98.

To optimise the quality and the user-friendliness of the system, the follow-ing concepts were included:

- dynamism, interactivity and rapid access to information
- continual evolution of the system in relation to new discoveries
- documentation (references) of all data

Table 9.1 Typical questions to be answered by Q-DIPS

Which substances have the highest affinity for an enzyme?
Which substances are substrates of an enzyme?
Where do the data come from?
How good is the evidence for a predicted interaction?
Which substances are likely to interact with a given substance?
Expected impact of an inhibitor on a substrate's kinetics?
Do predictions match published *in vivo* data?
What is the best administration profile to avoid an interaction?
What is the likelihood of drug interactions in a specific patient?
Choice of alternative drug(s) to avoid a potential interaction?

- multi-access to drugs and documentation
- evaluation by Q-DIPSs authors of the quality of the data
- prediction of *in vivo* impact on the basis of *in vitro* data.

The central module of the system is constituted by three dynamic tables, displaying information about interactions between drugs and specific cytochrome P450 isozymes. Metabolism, inhibition and induction data are determined in our laboratory or collected in the literature and their importance is semi-quantified (black/grey boxes) (Figure 9.1). Tables are continuously updated with new data, published or generated in our laboratory.

The application was first conceived to answer simple clinical questions related to cytochrome P450-mediated metabolism. For that purpose, we developed a 'clinical case' module, which gives the opportunity to build a specific table by selecting the administered drugs. This function allows a rapid qualitative evaluation of the risk associated with a multiple-drug prescription (Figure 9.2).

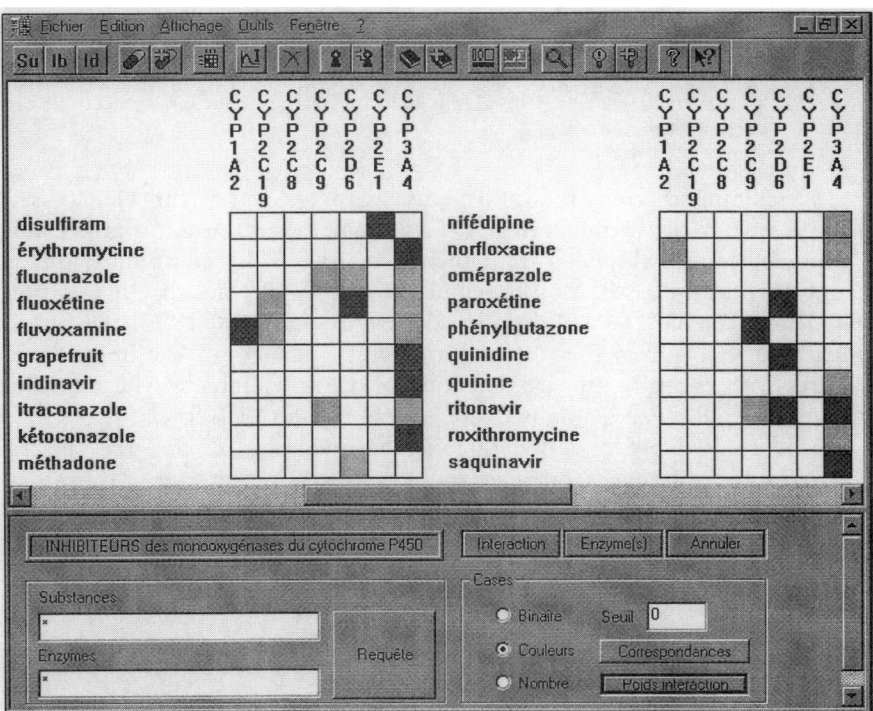

Figure 9.1 Partial illustration of the table listing inhibitors. Black box=strong inhibition, grey box=moderate inhibition.

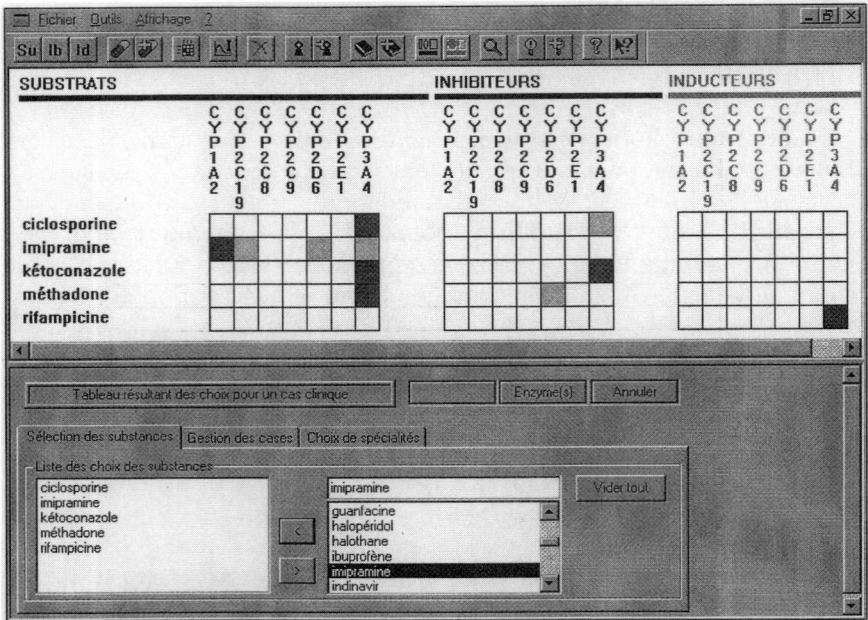

Figure 9.2 'Clinical case' module. The table is built by selecting appropriate drugs at the bottom of the interface.

To facilitate searches, the information is indexed so it can be accessed using a variety of search strategies. Generic names are used in tables and a module was developed to link them with the ATC (anatomical therapeutic chemical) classification developed by the World Health Organisation (Guidelines for ATC Classification and DDD Assignment, 1996). This tool, illustrated in Figure 9.3, is of major interest, in view of the importance progressively taken by this classification of drugs. Complete ATC classification with DDD (defined daily dose) is included in Q-DIPS.

As postulated before, all data must be documented, and the related bibliographic references (articles, books, abstracts, internet, laboratory data) made readily available. For each box, rapid access to the reference bibliography is possible by just clicking on it. A documentation module was also developed to manage all the references and allows one to perform searches by authors, drugs, enzymes, sources, years of publication and keywords (Figure 9.4).

Quantitative data related to a bibliographic reference can be checked at any time, as illustrated in Figure 9.5.

The *in vitro–in vivo* extrapolation module was built on the basis of concepts described above. Pharmacokinetic and enzymatic data are extracted from the database and included in predictive models. It is also possible to

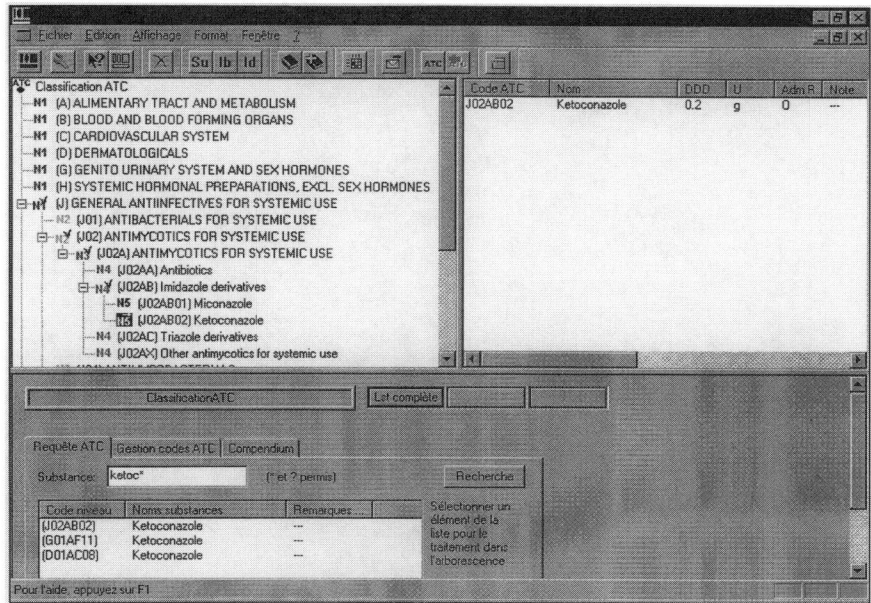

Figure 9.3 Anatomical therapeutic chemical (ATC) classification module.

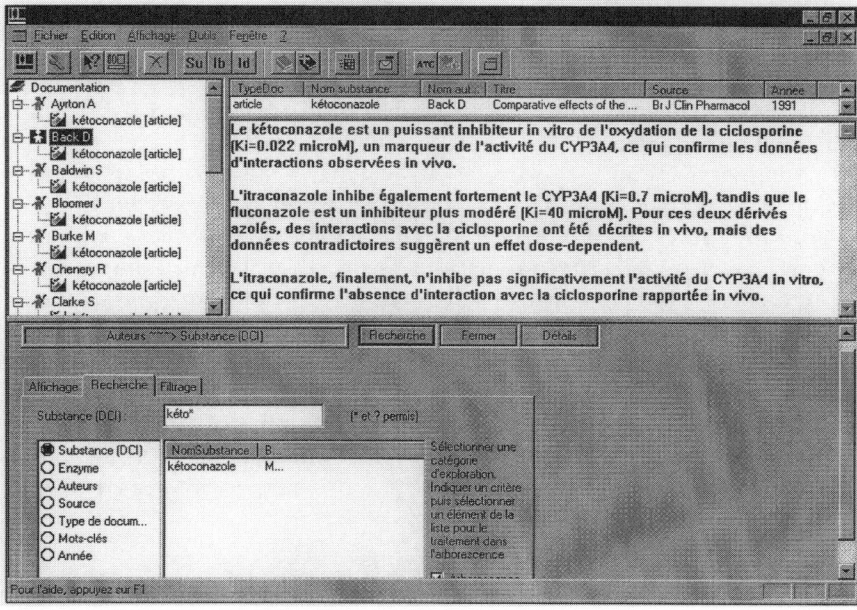

Figure 9.4 Documentation module. Detailed quantitative data are accessible for each set of documentation.

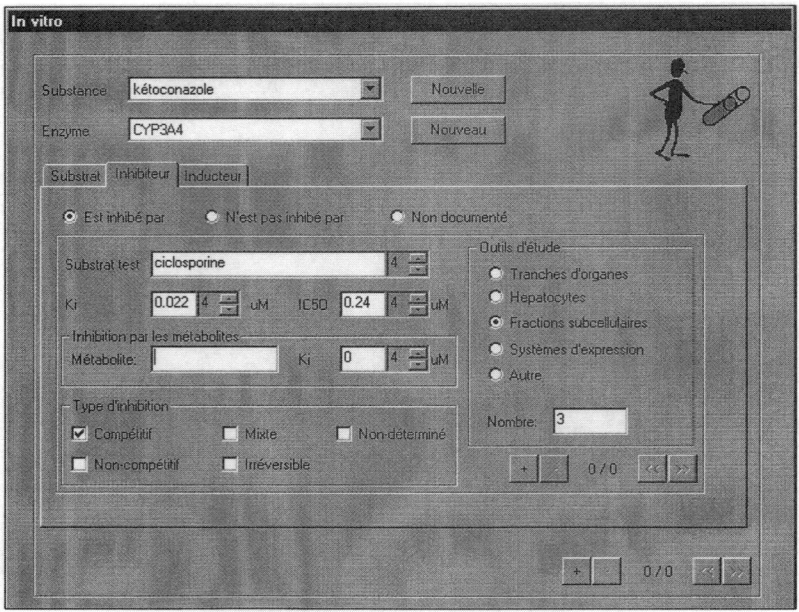

Figure 9.5 Example of quantitative data. *In vitro* inhibition of CYP3A4 by ketoconazole (Back *et al.*, 1991).

perform simulations with hypothetical data, with a view to test specific patient conditions or to make predictions when necessary values are missing. Predictions were performed for several drug families and their results will be described later.

In summary, Q-DIPS constitutes an original system, offering a multivariate and complete approach to drug-interaction problems, with global vision, rapid access to bibliographic data, quality assessment, quantitative data and *in vitro–in vivo* extrapolation. The access to a 'third dimension' – the references associated with each piece of information – constitutes a very useful and powerful source.

Major Q-DIPS developments for future years will be to update the data continuously in parallel with new discoveries, to pursue the validation of the pharmacokinetic models, to extend the system to other sources of metabolic (transferases, FMO, MAO) or renal interactions (P-glycoprotein) (Woodland *et al.*, 1998) and to diffuse the program to interested people, most probably by way of the internet.

Validation studies

Prediction studies were performed for several drug classes, using the extrapolation models described above. Enzymatic and pharmacokinetic data were mostly heterogeneous, either generated in our laboratory or published elsewhere. Results of prediction were compared for validation with published *in vivo* interaction data. As will be shown, *in vivo* data were:

- either very abundant, or very scarce or absent
- obtained either from large clinical studies or from isolated case reports
- sometimes contradictory

Results of predictions were compared quantitatively and after semi-quantification (Table 9.2).

Table 9.2 Semi-quantification of predicted potential of inhibition

Maximum inhibition index	Extent of inhibition
1–1.1	No inhibition
1.2	Very moderate
1.3–1.6	Moderate
1.7–2.5	Strong
>2.5	Very strong

Azoles antifungals

The inhibition potential of fluconazole, ketoconazole and itraconazole for CYP3A4 have been investigated (Bonnabry and Leemann, 1993) on the basis of published *in vitro* inhibition data (Back and Tjia, 1991). Results are summarised in Table 9.3.

For fluconazole and ketoconazole, predictions were in accordance with the known potential to inhibit CYP3A4. Ketoconazole effect was strong, but fluctuating, whereas the impact of fluconazole was lower, but more

Table 9.3 Prediction of drug interactions by antifungals with the simplest model

Drug	Administra-tion rate	Isozyme	K_i [μM]	I_{Imax}[a]	Predicted extent of inhibition	In vivo validation (semi quantitative)
Fluconazole	50–400 mg/day	CYP3A4	40	1.2–2.4	Moderate to strong, dose dependant	Yes
Itraconazole	2×200 mg/day	CYP3A4	0.7	1	No inhibition	No
Ketoconazole	2×200 mg/day	CYP3A4	0.022	8	Very strong, fluctuating	Yes

Note
[a] I_{Imax} = maximum inhibition index.

regular over time. Validation by comparison with published *in vivo* inter-action data confirmed these results. Indeed, cyclosporine daily dose had to be markedly reduced when ketoconazole was concomitantly administered (80% dose reduction; 200 mg ketoconazole b.i.d.) (First *et al.*, 1991), whereas the impact of fluconazole was smaller ($C_{pl[FLUC]}$ /C_{pl} ≈ 2; 200 mg/day fluconazole) (Canafax, 1991). The relation between dose and effect was particularly important for fluconazole, leading to a variable inter-action potential, as described in the literature (Lopez-Gil, 1993; Collignon *et al.*, 1989) and modelled in Q-DIPS (I_{Imax} from 1.2 to 2.4 for daily doses from 50 mg to 400 mg).

The prediction of an absence of *in vivo* CYP3A4 inhibition by itra-conazole was not confirmed by *in vivo* published studies, which suggested an interaction profile with ciclosporine nearly similar to fluconazole (McLachlan and Tett, 1998). The prediction of a low inhibition potential can be related to the very strong protein binding (f_u=0.002 (Grant and Clissold, 1989)) and to the consequently low free plasma concentrations. Two phenomena might intervene *in vivo* and explain the discrepancy between our *in vitro* prediction and the available *in vivo* evidence: a higher than expected active concentration of the antifungal at the enzymatic level (due to intrahepatocyte drug accumulation) and the contribution of the major active hydroxylated metabolite to the inhibition. No available data could actually resolve this question.

NSAIDs

CYP2C9 was identified in our laboratory as being the major determinant of diclofenac (Leemann *et al.*, 1993), (R)- and (S)-ibuprofen (Leemann *et al.*, 1994), lornoxicam (Bonnabry *et al.*, 1996a), mefenamic acid (Bonnabry *et al.*, 1994), piroxicam (Kondo *et al.*, 1992) and tenoxicam (Zhao *et al.*, 1992) elimination. The potential of all these drugs and phenylbutazone to inhibit this isozyme was investigated. Results of pre-dictions using the simplest case model are summarised in Table 9.4 and illustrated in Figure 9.6. A multiple inhibitor model was used for ibuprofen (two enantiomers) and piroxicam (pharmacokinetic and enzymatic data available for its major 5′-hydroxy metabolite).

Predictions were validated by comparison with *in vivo* data of inter-actions with oral anticoagulants (S-warfarin, S-acenocoumarol), typical substrates of CYP2C9 (Chan, 1995).

The very strong potential of phenylbutazone to inhibit CYP2C9 is well documented (Aggeler *et al.*, 1967; Lewis *et al.*, 1974; O'Reilly *et al.*, 1980; Banfield *et al.*, 1983), with a demonstrated inhibition of S-warfarin meta-bolism. The low potential of diclofenac (Michot and Ajdacic, 1975; Fitzgerald and Russel, 1981), ibuprofen (Thilo and Nyman, 1974; Penner and Abbrecht, 1975; Schulman and Henriksson, 1989) and tenoxicam

Table 9.4 Prediction of drug interactions by NSAIDs with the simplest model

Drug	Administra-tion rate	Isozyme	K_i [μM]	I_{Imax}^a	Predicted extent of inhibition	In vivo validation (semi quantitative)
Diclofenac	2×75 mg/day	CYP2C9	5.6	I	No inhibition	Yes
Ibuprofen[b]	3×600 mg/day	CYP2C9	40	I	No inhibition	Ye
Lornoxicam	2×8 mg/ day	CYP2C9	3.6	I	No inhibition	No
Mefenamic acid	3×500 mg/day	CYP2C9	7	1.5	Moderate	Yes, but few data
Phenylbutazone	300 mg/ day	CYP2C9	3	3.3	Very strong	Yes
Piroxicam	20 mg/ day	CYP2C9	54	I	No inhibition	Yes for CYP2C9
Tenoxicam	20 mg/day	CYP2C9	34	I	No inhibition	Yes

Notes
[a]I_{Imax}=maximum inhibition index.
[b]Multiple inhibitors model (both enantiomers).
[c]Multiple inhibitors model (5′OH-piroxicam).

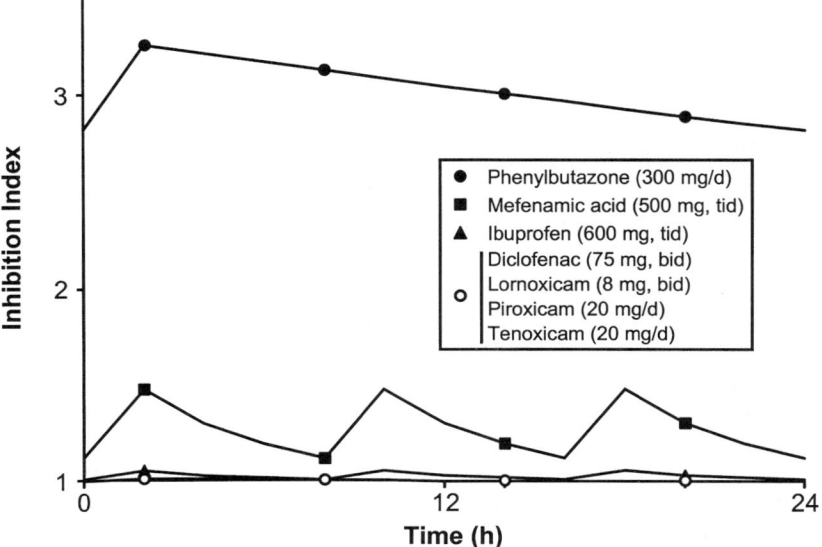

Figure 9.6 Prediction of CYP2C9 inhibition by NSAIDs with the simplest case model.

(Eichler *et al.*, 1992) to inhibit CYP2C9 has also been confirmed by clinical studies.

Mefenamic acid is generally considered as causing a moderate but significant pharmacokinetic interaction with oral anticoagulants, on the basis of a single and very old study (Holmes, 1967). Our predictions tend to confirm this potential, but complementary data are needed.

A low potential to inhibit CYP2C9 was also predicted for piroxicam, but several well documented case reports of interactions with oral anti-coagulants tend to contradict this result (Rhodes *et al.*, 1985; Mallet and Cooper, 1991; Desprez *et al.*, 1992). A clinical study performed in healthy volunteers confirmed an inhibition of R-acenocoumarol metabolism by a single 40 mg piroxicam dose, with a 50% increase of the AUC and a 37% decrease of the half-life (Bonnabry *et al.*, 1996b). No interaction was observed with S-acenocoumarol, which is practically completely metabo-lised by CYP2C9. Knowing that a large part of R-acenocoumarol metabolism is catalysed by unidentified isozymes (Hermans and Thijssen, 1993), this study confirms the results of our predictions. To summarise, piroxicam inhibits R-acenocoumarol metabolism, but probably not by way of CYP2C9 inhibition.

Lornoxicam was demonstrated to have an impact on the control of warfarin anticoagulation in twelve healthy volunteers (Ravic *et al.*, 1990), whereas our prediction suggests an absence of interaction. In view of the absence of enantiomeric data and its similarity with the chemical structure of piroxicam, a target other than CYP2C9 cannot be excluded. A study similar to that performed with piroxicam would be necessary to identify the mechanism involved definitively and to confirm the accuracy of the prediction.

SSRI antidepressants

Interactions due to inhibition of several cytochromes P450 isozymes by selective serotonin re-uptake inhibitor antidepressants are well known, with large differences between drugs. The inhibition potentials of citalopram, fluoxetine, fluvoxamine, paroxetine and sertraline for CYP1A2, CYP2C19, CYP2D6 and CYP3A4 were predicted on the basis of published *in vitro* inhibition data (Crewe *et al.*, 1992; Otton *et al.*, 1993; Rasmussen *et al.*, 1995; Kobayashi *et al.*, 1995; Von Moltke *et al.*, 1995). Since evidence of intrahepatocyte accumulation has been described in the literature (Von Moltke *et al.*, 1995), a model taking this feature into account was used, with a mean accumulation factor (α) of 20. For fluoxetine, the model also included the contribution of norfluoxetine, its major metabolite, as enzy-matic and pharmacokinetic data were available. Results are summarised in Table 9.5.

Table 9.5 Prediction of drug interactions by SSRI antidepressants with the intrahepatocytes accumulation model

Drug	Administration rate	Isozyme	K_i [μM]	I_{Imax}[a]	Predicted extent of inhibition	In vivo validation (semi quantitative)
Citalopram	40 mg/day	CYP1A2	100	1	No inhibition	Yes
		CYP2C19	87.3	1	No inhibition	Yes
		CYP2D6	5.1	1.5	Moderate	Yes
		CYP3A4	100	1	No inhibition	No data
Fluoxetine[b]	20 mg/day	CYP1A2	100	1	No inhibition	Yes
		CYP2C19	5.2 (1.1)[b]	1.3	Moderate	Yes
		CYP2D6	0.6 (0.43)[b]	2.2	Strong	Yes
		CYP3A4	24 (3.5)[b]	1.1	No inhibition	Contradictory data
Fluvoxamine	100 mg/day	CYP1A2	0.1	30	Very strong	Yes
		CYP2D6	8.2	1.4	Moderate	Yes
		CYP3A4	19	1.2	Very moderate	Yes
Paroxetine	20 mg/day	CYP1A2	50	1	No inhibition	Yes
		CYP2C19	7.5	1	No inhibition	Yes
		CYP2D6	0.15	1.8	Strong	Yes
		CYP3A4	100	1	No inhibition	Yes
Sertraline	50 mg/day	CYP1A2	100	1	No inhibition	Yes
		CYP2C19	2	1	No inhibition	Yes
		CYP2D6	0.7	1	No inhibition	No
		CYP3A4	100	1	No inhibition	Yes

Notes
[a] I_{Imax} = maximum inhibition index.
[b] Multiple inhibitors model (norfluoxetine).

On a semi-quantitative basis, most predictions were confirmed by *in vivo* studies of interactions. The very strong and specific potential of fluvoxamine to inhibit CYP1A2 is well known, whereas other SSRIs do not have significant impact on this isozyme (Jeppesen *et al.*, 1996a; Kashuba *et al.*, 1998; Ozdemir *et al.*, 1998). Quantitatively, our theoretical prediction overestimated the real effect of this drug, a five-fold decrease of CYP1A2-mediated caffeine metabolism being observed after a 100 mg/day administration of fluvoxamine for 8 days (Jeppesen *et al.*, 1996b). Reasons for this quantitative discrepancy remain unknown, but might be related to an overestimation of *in vitro* inhibition potential or *in vivo* free concentrations at the enzymatic site.

Moderate inhibition of CYP2C19 by fluoxetine, as well as the weak effects of citalopram and paroxetine, were confirmed by *in vivo* studies using S-mephenytoin as the probe substrate (Jeppesen *et al.*, 1996a). The low potential predicted for sertraline was also confirmed by an absence of inhibiting effect on diazepam metabolism, which is catalysed by CYP3A4 and CYP2C19 (Gardner, 1997). For fluvoxamine, a moderate impact on S-mephenytoin metabolism has been described (Jeppesen et al., 1996a; Xu et al., 1996), but this result could not be confirmed by in vitro-in vivo extrapolations, owing to the absence of published in vitro data of inhibition.

CYP2D6 inhibition by SSRIs is a major source of drug interaction. Results of our predictions are illustrated in Figure 9.7. The strong impact of paroxetine and fluoxetine is well described in the literature (Otton et al., 1993; Brosen et al., 1993; Alderman et al., 1997), but the potential of paroxetine was shown to be higher than fluoxetine. This relative under-estimation of the impact of paroxetine in the theoretical model (a five-fold decrease in desipramine clearance during paroxetine 20 mg/day treatment was observed (Jeppesen et al., 1996a)) might be related to the contribution of inhibiting metabolites, as modeled for the N-demethylated metabolite of fluoxetine. Moderate citalopram and fluvoxamine potentials of inhibition were confirmed semi-quantitatively (Jeppesen et al., 1996a) and quantitatively for the latter (Spigset et al., 1997; Kashuba et al., 1998). In vivo data described a moderate inhibition of CYP2D6 by sertraline (Alderman et al., 1997; Ozdemir et al., 1998), in contradiction with our predictions, but Solai et al. have observed a significant effect only with doses greater than 100 mg/day (Solai et al., 1997). This study also suggested a large

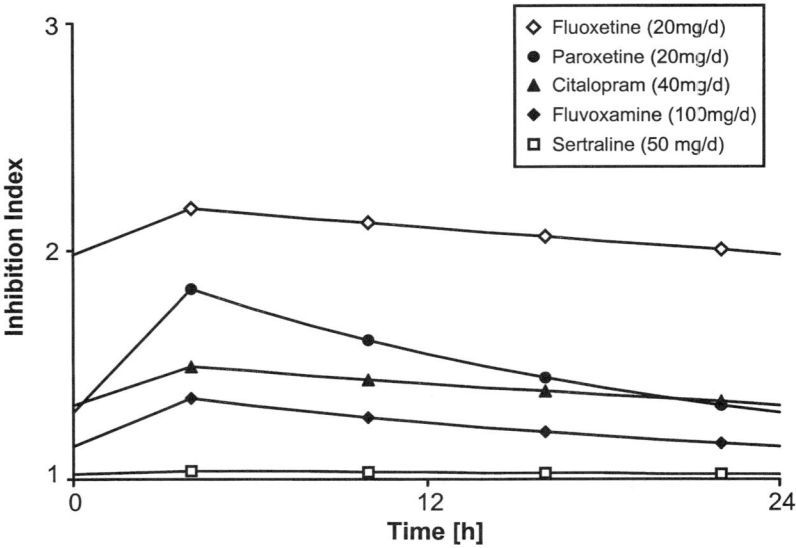

Figure 9.7 Prediction of CYP2D6 inhibition by SSRI antidepressants with the intrahepatocytes accumulation model ($\alpha = 20$).

interindividual variability in the occurrence of the interaction, which may partially explain the frequent contradictions existing in the literature in the description of *in vivo* interaction potentials.

The impact of SSRIs on CYP3A4 was predicted to be low, with only a very moderate effect of fluvoxamine. Results for fluvoxamine (Kashuba *et al.*, 1998), paroxetine (Martin *et al.*, 1997) and sertraline (Rapeport *et al.*, 1996; Gardner *et al.*, 1997) were confirmed, whereas prediction for citalopram was impossible to validate, due to the absence of *in vivo* studies. Data concerning fluoxetine were contradictory and therefore difficult to interpret: occurrence of a moderate drug interaction was suggested by case reports describing increased cyclosporin blood concentrations (Horton and Bonser, 1995) and terfenadine-dependent arrhythmias (Swims, 1993), as well as by a small clinical study reporting increased carbamazepine plasma concentrations (Grimsley *et al.*, 1991); in contrast, the absence of zolpidem pharmacokinetic alterations during concomitant fluoxetine administration was demonstrated in a clinical study involving 29 women (Allard *et al.*, 1998). Although definitive validation of the theoretical predictions has not been possible, clinical data suggest a moderate CYP3A4 inhibition appearing in some patients with higher fluoxetine doses. *In vitro* experiments demonstrated that the affinity of norfluoxetine for CYP3A4 was much higher than fluoxetine and, in consequence, plasma concentrations of this metabolite would be the major determinant of the interaction. As the polymorphic isozyme CYP2D6 contributes at least partially to the formation of norfluoxetine (Hamelin *et al.*, 1996), a variable impact on CYP3A4 activity is not surprising.

HIV protease inhibitors

The *in vitro* potential of four HIV protease inhibitors (indinavir, nelfinavir, ritonavir and saquinavir) to inhibit three major cytochrome P450 isozymes was investigated in our laboratory, using human liver microsomes (Rasca *et al.*, 1998). The values obtained were very similar to those previously published (Eagling *et al.*, 1997). Predictions were performed using the simplest case model and results are summarised in Table 9.6 (Bonnabry *et al.*, 1998).

On a semi-quantitative basis, CYP3A4 inhibition was adequately predicted by the model. Ritonavir and indinavir were very strong inhibitors, nelfinavir had a moderate impact and saquinavir did not display any significant potential of inhibition (Figure 9.8). Quantitatively, results for saquinavir (Hsu *et al.*, 1998) and nelfinavir (Lillibridge *et al.*, 1998) were validated, the latter being associated with a 27% decrease in the urinary recovery of 6β-hydroxycortisol, a result matching well with our prediction. To reflect the reality, the predicted inhibition potencies of indinavir and ritonavir should probably be crossed. Indeed, coadministration of saquinavir

Table 9.6 Prediction of drug interactions by HIV protease inhibitors with the simplest model

Drug	Administration rate	Isozyme	K_i [μM]	I_{Imax}[a]	Predicted extent of inhibition	In vivo validation (semi quantitative)
Indinavir	3×800 mg/day	CYP2C9	9	1.6	Moderate	No data
		CYP2D6	3.5	2.4	Strong	No data
		CYP3A4	0.15	34	Very strong	Yes
Nelfinavir	3×750 mg/day	CYP2C9	2.9	1	No inhibition	No data
		CYP2D6	2.5	1	No inhibition	No data
		CYP3A4	0.4	1.3	Moderate	Yes
Ritonavir	2×600 mg/day	CYP2C9	0.8	1.4	Moderate	Yes, but few data
		CYP2D6	0.7	1.4	Moderate	Yes, but few data
		CYP3A4	0.07	5.5	Very strong	Yes
Saquinavir	3×600 mg/day	CYP2C9	5.6	1	No inhibition	No data
		CYP2D6	4	1	No inhibition	No data
		CYP3A4	1.5	1	No inhibition	Yes

Note
[a]I_{Imax}=maximum inhibition index.

and indinavir 800 mg t.i.d. was associated with five- to eight-fold increase in AUC and C_{max} of saquinavir (McCrea et al., 1997), whereas ritonavir had a much larger impact (50–100-fold increase in saquinavir AUC) (Tseng and Foisy, 1997). The underestimation of ritonavir's inhibition index can be explained by the mechanism of inhibition, since irreversible inactivation of CYP3A4 has been precisely described for this HIV protease inhibitor (Koudriakova et al., 1998). An increase of the in vivo impact during chronic administration is therefore comprehensive, but difficult to model. For indinavir, the overestimation might be due to the inaccuracy of published plasma unbound fractions. This HIV protease inhibitor was described to be only 60% protein bound, against more than 98% for the others, although they all have similar chemical structures (Barry et al., 1997). Consequently, the plasma unbound concentrations and the inhibition potential might be overestimated. A moderate to strong potential to inhibit CYP2C9 and CYP2D6 was also predicted for indinavir, without any evidence of in vivo interactions, which tends to confirm this hypothesis. A strict and comparative measurement of indinavir protein binding would be necessary to re-evaluate its potential to inhibit cytochromes P450.

Moderate predicted inhibitions of CYP2C9 and CYP2D6 by ritonavir were confirmed in vivo, interactions with piroxicam and desipramine being

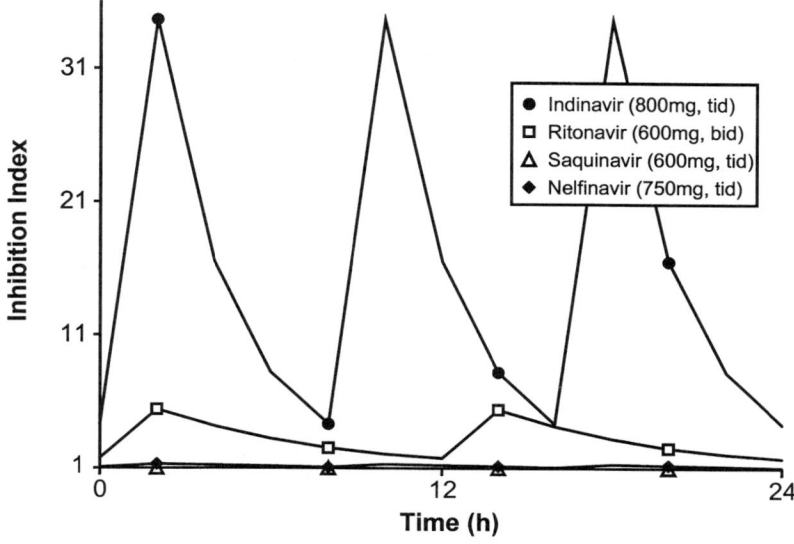

Figure 9.8 Prediction of CYP3A4 inhibition by HIV protease inhibitors with the simplest model.

mentioned by the manufacturer and also reported elsewhere (Tseng and Foisy, 1997).

Effects of HIV protease inhibitors on non-CYP3A4 isozymes are difficult to validate, owing to the lack of *in vivo* data. As a result, the validation cannot be completed, even when an absence of significant interaction is hypothesised.

HMG-CoA reductase inhibitors

Fluvastatin constitutes a good example of a thorough study, complete with the *in vitro* measurement of the potential of inhibition on three major human cytochrome P450 isozymes, the prediction of *in vivo* impact and the validation with a clinical study done on healthy volunteers. *In vitro* experiments showed a strong inhibition of CYP2C9 by both enantiomers (K_i=0.06 μmol/l for (+) and 0.28 mmol/l for (−)), whereas the affinity for CYP2D6 and CYP3A4 was very low (Transon *et al.*, 1996). As intra-hepatocytes accumulation was described for pravastatin (Yamazaki *et al.*, 1993; Ziegler and Hummelsiep, 1993) and lovastatin (Mahoney *et al.*, 1990), a model including this phenomenon was used, even if data specific to fluvastatin were absent. Predictions were done using pharmacokinetic data (free plasma concentrations for each enantiomers over time) from a published study including 37 patients (Smith *et al.*, 1991). Results are summarised in Table 9.7.

Table 9.7 Prediction of drug interactions by HMG-CoA reductase inhibitors with the intrahepatocytes accumulation and the multiple inhibitors (enantiomers) model

Drug	Administra-tion rate	Isozyme	K_i [μM]	$I_{Imax}{}^a$	Predicted extent of inhibition	In vivo validation (semi quantitative)
Fluvastatin	40 mg/day	CYP2C9	0.1	1.4	Moderate, short duration	Yes

Note
$^a I_{Imax}$ = maximum inhibition index.

A moderate and short inhibition of CYP2C9 was predicted by our model, with an estimated inhibition index of 1.4. A large interindividual variability of the effect was also observed, related to the large variability of plasma concentrations. The half-life of fluvastatin being short, the inhibition was shown to be transient and to disappear within a few hours (unpublished data).

A validation study (Transon *et al.*, 1995) evaluated the impact of fluvastatin administration (40 mg/day for 8 days) on diclofenac pharmacokinetics, a prototype CYP2C9 substrate, on fourteen healthy volunteers. Results were in accordance with the predictions, fluvastatin reducing the 0–4 h urinary metabolic ratio (4′hydroxydiclofenac/diclofenac) by about 35%, without effect on the 4–8 h collection. These results thereby confirmed the large interindividual variability.

Fluvastatin is therefore likely to interact with CYP2C9 substrates, at least in some individuals. A report of three cases of interactions in a twenty-five patient population taking warfarin and fluvastatin tends to confirm this prediction (Trilli *et al.*, 1996). Significant interactions are expected primarily when fluvastatin is administered simultaneously with high clearance CYP2C9 substrates (e.g. some oral anticoagulants such as acenocoumarol) or when fluvastatin elimination is impaired.

Global evaluation of validation studies

A global evaluation of the forty-two validation studies described above was done, to assess the ability of models to predict interaction potentials accurately. When the inhibition indexes were expressed in a semi-quantitative way, 91% of validated predictions were in agreement with *in vivo* data (Table 9.8). As these semi-quantitative evaluations give very useful information despite the complexity of the clinical context, this result suggests that the methodology is adequate and useful. When quantitative predictions are made, the accuracy decreases slightly to 79%; seven of the thirty-four validation studies giving inappropriate results.

Table 9.8 Validation studies: accuracy of predictions

Type of validation	Semi-quantitative		
Results of validation	Number	% of total	% of validated data
Good prediction	31	74	91
Bad prediction	3	7	9
Validation impossible (no data or contradictory data)	8	19	–
Total	42	100	100
Type of validation	Quantitative		
Results of validation	Number	% of total	% of validated data
Good prediction	27	64	79
Bad prediction	7	17	21
Validation impossible (no data or contradictory data)	8	19	–
Total	42	100	100

As shown in Table 9.8, 19% of studies remained unvalidated, due to an absence of *in vivo* data or to contradictory information. Most of these predictions correspond to situations where no inhibition was expected and this can partly explain why clinical studies were not performed.

As illustrated in these validation studies, many factors may contribute to the development of interactions. Unfortunately, some of them can generally not be taken into account in predictions (unknown or missing data) and unidentified mechanisms therefore account for most errors. The examples discussed before especially illustrated the following potential problems:

- Free concentrations at enzymatic sites are generally unknown and may differ from free plasma concentrations
- Metabolites may contribute to the interaction, but enzymatic and pharmacokinetic data are seldom determined
- Inactivation of enzymes may lead to a larger inhibition when the inhibitor is administered chronically; this mechanism is not frequently investigated *in vitro*
- Multiple biotransformation pathways increase the possibility for a substrate to be the target of an interaction; pathways are not always extensively and quantitatively identified.

Reliability and accuracy of data are major determinants of the quality of prediction and validation studies. This is particularly true for input data (K_i, f_u, C_{plasm}), but results of *in vivo* validation studies can also be poorly representative (very small clinical studies, case reports, administration of low doses, single dose studies).

Chronological factors have to be taken into consideration when the clinical impact of an inhibitor is evaluated. The occurrence of an interaction will possibly be avoided if a reversible inhibitor has a short half-life and the substrate is administered when the effect disappeared. Q-DIPS approach help predict this type of impact, as exemplified by the transient impact of CYP2C9 inhibition by fluvastatin. On the contrary, when the half-life of the inhibitor is large, the interaction will not be avoidable by a modification of the administration schedule.

The coefficient of correlation between inhibition constants and maximum inhibition indexes was low ($r = -0.2$), even when validated predictions were only used. This confirms the poor predictability of *in vivo* drug interactions on the sole basis of K_i values and it totally justifies the development of prediction systems such as Q-DIPS.

Conclusions

As the occurrence of drug interactions is a major problem in many patient situations, the usefulness of extrapolation techniques is well-defined. At present, major limitations are not due to failure of extrapolation techniques, but to the absence of complete data for input (intrahepatocytes accumulation, enzymatic and pharmacokinetic data for metabolites). Without all of these, predictions are difficult to perform with any degree of certainty. In future years, these parameters will certainly be more systematically investigated and accurate predictions will therefore be easier.

It would be interesting to separate factors influencing the occurrence of drug interactions better. For this, three major typical scenarios should especially be studied: (1) the theoretical evaluation of drug interactions between two or several drugs (without patient or treatment contexts); (2) the consideration of treatment parameters (drug administration, doses, chronology); and (3) the inclusion of individualised patient data (real plasma concentrations, renal clearance).

Beside their clinical applications, prediction systems have a great interest for research and development purposes, as they can help select and design clinical studies useful to perform in man.

Numerous validation studies have shown the interest and the performance of the Q-DIPS approach and have allowed the determination of major sources of discrepancy. In the future, validation will continue, with a particular interest for drugs with well documented enzymatic and pharmacokinetic data.

Acknowledgements

This work was supported by the National Swiss Research Foundation (32–36600.92).

References

Aggeler, P. A., O'Reilly, R. A., Leong, L. and Kowitz, P. E. (1967) 'Potentiation of anticoagulant effect of warfarin by phenylbutazone', *N. Engl. J. Med.* **276**: 496–501.

Alderman, J., Preskorn, S. H., Greenblatt, D. J., Harrison, W., Penenberg, D., Allison, J. and Chung, M. (1997) 'Desipramine pharmacokinetics when co-administered with paroxetine or sertraline in extensive metabolizers', *J. Clin. Psychopharmacol.* **17**: 284–91.

Allard, S., Sainata, S., Roth-Schechter, B. and MacIntyre, J. (1998) 'Minimal interaction between fluoxetine and multiple-dose zolpidem in healthy women', *Drug Metab. Dispos.* **26**: 617–22.

Anonymous (1996) 'Guidelines for ATC classification and DDD assignment', 1st edn, Oslo: WHO Collaborating Center for Drug Statistics Methodology.

Back, D. J. and Tjia, J. F. (1991) 'Comparative effects of the antimycotic drugs ketoconazole, fluconazole, itraconazole and terbinafine on the metabolism of cyclosporin by human liver microsomes', *Br. J. Clin. Pharmacol.* **32**: 624–6.

Banfield, C., O'Reilly, R. A., Chan, E. and Rowland, M. (1983) 'Phenylbutazone–warfarin interaction in man: further stereochemical and metabolic consider-ations', *Br. J. Clin. Pharmacol.* **16**: 669–75.

Barry, M., Gibbons, S., Back, D. and Mulcahy, F. (1997) 'Protease inhibitors in patients with HIV disease, clinically important pharmacokinetic considerations', *Clin. Pharmacokinet.* **32**: 194–209.

Bertz, R. J., and Grannenman, G. R. (1997) 'Use of in vitro and in vivo data to estimate the likelihood of metabolic pharmacokinetic interactions', *Clin. Pharmacokinet.* **32**: 210–58.

Bonnabry, P., Desmeules, J., Rudaz, S., Leemann, T., Veuthey, J. L. and Dayer, P. (1996b) 'Stereoselective interaction between piroxicam and acenocoumarol', *Br. J. Clin. Pharmacol.* **41**: 525–30.

Bonnabry, P. and Leemann, T. (1993) 'Prédiction rationnelle des interactions médicamenteuses avec les nouveaux antifongiques systémiques', *Méd. et Hyg.* **51**: 1046–50.

Bonnabry, P., Leemann, T. and Dayer, P. (1994) 'Biotransformation by hepatic P450TB (CYP2C) controls mefenamic acid elimination', *Clin. Pharmacol. Ther.* **55**: 139.

Bonnabry, P., Leemann, T. and Dayer, P. (1996a) 'Role of human liver microsomal CYP2C9 in the biotransformation of lornoxicam', *Eur. J. Clin. Pharmacol.* **49**: 305–8.

Bonnabry, P., Rasca, A. F., Leemann, T. and Dayer, P. (1998) 'Prediction of in vivo impairment of cytochrome P450–mediated metabolism by HIV protease inhibitors', Geneva: 12th World AIDS Conference, p. 91.

Bonnabry, P., Sievering, J., Leemann, T. and Dayer, P. (1997) 'Approche systé-matique des interactions au niveau métabolique: les nouveaux antidépresseurs', *Méd. et Hyg.* **55**: 834–42.

Bonnabry, P., Sievering, J, Leemann, T. and Dayer, P. (1999) 'Quantitative drug interactions prediction system (Q-DIPS): a computer-based prediction and management support system for drug metabolism interactions', *Eur. J. Clin. Pharmacol.* **55**: 341–7.

Brosen, K., Hansen, J. G., Nielsen, K. K., Sindrup, S. H. and Gram, L. F. (1993) 'Inhibition by paroxetine of desipramine metabolism in extensive but not in poor metabolizers of sparteine', *Eur. J. Clin. Pharmacol.* **44**: 349–55.

Canafax, D. M., Graves, N. M., Hilligoss, D. M., Carleton, B. C., Gardner, M. J. and Matas, A. J. (1991) 'Interaction between cyclosporine and fluconazole in renal allograft recipients', *Transplantation* **51**: 1014–8.

Chan, T. Y. (1995) 'Adverse interactions between warfarin and nonsteroidal antiinflammatory drugs: mechanisms, clinical significance, and avoidance', *Ann. Pharmacother.* **29**: 1274–83.

Collignon P., Hurley, B. and Mitchell, D. (1989) 'Interaction of fluconazole with ciclosporin', *Lancet* **1**: 1262.

Crewe, H. K., Lennard, M.S., Tucker, G. T., Woods, F. R. and Haddock, R. E. (1992) 'The effects of selective serotonin re-uptake inhibitors on cytochrome P450 2D6 (CYP2D6) activity in human liver microsomes', *Br. J. Clin. Pharmacol.* **34**: 262–5.

Desprez, D., Blanc, P., Larrey, D. and Michel, H. (1992) 'Hémorragie digestive favorisée par une hypocoagulation excessive due à une interaction médicamenteuse piroxicam-antagoniste de la vitamine K'. *Gastroenterol. Clin. Biol.* **16**: 906–7.

Eagling, V. A., Back, D. J. and Barry, M. G. (1997) 'Differential inhibition of cytochrome P450 isoforms by the protease inhibitors ritonavir, saquinavir and indinavir', *Br. J. Clin. Pharmacol.* **44**: 190–4.

Eichler, H. G., Jung, M., Kyrle, P. A., Rotter, M. and Korn, A. (1992) 'Absence of interaction between tenoxicam and warfarin', *Eur. J. Clin. Pharmacol.* **42**: 227–9.

First, M. R., Schroeder, T. J., Alexander, J. W., Stephens, G. W., Weiskittel, P., Myre, S. A. and Pesce, A. J. (1991) 'Cyclosporine dose reduction by ketoconazole administration in renal transplant recipients', *Transplantation* **51**: 365–70.

Fitzgerald, D. E. and Russell, J. G. (1981) 'Voltarol and warfarin, an interaction?', in *Current Themes in Rheumatology*, Northampton: Cambridge Medical Publications.

Gardner, M. J., Baris, B. A., Wilner, K. D. and Preskorn, S. H. (1997) 'Effect of sertraline on the pharmacokinetics and protein binding of diazepam in healthy volunteers', *Clin. Pharmacokinet.* **32** (Suppl. 1): 43–9.

Grant, S. M. and Clissold, S. P. (1989) 'Itraconazole: a review of its pharmacodynamic and pharmacokinetic properties, and therapeutic potential in superficial and systemic mycoses', *Drugs* **37**: 310–44.

Grimsley, S. R., Jann, M. W., Carter, J. G., D'Mello, A. P. and D'Souza, M. J. (1991) 'Increased carbamazepine plasma concentrations after fluoxetine coadministration', *Clin. Pharmacol. Ther.* **50**: 10–15.

Guengerich, F. P. (1995) 'Human cytochromes P450 enzymes', in P. R. Ortiz de Montellano (ed.) *Cytochrome P450, Structure, Mechanism and Biochemistry*, New York, London: Plenum Press, pp. 473–535.

Guengerich, F. P. (1997) 'Role of cytochrome P450 enzymes in drug–drug interactions', *Adv. Pharmacol.* **43**: 7–35.

Hamelin, B. A., Turgeon, J., Vallee, F., Belanger, P. M., Paquet, F. and Le Bel, M. (1996) 'The disposition of fluoxetine but not sertraline is altered in poor metabolizers of debrisoquine', *Clin. Pharmacol. Ther.* **60**: 512–21.

Hermans, J. J. and Thijssen, H. H. (1993) 'Human liver microsomal metabolism of the enantiomers of warfarin and acenocoumarol: P450 isozyme diversity determines the differencies in their pharmacokinetics', *Br. J. Clin. Pharmacol.* **110**: 482–90.

Holmes, E. L. (1967) 'Mefenamic acid, IV. Toleration by normal human subjects', *Ann. Phys. Med.* **9** (Suppl.): 36–49.

Horton, R. C. and Bonser, R. S. (1995) 'Interaction between cyclosporin and fluoxetine', *Br. Med. J.* **311**: 422.

Hsu, A., Granneman, G. R., Cao, G., Carothers, L., El-Shourbagy, T., Baroldi, P., Erdman, K., Brown, F., Sun, E. and Leonard, J. M. (1998) 'Pharmacokinetic interactions between two human immunodeficiency virus protease inhibitors, ritonavir and saquinavir', *Clin. Pharmacol. Ther.* **63**: 453–64.

Ito, K., Iwatsubo, T., Kanamitsu, S., Nakajima, Y. and Sugiyama, Y. (1998) 'Quantitative prediction of in vivo drug clearance and drug interactions from in vitro data on metabolism, together with binding and transport', *Annu. Rev. Pharmacol. Toxicol.* **38**: 461–99.

Jeppesen, U., Gram, L. F., Vistisen, K., Loft, S., Poulsen, H. E. and Brosen, K. (1996a) 'Dose-dependent inhibition of CYP1A2, CYP2C19 and CYP2D6 by citalopram, fluoxetine, fluvoxamine and paroxetine', *Eur. J. Clin. Pharmacol.* **51**: 73–8.

Jeppesen, U., Loft, S., Poulsen, H. E. and Brosen, K. (1996b) 'A fluvoxamine-caffeine interaction study', *Pharmacogenetics* **6**: 213–22.

Kashuba, A. D., Nafziger, A. N., Kearns, G. L., Leeder, J. S., Gotschall, R., Rocci, M. L., Kulawy, R. W., Beck, D. J. and Bertino, J. S. (1998) 'Effect of fluvoxamine therapy on the activities of CYP1A2, CYP2D6 and CYP3A as determined by phenotyping', *Clin. Pharmacol. Ther.* **64**: 257–68.

Kedderis, G. L. (1997) 'Extrapolation of in vitro enzyme induction data to humans in vivo', *Chem-Biol. Inter.* **107**: 109–21.

Kobayashi, K., Yamamoto, T., Chiba, K., Tani, M., Ishizaki, T. and Kuroiwa, Y. (1995) 'The effects of selective reuptake inhibitors and their metabolites on S-mephenytoin 4′-hydroxylase activity in human liver microsomes', *Br. J. Clin. Pharmacol.* **40**: 481–5.

Kondo, M., Leemann, T. and Dayer, P. (1992) 'Piroxicam 5′-hydroxylation is catalyzed by human liver cytochrome P450TB (CYP2C)', *Experientia* **48**: A7.

Koudriakova, T., Iatsimirskaia, E. and Utkin, I. (1998) Metabolism of the human immunodeficiency virus protease inhibitors indinavir and ritonavir by human intestineal microsomes and expressed cytochrome P4503A4/3A5: mechanism-based inactivation of cytochrome P4503A by ritonavir', *Drug Metab. Dispos.* **26**: 552–61.

Le Blanc, G. A. (1994) 'Hepatic vectorial transport of xenobiotics', *Chem-Biol. Inter.* **90**: 101–20.

Leemann, T., Transon, C. and Dayer, P. (1993) 'Cytochrome P450TB (CYP2C): a major monooxygenase catalysing diclofenac 4′-hydroxylation in human liver', *Life Sci.* **52**: 29–34.

Leemann, T., Bonnabry, P. and Dayer, P. (1994) 'Stereo- and nonstereoselective oxidation by P450TB (CYP2C9: the major elimination pathway of (±)-ibuprofen', *Clin. Pharmacol. Ther.* **55**: 208.

Leemann, T. and Dayer, P. (1995) 'Quantitative prediction of in vivo drug metabolism and interactions from in vitro data', in G. M. Pacifici, and G. N. Fracchia (ed.) *Advances in drug matabolism in man*, Luxembourg: European Commission, pp.783–830.

Lewis, R. L., Trager, W. F. and Chan, K. K. (1974) 'Warfarin, stereochemical aspects of its metabolism and the interaction with phenylbutazone', *J. Clin. Invest.* **53**: 1607–17.

Lillibridge, J. H., Liang, B. H., Kerr, B. M., Webber, S., Quart, B., Shetty, B. V. and Lee, C. A. (1993) 'Characterization of the selectivity and mechanism of human cytochrome p450 inhibition by the human immunodeficiency virus-protease inhibitor nelfinavir mesylate', *Drug Metab. Dispos.* **26**: 609–16.

Lopez-Gil, J. A. (1993) 'Fluconazole–cyclosporine interaction: a dose-dependent effect?', *Ann. Pharmacother.* **27**: 427–30.

McCrea, J., Buss, N. and Stone, J. (1997) 'Indinavir-saquinavir single dose pharmacokinetic study', 4th National Conference on Retroviruses and Opportunistic Infections, Washington DC.

McLachlan, A. J. and Tett, S. E. (1998) 'Effect of metabolic inhibitors on cyclosporine pharmacokinetics using a population approach', *Ther. Drug Monit.* **20**: 390–5.

Mahoney, E. M., Child, M. J. and Smith-Monroy, C. A. (1990) 'Differential transport of pravastatin and lovastatin by hepatocytes and fibroblasts', *Circulation* **82**: abstract 23.

Mallet, L. and Cooper, J. W. (1991) 'Prolongation of prothrombine time with the use of piroxicam and warfarin', *Can. J. Hosp. Pharm.* **44**: 93–4.

Martin, D. E., Zussman, B. D., Everitt, D. E., Benincosa, L. J., Etheredge, R. C. and Jorkasky, D. K. (1997) 'Paroxetine does not affect the cardiac safety and pharmacokinetics of terfenadine in healthy adult men', *J. Clin. Psychopharmacol.* **17**: 451–9.

Meijer, D. K., Mol, W. E., Müller, M. and Kurz, G. (1990) 'Carrier-mediated transport in the hepatic distribution and elimination of drugs, with special reference to the category of organic cations', *J. Pharmacokinet. Biopharm.* **18**: 35–70.

Michot, F. and Ajdacic, K. (1975) 'A double-blind clinical trial to determine if an interaction exists between diclofenac sodium and the oral anticoagulant acenocoumarol (Nicoumalone)', *J. Int. Med. Res.* **3**: 153–7.

Nakasa, H., Nakamura, H., Ono, S., Tsutsui, M., Kiuchi, M., Ohmori, S. and Kitada, M. (1998) 'Prediction of drug–drug interactions of zonisamide metabolism in humans from in vitro data', *Eur. J. Clin. Pharmacol.* **54**: 177–83.

Nelson, D. R., Koymans, L., Kamataki, T., Stegeman, J. J., Feyereisen, R., Waxman, D. J., Waterman, M. R., Gotoh, O., Coon, M. J., Estabrook, R. W., Gunsalus, I. C. and Nebert, D. W. (1996) 'P450 superfamily: update on new sequence, gene mapping, accession number and nomenclature', *Pharmacogenetics* **6**: 1–42.

Obach, R. S. (1997) 'Nonspecific binding to microsomes: impact on scale-up of in vitro intrinsic clearance to hepatic clearance as assessed through examination of warfarin, imipramine and propranolol', *Drug Metab. Dispos.* **25**: 1359–69.

O'Reilly, R. A., Trager, W. F., Motley, C. H. and Howald, W. (1980) 'Stereoselective interaction of phenylbutazone with $[^{12}C/^{13}C]$ warfarin pseudoracemates in man', *J. Clin. Invest.* **65**: 746–53.

Otton, S. V., Wu, D., Joffe, R. T., Cheung, S. W. and Sellers, E. M. (1993) 'Inhibition by fluoxetine of cytochrome P450 2D6 activity', *Clin. Pharmacol. Ther.* **53**: 401–9.

Ozdemir, V., Naranjo, C. A., Herrmann, N., Shulman, R. W., Sellers, E. M., Reed, K. and Kalow, W. (1998) 'The extent and determinants of changes in CYP2D6 and CYP1A2 activities with therapeutic doses of sertraline', *J. Clin. Psychopharmacol.* **18**: 55–61.

Penner, J. A. and Abbrecht, P. H. (1975) 'Lack of interaction between ibuprofen and warfarin', *Curr. Ther. Res.* **18**: 862–71.

Rapeport, W. G., Williams, S. A., Muirhead, D. C., Dewland, P. M., Tanner, T. and Wesnes, K. (1996) 'Absence of sertraline-mediated effect on the pharmacokinetics and pharmacodynamics of carbamazepine', *J. Clin. Psychiatry* **57** (Suppl. 1): 20–3.

Rasca, A. F., Bonnabry, P. and Dayer, P. (1998) 'In vitro inhibition of cytochrome P450 2D6 and 3A4 by HIV protease inhibitors', 12th World AIDS Conference, Geneva, p. 90.

Rasmussen, B. B., Mäenpää, J., Pelkonen, O., Loft, S., Poulsen, H. E., Lykkesfeldt, J. and Brosen K. (1995) 'Selective serotonin reuptake inhibitors and theophylline metabolism in human liver microsomes: potent inhibition by fluvoxamine', *Br. J. Clin. Pharmacol.* **39**: 151–9.

Ravic M., Johnston, A., Turner, P. and Ferber, H. P. (1990) 'A study of the interaction between lornoxicam and warfarin in healthy volunteers', *Hum. Exp. Toxicol.* **9**: 413–4.

Rhodes, R. S., Rhodes, P. J., Klein, C. and Sintek, C. D. (1985) 'A warfarin–piroxicam drug interaction', *Drug Intell. Clin. Pharm.* **19**: 556–8.

Rodrigues, A. D. and Wong, S. L. (1997) 'Application of human liver microsomes in metabolism-based drug–drug interactions: in vitro–in vivo correlations and the Abbott laboratories experience', *Adv. Pharmacol.* **43**: 65–101.

Schulman, S. and Henriksson, K. (1989) 'Interaction of ibuprofen and warfarin on primary haemostasis', *Br. J. Rheumatol.* **28**: 46–9.

Smith, H. T., Hsuan, F. and Troendle, A. J. (1991) 'A study to investigate the effect of gender and age on the steady-state pharmacokinetics of fluvastatin in patients; amendment no. 5. Study report 303–293', Sandoz Research Institute, East Hanover, NJ, USA.

Solai, L. K., Mulsant, B. H., Pollock, B. G., Sweet, R. A., Rosen, J., Yu, K. and Reynolds, C. F. (1997) 'Effect of sertraline on plasma nortriptyline levels in depressed elderly', *J. Clin. Psychiatry* **58**: 440–3.

Spigset, O., Granberg, K., Hagg, S., Norstrom, A. and Dahlqvist, R. (1997) 'Relationship between fluvoxamine pharmacokinetics and CYP2D6/CYP2C19 phenotype polymorphisms', *Eur. J. Clin. Pharmacol.* **52**: 129–33.

Swims, M. P. (1993) 'Potential terfenadine–fluoxetine interaction', *Ann. Pharmacother.* **27**: 1404.

Thilo, D. and Nyman, D. (1974) 'A study of the effects of the anti-rheumatic drug ibuprofen (Brufen) on patients being treated with the oral anticoagulant phenprocoumon (Marcoumar)', *J. Int. Med. Res.* **2**: 276–8.

Transon, C., Leemann, T. and Dayer, P. (1996) 'In vitro comparative inhibition profiles of major human drug metabolising cytochrome P450 isozymes (CYP2C9, CYP2D6 and CYP3A4) by HMG-CoA reductase inhibitors', *Eur. J. Clin. Pharmacol.* **50**: 209–15.

Transon, C., Leemann, T., Vogt, N. and Dayer, P. (1995) 'In vivo inhibition profile of cytochrome P450TB (CYP2C9) by (±)-fluvastatin', *Clin. Pharmacol. Ther.* **58**: 412–7.

Trilli, L. E., Kelley, C. L., Aspinall, S. L. and Kroner, B. A. (1996) 'Potential interactions between warfarin and fluvastatin. Ann. Pharmacother', 30: 1399–1402.

Tseng A. L. and Foisy, M. M. (1997) 'Management of drug interactions in patients with HIV', *Ann. Pharmacother.* 31: 1040–58.

Von Moltke, L. L., Greenblatt, D. J., Cotreau-Bibbo, M. M., Harmatz, J. S. and Shader, R.I. (1994) 'Inhibitors of alprazolam metabolism in vitro: effect of serotonin-reuptake-inhibitor antidepressants, ketoconazole and quinidine', *Br. J. Clin. Pharmacol.* 38: 23–31.

Von Moltke, L. L., Greenblatt, D. J., Court, M. H., Duan, S. X., Harmatz, J. S. and Shader, R.I. (1995) 'Inhibition of alprazolam and desipramine hydroxylation in vitro by paroxetine and fluvoxamine: comparison with other selective serotonin reuptake inhibitor antidepressants', *J. Clin. Psychopharmacol.* 15: 125–31.

Von Moltke, L. L., Greenblatt, D. J., Schmider, J., Wright, C. E., Harmatz, J. S. and Shader, R. I. (1998) 'In vitro approaches to predicting drug interactions in vivo', *Biochem. Pharmacol.* 55: 113–22.

Woodland, C., Ito, S. and Koren, G. (1998) 'A model for the prediction of digoxin-drug interactions at the renal tubular cell level', *Ther. Drug Monit.* 20: 134–8.

Wrighton, S. A. and Stevens, J. C. (1992) 'The human hepatic cytochromes P450 involved in drug metabolism', *Crit. Rev. Toxicol.* 22: 1–21.

Xu, Z. H., Xie, H. G. and Zhou, H. H. (1996) 'In vivo inhibition of CYP2C19 but not CYP2D6 by fluvoxamine', *Br. J. Clin. Pharmacol.* 42: 518–21.

Yamazaki, M., Suzukui, H., Hanano, M., Tokui, T., Komai, T. and Sugiyama, Y. (1993) 'Na+-dependent multispecific anion transporter mediates active transport of pravastatin into rat liver', *Am. J. Physiol.* 264: G36–G44.

Yamazaki, M., Suzuki, Y., Iga, T. and Hanano, M. (1992) 'Uptake of organic anions by isolated rat hepatocytes. A classification in terms of ATP-dependency', *J. Hepatology* 14: 41–7.

Zhao, J., Leemann, T. and Dayer, P. (1992) 'In vitro oxidation of oxicam NSAIDS by a human liver cytochrome P450', *Life Sci.* 51: 575–81.

Ziegler, K. and Hummelsiep, S. (1993) 'Hepatoselective carrier–mediated sodium-independent uptake of pravastatin and pravastatin-lactone', *Biochim. Biophys. Acta.* 1153: 23–33.

Chapter 10

Interindividual variation of P450 enzymes *in vitro* and its causes

O. Pelkonen, A. R. Boobis, P. Kremers,
M. Ingelman-Sundberg and A. Rane

Introduction

Interindividual variation in the activities of drug-metabolising enzymes is one of the principal determinants of variability in the outcome of drug therapy, adverse drug reactions and drug interactions. Furthermore, it complicates extrapolations during drug development, dose titration during clinical trials and is often behind morbidity and mortality in drug treatment.

Nowadays, preclinical documentation of *in vitro* metabolism is needed in drug development, as well as for approval of new drugs. Quantitative information on clearance, as well as qualitative information on metabolism, are considered useful. The variability in drug metabolism is predominantly caused by genetic and environmental influences on the enzymes. Both of these aspects may be studied *in vitro* with enzyme-specific methods.

Any adverse drug reaction may be elicited by the parent drug, or by a metabolite. Information on the pattern of metabolism and relative rates of the different pathways may help elucidate the causative role of the metabolites in these reactions. Such studies may also cast light on the mechanisms of metabolic interactions. This is particularly important to investigate when other drugs are likely to be co-used in target groups of patients.

Because P450 enzymes are the principal rate-limiting enzymes in the metabolism of most pharmaceuticals, it is of utmost importance to characterise factors causing interindividual variation in activities catalysed by various P450 enzymes. More general aspects of hereditary factors have been dealt with in previous chapters (Kalow and Tang, 1991) and here we present what is known about interindividual variation of various P450 enzymes and the factors causing this variation.

Basically, two different sources for experimentally measured variability can be identified, namely technical and biological. These two sources correspond roughly to "artificial" and "genuine" variability. For this reason, we first cover some technical and methodological aspects of measuring drug metabolising enzymes in human samples and only after this deal with the individual CYP enzymes and causes for their variation. Finally, we briefly discuss some aspects of *in vitro–in vivo* extrapolation.

Methodological considerations in *in vitro* studies

The metabolism of a drug can have important consequences on its therapeutic effect or its toxicity. For this reason, early assessment of metabolic pathways in man is a necessity to evaluate the effects of interindividual variations in drug response and metabolism. To address these issues, *in vitro* techniques based on human material are currently being used. They appear to be particularly useful in the selection and development processes of new drugs and very effective in the assessment of human risk and potential drug–drug or drug–xenobiotic interactions.

Microsomes

Microsomes, a subcellular preparation made from endoplasmic reticulum membranes, are one of the most universally used *in vitro* models. Microsomes contain the phase I enzymes, namely all the drug-metabolising P450s, and some phase II enzymes such as UDP-glucoronosyltransferase. Microsomes are considered a practical enzyme source as they may be kept at −80°C for years without any loss of activity (Beaune *et al.*, 1986, Shimada *et al.*, 1994; Boobis *et al.*, 1998; Pearce *et al.*, 1996b). They constitute a simple experimental model and help provide rapid and precise answers to specific questions regarding drug metabolism.

Microsomes are particularly useful for the study of metabolic routes, for the production of metabolites, for the identification of the enzyme concerned and for inhibition studies including identification and characterisation of inhibitors and the study of their mechanisms of action (Boobis *et al.*, 1999; Pelkonen *et al.*, 1998). They cannot be used to study the effect of inducers, unless they are prepared from induced animals.

Generally, microsomes produce primary metabolites. This is convenient in identifying phase I products, even those produced in small amounts or rapidly converted *in vivo* by phase II enzymes or via spontaneous rearrangement of an unstable chemical structure. However, studies on microsomes may lead to an overestimation of the yield of phase I metabolites. For this reason, it is possible that some metabolites observed after incubation of a drug in the presence of microsomes are never encountered during an *in vivo* study.

Microsomes from different tissues, animal species and induced animals as well as from human tissues are now commercially available. They are usually characterised and their content of P450 and phase I enzymes provided. These "new reagents" are currently being used in drug development studies and in new approaches such as high throughput screening.

When dealing with human liver microsomes, it must be kept in mind that their activity may vary by a factor of up to 30–100 between two donors as the result of genotype, drug and medication background or nutritional and environmental exposure (Beaune *et al.*, 1986; Shimada *et al.*, 1994; Boobis *et al.*, 1998; Edwards *et al.*, 1998).

A possible difficulty in extrapolating results obtained on microsomes is linked to the shape of microsomal membranes and to the incubation conditions used:

- During the preparation process, endoplasmic reticulum membranes are disrupted and reconstituted into small vesicles which may behave differently from the original membrane
- Artificial amounts (saturating amounts) of cofactors and of substrates are used
- Access of the substrate to and release of the metabolites from the catalytic site may be different in microsomes; this also applies to the electron flow from NADPH to the enzyme, although this may not be a major problem for most P450 enzymes (Edwards *et al.*, 1991).

Human hepatocytes in suspension and in culture

Important progress has been made in hepatocyte culture during the last 10 years. It is based on different experimental approaches, coculture, use of matrigel matrices, collagen coating of dishes, etc., and allows reproducible culture conditions and maintenance of expression of drug-metabolising enzymes (Gomez-Lechon *et al.*, 1997; Guillouzo, 1998). It has even become possible to freeze and store hepatocytes for later use (Li *et al.*, 1997).

Consequently, banks of characterised (genotyped, phenotyped, etc.) human liver cells are becoming a reality and may contribute to better use of this material during drug development. Unlike microsomes, hepatocytes permit the measurement of toxic effects, of induction (Maurel, 1996; Morel *et al.*, 1990; Mattes and Li, 1997) and of drug metabolism resulting from both phase I and phase II enzymes (Ferrini *et al.*, 1997).

When used for metabolic studies, hepatocytes in suspension or culture provide results that reflect the integrated effects of both phase I and phase II enzymes, controlled or at least modulated by the cellular biosynthesis of the necessary cofactors and by the intracellular organisation. In intact cells, where both phase I and phase II enzymes are present and active, drug metabolism is, in principle, closer to the *in vivo* situation.

As with microsomes, by using a set of hepatocytes from different individuals it is possible to examine variability in a given enzyme. It is also possible to select samples corresponding to a particular genotype or phenotype.

Liver slices

Liver slices offer the advantage of keeping much of the tissue organisation and the possible intercellular communications intact (Lake et al., 1996). However, slices cannot be maintained metabolically active for more than a few hours, although under appropriate conditions slices can survive for 48 h. The outer cell layer is usually damaged by the slicing process and the innermost cells may become hypoxic. Several authors (Silva et al., 1998) have developed methods enabling these slices to be frozen and thawed as needed, without exaggerated loss of activity.

Recombinant enzyme systems

Several transforming methods and different types of genetically transformed cells are currently available. Their main advantage lies in their expressing human enzymes and in their frequent use as a source of "purified" enzymes. They are particularly useful to address specific questions on the potential role of a given enzyme and to perform inhibition and mechanistic studies. They are most often used to verify whether a given enzyme is able to perform, and to what extent, a given reaction.

From the isolated observation that a recombinant drug-metabolising enzyme is able to metabolise a given drug one cannot infer that the metabolic reaction is supported by this enzyme in vivo. In the P450 field, absolute substrate specificity does not exist and an exhaustive kinetic analysis is necessary to interpret the results correctly. In addition, it is difficult to define optimal reaction conditions with these enzymatic preparations.

Several cell lines have been considered as possible models for drug metabolism and induction studies (Daujat et al., 1996). Unfortunately and for various reasons, most of the available cell lines are unable to express the different CYP genes. This disadvantage can be partly overcome by co-transfecting these cells (Gonzalez and Korzekwa, 1995).

What to measure in in vitro systems?

Measures of cDNA

The identification of and/or search for specific genes using existing cDNA probes makes it possible to compare tissues, individuals or even species on the basis of their genotype. However, the presence of a given dose does not guarantee its expression. Moreover, the sensitivity of the PCR and hybridisation techniques can yield positive results with very limited amounts of genetic material. Particularly in the CYP field, cross-reactions may often occur, as considerable sequence homology exists between the different forms.

Measures of mRNA

Measurement of mRNAs corresponding to a particular enzyme is often used to evaluate expression, particularly changes in expression such as following exposure to an inducing agent. This can be a useful, rapid and very sensitive method, providing the appropriate probes are used. Nowadays, some of the probes for CYP enzymes are commercially available. The techniques for mRNA extraction, hybridisation and measurement are now in routine use in many laboratories (Andersson *et al.*, 1998). The techniques can be used to measure mRNA in cultured cells or in tissues and to determine the extent of induction after exposure to possible inducers. It can provide a rapid and convenient approach to screen a large number of samples for several different products, in cultured cells, in order to detect potent inducers of a given P450. It must, however, be remembered that some compounds are able to increase a particular P450 activity without increasing the synthesis of the corresponding mRNA; other mechanisms may be involved. Therefore, for a correct interpretation it is necessary to know the relationship between gene expression and the function of the gene product.

Determination of protein

Various immunological assays, among which the Western blot technique is probably the most used, have been developed to detect and quantify the different P450 isozymes. These methods are practical, rapid and easy to perform, but are completely dependent on the quality and specificity of the antibodies used. A large variety of antibodies, including monoclonals, are available and widely used. It must however be kept in mind that in many cases their specificity has never been extensively characterised and that cross-reactions between different CYPs are rather common. Moreover, the specificity of these antibodies may vary from one animal species to the other. An antibody, prepared against a rat liver enzyme may react differently with the corresponding human enzyme (Edwards *et al.*, 1998).

Another difficulty arising during these approaches concerns quantification. It is difficult to prepare a true calibration curve since, most often, the reference molecule, i.e. the measured CYP, is not available in a pure form at a precisely known concentration. This problem can be overcome by using antibodies raised against peptides corresponding to suitable sequences of the target P450, and then using a peptide-conjugate as a standard for immunoquantification (Edwards *et al.*, 1998).

Determination of enzymatic activities

Measurement of enzymatic activities is, in some cases, more difficult to perform than the two preceding types of measure, but constitute nevertheless the most informative assay. An enzymatic activity can, indeed, be expressed only by a complete and intact enzyme and remains, therefore, the only effective functional proof for the methodological model chosen.

The difficulty arises most often from the methods available to measure the products arising from the metabolic activity. This is linked both to the analytical methods available and to the substrates used to characterise a given enzyme. Nowadays, most enzymatic activities are measured via a colorimetric, spectrophotometric, fluorimetric, radiometric or HPLC assay, but recently highly sensitive and specific mass spectrometric methods have also become available. It is critical to define the specificity, sensitivity, and reproducibility of the employed analytical method.

In recent years, new substrates have been developed in order to increase both the specificity and the sensitivity of the assays (Crespi *et al.*, 1997). It is highly probable that, under the demands of the new high throughput screening approach, new fluorimetric and eventually luminescent assays will be rapidly developed leading to development of sensitive assays designed for large-scale measures in a small volume of incubation.

Specificity of substrates and inhibitors remains a major problem when studying the relative contribution or characterising the different CYPs (Eagling *et al.*, 1997). Several review articles have been published on this subject (e.g. Rendic and Di Carlo, 1997; Pelkonen *et al.*, 1998); these reviews and many more similar provide a large number of references containing information on substrates, inhibitors and inducers of the different P450s. Knowledge of substrates, inhibitors and inducers of the CYP enzymes assists in predicting clinically significant drug interactions.

Need for validation of both experimental models and assays

The main problem in using *in vitro* systems for predicting drug metabolism or drug interactions is that none of them has been properly validated. Therefore, it is advisable to combine results from several *in vitro* approaches, based on different models in order to obtain reliable and interpretable results. Cross-confirmations using different approaches is still primordial in this field, mainly when these results are used for supporting drug registration. The optional approach is to validate *in vitro* methods employing human tissue with functional probe drugs or therapeutic drugs used *in vivo* in the same patients (Säwe *et al.*, 1985).

A few interlaboratory comparisons of the assessment of P450 activities have been published (Boobis *et al.*, 1998; Kremers, 1999). They usually indicate large differences in results obtained from one laboratory to the other. There may be different reasons for this:

• Variation in the quality of the biological material (quality of collected tissues, prepared cells or microsomes, storage conditions, etc.)

- Differences in the incubation parameters (substrate and solvent concentration, concentration of cofactors, buffer, volume) (see Hickman *et al.*, 1998)
- Differences in the analytical technique used to quantify the reaction products.

However, these reports also indicate that, once a consensus is obtained on common experimental protocol, inter-laboratory variation is considerably reduced, indicating that its origin is essentially methodological.

The introduction of good laboratory practice (GLP) in drug development will necessarily also have to be applied in metabolic work and include validation and inter-laboratory comparisons for all these assays at some point in time. The validation process is expected not only to improve the methodology used, but also to allow a better inter-laboratory comparison and quality control.

Relative amounts and variation in total P450 and various CYP forms *in vitro*

Liver

Liver displays variability in the amounts of P450 enzymes at several levels:

- The absolute amounts of total P450 and various CYP enzymes may vary from one individual to another
- Relative amounts, i.e. the profile of CYP enzymes may differ in different individuals
- Both the amount of total P450, as well as that of different CYP enzymes vary according to the location in the hepatic lobule.

Usually the first aspects are taken into consideration when assessing the variability of CYP enzymes in the liver, but the third case, intralobular variability, is also of importance. It is clear that the location dictates, at least to a certain extent, the exposure of an individual cell to a drug or any other chemical. The toxicological consequences, in particular may be profoundly dependent on spatial differences in the concentrations of CYP enzymes.

For obvious reasons, measurements of total P450 content, as well as those of individual CYP enzymes, have usually been made in the microsomal fraction. Less common are studies in homogenate or isolated hepatocytes, or in liver slices. Some semiquantitative or qualitative information with respect to individual CYP enzymes will be given in later sections, but here we try to give an overview of absolute and relative amounts of various CYP enzymes in human liver microsomes, as measured by immunochemical means. These methods have some drawbacks as discussed above, but they can give some information about relative amounts of various CYP enzymes.

It has become rather common practice to use the relative liver microsomal amounts of P450 enzymes as measured by Shimada *et al.* (1994) in various calculations, for example when activities measured in heterologously expressed enzyme systems have been "upscaled" to the microsomes or the whole liver. In Table 10.2, the original results of Shimada *et al.* (1994) have been tabulated, together with some later results on the concentrations of various CYP enzymes in human liver. Some interesting conclusions can be made on the basis of these results:

- Although the amounts of CYP2C and 3A subfamilies are certainly quantitatively most abundant, their relative amounts seem to differ in different studies.
- It seems that the amounts of some less abundant subfamilies, CYP2A and CYP2B, are higher in later studies than in the survey of Shimada *et al.* (1994).
- On the basis of immunoquantification studies alone, it is difficult to say whether there is any real polymorphism in the expression of CYP2B6 or CYP3A5 in human liver microsomes.

Another approach to variability in CYP enzymes in human liver microsomes is to look at CYP-specific activities. A list of more or less CYP-

---

Table 10.1 Principal applications of the different *in vitro* models

Microsomes serve the following functions
    Search for primary metabolites
    Metabolic pathway
    Identification of metabolites
    Elucidation of metabolite structure
    Detection of unstable or transient metabolites
    Drug–drug interaction: inhibition studies
    Mechanism of reaction
    Identification of the responsible enzyme (CYP)

Hepatocytes/slices are used in the following areas
    Search for all metabolites
    Rates of metabolism, Cl_{int}
    Drug–drug interaction: induction
    Toxic effects: viability functions
    Histological evaluation

Expression systems are used for
    Identification of concerned enzyme
    Interactions at the enzyme level: inhibition studies
    Comparison of different potential substrate/inhibitors: affinity

Table 10.2 Nominal specific content and variability of CYP proteins in human liver microsomes

Protein	Shimada et al, 1994 pmol/mg protein	Gentest Corp[a] pmol/mg protein	Lasker et al, 1998 pmol/mg protein	Wrighton et al, 1996 fold-variation	Remarks
Total P450	344±167	534	255±17	5	
CYP1A1					negligible
CYP1A2	42±23 (12.7±6.2)	45 (8.0)		3	
CYP2A6	14±13 (4.0±3.2)	68 (13)		23	deletion alleles
CYP2B6	1±2 (0.2±0.3)	39 (7.0)			(deletions?)
Total CYP2C	60±27 (18.2±6.7)	[179 (34)]	[119]		
CYP2C8		64 (12)	12±12	6	
CYP2C9		96 (18)	89±36	5	
CYP2C18					negligible
CYP2C19		19 (4.0)	18±14	10	deletion alleles
CYP2D6	5±4 (1.5±1.3)	10 (2.0)		10	deletion alleles
CYP2E1	22±12 (6.6±2.9)	49 (9.0)		6	
Total CYP3A	96±51 (28.8±10.4)	[109 (20.2)]		5	
CYP3A4		108 (20)			
CYP3A5		1.0 (0.2)		present 3/14	
CYP3A7					negligible

Note
[a] A pool of twelve livers.

specific substrates and reactions is presented in Table 10.3, with an estimation of maximum variability in activity. However, one should not regard this variability as absolute, because obviously it is dependent on a large number of potential factors, including nature of population, genetic, host and environmental factors, technical matters and so on. Estimation of quantitative contributions of various factors to the overall variability is extremely difficult and has not been attempted to any significant extent with any one of these CYP-specific substrates and reactions.

Extrahepatic tissues

Most extrahepatic tissues contain variable complements of CYP enzyme (Raunio et al., 1995). Except intestine, and maybe lungs, these enzymes are

Table 10.3 Variability in the in vitro metabolism of compounds displaying a high degree of CYP-enzyme specificity (for more extensive references, see Pelkonen et al., 1998)

Enzyme(s)	Preferred substrate and reaction	"Typical" variation (fold)[a]	Maximal variation (fold)[a]	Remarks
CYP1A2	phenacetin O-deethylation	18	100	
	ethoxyresorufin O-deethylation	8–18	50	
CYP2A6	coumarin 7-hydroxylation	23–28	164	null alleles
CYP2C8	taxol hydroxylation	>10	large	
CYP2C9	tolbutamide methylhydroxylation	5	100	
	diclofenac hydroxylation	15	40	
	S-warfarin 7-hydroxylation		50	
CYP2C19	S-mephenytoin-4-hydroxylation	7	large (>155)	null alleles
	omeprazole oxidation	10	large (>50)	null alleles
CYP2D6	dextromethorphan O-deethylation	30	large (>80)	null alleles
	bufuralol 1'-hydroxylation	5–18	large (>80)	null alleles
CYP2E1	chlorzoxazone 6-hydroxylation	10	20	
	aniline 4-hydroxylation	6	50	
CYP3A4	testosterone 6β-hydroxylation	10	50	
	midazolam 1'-hydroxylation	10	30	
	nifedipine dehydrogenation	8	100	
	erythromycin N-demethylase	15	50	

Notes

[a] Fold-variation are approximate only: "typical" variation refers to values for individuals with no known "extreme" CYP-affecting factors in the history; maximal variation refers to values for individuals with known affecting factors (e.g. cigarette smoking, inducers, severe liver disease, etc).

Various activities measured in human liver banks of variable sizes (14 to 60 individuals) have been reported in the following papers: Shimada et al., 1994; Bourrie et al., 1996; Wrighton et al., 1996: Transon et al., 1996).

thought to have a more important role in toxic reactions rather than in overall metabolic clearance of drugs. This subject is not elaborated further here, but the reader may consult some review articles for further information.

Factors causing variation of individual CYPs

In this section we deal with all the major and some minor CYP enzymes expressed in human liver. Obviously it is impossible to cover the extensive literature on the subject in detail. We have tried to give some indication of the major factors causing variability of each enzyme at the levels of mRNA, protein and associated activities. Some of the difficulties in the measurement of each enzyme at mRNA, protein and activity levels have been discussed above. However, it is worth pointing out, that compiling a list of substrates for each enzyme with some quantitative information about the role of this particular enzyme in the metabolism of a given substrate would be an enormous and probably impossible task and is not attempted here.

CYP1 family

CYP1A1

Most studies have shown that CYP1A1 is not normally expressed in liver, determined at the mRNA, protein or activity level (Andersen et al., 1998; Edwards et al., 1998; Turesky et al., 1998). However, in studies using a cross-reacting monoclonal antibody raised against fish (Scup) CYP1A, it has been reported that most human liver samples express low but detectable amounts of CYP1A1 (Drahushuk et al., 1998). CYP1A1 is the most important inducible enzyme in lung (Willey et al., 1997), skin (Sadek and Allen-Hoffmann, 1994), colon (Fontana et al., 1999) and perhaps other tissues. CYP1A1 is also expressed in lymphocytes (Landi et al., 1994; Jacquet et al., 1997). Lymphocytes are easily isolated and cultured in vitro. CYP1A1 is considered a major catalyst in the biotransformation of a number of procarcinogens into mutagenic/carcinogenic compounds. There is considerable overlap in substrate specificity between CYP1A1 and the other members of the CYP1 family, CYP1A2 and CYP1B1. Although CYP1A1 can be inhibited selectively by some compounds, such as alpha-naphthoflavone, these also inhibit CYP1A2.

CYP1A1 in extrahepatic tissues is highly inducible by various environmental products, polycyclic aromatic hydrocarbons, polychlorinated biphenyls, dioxins as well as by cigarette smoke. The hepatic enzyme does not appear to be induced at normal environmental levels of these compounds. However, at high levels of exposure induction does occur.

CYP1A1 mRNA levels, measured in peripheral lymphocytes, have been used as a biomarker of exposure to PAH and dioxin derivatives (Vanden Heuval *et al.*, 1993). In this respect, mRNA determination is certainly the easiest and most sensitive parameter to evaluate CYP1A1 induction. In fact, the amount of CYP1A1 present in lymphocytes is relatively low and creates numerous problems when enzymatic activity or specific apoprotein has to be measured.

A hyperinducible phenotype has been described for this enzyme and its association with the incidence of lung cancer has been suggested (Jacquet *et al.*, 1996; Hirvonen, 1999). Two point mutations have been observed on the CYP1A1 gene:*Msp*I corresponding to a point mutation some 300 bp downstream of the CYP1A1 in the 3′ flanking region; an Ile/Val substitution at residue 462 in the heme binding region. The *Msp*I polymorphism is claimed to be associated with the increased risk of lung cancer in a Japanese population (Hayashi *et al.*, 1991); in Caucasians no significant correlation was found between the presence of the M2 allele and hyperinducibility or with cancer risk. The only positive correlation found was between hyperinducibility and cancer risk (Jacquet *et al.*, 1996). The frequency of the *Msp*I M2 allele is approximately 10% in the Caucasian population. Approximately 8% of a healthy population and 24% of lung cancer patients are hyperinducible for CYP1A1.

CYP1A2

CYP1A2 expression is largely restricted to the liver, where it represents, on average, about 12% of total hepatic P450 content (Shimada *et al.*, 1994). However, it plays a key role in the metabolism of a range of dietary chemicals, environmental contaminants and a number of drugs. It is inducible by many environmental agents, but by very few drugs. To date, there are no established genetic polymorphisms affecting its activity.

VARIABILITY OF PROTEIN AND MRNA

CYP1A2 expression has been detected in almost all liver samples studied, at both the mRNA and protein level (Edwards *et al.*, 1998; Kahn *et al.*, 1985; Shimada *et al.*, 1994). However, expression exhibits large interindividual variability, ranging from 10 to 250 pmoles/mg protein (Edwards *et al.*, 1998; Shimada *et al.*, 1994; Schweikl *et al.*, 1993; Turesky *et al.*, 1998).

VARIABILITY OF FORM-SPECIFIC ACTIVITY/ACTIVITIES

The activity of CYP1A2 *in vitro* can be assessed by measuring high affinity phenacetin O-deethylase (Sesardic *et al.*, 1988) or caffeine N3-demethylase (Butler *et al.*, 1989) activity. Both activities are relatively specific for

CYP1A2 in liver. The O-dealkylation of some of the alkoxyresorufins can also be used to assess the activity of CYP1A2 in liver (Burke *et al.*, 1994), particularly ethoxyresorufin O-deethylation (EROD) (Tassaneeyakul *et al.*, 1993). Caffeine N3-demethylation can be assessed *in vivo* by determining the ratio of the appropriate urinary metabolites (Kalow and Tang, 1991; Rostami-Hodjegan *et al.*, 1996; Nordmark *et al.*, 1999). However, the ratio most accurately reflecting CYP1A2 activity has been the subject of some debate (Miners and Birkett, 1996; Notarianni *et al.*, 1995; Tang *et al.*, 1994), and several different ratios have been used in population studies (Butler *et al.*, 1992; Nordmark *et al.*, 1999). CYP1A2-dependent activity shows considerable interindividual variation, both *in vitro* and *in vivo*, with a 180-fold (Sesardic *et al.*, 1988) and six-fold (Schrenk *et al.*, 1998) range, respectively. The extent to which activity varies *in vivo* depends on the choice of substrate. Whilst in non-smokers the CYP1A2-dependent caffeine metabolic ratio varies six-fold (Schrenk *et al.*, 1998), the intrinsic clearance of phenacetin varies approximately ten-fold (Kahn *et al.*, 1985). Substantial intra-individual variation of the CYP1A2 urinary metabolic ratio has also been noted (Nordmark *et al.*, 1999).

OTHER SUBSTRATES/ACTIVITIES

CYP1A2 is involved in the metabolism of a large number of environmental and dietary chemicals, in some cases converting them into toxic or carcinogenic intermediates (Guengerich, 1995; Guengerich *et al.*, 1999). Amongst important substrates are heterocyclic aromatic amines (e.g. PhIP) (McManus *et al.*, 1990; Zhao *et al.*, 1994), aromatic amines (e.g. aminobiphenyl) (Butler *et al.*, 1989), aflatoxin B_1 (Gallagher *et al.*, 1994), dietary flavonoids (Doostdar *et al.*, 2000) and several drugs of different chemical classes and structures (Guengerich, 1995). These include minor analgesics such as paracetamol (Manyike *et al.*, 2000) and other arylamides (Liu *et al.*, 1991), anti-depressants (e.g. clozapine) (Eiermann *et al.*, 1997), other CNS active agents (e.g. tacrine) (Spaldin *et al.*, 1995), methylxanthines (Fuhr *et al.*, 1993), cardiovascular drugs (e.g. propranolol (Masubuchi *et al.*, 1994), mexilitine (Nakajima *et al.*, 1998)), oral contraceptive steroids (estradiol) (Yamazaki *et al.*, 1998) and several others (e.g. chlorzoxazone) (Ono *et al.*, 1995).

ENVIRONMENTAL/HOST FACTORS

CYP1A2 is selectively and potently inhibited by furafylline (Sesardic *et al.*, 1990a). Fluvoxamine is also a relatively selective inhibitor of the enzyme (Jeppesen *et al.*, 1996). Other inhibitors, with less selectivity, include alpha-naphthoflavone (Tassaneeyakul *et al.*, 1993), several dietary flavonoids (Zhai *et al.*, 1998), a number of fluoroquinolone antibiotics (e.g. enoxacin)

(Fuhr *et al.*, 1992) and various other drugs which tend also to inhibit other forms of P450 to a greater or lesser extent (e.g. methimazole (Guo *et al.*, 1997), methoxsalen (Ono *et al.*, 1995).

CYP1A2 is inducible by many of the compounds that induce CYP1A1, including polycyclic aromatic hydrocarbons (Sesardic *et al.*, 1990b), polyhalogenated aromatic hydrocarbons (Lake *et al.*, 1996), dioxins (Xu *et al.*, 2000) and indoles contained in cruciferous vegetables (Schrenk *et al.*, 1998). A number of dietary and environmental sources contain polycyclic aromatic hydrocarbons at levels sufficient to induce CYP1A2. These include cigarette smoke (Sesardic *et al.*, 1990b), pyrolysed and charcoal-grilled food (Pantuck *et al.*, 1976). A limited number of drugs can cause modest induction of CYP1A2, including omeprazole (Rost *et al.*, 1992) and related compounds (Andersson *et al.*, 1998) and fluparoxan (Beresford et al., 1997).

Induction of CYP1A2 involves at least two different mechanisms. The 5′-upstream region of the gene contains elements (Quattrochi *et al.*, 1994) responsive to the AH receptor/ARNT complex (Li *et al.*, 1998), just as CYP1A1 (Kress *et al.*, 1998) and CYP1B1 (Tang *et al.*, 1996). However, induction also requires the correct balance of co-activators, and the absence of co-repressors or silencers (Xu *et al.*, 2000), as induction is tissue-specific, being confined largely to the liver (Quattrochi and Tukey, 1989; Sesardic *et al.*, 1990b). There is also evidence that CYP1A2 levels can be increased by protein stabilisation (Werlinder *et al.*, 2000). Induction varies between individuals (Landi *et al.*, 1999), but has been difficult to study in detail, due to the absence of suitable *in vitro* and *in vivo* models (Li *et al.*, 1998). Omeprazole appears to induce CYP1A2 by a novel mechanism involving ligand-independent activation of the Ah receptor (Backlund *et al.*, 1997; Daujat *et al.*, 1992).

GENETIC FACTORS

Despite the considerable interindividual variability that exists in the expression of CYP1A2, until recently there was no known genetic basis for this. Indeed, in studies by Nakajima *et al.* (1994) and by Welfare *et al.* (1999) no evidence for a genetic basis could be found, either in the coding region or in the 5′-untranslated region, to underlie the extremes of CYP1A2 activity found within the populations studied. However, in the last couple of years there have been reports of several mutations of the CYP1A2 gene. Nakajima *et al.* (1999) identified a point mutation in the 5′-upstream region of the CYP1A2 gene in Japanese subjects, which appears to result in reduced expression of the enzyme. In a study of Caucasian subjects by Sachse *et al.* (1999) a mutation of CYP1A2 was found in intron 1. From studies *in vivo*, this mutation appears to be associated with increased inducibility of CYP1A2. The extent to which interindividual variation in the expression and inducibility of CYP1A2 is due to these and other genetic polymorphisms remains to be determined.

EXPRESSION IN EXTRAHEPATIC TISSUES

The expression and inducibility of CYP1A2 are confined largely to the liver (Sesardic *et al.*, 1990b; Windmill *et al.*, 1997). There are reports of detectable levels of CYP1A2 mRNA or apoprotein in other tissues (Ding *et al.*, 2000; Foster *et al.*, 1993), but the metabolic significance of this appears to be very low. When the CYP1A2 gene was "knocked out" in the mouse the phenotype was apparent primarily in the liver (Liang *et al.*, 1996). The hepatic-specific expression of CYP1A2 has implications for studies in isolated cells, which should be liver-derived. Even in studies of induction by transfection of upstream region of the CYP1A2 gene, it is necessary to use liver-derived cell lines, to ensure that the necessary co-activators are present (Quattrochi and Tukey, 1989).

CYP1B1

The CYP1B1 enzyme was recently discovered as the product of the CYP1B1 gene mapping to chromosome 2 in man (Sutter *et al.*, 1994). The CYP1B1 cDNA had previously been cloned from keratinocyte cell lines and was discovered on the basis of its inducibility by TCDD (Sutter *et al.*, 1991). It has a 40–41% homology with human CYP1A1 and CYP1A2 (Sutter *et al.*, 1994). The endogenous function of the enzyme is incompletely understood, but its rich location in glandular tissues in experimental animals (Otto *et al.*, 1992), human placenta (Hakkola *et al.*, 1997), human embryonic adrenal gland (Juchau *et al.*, 1998) and prostate (Finnström N, Rane A *et al.*, unpublished observations) suggests a role in the metabolism of steroids.

VARIABILITY OF PROTEIN AND MRNA

First of all, the level of gene expression and enzyme concentration in the liver is very low or absent. The gene is, however, highly expressed in a multitude of other human organs including kidney, brain, lymphocytes, endometrium, placenta, fetal adrenal glands, lung, brain and kidney (Sutter *et al.*, 1994; Hakkola *et al.*, 1997). In addition, the prostate consistently contains high levels of the CYP1B1 specific mRNA (Finnström N, Rane A *et al.*, unpublished observations). The variation in CYP1B1 mRNA was very small in prostate specimens from twenty-four individuals. All specimens contained the CYP1B1 transcript at levels higher than any other CYP-specific transcript. In contrast to other CYP specific mRNAs, CYP1B1 mRNA is measurable in blood in almost all individuals (Finnström N, Rane A *et al.*, unpublished observations).

VARIABILITY OF ACTIVITIES

Estradiol is a major candidate substrate for CYP1B1. Different lines of evidence suggest that the estradiol 4-hydroxylase is catalysed by CYP1B1

(Spink *et al.*, 1994; Liehr *et al.*, 1995). This presumed role of the enzyme is consonant with its expression in myometrium (Hakkola *et al.*, 1997). Further support for an endocrine steroid metabolism function was given by the recent observation that blood of pregnant women contains considerably higher CYP1B1-specific mRNA levels in pregnancy than after (Lind AB, Rane A *et al.*, unpublished observations).

The CYP1B1 enzyme has also been shown to catalyse the activation of several procarcinogens. Therefore, it was suggested that the enzyme may have a role in carcinogenesis, particularly in extra-hepatic organs (Shimada *et al.*, 1996).

ENVIRONMENTAL FACTORS

Unlike CYP1A1, which is highly variable in placenta and some other extrahepatic tissues because of induction by ubiquitous polycyclic hydrocarbons, CYP1B1 is virtually unaffected by such chemical exposure (Hakkola *et al.*, 1997). Therefore, the variation in the CYP1B1 mRNA level is much lower in this organ. Otherwise, virtually nothing is known about environmental or host factors affecting CYP1B1.

GENETIC FACTORS

The recent discovery of different frameshift mutations in the CYP1B1 gene (Stoilov *et al.*, 1997) has triggered the interest in the functional consequences of this mutation, and the cancer risk association of the alleles and genotypes. Only scarce information on these aspects has been published so far. However, Stoilov *et al.* (1997) suggested CYP1B1 to be a candidate gene for congenital glaucoma associated with the GLC3A locus on chromosome 2. Therefore, CYP1B1 may have a role in the metabolism of oxidized growth-effector molecules.

CYP2A subfamily

The *CYP2A6* gene is one of the three members in the human CYP2A gene subfamily, the other members being CYP2A7 and CYP2A13 (Fernandez-Salguero and Gonzales, 1995; Raunio *et al.*, 2001). CYP2A6 is the best-characterised enzyme in the CYP2A subfamily (Pelkonen *et al.*, 1993). It appears that CYP2A7 is non-functional, but CYP2A13 is highly expressed and catalytically active at least in olfactory mucosa (Gu *et al.*, 2000).

VARIABILITY OF PROTEIN AND MRNA

Large interindividual differences exist at the CYP2A6 apoprotein and mRNA levels (see Pelkonen *et al.*, 1993; Pelkonen and Raunio, 1995). In immunoblotting experiments using purified human CYP forms as standards,

CYP2A6 protein constitutes 1–10% of the total liver CYP content (Table 10.2; Yun *et al.*, 1991; Shimada *et al.*, 1994; Imaoka *et al.*, 1996). CYP2A6 mRNA expression has been investigated by RT-PCR (Hakkola *et al.*, 1994, 1996). There are seemingly large differences, but real quantitation has not been performed. However, it is clear that rather large interindividual variation exists in both CYP2A6 mRNA and protein levels in human liver.

VARIABILITY OF FORM-SPECIFIC ACTIVITY/ACTIVITIES

Coumarin 7-hydroxylation seems to be one of the most specific probes for any CYP available, since no other human CYP form has the capacity to catalyse coumarin 7-hydroxylation to a significant degree (Waxman *et al.*, 1991). CYP2A6 is a high-affinity coumarin 7-hydroxylating enzyme (Pelkonen and Raunio, 1995; Chang and Waxman, 1996). Interindividual variability of the activity is very large, up to about 100-fold in some studies (see Pelkonen *et al.*, 2000), but many studied populations have been unselected and included individuals with various diseases and modifying influences.

OTHER SUBSTRATES/ACTIVITIES

CYP2A6 has also been shown to catalyse the metabolism of several pharmaceuticals, as well as compounds that are of toxicological significance, such as nitrosamines and aflatoxin B_1 (see Pelkonen *et al.*, 1997, 2000; Raunio *et al.*, 1999). Except for coumarin and, perhaps, nicotine, there is currently very little knowledge about the quantitative importance of CYP2A6 in the metabolism of the known CYP2A6 substrates. However, it would be of considerable importance to know the contribution of CYP2A6 in the metabolism of various substrates, because it is then possible to envisage whether the variability of CYP2A6 and factors causing it has any role in the variability of kinetics or biological effects of the studied substance.

Nicotine is, because of its widespread use, an especially interesting substrate. The inactivation of nicotine via C-oxidation to cotinine is mediated to a major extent by CYP2A6 (Cashman *et al.*, 1992; Nakajima *et al.*, 1996a, 1996b), and also the 3′-hydroxylation of cotinine is mediated by CYP2A6. Thus, any inter-individual variations in CYP2A6 levels may affect nicotine inactivation rates and possibly also smoking patterns. Also numerous other agents of toxicological interest are substrates for CYP2A6 enzyme (see Raunio *et al.*, 1999).

ENVIRONMENTAL/HOST FACTORS

Very little is known about the inducibility and regulation of CYP2A6, but studies on the mouse orthologue, CYP2A5, have revealed novel pathways for induction by a large number of chemical agents and biological conditions (see Pelkonen et al., 1995, 1997). Taken together, available studies indicate that murine CYP2A5 is regulated in a very complex manner, possibly involving several independent cellular pathways.

Studies with primary human hepatocytes have shown that at least phenobarbital and rifampicin are capable of inducing CYP2A6 (Dalet-Beluche et al., 1992). On the basis of in vivo studies, it is possible that anti-epileptic drugs (carbamazepine, clonazepam, phenobarbital and phenytoin), fibrosis, infestation of the liver with Opisthorchiasis viverrini, and chronic HBV infection enhance coumarin 7-hydroxylation (Satarug et al., 1996). It is also shown that coumarin 7-hydroxylation is decreased in severe alcohol-induced liver cirrhosis (Sotaniemi et al., 1995), but the significance of other environmental and host factors is currently unknown.

GENETIC FACTORS

Polymorphisms of CYP2A6 are under intensive investigation at the present time. Earlier, two mutant alleles of the CYP2A6 gene were reported, i.e. CYP2A6*2 and CYP2A6*3 (Fernandez-Salguero et al., 1995). CYP2A6*2 has a point mutation in codon 160 leading to a Leu-His amino acid change and to a defective enzyme incapable of coumarin 7-hydroxylation (Yamano et al., 1990). Later studies have indicated that the mutant CYP2A6*3 allele is an artefact (Oscarson et al., 1998, 1999a; Chen et al., 1999). Two deletion alleles have also been uncovered, both resulting in a lack of coumarin 7-hydroxylation activity (Oscarson et al., 1999b). In addition, two to three additional variant alleles have been identified (see http://www.imm.ki.se/CYPalleles/). In addition, evidence has been given for the existence of subjects carrying alleles with duplicated CYP2A6 genes (Rao et al., 2000) with higher capacity for nicotine metabolism. The frequency of variant alleles studied thus far is rather low in Caucasian populations, i.e. a few percent, but the incidence of the CYP2A6*4 allele having a gene deletion is high in Oriental populations (Oscarson et al., 1999b). The apparent higher number of variant alleles in the Japanese is consistent with the recent observation that a higher percentage of Japanese lack hepatic coumarin 7-hydroxylation compared with Caucasians (Shimada et al., 1996).

EXPRESSION OF CYP2A GENES IN EXTRAHEPATIC TISSUES

With the aid of gene-specific RT-PCR, several tissues have been screened for the presence or absence of CYP2A transcripts (Koskela et al., 1999). Transcripts for all three genes (CYP2A6, CYP2A7 and CYP2A13) were found in liver. CYP2A6 was the most abundant form, followed by CYP2A7, and very little CYP2A13 mRNA was present. In comparison with liver, nasal mucosa contained a low amount of CYP2A6 and a relatively high level of CYP2A13 transcripts. Kidney, duodenum, lung, alveolar macrophages, peripheral lymphocytes, placenta and uterine endometrium were negative for all transcripts (Koskela *et al.*, 1999).

CYP2B subfamily

CYP2B6 is one of the less well characterised P450 enzymes in the human liver. The exact percentage of the total hepatic P450 is difficult to give because the immunochemically measured variation is very large, up to 100-fold, ranging from 0.7 to 71.1 pmol/mg microsomal protein (Ekins *et al.*, 1997, 1998, 1999). On the basis of earlier studies it was hypothesised that CYP2B6 shows polymorphism, i.e. only a small percentage of the individuals express the enzyme. However, with more sensitive methods it seems that a large majority of the individuals express both CYP2B6 mRNA and protein (Czerwinski *et al.*, 1994; Hakkola *et al.*, 1994).

S-mephenytoin N-demethylation to nirvanol has been suggested to be a CYP2B6-specific probe activity (Ekins *et al.*, 1998). In contrast, some 7-ethoxycoumarin derivatives (especially 7-ethoxy-4-trifluoromethylcoumarin), which were earlier claimed to be specific, in later studies have actually been shown to be metabolised by multiple CYP enzymes (Code *et al.*, 1997; Ekins *et al.*, 1997). Variability of these activities has been shown to be large, several ten-fold in populations containing from ten to forty individuals. When testosterone is used as a substrate with the expressed CYP2B6, only 16ß-hydroxylation was observed (Ekins and Wrighton, 1999). CYP2B6 seems to be involved in cyclophosphamide hydroxylation (Roy *et al.*, 1999).

Not much is known about environmental and genetic factors regulating the expression of CYP2B6. The immunochemically measured protein concentration was three times higher in Caucasians than in Chinese, suggesting differences between these two populations in genetic background or in dietary and/or environmental factors (Kim *et al.*, 1997). In cultured human hepatocytes, CYP2B6 is induced by phenobarbital, rifampicin and dexamethasone (Strom *et al.*, 1996).

CYP2C subfamily

The human genome has been shown to contain at least four genes belonging to the CYP2C subfamily (Goldstein and de Morais, 1994) and at least CYP2C8, 2C9 and 2C19 have been shown to be expressed significantly in the liver. The expression of CYP2C18 is particularly low (or absent) in human liver and we do not deal with it further here. The relative metabolic roles of the different hepatic enzymes are still rather poorly defined. There are some indications of the expression of CYP2C enzymes in other tissues (see Raunio *et al.*, 1995; Miners and Birkett, 1998).

CYP2C8

CYP2C8 has been purified from human liver and cDNA has been cloned (see Goldstein and de Morais, 1994). It has a role in the metabolism of endogenous substances like retinol and retinoic acid and drugs such as benzphetamine. Tolbutamide is also metabolised by CYP2C8, although the affinity of tolbutamide for this isoenzyme is clearly lower than for CYP2C9 (Lasker et al., 1998). There are discrepant results as to the amount of CYP2C8 in human liver microsomes (see Table 10.2).

Taxol 6-hydroxylation has been used as a CYP2C8-specific marker activity in vitro. It displays rather large interindividual variability, up to twenty-fold (see Table 10.3). Otherwise this enzyme belongs to the less well characterised P450 enzymes in human liver.

CYP2C9

VARIABILITY OF PROTEIN AND MRNA

CYP2C9 is a major component of the human CYP2C pool (Miners and Birkett, 1998), accounting for approximately 20% of total P450 in liver microsomes (see Table 10.2).

VARIABILITY OF CYP-ASSOCIATED ACTIVITIES

There are a number of substrates that are metabolised predominantly by CYP2C9. Good correlation has been found between CYP2C9 level and tolbutamide methyl hydroxylation, this substrate seemingly specific both in vitro and in vivo (Yamazaki et al., 1997; Inoue et al., 1997). Other more or less enzyme-specific substrates for CYP2C9 include fluoxetine, losartan, phenytoin, S-warfarin and several NSAIDs (Goldstein and de Morais, 1994). Variability of these activities seems to be large, several ten-fold at the maximum (see Table 10.3).

ENVIRONMENTAL/HOST FACTORS

CYP2C9 may be induced by several drugs such as rifampicin, phenobarbital and ethanol (Miners and Birkett, 1998). Among a series of selective serotonin reuptake inhibitors, only fluvoxamine appeared as an effective CYP2C9 inhibitor, both in vitro and in vivo (Hemeryck et al., 1999). Using 3D-/4D-QSAR analysis, Ekins et al. (2000) were able to define models of the CYP2C9 active site allowing prediction of drug–drug interactions. The substrate binding site of CYP2C9 has been studied by Poli-Scaife et al. (1997), who were able to propose a structure–activity-based molecular model accounting for the three-dimensional positioning of the substrates in the active site of the enzyme. In general, these sorts of in silico approaches are currently becoming more and more refined.

GENETIC FACTORS

Polymorphism in the coding region of CYP2C9 produces variants at amino acid residues 144 (Arg/Cys) and 359 (Ile/Leu). Individuals homozygous for Leu359 have markedly reduced enzymatic activity, although the frequency of this allele is relatively low. This reduced activity seems to be of importance *in vivo* for the elimination rate of warfarin (Steward *et al.*, 1997). Three major CYP2C9 alleles termed *1, *2 and *3 with respective allele frequencies of 0.79, 0.125 and 0.085 have been described and a PCR-based method developed for predicting the phenotype (Stubbins *et al.*, 1996).

CYP2C19

VARIABILITY OF PROTEIN AND MRNA

The human liver CYP2C19 content is approximately five times lower than the CYP2C9 content (see Table 10.2).

VARIABILITY OF CYP2C19-ASSOCIATED ACTIVITIES

CYP2C19 is best characterised both *in vitro* and *in vivo* by S-mephenytoin 4′-hydroxylation or omeprazole 5-hydroxylation (Andersson *et al.*, 1993). In PM individuals, both activities are extremely low and this alone results in huge interindividual variability in the metabolic rate of these two substrates. However, in EM individuals, the variability is also large, several ten-fold, in the metabolism of these substrates, indicating that other than genetic factors affect the activities.

ENVIRONMENTAL/HOST FACTORS

CYP2C19 is inducible by carmabazepine and norethindrone (Goldstein and de Morais, 1994). Otherwise, very little is known about environmental and host factors affecting CYP2C19.

GENETIC FACTORS

Genetic polymorphism in the metabolism of mephenytoin and other clinically important drugs has been attributed to variant CYP2C19 alleles. Recent studies have demonstrated that the polymorphism is due to at least two major and several minor variant alleles of CYP2C19 (Goldstein and de Morais, 1994). Approximately 3% of Caucasians, 4–7% of Negroids and 15–20% of Orientals are poor metabolisers of S-mephenytoin, their CYP2C19 enzyme being inactive.

CYP2D6

CYP2D6 enzyme is mainly distributed in the endoplasmic reticulum of hepatocytes and accounts for only a small percentage (about 4%) of all hepatic P450s, but its role in drug metabolism is considerably more important than its relative content. In the late 1970s it was found that the drugs debrisoquine and sparteine were polymorphically metabolised. Using bufuralol as a marker substrate the human enzyme, catalysing debrisoquine hydroxylation, could be purified (Gut *et al.*, 1986) and the cDNA was cloned in 1988 (Gonzalez *et al.*, 1988) with the use of antibodies raised against the rat CYP2D1 enzyme. The major genetic cause for the lack of enzyme activity was described in 1988–1990 (Skoda *et al.*, 1988; Heim and Meyer, 1990) and the phenomenon of stable *CYP2D6* gene duplication and amplification in 1993 (Johansson *et al.*, 1993).

VARIABILITY OF MRNA AND PROTEIN

Because of a large number of various CYP2D6 alleles (see below) with variable outcomes in terms of mRNA, protein and associated activities, it is too optimistic to expect a perfect correlation between these parameters. Because some alleles produce labile mRNAs and also the stability of some CYP2D6 protein species is poor, it is not possible to get reliable correlations. Furthermore, at least in some tissues multiple CYP2D6-associated mRNAs are detectable. Studies on the expression of various mRNAs in heterologous expression systems have provided a great deal of data to solve the above problems.

Because of the above-mentioned complexities, the significance of CYP2D6 mRNA expression in various extrahepatic tissues is still under debate. With RT-PCR technique it is possible to demonstrate the presence of CYP2D6-like mRNA sequences in various tissues, including lungs and respiratory tract, lymphocytes, etc., but whether the expression leads to production of active protein, is in most instances not known. Discrepant results have been obtained (see Raunio *et al.*, 1995).

VARIABILITY OF FORM-SPECIFIC ACTIVITIES

In *in vitro* systems, bufuralol 1′-hydroxylation, debrisoquine 4-hydroxylation, sparteine oxidation and dextromethorphan O-demethylase have been used as CYP2D6-specific activities, the last three also as *in vivo* probes (Streetman *et al.*, 2000). Very little activity of any one of these probes can be seen in samples from homozygous poor metabolisers. In samples from individuals carrying one or more active alleles, variabilities of these activities are large, several ten-fold (see Table 10.3). The extent to which non-genetic host factors (e.g. disease effects) or genetic factors (heterozygosity, gene dose, variously active alleles, etc.) contribute to the variability has not been rigorously evaluated.

OTHER SUBSTRATES/ACTIVITIES

CYP2D6 substrates are lipophilic bases with a protonable nitrogen atom. The hydroxylation reaction takes place at a distance of 5 or 7 Å from the nitrogen atom. Site-directed mutagenesis experiments indicate that Asp301 is the negatively charged amino acid responsible for binding to the substrate nitrogen. Besides this amino acid, Ser304, Thr309 and Val370 also appear to be involved in substrate binding (de Groot *et al.*, 1997). A large number of clinically important drugs are substrates for CYP2D6.

CYP2D6 has a very high affinity for alkaloids (Fonne-Pfister and Meyer, 1988). No endogenous substrate is known. Since no adverse or deleterious phenotype has been described among subjects lacking CYP2D6, one might conclude that the enzyme has no major endogenous function. A role for metabolism of some neurotransmitters has been suggested. It is likely that the enzyme has had a major role in the metabolism of environmental food constituents, in particular alkaloids.

ENVIRONMENTAL/HOST FACTORS

The enzyme expression is, as compared with other hepatic xenobiotic metabolising P450s, not regulated by any known environmental agent and is not inducible by known hormones. The absence of environmental inducibility and the ability of the enzyme to bind and probably metabolise plant toxins has led to the hypothesis that inducibility in response to dietary stress in the past instead has occurred by preservation of alleles with *CYP2D6* gene duplication and gene amplification, causing higher amounts of expressed enzyme. The gene dosage effect *in vivo* is high (Ingelman-Sundberg *et al.*, 1999). Interestingly, however, CYP2D6 activity varies with the female reproductive phases. Increase of the enzyme activity has been noted, as assessed in pharmacokinetic studies of CYP2D6 substrates during and after human pregnancy. Thus, the apparent oral clearance of metoprolol increases 300–400% during pregnancy (Högstedt *et al.*, 1983, 1985). An endocrine effect of pregnancy on metabolic ratios reflecting the CYP2D6 activity has subsequently been demonstrated with dextromethorphan as a probe drug (Wadelius *et al.*, 1997). These suggest a role of the enzyme in the metabolism of estrogens or progestogens.

GENETIC FACTORS

The *CYP2D6* gene is localised at chromosome 22q13.1. The locus contains two neighboring pseudogenes, *CYP2D7* and *CYP2D8* (Heim and Meyer, 1990). The evolution of the human *CYP2D* locus has involved elimination of three genes and inactivation of two (*CYP2D7P* and *CYP2D8P*) and partial inactivation of one (*CYP2D6*). Rodents have kept five active genes, probably for dietary reasons. At present more than sixty known different polymorphic *CYP2D6* alleles are known (see: http://www.imm.ki.se/

CYPalleles) causing absent, decreased, altered or increased enzyme activity. The most common variant alleles distributed in different ethnic groups are listed in Table 10.4. Genotyping for the five most frequently distributed mutations can predict the phenotype by about 95–98% accuracy.

There are important interethnic differences in the distribution of the variant alleles. The inactivating CYP2D6*3, CYP2D6*4 and CYP2D6*6 alleles are mainly seen in Caucasians, whereas the allele having a gene deletion (CYP2D6*5) is evenly distributed in the world. In Asia, a gene with a Pro34Ser mutation is the most common allele, causing reduced but not abolished CYP2D6 activity. Among Black people, in, for example, Zimbabwe and the US, the CYP2D6*17 allele is very common causing an enzyme with altered substrate specificity with a generally reduced capacity for metabolism of substrates.

Ultrarapid metabolisers often have multiple active gene copies of mainly the CYP2D6*2 type. At present alleles carrying 0, 1, 2, 3, 4, 5 and 13 CYP2D6 gene copies have been identified (see Ingelman-Sundberg et al., 1999). These alleles are stably inherited from generation to generation.

CLINICAL IMPLICATIONS

Subjects with multiple gene copies will metabolise drugs more rapidly and therapeutic plasma levels will not be achieved at ordinary drug dosages. Individuals lacking functional CYP2D6 genes metabolise selective CYP2D6 substrates at a lower rate, particularly antidepressants and neuroleptics. The CYP2D6 genotype has been successfully shown to predict the clearances of, for example, the antidepressants desipramine, fluvoxamine, fluoxetine, mexiletine, mianserin, nortryptiline, paroxetine and citalopram, as well as the clearance of the neuroleptics perphenazine and

Table 10.4 The major human polymorphic CYP2D6 alleles and their global distribution

Major variant alleles	Mutation	Consequence	Allele frequencies (%)			
			Caucasians	Asians	Black Africans	Ethiopians and Saudi Arabians
CYP2D6*2xn	gene duplication /multiduplication	increased enzyme activity	1–5	0–2	2	10–16
CYP2D6*4	defective splicing	inactive enzyme	12–21	1	2	1–4
CYP2D6*5	gene deletion	no enzyme	2–7	6	4	1–3
CYP2D6*10	P34S, S486T	unstable enzyme	1–2	51	6	3–9
CYP2D6*17	T107I, R296C, S486T	reduced affinity for substrates	0	ND	34	3–9

Notes
For a complete list, see http://www.imm.ki.se/cypalleles/cyp2d6.htm
ND=not determined.

zuclopenthixol and the competitive muscarinic receptor antagonist toltero-dine (see Ingelman-Sundberg *et al.*, 1999). Adverse effects due to elevated drug plasma levels occur more frequently in cases where the drug clearance is dependent on CYP2D6. A lack of CYP2D6 enzyme results in reduced drug therapy effectiveness for drugs that are bioactivated by CYP2D6. Examples of this include tramadol and codeine (Ingelman-Sundberg *et al.*, 1999).

CYP2D6 IN MOLECULAR EPIDEMIOLOGY

The CYP2D6 phenotype and genotype has been investigated with respect to the risk of suffering from different diseases. Investigators have evaluated hypotheses whether the PM phenotype predispose for diseases besides melanoma, lung, breast, anogenital, basal cell, aerodigestive tract, oral, prostate, pancreatic and bladder cancer, also with Parkinsonism, Alzheimer's disease, optic neuropathy, tremor, hair color, neuroleptic malignant syn-drome, smoking behavior, opiate dependence, tardive dyskinesia, tremor, hematological neoplasias, and Lewy body disease, etc., but no established relation has hitherto been found.

CYP2E1

The *CYP2E* subfamily has evolved relatively recently, compared with, for example, *CYP3* and *CYP4* and only been described in mammals. There is only one gene in the *CYP2E* locus in humans containing nine exons and locating to chromosomes 10q24.3-qter (see Ronis *et al.*, 1996). CYP2E1 is constitutively expressed in the liver, where the highest concentration is found in the centrilobular region with highest concentration in the four to five layers of hepatocytes surrounding the terminal hepatic venules (Ingelman-Sundberg *et al.*, 1988). In general CYP2E1 accounts for approximately 8% of the total P450 in liver (see Table 10.2).

In any discussion of CYP2E1 variability, the complex regulation of its expression has to be kept in mind. In general, many factors affect the expression of CYP2E1 and the control is exerted at the transcriptional, mRNA, translational and post-translational level. The endogenous regula-tion of CYP2E1 is similar to that of other gluconeogenetic enzymes which includes repression of enzyme expression during well-fed conditions and increased expression during starvation and diabetes. Studies in experimental animals have demonstrated increases of CYP2E1 either at transcriptional or post-transcriptional level in chemically induced diabetes and starvation (Johansson *et al.*, 1990; see Ronis *et al.*, 1996). On the other hand, insulin treatment causes a decrease of the CYP2E1 protein in chemically induced diabetes, probably by accelerating the mRNA turnover (de Waziers *et al.*, 1995). The expression of CYP2E1 is also regulated by different cytokines.

Similar to other P450s such as CYP1A2, CYP2C and CYP3A, the level of CYP2E1 is decreased by, for example, IL-1, IL-6 and TNF-α in primary culture of human hepatocytes (Abdel-Razzak *et al.*, 1993). By contrast, IL-4 induces the expression of CYP2E1 at least in primary hepatocytes (Abdel-Razzak *et al.*, 1993).

VARIABILITY OF PROTEIN AND MRNA

The interindividual variability in CYP2E1 expression in human liver is about twenty-fold (Ekström *et al.*, 1989). However, because of the complex regulation at various levels of expression, it is difficult to judge whether the changes at mRNA or protein level are actually reflected into the catalytic activity.

VARIABILITY OF FORM-SPECIFIC ACTIVITY/ACTIVITIES

Chlorzoxazone 6-hydroxylation is currently the preferred method to measure CYP2E1 activity in liver microsomes (Peter *et al.*, 1990). Also CYP1A1 and CYP1A2 catalyse the reaction (Ono *et al.*, 1995), but it seems that K_m values are higher and turnover numbers lower than with CYP2E1 and consequently, their contribution to chlorzoxazone 6-hydroxylation is relatively small. Furthermore, the amount of CYP1A1 is very low in the liver (<1 pmol/mg protein). There are some *in vivo* observations that chlorzoxazone 6-hydroxylation activity is increased in liver microsomes after heavy alcohol drinking and upon the administration of isoniazid, and decreased by disulfiram and obesity, whereas no effect has been seen by cigarette smoking (polycyclic aromatic hydrocarbons) and anti-epileptic drugs. Similar changes have been observed in *in vivo* studies on alcoholics, obese subjects and other patients (see Streetman *et al.*, 2000).

OTHER SUBSTRATES/ACTIVITIES

CYP2E1 has very broad substrate specificity. More than seventy different chemicals with diverse structures have been identified to be metabolised by CYP2E1 (Ronis *et al.*, 1996). In general most CYP2E1 substrates are small and hydrophobic in character. Many of the substrates exert a high affinity to the enzyme. Among the substrates are alcohols/ketones/aldehydes (ethanol, glycerol, 1-butanol, 1-propanol, acetone, acetaldehyde), aromatic compounds (benzene, aniline, phenol, toluene, acetaminophen), halogenated alkanes or alkanes (chloroform, carbon tetrachloride, vinyl chloride, vinyl carbamate, halothane, enflurane and pentane), anesthetics (ether, enflurane and halothane), drugs (chlorzoxazone and acetaminophen) and carcinogens (nitrosamines and azo carcinogens). The endogenous substrate for CYP2E1 is most likely acetone, but also other endogenous substrates such as the lipid peroxidation products pentane and hexane, as well as fatty acids are likely (see Ronis *et al.*, 1996).

ENVIRONMENTAL AND HOST FACTORS

The onset of CYP2E1 expression is apparently at birth. Several investigators have failed to detect CYP2E1 mRNA and protein in fetal liver by Northern and Western blotting analysis, as well as by RT-PCR (see Hakkola *et al.*, 1998), whereas Carpenter *et al.* (1996) using RNase protection assay, RT-PCR and immunoblotting provided evidence for the presence of CYP2E1 in fetal liver. In rats, significant levels of CYP2E1 mRNA are detectable within a few hours after birth and increase until a plateau level is reached at about 12 days of age. The onset of transcriptional activation correlates with the demethylation of cytosine residues in the 5′-flanking region of the gene (Umeno *et al.*, 1988).

Many of the CYP2E1 substrates are also inducers of the enzymes. The inducers commonly used in experimental animals are ethanol, acetone, isoniazid, pyridine and pyrazole. Among these, pyridine, acetone and isoniazid have been described to increase the translation efficiency of the CYP2E1 mRNA (see Ronis *et al.*, 1996). It has been demonstrated that post-translational regulation of CYP2E1 is the major mechanism for induction caused by most CYP2E1 substrates. Measurement of CYP2E1 turnover *in vivo* in rats chronically treated with acetone (Song *et al.*, 1989) and experiments *in vitro* using hepatocyte culture systems (Eliasson *et al.*, 1988), demonstrated that CYP2E1 inducers such as acetone, ethanol, 4-methylpyrazole and imidazole increase the CYP2E1 level by protein stabilisation. In the absence of inducers, CYP2E1 is degraded in a biphasic fashion with a short half-life of 7 h and a longer half-life of 37 h. However, after chronic acetone administration, the rapid phase of degradation is abolished. The substrate binding has been shown to protect CYP2E1 from phosphorylation at Ser-129, and subsequent degradation (Eliasson *et al.*, 1990). The rapid degradation of CYP2E1 might be partly due to covalent modifications by the radicals produced by CYP2E1 or to other changes during catalytic cycling. In fact, the inhibition of electron supply from NADPH-cytochrome P450 stabilizes the protein (Zhukov *et al.*, 1999).

GENETIC FACTORS

In comparison to many other P450s important for metabolism of xenobiotics, the human *CYP2E1* gene has been found to be relatively well conserved (Rannug *et al.*, 1995). This might be suggested to be inherent in the capability of the gene product to metabolise ketone bodies which presumably makes the enzyme of physiological importance during periods of starvation and thus of importance for selection.

Initially, several polymorphisms in human *CYP2E1* gene were detected by RFLP by various restriction enzymes (see Ronis *et al.*, 1996; Carriere *et al.*, 1996). In these polymorphisms (currently termed *CYP2E1*1B*, *CYP2E1*5B* and *CYP2E1*6*) the mutations have been shown to locate in either introns or in the 5′-flanking region. There are contradictory results as to whether these polymorphisms correlate to the *in vitro* transcriptional rate. The incidence of these polymorphisms has been investigated in relation to different types of cancer, alcoholic liver disease and to alcoholism. However, the results are controversial and no firm conclusions can be drawn.

A polymorphic 100 bp insertion was found in the 5′-flanking region of the *CYP2E1* gene in some individuals by using RFLP analysis with different restriction enzymes. The region was limited to a 600 bp region, −2270 to −1672 (McCarver *et al.*, 1998). The insertion was associated with increased chlorzoxazone hydroxylation in obese patients and subjects drinking ethanol in a relatively small number of subjects. The basis for the insertion polymorphism was shown to be repeat sequence present in five, six or eight copies (Hu *et al.*, 1999).

SSCP screening of 200 individuals of Chinese and Caucasian origin revealed very few variant alleles with functional mutations. Indeed only three subjects exhibited a *CYP2E1* gene with an altered open reading frame and two variant alleles, *CYP2E1*2* with Arg76His and CYP2E1*3 with Val 389Ile was found. The CYP2E1*2 allele was found to cause only 40% of the activity of the CYP2E1*1 allele, when expressed in COS 1 cells (Hu *et al.*, 1997).

Several mutations in the *CYP2E1* gene have been identified recently, at positions −316 (A to G), −297 (T to A), −35 (G to T), 1107 (G to C; intron 1), 4804 (G to A Val179Ile; exon 4) and 10157 (C to T; exon 8) (Fairbrother *et al.*, 1998). The allele frequencies were low (0.013 to 0.052), with the exception of −297 (T to A), which had an allele frequency of 0.20. A reporter gene containing both G(−35)T/T(−297)A mutations had a 1.8-fold and 2.5-fold higher luciferase activity compared with the wild-type and T(−297)A only, respectively, whereas the rest of the mutations have no functional significance for CYP2E1 expression (Fairbrother *et al.*, 1998).

EXPRESSION OF CYP2E1 GENE IN EXTRAHEPATIC TISSUES

In addition to liver, CYP2E1 is expressed in extrahepatic tissues, e.g. kidney, nasal mucosa, gastrointestinal tract, testis and lymphocytes (Ronis *et al.*, 1996). CYP2E1 is also found in small amounts in rat and human brain, mainly in the neurons of the hippocampus, substantia nigra and striatum, as well as in endothelial cells and some glial cells (see Raunio *et al.*, 1995). It seems probable that CYP2E1 is induced in some extrahepatic tissues, but the significance of extrahepatic activity in the kinetics of drugs *in vivo* is not clear (Shimizu *et al.*, 1990).

CYP3A subfamily

In humans, three members of the CYP3A subfamily, the only subfamily in family 3, have been characterised. These are CYP3A4, CYP3A5 and CYP3A7. Initial reports suggested the existence of a fourth member of this subfamily, designated CYP3A3. However, careful examination of the sequence has shown that this is not the product of a separate gene locus (see Guengerich, 1999). Very recently, Strobel and Nelson (in Nelson, 2000) have identified a fourth member of this subfamily, CYP3A43 (GenEMBL AC011904 8902-46787). CYP3A4 is expressed at high, but variable, levels in liver and small intestine. CYP3A5 is expressed at lower levels in liver, but exhibits a wider tissue distribution than CYP3A4. CYP3A7 is a fetal form, that is not significantly expressed in the adult. CYP3A4 is highly dependent. To date, no generic polymorphism has been identified to account for the wide interindividual variation that occurs in the expression of these enzymes.

CYP3A4

CYP3A4 is, both in terms of content and number of drugs metabolised, the major form of P450 in the liver (Guengerich, 1995; Shimada et al., 1994). It also metabolises a range of dietary and endogenous substrates. CYP3A4 is highly inducible by a range of drugs and other chemicals. Although exhibiting large interindividual variation in its expression and inducibility, no genetic polymorphism has yet been found to account for this.

VARIABILITY OF PROTEIN AND MRNA

CYP3A4 mRNA and apoprotein have been found in all human liver samples studied to date (Edwards et al., 1998; Shimada et al., 1994; Wolbold et al., 2000). This suggests that CYP3A4 is required to metabolise a substrate of some importance, or at least until relatively recently, in evolutionary terms. In immunoblotting studies, CYP3A4 accounts for up to 30%, on average, of total hepatic P450 (Shimada et al., 1994). However, there is very large interindividual variability in expression, with hepatic microsomal apoprotein content varying by forty to fifty-fold (Edwards et al., 1998; Shimada et al., 1994; Tateishi et al., 1999; Wolbold et al., 2000). Studies at the mRNA level similarly show extensive variability (Sumida et al., 1999).

VARIABILITY OF FORM-SPECIFIC ACTIVITY/ACTIVITIES

Several substrates specific for CYP3A4 (and CYP3A5) have been identified, but their study is complicated by the unusual kinetics of the enzyme (Guengerich, 1995). It has recently been established that the active site of

CYP3A4 may accommodate two molecules (of either the same or different compounds) and that these influence the kinetics of the other, some compounds causing positive cooperativeness, homotropic and heterotropic cooperativeness, respectively (Harlow and Halpert, 1998). As the ability to cause such an effect varies with the compound, this can make correlation studies of activity and inhibitory potency very difficult, and sometimes impossible. The solution most often recommended is to use a number of different substrates, falling into three or four different groups (Kenworthy et al., 1999).

Additional complications exist in studying the activity of CYP3A4 in vivo, due to the extensive expression of the enzyme in the small intestine (see below) and the overlap in specificity of substrates for CYP3A4 with P-glycoprotein (Wacher et al., 1995). These factors confound the interpretation of metabolic data obtained following the oral administration of substrates for CYP3A4.

Widely used probe substrates for CYP3A4 include midazolam (1′-hydroxylation) (Kronbach et al., 1989), erythromycin (N-demethylation) (Wrighton et al., 1990). cortisol (6β-hydroxylation) (in vivo) (Ged et al., 1989) and testosterone (6β-hydroxylation) (in vitro) (Waxman et al., 1988). Studies both in vitro and in vivo using such substrates have shown large interindividual variation in CYP3A4-dependency. However, whereas variation ranged up to fifty-fold in vitro, activity (Iyer and Sinz, 1999; Sumida et al., 1999) as with many other P450 enzymes, variation is less marked in vivo (Schellens et al., 1988), approximately five-fold with some substrates (Kinirons et al., 1999). The reasons for this are not clear, but possibly reflect the contribution of non-CYP3A4-dependent elimination in vivo together with some of the other confounding factors discussed above.

OTHER SUBSTRATES/ACTIVITIES

CYP3A4 metabolises a very large number of drugs, other xenobiotic chemicals and endogenous compounds (Li et al., 1995). Hence, no attempt will be made here to provide a comprehensive list. A recent review by Guengerich (1999) provides a relatively up to date list of drugs metabolised by CYP3A4.

CYP3A4 plays a pivotal role in determining the duration and intensity of action of such drugs as cyclosporin A (Aoyama et al., 1989), HIV protease inhibitors (e.g. saquinivir) (Fitzsimmons and Collins, 1997), macrolide antibiotics (e.g. erythromycin) (Wrighton et al., 1990), dihydropyridine calcium antagonists (e.g. nifedipine) (Guengerich et al., 1986), HMGCo reductase inhibitors (e.g. atorvastatin) (Prueksaritanont et al., 1999), benzimidazoles (e.g. lansoprazole) (Pearce et al., 1996a), non-sedative antihistamines (e.g. astemizole) (Woosley, 1996), benzodiazepines (e.g. midazolam) (Gorski et al., 1994), and the anti-convulsant, carbamazepine

(Kerr *et al.*, 1994). In general, the metabolism of such drugs shows wide interindividual variation and is affected by inducers and inhibitors of CYP3A4 (see below).

CYP3A4 also plays a role in the metabolism of dietary and environmental chemicals, the full extent of which has yet to be determined. Substrates include flavanoids (Shou *et al.*, 1994), mycotoxins such as aflatoxin B$_1$ (Shimada and Guengerich, 1989), numerous pesticides (e.g. parathion) (Butler and Murray, 1997), a number of food additives and even non-ionic detergents such as Triton N-101 (Hosea and Guengerich, 1998) and perhaps even certain oligopeptides such as some enkephalins (see Guengerich, 1999).

ENVIRONMENTAL/HOST FACTORS

CYP3A4 can be inhibited by a number of drugs and other exogenous chemicals (Thummel and Wilkinson, 1998). Amongst potent, relatively selective inhibitors of this enzyme are azole antifungal agents such as ketoconazole (Back and Tjia, 1991; von Moltke et al., 1996), macrolide antibiotics such as troleandomycin (Marre *et al.*, 1993; Pichard *et al.*, 1990), HIV protease inhibitors such as saquinavir (Eagling *et al.*, 1997; Kumar *et al.*, 1996), antidepressants such as fluoxetine (Ring *et al.*, 1995), 17α-ethinyl substituted steroids such as gestodene (Guengerich, 1990) and the furanocoumarin, 6′, 7′-dihydroxybergamottin, found in grapefruit juice (Edwards *et al.*, 1996). Many of these compounds produce inhibition by forming tightly-bound complexes with the enzyme or serve as mechanism-based inhibitors (Thummel and Wilkinson, 1998). As a consequence, inhibition may take some time to reach a maximum, and potency *in vivo* may be greater than predicted simply from the K$_i$ determined *in vitro* (see Thummel and Wilkinson, 1998). In addition, recovery from inhibition is often prolonged, as enzyme resynthesis may be necessary. The possibility of cooperative stimulation of CYP3A4 activity was discussed above. One compound that is particularly potent in this respect is α-naphthoflavone, at least *in vitro* (Shou *et al.*, 1994). The extent that such enhancement of activity occurs *in vivo* is not known (see Guengerich, 1999).

The presence of a potent inhibitor of CYP3A4 in grapefruit juice has been demonstrated to influence the bioavailability and hepatic elimination of substrates for this enzyme following dietary consumption of grapefruit juice (Bailey *et al.*, 1998; Clifford *et al.*, 1997). However, it appears that it takes several days of such consumption before inhibition of the hepatic enzyme is apparent (Kivistö *et al.*, 1999). In contrast, the intestinal enzyme is readily inhibited by the consumption of even a single dose of grapefruit juice (Schmiedlin-Ren *et al.*, 1997).

CYP3A4 is inducible by several different classes of compound, both therapeutic agents and dietary chemicals (Maurel, 1996). Amongst drugs that can induce CYP3A4 are certain macrolide antibiotics, although in this case the induced enzyme may be inhibited by the antibiotic (Watkins *et al.*, 1985), rifamycins such as rifampicin (Backman *et al.*, 1996; Roots *et al.*, 1979), anticonvulsants such as carbamazepine (Ogg *et al.*, 1999; Roots *et al.*, 1979) and glucocorticoids such as dexamethasone, although these appear to be only weak inducers in humans (Villikka *et al.*, 1998; Watkins *et al.*, 1985). A recent intriguing observation was that the natural plant remedy St John's Wort contains a potent inducer of CYP3A4 (Moore *et al.*, 2000).

Induction of hepatic CYP3A4 can markedly affect the metabolism and kinetics of substrates for this enzyme. However, the implications of hepatic induction *in vivo* are often confounded by effects on the intestinal enzyme (see below). In general, if intrinsic clearance is not hepatic blood-flow dependent (i.e. less than 1000–1500 ml/min), induction of CYP3A4 in liver will increase systemic metabolism and elimination. When intrinsic clearance is ≥1500 ml/min, induction of hepatic CYP3A4 may contribute to reduced presystemic elimination, depending upon the extent of any intestinal elimination (Wilkinson and Shand, 1975).

Until relatively recently, there was little information on the mechanism of induction of CYP3A4. However, the identification of the pregnane X receptor (PXR) in 1998 (Lehmann *et al.*, 1998), has dramatically increased our understanding of this system. PXR is an orphan nuclear receptor, belonging to the steroid receptor superfamily. On binding of an inducer ligand, the inducer-receptor dimerises with the retinoic acid X receptor (RXR) and the dimer binds to a cognate 5′-upstream response element on the *CYP3A4* gene, resulting in transcriptional activation (Honkakoski and Negishi, 2000; Kliewer *et al.*, 1999). Examination of the upstream region of the *CYP3A4* gene has revealed binding sites for a number of transcription factors including AP-3, hepatocyte nuclear factor-4 and -5 and a glucocorticoid response element (GRE) (Hashimoto *et al.*, 1993). The role that these play in regulating CYP3A4 expression, if any, has yet to be determined.

GENETIC FACTORS

As indicated above, there is considerable interindividual variation in the expression and activity of CYP3A4 in human liver. However, the basis for this variability has yet to be established. Until relatively recently, there were no known polymorphisms of CYP3A4. Over the last couple of years, polymorphisms in both the coding region and the 5′-upstream regulatory region have been reported. The first of these involves a −290 A to G transition in the non-coding upstream region, giving rise to an allele designated CYP3A4*1B (CYP3A4-V) (Rebbeck *et al.*, 1998). The allele is significantly more common amongst African Americans (~30% homozygous for the mutant allele; allele frequency 55%) than in other ethnic groups including White Americans (allele frequency 3.6%), Hispanic Americans (allele frequency 9.3%), Chinese Americans (allele frequency 0%) or Japanese Americans (allele frequency 0%) (Ball *et al.*, 1999; Sata *et al.*, 2000). The mutation occurs in the so-called nifedipine specific element (NFSE), which may comprise a promoter site for the gene (Walker *et al.*, 1998). There have been reports of an association between the CYP3A4*1B genotype and certain pathological conditions, such as prostate cancer (Paris *et al.*, 1999; Rebbeck *et al.*, 1998) and some leukemias (Felix *et al.*, 1998). However, no effect of the mutation has been found on the metabolism of CYP3A4-dependent substrates either *in vivo* or *in vitro*, or on the level of expression of CYP3A4 (Ball *et al.*, 1999; Westlind *et al.*, 1999).

Even more recently, the first report of a polymorphism in the coding region of CYP3A4 has appeared. Two mutations have been identified. In the CYP3A4*2 allele, there is a Ser222Pro change in exon 7 (Sata *et al.*, 2000) and in the CYP3A4*3 allele, there is a Met445Thr change in exon 12 (Sata *et al.*, 2000). The CYP3A4*2 allele was present in Caucasians with a frequency of 2.7%, but was not detected in Black or Chinese subjects. In contrast, the CYP3A4*3 allele was identified in a single Chinese subject. CYP3A4*2 codes for a protein with altered specificity to that of the wild type (Sata *et al.*, 2000). Whilst the intrinsic clearance of nifedipine oxidation was reduced, that of testosterone was not. The functional consequences of the CYP3A4*3 allele, in which the mutation occurs in the conserved heme-binding domain, have yet to be determined.

The frequency of occurrence and functional consequences of the CYP3A4 alleles identified to date are such that they cannot account for the majority of the variability seen in the expression and activity of this enzyme.

EXPRESSION IN EXTRAHEPATIC TISSUES

CYP3A4 is primarily a hepatic enzyme, where it comprises up to 30% of total P450 content (Shimada *et al.*, 1994). However, expression is found in certain other tissues. Studies of mRNA and/or apoprotein expression have established that CYP3A4 is expressed in: gallbladder-derived biliary epithelial cells (mRNA and apoprotein) (Lakehal *et al.*, 1999), pancreas (apoprotein) (Kolars *et al.*, 1994), small intestine (mRNA and apoprotein) (Kolars *et al.*, 1994; McKinnon *et al.*, 1995), kidney (mRNA and apoprotein, <40% of samples) (Haehner *et al.*, 1996; Schuetz *et al.*, 1992), breast tissue (mRNA, most samples) (Huang *et al.*, 1996), peripheral lung and bronchial tissue (mRNA and apoprotein, a few samples) (Anttila *et al.*, 1997). CYP3A4 is not expressed in: oesophageal mucosa (mRNA) (Lechevrel *et al.*, 1999), kidney (mRNA and apoprotein, >60% of samples) (Schuetz *et al.*, 1992; Haehner *et al.*, 1996), neutrophils and other peripheral blood white cells (mRNA and apoprotein) (Janardan *et al.*, 1996), peripheral lung and bronchial tissue (mRNA and apoprotein, most samples) (Anttila *et al.*, 1997), gastric mucosa (mRNA and apoprotein) (Yokose *et al.*, 1998), colon (mRNA and apoprotein, some studies) (Gervot *et al.*, 1996; McKinnon *et al.*, 1995).

In human lung, CYP3A4 mRNA and apoprotein could be detected in the epithelium of less than 20% of the samples, and was confined to bronchial glands, bronchiolar columnar and terminal epithelium, type II alveolar epithelium and also in alveolar macrophages (Anttila *et al.*, 1997). In the small intestine, CYP3A4 is expressed at high levels, 50% of hepatic content and 70% of total P450 present (Kolars *et al.*, 1994; McKinnon *et al.*, 1995). Apoprotein content increases slightly from the duodenum to the jejunum and then decreases considerably towards the ileum (Zhang *et al.*, 1999). Expression in small intestinal epithelium occurs particularly in the apical region of mature enterocytes at the tips of the microvilli (Zhang *et al.*, 1999). Little or no CYP3A4 can be found in the colon (Gervot *et al.*, 1996). In those kidney samples in which CYP3A4 can be detected, it is found mainly in the collecting ducts (Haehner *et al.*, 1996).

CYP3A5

CYP3A5 is expressed at lower levels than CYP3A4 in liver, but has a wider tissue distribution. Its specificity is similar to that of CYP3A4, but generally it is less active. If CYP3A5 is inducible, its response is more blunted than that of CYP3A4.

VARIABILITY OF PROTEIN AND MRNA

Initial reports, and even some recent ones, suggested that CYP3A5 was expressed in only a small number of liver samples (Aoyama *et al.*, 1989; Shuetz *et al.*, 1989; Tateishi *et al.*, 1999; Wrighton *et al.*, 1989). However, more recent studies, using sensitive specific antibodies have established that CYP3A5 is expressed in almost all samples, albeit with low levels in approximately 75% of the samples (Edwards *et al.*, 1998). mRNA was also detectable in all samples, with considerable inter-individual variability (Jounaidi *et al.*, 1996). Hepatic CYP3A5 mRNA and apoprotein content vary by fifty-fold or more (Edwards *et al.*, 1998; Jounaidi *et al.*, 1996), although as indicated, the above samples appear to segregate into two groups, amongst which variability is less. In samples with higher levels of expression, apoprotein content varies approximately five-fold (Jounaidi *et al.*, 1996; Tateishi *et al.*, 1999).

VARIABILITY OF FORM-SPECIFIC ACTIVITY/ACTIVITIES

No form-specific substrates for CYP3A5 are known (see Guengerich, 1999). In general, CYP3A5 shows similar specificity to CYP3A4, although it tends to be less active (Ohmori *et al.*, 1998b). However, there are some differences, as indicated below. Given the absence of suitable substrates, it has not been possible to establish the extent of interindividual variability in the activity of this enzyme.

OTHER SUBSTRATES/ACTIVITIES

The substrate specificity of CYP3A5 has not been as extensively studied as that of CYP3A4. CYP3A5 appears to metabolise most of the substrates metabolised by CYP3A4, but there are some important differences (Guengerich, 1999). For example, neither quinidine nor erythromycin appear to be a substrate for CYP3A5 (Aoyama *et al.*, 1989; Wrighton *et al.*, 1990). Of the three primary metabolites of cyclosporin A produced by CYP3A4, only one is produced by CYP3A5 (Aoyama *et al.*, 1989). As indicated above, for those substrates metabolised by both CYP3A4 and CYP3A5, the latter enzyme is generally the less active (Ohmori *et al.*, 1998b). For example, CYP3A5 is less than 20% as active as CYP3A4 at catalysing the N-debutylation of halofantrine (Baune *et al.*, 1999). Similarly, CYP3A5 has both a lower affinity and a lower V_{max} towards indinavir than CYP3A4 (resulting in a fifteen-fold lower Cl_I than that of CYP3A4), whilst producing a different metabolic profile (Koudriakova *et al.*, 1998). CYP3A5 is also much less active towards irinotecan than CYP3A4 (Santos *et al.*, 2000). In addition, the metabolic profile of irinotecan with CYP3A5 differed markedly from that with CYP3A4, with a number of metabolites formed by one enzyme not being produced by the other (Santos *et al.*, 2000). However, CYP3A5 is not always less active than CYP3A4. For example, the 1′-hydroxylation of midazolam is two-fold greater with CYP3A5 than with CYP3A4 (Gorski *et al.*, 1994) and CYP3A5 is more active in catalysing the N-demethylation of oxybutynin (Lukkari *et al.*, 1998). The rate of 4-hydroxylation of midazolam by CYP3A5 is similar to that by CYP3A4 (Gorski *et al.*, 1994) as are the kinetics of metabolism of ritonavir (Koudriakova *et al.*, 1998).

ENVIRONMENTAL/HOST FACTORS

CYP3A5 appears to be inhibited by many of the compounds that inhibit CYP3A4, although detailed information is lacking (Ohmori *et al.*, 1998b). Ketoconazole is a slightly less potent inhibitor of CYP3A5 than CYP3A4 (Gibbs *et al.*, 1999). Similarly, fluconazole was less potent towards CYP3A5 (Gibbs *et al.*, 1999). Itraconazole was also a less potent inhibitor of CYP3A5 than CYP3A4 (Gibbs *et al.*, 1999). The potency of triacetyloleandomycin was similar with the two enzymes (Ohmori *et al.*, 1998b). Although the inducibility of CYP3A5 has been studied much less than that of CYP3A4, the available evidence would suggest that it is much less inducible, if at all, at least to the types of inducer that increase the expression of CYP3A4, such as rifampicin (Chang *et al.*, 1997; Schuetz *et al.*, 1993b; Wrighton *et al.*, 1989). The consensus binding site for PXR:RXR in the 5′-upstream region of CYP3A5 is similar to, but distinct from that for CYP3A4, which might explain the reduced/absent inducibility of the former enzyme. There is evidence that CYP3A5 may be inducible by glucocorticoids (Hukkanen *et al.*, 2000), via the glucocorticoid receptor and an upstream GRE (Schuetz *et al.*, 1996).

GENETIC FACTORS

Little is known about genetic factors affecting the expression or activity of CYP3A5. There has been one report of a C to A point mutation at position 1280 in exon 11, leading to a change in Thr 298 to alanine (Jounaidi *et al.*, 1996). The functional consequences of this mutation are not known. Two out of five liver samples in which CYP3A5 expression was not detectable carried the mutation. The extent to which this mutation explains the bimodal distribution of CYP3A5 expression in human liver, if at all, has yet to be established. Recently, Paulussen *et al.* (2000) identified an allele containing linked mutations at T −369G and A −45G, which are located in transcriptional regulatory elements. These mutations were shown to be associated with increased expression of the *CYP3A5* gene, and may be responsible for the polymorphic expression of this enzyme.

EXPRESSION IN EXTRAHEPATIC TISSUES

Unlike CYP3A4, CYP3A5 is expressed in a wide range of tissues, in many of which it is the predominant member of the CYP3A subfamily present. These include (for both mRNA and apoprotein levels) lung (Anttila *et al.*, 1997), oesophagus (Lechvrel *et al.*, 1999), stomach (Kolars *et al.*, 1994), colon (Gervot *et al.*, 1996), kidney (Haehner *et al.*, 1996; Schuetz *et al.*, 1992), peripheral blood white cells (particularly neutrophils) (Janardan *et al.*, 1996), the anterior pituitary gland (Murray *et al.*, 1995) and gallbladder-derived biliary epithelial cells (Lakehal *et al.*, 1999). CYP3A5 mRNA has also been found in breast tissue (Huang *et al.*, 1996). Reports on the expression of CYP3A5 in the small intestine are somewhat inconsistent, but levels are certainly lower than those of CYP3A4 (Kivistö *et al.*, 1996; Kolars *et al.*, 1992; Lown *et al.*, 1994; McKinnon *et al.*, 1995; Zhang *et al.*, 1999).

Recently, it has been reported that prostate expresses a form of CYP3A5 with a unique 5′-untranslated region (Yamakoshi *et al.*, 1999). This may control specific regulation of this P450 in the prostate, although no further details are available.

In lung, CYP3A5 apoprotein is found in ciliated and mucous cells of the bronchial wall, bronchial glands, bronchiolar columnar and terminal cuboidal epithelium, type I and type II alveolar epithelium, vascular and capillary epithelium and alveolar macrophages (Anttila *et al.*, 1997). In the kidney, CYP3A5 is expressed most prominently in the proximal tubular epithelial cells (Murray *et al.*, 1999). As in the liver, expression of CYP3A5 in the kidney appears to be bimodal, with 4/27 high activity samples (Haehner *et al.*, 1996).

Whilst CYP3A5 expression predominates in the stomach and colon, in the small intestine the major form of CYP3A present is CYP3A4 (Zhang *et al.*, 1999). Nevertheless, in several studies, both CYP3A5 mRNA and apoprotein could be detected in the small intestine. However, levels were much lower than those of CYP3A4 (Kivistö *et al.*, 1996; Kolars *et al.*, 1992; Lown *et al.*, 1994; McKinnon *et al.*, 1995; Zhang *et al.*, 1999).

CYP3A7

CYP3A7 is expressed at high levels in fetal liver during development, but appears to be expressed little if at all in the adult (Greuet *et al.*, 1996; Schuetz *et al.*, 1994; Tateishi *et al.*, 1999). It metabolises both endogenous and exogenous compounds. CYP3A7 is inducible by compounds that induce CYP3A4.

VARIABILITY OF PROTEIN AND MRNA

There is very little information on interindividual variation in the expression of CYP3A7. In one study, in which it was reported that CYP3A7 apoprotein could be detected in adult liver, levels varied by forty-fold (Tateishi *et al.*, 1999). In contrast, variability in fetal liver is reportedly much less, one study indicating <2.5-fold variation amongst samples (Schuetz *et al.*, 1994). These studies are difficult to compare because of confounding factors related to post-mortem changes and handling of the material before and after collection/freezing. The fetal age may also be difficult to assess precisely, as well as the clinical features of the mother.

VARIABILITY OF FORM-SPECIFIC ACTIVITY/ACTIVITIES

CYP3A7 catalyses the 1'- and 4'-hydroxylation of midazolam (Gillam *et al.*, 1997; Gorski *et al.*, 1994). Although the activities are approximately five-fold lower than those of CYP3A4 (Gillam *et al.*, 1997), they can be used as marker activities for CYP3A7 in samples, such as fetal liver, in which no other member of the CYP3A subfamily is expressed (Schuetz *et al.*, 1994). There was a ten-fold variation in both of these activities amongst fetal samples (Gorski *et al.*, 1994).

OTHER SUBSTRATES/ACTIVITIES

CYP3A7 metabolises many of the substrates metabolised by CYP3A4, albeit with significant differences in activity (Gillam *et al.*, 1997). CYP3A7 catalyses the 16α-hydroxylation of dehydroepiandrosterone and of its 3-sulphate much more actively than either CYP3A4 or CYP3A5 (Lacroix *et al.*, 1997; Ohmori *et al.*, 1998b). CYP3A7 has similar activity to CYP3A4 and CYP3A5 at catalysing the N-demethylation of ethylmorphine and erythromycin (Gillam *et al.*, 1997). In contrast, CYP3A7 was less active than CYP3A4 at 6β-hydroxylation of testosterone, the 10,11-epoxidation of carbamazepine, the reduction of zonisamide (Ohmori *et al.*, 1998b) and the oxidation of nifedipine (Gillam *et al.*, 1997). CYP3A7 catalyses the 6β-hydroxylation of cortisol at a similar rate to that which it catalyses the 6β-hydroxylation of testosterone (Ohmori *et al.*, 1998a). CYP3A7 also catalyses benzyloxyresorufin O-debenzylation (Yang *et al.*, 1994). There is evidence that CYP3A7 has similar activity to CYP3A4 in catalysing the oxidative activation of mycotoxins such as aflatoxin B_1 and sterigmatocystin (Gillam *et al.*, 1997; Hashimoto *et al.*, 1995a) and hydrocarbons such as benzo[a]pyrene 7,8-diol and 6-aminochrysene (Gillam *et al.*, 1997). CYP3A7 also appears to catalyse the N-hydroxylation of heterocyclic aromatic amines such as MeIQx at rates which may be similar to those of CYP3A4 (Gillam *et al.*, 1997; Hashimoto *et al.*, 1995b). Unlike CYP3A4 and CYP3A5, CYP3A7 was inactive towards irinotecan (Santos *et al.*, 2000).

ENVIRONMENTAL/HOST FACTORS

CYP3A7 is inhibited by some of the compounds that inhibit CYP3A4 and CYP3A5, although there are differences in the specificity of inhibition. For example, triazolam inhibited the 6β-hydroxylation of testosterone by CYP3A7, but not by CYP3A4 (Ohmori *et al.*, 1998b). Triacetyloleando-mycin, a diagnostic inhibitor of CYP3A4, inhibited the activity of CYP3A7 whilst alpha-naphthoflavone stimulated activity (Hashimoto *et al.*, 1995a; Yang *et al.*, 1994), although Ohmori *et al.* (1995b) found no inhibition of CYP3A7 with triacetyloleandomycin.

CYP3A7 appears to exhibit similar inducibility to CYP3A4 (Schuetz *et al.*, 1993b). The 5′-upstream region of the CYP3A7 gene possesses a similar PXR responsive promoter to CYP3A4, and is inducible by rifampicin and clotrimazole (Pascussi *et al.*, 1999). Interestingly, whilst CYP3A7 mRNA was induced by rifampicin in cultured adult hepatocytes, the corresponding protein remained undetectable (Greuet *et al.*, 1996).

GENETIC FACTORS

To date, there have been no reports of variant alleles of CYP3A7.

EXPRESSION IN EXTRAHEPATIC TISSUES

CYP3A7 is expressed primarily in fetal hepatic tissue, particularly when analysed at the protein level (Greuet et al., 1996; Kitada et al., 1985a; Schuetz et al., 1994). The highest levels of CYP3A protein are found in fetal liver, where it accounts for 30–50% of the total P450 present (Wrighton and Vandenbranden, 1989). Expression is detectable very early on, in the embryonic stage (Yang et al., 1994). Levels vary with gestational age, and are reportedly greatest during the first week after birth (Lacroix et al., 1997). Thereafter, levels decline to very low to undetectable in adult liver (Lacroix et al., 1997; de Wildt et al., 1999). Some, though not all, recent reports suggest that CYP3A7, at levels approximately 5–20% of those of CYP3A4, can be detected in the majority of adult liver samples (Greuet et al., 1996; Schuetz et al., 1994; Tateishi et al., 1999). The decline in CYP3A7 after birth is paralleled by an increase in CYP3A4 expression such that the total CYP3A content of the liver remains relatively constant (Lacroix et al., 1997; de Wildt et al., 1999).

In addition to fetal liver, CYP3A7 expression has been reported in fetal adrenal (apoprotein) (Kitada et al., 1985b), placenta (mRNA and apoprotein) (Schuetz et al., 1993a), adult endometrium (mRNA and apoprotein) (Schuetz et al., 1993a), adult liver (mRNA and apoprotein; most samples) (Schuetz et al., 1994; Tateishi et al., 1999), gallbladder-derived biliary epithelial cells (mRNA, very low levels) (Lakehal et al., 1999) and adult kidney (mRNA) (Murray et al., 1999). There are unconfirmed reports of low CYP3A7 expression in fetal lung, kidney, spleen and thymus (Ladona et al., 1988).

Endometrial expression of CYP3A7 increases in pregnancy (twelve-fold) (Schuetz et al., 1993a). Both endometrial and placental levels appear to increase from the first to the second trimester of pregnancy, declining to undetectable levels by full term (Schuetz et al., 1993a). Even at their maximum, levels of CYP3A7 in placenta are very low (Hakkola et al., 1996; Schuetz et al., 1993a). In adult kidney, expression was restricted largely to the proximal epithelial cells (Murray et al., 1999).

There is some evidence that the expression of CYP3A7 is increased in certain types of cancer, including hepatocellular carcinoma (Kondah et al., 1999).

No detectable expression of CYP3A7 was found in embryonic lung (apoprotein) (Yang et al., 1994), embryonic kidney (apoprotein) (Yang et al., 1994), embryonic heart (apoprotein) (Yang et al., 1994), embryonic adrenal (apoprotein) (Yang et al., 1994), embryonic brain (apoprotein) (Yang et al., 1994), adult lung (mRNA and apoprotein) (Anttila et al., 1997), peripheral blood white cells (mRNA and apoprotein) (Janardan et al., 1996), adult stomach, jejunum, colon and pancreas (mRNA and apoprotein) (Kolars et al., 1994) and adult duodenum (mRNA) (Kivistö et al., 1996).

Extrapolation from *in vitro* to *in vivo*

Although this chapter deals with *in vitro* variability of CYP-associated drug metabolism in humans, it might be useful to consider to what extent and how this variability is reflected in *in vivo* metabolic elimination of drugs. Here we give only some basic considerations and a few examples; for a more detailed treatment of the subject, the reader is referred to some recent review articles (Rodriguez, 1994; Pelkonen *et al.*, 1998; Boobis, 1999).

In vitro studies of metabolism may include information on metabolism pattern, rates of metabolism for individual pathways, *in vitro* metabolic ratios, inhibitory effects on enzyme pathways, etc. As discussed below, this information may be compared with data from *in vivo* studies on drug kinetics. The *in vivo* kinetics may be documented by estimation of elimination rate constants, clearance rates, steady-state levels, metabolic ratios in blood and urine, etc. In addition, studies on panels of pharmacogenetic phenotypes may be performed and compared with pharmacogenetic information obtained from *in vitro* studies.

The relation between clearance (Cl) and the elimination rate constant (k) is described as:

$$Cl = k \times V_d \tag{1}$$
where V_d = volume of distribution.

The relation between Cl, intrinsic metabolic clearance (Cl_i), blood flow (Q), and extraction ratio (E) is given by the following expressions (Rowland *et al.*, 1973; Wilkinson and Shand, 1975):

$$Cl = Q \times E \tag{2}$$
$$Cl = Q \times [Cl_i/Cl_i + Q] \tag{3}$$

From equation 3 it is obvious that high or low values for Cl_i will simplify the equation. Thus, for high clearance drugs

$$Cl = Q \tag{4}$$

whereas for low clearance drugs,

$$Cl = Cl_i \tag{5}$$

How is quantitative information on clearance obtained *in vitro*? According to Michaelis–Menten expression for velocity of an enzyme reaction:

$$V = V_{max} \times [S]/K_m + [S] \tag{6}$$

When [S] is considerably lower than the value of K_m, which is the case in most therapeutic situations, equation (6) reduces to:

$$V = V_{max} \times [S]/K_m \tag{7}$$

In this situation, which prevails for most drugs under *in vivo* conditions, Cl_i (intrinsic metabolic clearance) may be expressed as a rate constant for the first order reaction:

$$v/[S] = V_{max}/K_m \tag{8}$$

V_{max}/K_m is expressed as volume/time and has been compared with data on Cl_i obtained *in vivo* in pharmacokinetic investigations.

Below follow a few examples where successful estimations of *in vivo* clearance, or hepatic extraction ratio have been made from *in vitro* metabolic data.

In one of the earliest studies on *in vitro/in vivo* extrapolation (Rane *et al.*, 1977) a good prediction of the extraction ratio (E) in the isolated perfused rat liver was demonstrated for a series of drugs belonging to three categories with high, medium, and low extraction ratios, respectively. Estimates of V_{max}/K_m (Cl_i) for these drugs were made from enzyme kinetics data in liver microsomes. The predicted E was calculated as $E_{predicted} = [Cl_i/Cl_i + Q]$. A high degree of correlation between $E_{predicted}$ and $E_{observed}$ ($r = 0.988$) was observed. This study demonstrated that it is possible to classify drugs on the basis of *in vitro* data into different categories in respect of their extraction ratios.

Recently, Carlile *et al.* (1998) investigated the relative importance of V_{max} and K_m in the Cl_i expression for different drug substrates of CYP2C9. Their V_{max} and K_m varied approximately between four- and twenty-fold. The relative Cl_i p/o, which indicates the ratio between predicted *in vitro* and observed *in vivo* estimate of Cl_i, correlated well with K_m for the different drugs ($r = 0.96$). On the other hand, Cl_i p/o did not correlate with V_{max} ($r = -0.21$). This study demonstrates the complex relation that exists between *in vitro* and *in vivo* estimates of the same pharmacokinetic parameters.

Qualitative information of *in vivo* drug kinetics may also be obtained *in vitro* in tissue preparations. Mortimer *et al.* (1990) studied the *in vitro* metabolism of codeine and dextromethorphan in human liver preparations from several individuals. Panels of extensive and poor metabolisers of dextromethorphan were included. Both probe drugs are metabolised by CYP2D6, and this enzyme was quantitated by Western blotting using a monoclonal antibody. The O-demethylation of codeine correlated highly with the O-demethylation of dextromethorphan. In addition, there was a high correlation ($r = 0.95$) between the rates of O-demethylation and CYP2D6 band intensity in Western blots. It was concluded that codeine

Table 10.5 Useful information about in vitro metabolism of drugs and new chemical
entities for the prediction of in vivo behavior of these substances

Type of in vitro information	Usefulness
Individual enzyme assignment for each metabolic pathway	Prediction of variability and interactions at an enzyme level Prediction of role of polymorphisms
Metabolic pattern	Prediction of role of various pathways to kinetic behavior
Organ/tissue-specific enzyme and metabolic data	Prediction of kinetic behavior in patients with specific organ diseases Prediction of metabolism in target organs
Michaelis–Menten kinetic parameters (V_{max}, K_m)	Prediction of in vivo clearance (in the same organ)

may be used as a probe drug for *in vitro* identification of extensive and poor metabolisers.

In summary, several models for *in vitro* to *in vivo* prediction have been tested and described. Quantitative *in vitro* estimates of Cl_i are predictive of the hepatic extraction ratio, at least for several drugs that are oxidised. Metabolic ratios observed *in vitro* are predictive of the corresponding ratios *in vivo*. Finally, metabolism patterns in microsomal preparations and isolated cells may be predictive of the pattern of metabolism in isolated cells and *in vivo*, respectively. Further exploration of other drugs in this respect should increase our knowledge of the prediction models and their usefulness in drug metabolism research. This review ends with an appropriate Table which summarises the usefulness of *in vitro* data for prediction of *in vivo* metabolism and kinetics (Table 10.5).

References

Abdel-Razzak, Z., Loyer, P., Fautrel, A., Gautier, J. C., Corcos, L., Turlin, B., Beaune, P. and Guillouzo, A. (1993) 'Cytokines down-regulate expression of major cytochrome P-450 enzymes in adult human hepatocytes in primary culture', *Mol. Pharmacol.* 44: 707–15.

Andersen, M. R., Farin, F. M. and Omiecinski, C. J. (1998) 'Quantification of multiple human cytochrome P450 mRNA molecules using competitive reverse transcriptase-PCR', *DNA Cell Biol.* 17: 231–8.

Andersson, T., Holmberg, J., Rohss, K. and Walan, A. (1998) 'Pharmacokinetics and effect on caffeine metabolism of the proton pump inhibitors, omeprazole, lansoprazole, and pantoprazole', *Br. J. Clin. Pharmacol.* 45: 369–75.

Andersson, T., Miners, J. O., Veronese, M. E., Tassaneeyakul, W., Meyer, U. A. and Birkett, D. J. (1993) 'Identification of human liver cytochrome P450 isoforms mediating omeprazole metabolism', *Br. J. Clin. Pharmacol.* 36: 521–30.

Anttila, S., Hukkanen, J., Hakkola, J., Stjernvall, T., Beaune, P., Edwards, R. J., Boobis, A. R., Pelkonen, O. and Raunio, H. (1997) 'Expression and localization of CYP3A4 and CYP3A5 in human lung', *Am. J. Respir. Cell Mol. Biol.* **16**: 242–9.

Aoyama, T., Yamano, S., Waxman, D. J., Lapenson, D. P., Meyer, U. A., Fischer, V., Tyndale, R., Inaba, T., Kalow, W., Gelboin, H. V. and Gonzalez, F. J. (1989) 'Cytochrome P-450 hPCN3, a novel cytochrome P-450 IIIA gene product that is differentially expressed in adult human liver. cDNA and deduced amino acid sequence and distinct specificities of cDNA-expressed hPCN1 and hPCN3 for the metabolism of steroid hormones and cyclosporine', *J. Biol. Chem.* **264**: 10388–95.

Back, D. J. and Tjia, J. F. (1991) 'Comparative effects of the antimycotic drugs ketoconazole, fluconazole, itraconazole and terbinafine on the metabolism of cyclosporin by human liver microsomes', *Br. J. Clin. Pharmacol.* **32**: 624–6.

Backlund, M., Johansson, I., Mkrtchian, S. and Ingelman-Sundberg, M. (1997) 'Signal transduction-mediated activation of the aryl hydrocarbon receptor in rat hepatoma H4IIe cells', *J. Biol. Chem.* **272**: 31755–63.

Backman, J. T., Olkkola, K. T. and Neuvonen, P. J. (1996) 'Rifampin drastically reduces plasma concentrations and effects of oral midazolam', *Clin. Pharmacol. Ther.* **59**: 7–13.

Bailey, D. G., Malcolm, J., Arnold, O. and Spence, J. D. (1998) 'Grapefruit juice–drug interactions', *Br. J. Clin. Pharmacol.* **46**: 101–10.

Ball, S. E., Scatina, J., Kao, J., Ferron, G. M., Fruncillo, R., Mayer, P., Weinryb, I., Guida, M., Hopkins, P. J., Warner, N. and Hall, J. (1999) 'Population distribution and effects on drug metabolism of a genetic variant in the 5′ promoter region of CYP3A4', *Clin. Pharmacol. Ther.* **66**: 288–94.

Baune, B., Flinois, J. P., Furlan, V., Gimenez, F., Taburet, A. M., Becquemont, L. and Farinotti, R. (1999) 'Halofantrine metabolism in microsomes in man: major role of CYP 3A4 and CYP 3A5', *J. Pharm. Pharmacol.* **51**: 419–26.

Beaune, P. H., Kremers, P. G., Kaminsky, L. S., De Graeve, J., Albert, A. and Guengerich, F. P. (1986) 'Comparison of monooxygenase activities, and cytochrome P-450 isozyme concentrations in human liver microsomes', *Drug Metab. Dispos.* **14**: 437–42.

Beresford, A. P., Ellis, W. J., Ayrton, J., Johnson, M. A. and Lewis, D. F. (1997) 'Cytochrome P4501A (CYP1A) induction in rat and man by the benzodioxino derivative, fluparoxan', *Xenobiotica* **27**: 159–73.

Boobis, A. R. (1999) 'Changing the in vivo extrapolation of in vitro drug metabolism data from fantasy to reality', in, A. R. Boobis, P. Kremers, O. Pelkonen and K. Pithan (eds) *Drug Metabolism in Man*, Luxembourg, EUR 18569, pp. 1–35.

Boobis, A. R., Kremers, P., Pelkonen, O. and Pithan, K. (eds) (1999) *European Symposium on the Prediction of Drug Metabolism in Man: Progress and Problems.* Luxembourg, EUR 18569, 332 pp.

Boobis, A. R., McKillop, D., Robinson, D. T., Adams, D. A. and McCormick, D. J. (1998) 'Interlaboratory comparison of the assessment of P450 activities in human hepatic microsomal samples', *Xenobiotica* **28**: 493–506.

Bourrie, M., Meunier, V., Berger, Y. and Fabre, G. (1996) 'Cytochrome P450 isoform inhibitors as a tool for the investigation of metabolic reactions catalyzed by human liver microsomes', *J. Pharmacol. Exp. Therap.* **277**: 321–32.

Burke, M. D., Thompson, S., Weaver, R. J., Wolf, C. R. and Mayer, R. T. (1994) 'Cytochrome P450 specificities of alkoxyresorufin O-dealkylation in human and rat liver', *Biochem. Pharmacol.* **48**: 923–36.

Butler, A. M. and Murray, M. (1997) Biotransformation of parathion in human liver: participation of CYP3A4 and its inactivation during microsomal parathion oxidation', *J. Pharmacol. Exp. Ther.* 280: 966–73.

Butler, M. A., Iwasaki, M., Guengerich, F. P. and Kadlubar, F. F. (1989) 'Human cytochrome P-450PA (P-450IA2), the phenacetin O-deethylase, is primarily responsible for the hepatic 3-demethylation of caffeine and N-oxidation of carcinogenic arylamines', *Proc. Natl. Acad. Sci. USA* 86: 7696–700.

Butler, M. A., Lang, N. P., Young, J. F., Caporaso, N. E., Vineis, P., Hayes, R. B., Teitel, C. H., Massengill, J. P., Lawsen, M. F. and Kadlubar, F. F. (1992) 'Determination of CYP1A2 and NAT2 phenotypes in human populations by analysis of caffeine urinary metabolites', *Pharmacogenetics* 2: 116–27.

Carlile, D. J., Bayliss, M. K. and Houston, J. B. (1998) 'Prediction of intrinsic clearance of CYP2C9 substrates in man using hepatic microsomes: importance of Km', *Br. J. Clin. Pharmacol.* 45: 512–3.

Carpenter, S. P., Lasker, J. M. and Raucy, J. L. (1996) 'Expression, induction, and catalytic activity of the ethanol-inducible cytochrome P450 (CYP2E1) in human fetal liver and hepatocytes', *Mol. Pharmacol.* 49: 260–8.

Carriere, V., Berthou, F., Baird, S., Belloc, C., Beaune, P. and de Waziers, I. (1996) 'Human cytochrome P450 2E1 (CYP2E1): from genotype to phenotype', *Pharmacogenetics* 6: 203–11.

Cashman, J. R., Park, S. B., Yang, Z.-C., Wrighton, S. A., Jacob, P. and Benowitz, N. L. (1992) 'Metabolism of nicotine by human liver microsomes: stereoselective formation of trans-nicotine N'-oxide', *Chem. Res. Toxicol.* 5: 639–46.

Chang, T. K. H. and Waxman, D. J. (1996) 'The CYP2A subfamily', in, C. Ioannides (ed.) *Cytochromes P450. Metabolic and Toxicological Aspects*, Boca Raton: CRC Press, pp. 99–134.

Chang, T. K., Yu, L., Maurel, P. and Waxman, D. J. (1997) 'Enhanced cyclophosphamide and ifosfamide activation in primary human hepatocyte cultures: response to cytochrome P-450 inducers and autoinduction by oxazaphosphorines', *Cancer Res.* 57: 1946–54.

Chen, G.-F., Tang, Y. M., Green, B., Lin, D.-X., Guengerich, F. P., Daly, A. K., Caporaso, N. E. and Kadlubar, F. F. (1999) 'Low frequency of CYP2A6 gene polymorphism as revealed by a one-step polymerase chain reaction method', *Pharmacogenetics* 9: 327–32.

Clifford, C. P., Adams, D. A., Murray, S., Taylor, G. W., Wilkins, M. R., Boobis, A. R. and Davies, D. S. (1997) 'The cardiac effects of terfenadine after inhibition of its metabolism by grapefruit juice', *Eur. J. Clin. Pharmacol.* 52: 311–5.

Code, E. L., Crespi, C. L., Penman, B. W., Gonzalez, F. J., Chang, T. K. and Waxman, D. J. (1997) 'Human cytochrome P4502B6: interindividual hepatic expression, substrate specificity, and role in procarcinogen activation', *Drug Metab. Dispos.* 25: 985–93.

Crespi, C. L., Miller, V. P. and Penman, B. W. (1997) 'Microtiter plate assays for inhibition of human drug metabolizing cytochrome P450', *Anal. Biochem.* 248: 188–90.

Czerwinski, M., McLemore, T., Gelboin, H. and Gonzalez, F. (1994) 'Quantification of CYP2B7, CYP4B1, and CYPOR messenger RNAs in normal human lung and lung tumors', *Cancer Res.* 54: 1085–91.

Dalet-Beluche, I., Boulenc, X., Fabre, G., Maurel, P. and Bonfils, C. (1992) 'Purification of two cytochrome P450 isozymes related to CYP2A and CYP3A gene families from monkey (baboon, Papio papio) liver microsomes. Cross reactivity with human forms', *Eur. J. Biochem.* **204**: 641–8.

Daujat, M., Charrasse, S., Fabre, I., Lesca, P., Jounaidi, Y., Larroque, C., Poellinger, L. and Maurel, P. (1996) 'Induction of CYP1A1 gene by benzimidazole derivatives during Caco-2 cell differentiation. Evidence for an aryl-hydrocarbon receptor-mediated mechanism', *Eur. J. Biochem.* **237**: 642–52.

Daujat, M., Peryt, B., Lesca, P., Fourtanier, G., Domergue, J. and Maurel, P. (1992) 'Omeprazole, an inducer of human CYP1A1 and 1A2 is not a ligand for the Ah receptor', *Biochem. Biophys. Res. Commun.* **188**: 820–5.

de Groot, M. J., Bijloo, G. J., Martens, B. J., van Acker, F. A. and Vermeulen, N. P. (1997) 'A refined substrate model for human cytochrome P450 2D6', *Chem. Res. Toxicol.* **10**: 41–8.

de Waziers, I., Garlatti, M., Bouguet, J., Beaune, P. H. and Barouki, R. (1995) 'Insulin down-regulates cytochrome P450 2B and 2E expression at the post-transcriptional level in the rat hepatoma cell line', *Mol. Pharmacol.* **47**: 474–9.

de Wildt, S. N., Kearns, G. L., Leeder, J. S. and van den Anker, J. N. (1999) 'Cytochrome P450 3A: ontogeny and drug disposition', *Clin. Pharmacokinet.* **37**: 485–505.

Ding, X., Zhuo, X., Zhang, J. and Zhang, Q.-Y. (2000) 'Nuclear factors involved in the control of CYP1A2 and CYP2A genes in the olfactory mucosa', Abstracts of 13th International Symposium on Microsomes and Drug Oxidations, Stresa, Italy, Abstr. S10-4: 77.

Doostdar, H., Burke, M. D. and Mayer, R. T. (2000) 'Bioflavonoids: selective substrates and inhibitors for cytochrome P450 CYP1A and CYP1B1', *Toxicology* **144**: 31–8.

Drahushuk, A. T., McGarrigle, B. P., Larsen, K. E., Stegeman, J. J. and Olson, J. R. (1998) 'Detection of CYP1A1 protein in human liver and induction by TCDD in precision-cut liver slices incubated in dynamic organ culture', *Carcinogenesis* **19**: 1361–8.

Eagling, V. A., Back, D. J. and Barry, M. G. (1997) 'Differential inhibition of cytochrome P450 isoforms by the protease inhibitors: ritonavir, saquinavir and indinavir', *Br. J. Clin. Pharmacol.* **44**: 190–4.

Edwards, D. J., Bellevue, F. H. 3rd and Woster, P. M. (1996) 'Identification of 6′,7′-dihydroxybergamottin, a cytochrome P450 inhibitor, in grapefruit juice', *Drug Metab. Dispos.* **24**: 1287–90.

Edwards, R. J., Adams, D. A., Watts, P. S., Davies, D. S. and Boobis, A. R. (1998) 'Development of a comprehensive panel of antibodies against the major xenobiotic metabolising forms of cytochrome P450 in humans', *Biochem. Pharmacol.* **56**: 377–87.

Edwards, R. J., Murray, B. P., Singleton, A. M. and Boobis, A. R. (1991) 'The orientation of cytochromes P450 in the endoplasmic reticulum', *Biochemistry* **30**: 71–6.

Eiermann, B., Engel, G., Johansson, I., Zanger, U. M. and Bertilsson, L. (1997) 'The involvement of CYP1A2 and CYP3A4 in the metabolism of clozapine', *Br. J. Clin. Pharmacol.* **44**: 439–46.

Ekins, S., Bravi, G., Binkley, S., Gillespie, J. S., Ring, B. J., Wikel, J. H. and Wrighton, S. A. (2000) 'Three and four dimensional quantitative structure activity relationship (3D/4D-QSAR) analyses of CYP2C9 inhibitors', *Drug Metab. Dispos.* **28**: 994–1002.

Ekins, S., Bravi, G., Ring, B. J., Gillespie, T. A., Gillespie, J. S., Vandenbranden, M., Wrighton, S. A. and Wikel, J. H. (1999) 'Three-dimensional quantitative structure activity relationship analyses of substrates for CYP2B6', *J. Pharmacol. Exp. Ther.* 288: 21–9.

Ekins, S., Vandenbranden, M., Ring, B. J., Gillespie, J. S., Yang, T. J., Gelboin, H. V. and Wrighton, S. A. (1998) 'Further characterization of the expression in liver and catalytic activity of CYP2B6', *J. Pharmacol. Exp. Ther.* 286: 1253–9.

Ekins, S., Vandenbranden, M., Ring, B. J. and Wrighton, S. A. (1997) 'Examination of purported probes of human CYP2B6', *Pharmacogenetics* 7: 165–79.

Ekins, S. and Wrighton, S. A. (1999) 'The role of CYP2B6 in human xenobiotic metabolism', *Drug Metab. Rev.* 31: 719–54.

Ekstrom, G., von Bahr, C. and Ingelman-Sundberg, M. (1989) 'Human liver microsomal cytochrome P-450IIE1. Immunological evaluation of its contribution to microsomal, ethanol oxidation, carbon tetrachloride reduction and NADPH oxidase activity', *Biochem. Pharmacol.* 38: 689–93.

Eliasson, E., Johansson, I. and Ingelman-Sundberg, M. (1988) 'Ligand-dependent maintenance of ethanol-inducible cytochrome P-450 in primary rat hepatocyte cell cultures', *Biochem. Biophys. Res. Commun.* 150: 436–43.

Eliasson, E., Johansson, I. and Ingelman-Sundberg, M. (1990) 'Substrate-, hormone, and cAMP-regulated cytochrome P450 degradation', *Proc. Natl. Acad. Sci. USA* 87: 3225–9.

Fairbrother, K. S., Grove, J., de Waziers, I., Steimel, D. T., Day, C. P., Crespi, C. L. and Daly, A. K. (1998) 'Detection and characterization of novel polymorphisms in the CYP2E1 gene', *Pharmacogenetics* 8: 543–52.

Felix, C. A., Walker, A. H., Lange, B. J., Williams, T. M., Winick, N. J., Cheung, N. K., Lovett, B. D., Nowell, P. C., Blair, I. A. and Rebbeck, T. R. (1998) 'Association of CYP3A4 genotype with treatment-related leukemia', *Proc. Natl. Acad. Sci. USA* 95: 13176–81.

Fernandez-Salguero, P. and Gonzalez, F. J. (1995) 'The CYP2A gene subfamily: species differences, regulation, catalytic activities and role in chemical carcinogenesis', *Pharmacogenetics* 5: S123–8.

Fernandez-Salguero, P., Hoffman, S. M. G., Cholerton, S., Mohrenweiser, H., Raunio, H., Rautio, A., Pelkonen, O., Huang, J., Evans, W. E., Idle, J. R. and Gonzalez, F. J. (1995) 'A genetic polymorphism in coumarin 7-hydroxylation: sequence of the human CYP2A genes and identification of variant CYP2A6 alleles', *Am. J. Hum. Genet.* 57: 651–60.

Ferrini, J. B., Pichard, L., Domergue, J. and Maurel, P. (1997) 'Long term primary cultures and human hepatocytes', *Chem.-Biol. Interact.* 107: 31–45.

Fitzsimmons, M. E. and Collins, J. M. (1997) 'Selective biotransformation of the human immunodeficiency virus protease inhibitor saquinavir by human small-intestinal cytochrome P4503A4: potential contribution to high first-pass metabolism', *Drug Metab.* Dispos. 25: 256–66.

Fonne-Pfister, R. and Meyer, U. A. (1988) 'Xenobiotic and endobiotic inhibitors of cytochrome P-450dbl function, the target of the debrisoquine/sparteine type polymorphism', *Biochem. Pharmacol.* 37: 3829–35.

Fontana, R. J., Lown, K. S., Paine, M. F., Fortlage, L., Santella, R. M., Felton, J. S., Knize, M. G., Greenberg, A. and Watkins, P. B. (1999) 'Effects of a chargrilled meat diet on expression of CYP3A, CYP1A, and P-glycoprotein levels in healthy volunteers', *Gastroenterology* 117: 89–98.

Foster, J. R., Idle, J. R., Hardwick, J. P., Bars, R., Scott, P. and Braganza, J. M. (1993) 'Induction of drug-metabolizing enzymes in human pancreatic cancer and chronic pancreatitis', *J. Pathol.* 169: 457–63.

Fuhr, U., Anders, E. M., Mahr, G., Sorgel, F. and Staib, A. H. (1992) 'Inhibitory potency of quinoline antibacterial agents against cytochrome P450IA2 activity in vivo and in vitro', *Antimicrob. Agents Chemother.* 36: 942–8.

Fuhr, U., Doehmer, J., Battula, N., Wolfel, C., Flick, I., Kudla, C., Keita, Y. and Staib, A. H. (1993) 'Biotransformation of methylxanthines in mammalian cell lines genetically engineered for expression of single cytochrome P450 isoforms. Allocation of metabolic pathways to isoforms and inhibitory effects of quinolones', *Toxicology* 82: 169–89.

Gallagher, E. P., Wienkers, L. C., Stapleton, P. L., Kunze, K. L. and Eaton, D. L. (1994) 'Role of human microsomal and human complementary DNA-expressed cytochromes P4501A2 and P4503A4 in the bioactivation of aflatoxin B1', *Cancer Res.* 54: 101–8.

Ged, C., Rouillon, J. M., Pichard, L., Combalbert, J., Bressot, N., Bories, P., Michel, H., Beaune, P. and Maurel, P. (1989) 'The increase in urinary excretion of 6 beta-hydroxycortisol as a marker of human hepatic cytochrome P450IIIA induction', *Br. J. Clin. Pharmacol.* 28: 373–87.

Gervot, L., Carrière, V., Costet, P., Cugnenc, P.-H., Berger, A., Beaune, P. H. and de Waziers, I. (1996) 'CYP3A5 is the major cytochrome P450 3A expressed in human colon and colonic cell lines', *Environ. Toxicol. Pharmacol.* 2: 381–8.

Gervot, L., Rochat, B., Gautier, J. C., Bohnenstengel, F., Kroemer, H., de Berardinis, V., Martin, H., Beaune, P. and de Waziers, I. (1999) 'Human CYP2B6: expression, inducibility and catalytic activities', *Pharmacogenetics* 9: 295–306.

Gibbs, M. A., Thummel, K. E., Shen, D. D. and Kunze, K. L. (1999). Inhibition of cytochrome P-450 3A (CYP3A) in human intestinal and liver microsomes: comparison of Ki values and impact of CYP3A5 expression', *Drug Metab. Dispos.* 27: 180–7.

Gillam, E. M., Wunsch, R. M., Ueng, Y. F., Shimada, T., Reilly, P. E., Kamataki, T. and Guengerich, F. P. (1997) 'Expression of cytochrome P450 3A7 in Escherichia coli: effects of 5′ modification and catalytic characterization of recombinant enzyme expressed in bicistronic format with NADPH-cytochrome P450 reductase', *Arch. Biochem. Biophys.* 346: 81–90.

Goldstein, J. A. and de Morais, S. M. F. (1994) 'Biochemistry and molecular biology of the human CYP2C subfamily', *Pharmacogenetics* 4: 285–99.

Gomez-Lechon, M. J., Donato, M. T., Ponsoda, X., Ricardo, F., Trullenque, R. and Castell, I. V. (1997) 'Isolation, culture and use of human hepatocytes in drug research', in, J. V. Castell and M. Gomez-Lechon (eds) *In Vitro Methods in Pharmaceutical Research*, New York: Academic Press, pp. 129–54.

Gonzalez, F. J. and Korzekwa, K. R. (1995) 'Cytochrome P450 expression systems', *Ann. Rev. Pharmacol. Toxicol.* 35: 369–90.

Gonzalez, F. J., Skoda, R. C., Kimura, S., Umeno, M., Zanger, U. M., Nebert, D. W., Gelboin, H. V., Hardwick, J. P. and Meyer, U. A. (1988) 'Characterization of the common genetic defect in humans deficient in debrisoquine metabolism', *Nature* **331**: 442–6.

Goodwin, B., Hodgson, E. and Liddle, C. (1995) 'The orphan human pregnane X receptor mediates the transcriptional activation of CYP3A4 by rifampicin through a distal enhancer module', *Mol. Pharmacol.* **56**: 1329–39.

Gorski, J. C., Hall, S. D., Jones, D. R., Vandenbranden, M. and Wrighton, S. A. (1994) 'Regioselective biotransformation of midazolam by members of the human cytochrome P450 3A (CYP3A) subfamily', *Biochem. Pharmacol.* **47**: 1643–53.

Greuet, J., Pichard, L., Bonfils, C., Domergue, J. and Maurel, P. (1996) 'The fetal specific gene CYP3A7 is inducible by rifampicin in adult human hepatocytes in primary culture', *Biochem. Biophys. Res. Commun.* **225**: 689–94.

Gu, J., Su, T., Chen, Y., Zhang, Q. Y. and Ding, X. (2000) 'Expression of biotransformation enzymes in human fetal olfactory mucosa: potential roles in developmental toxicity', *Toxicol. Appl. Pharmacol.* **165**: 158–62.

Guengerich, F. P. (1990) 'Mechanism-based inactivation of human liver microsomal cytochrome P-450 IIIA4 by gestodene', *Chem. Res. Toxicol.* **3**: 363–71.

Guengerich, F. P. (1995) 'Human cytochrome P-450 enzymes', in P. R. Ortiz de Montellano (ed.) *Cytochrome P-450*, New York: Plenum Press, pp. 473–535.

Guengerich, F. P. (1999) 'Cytochrome P-450 3A4: regulation and role in drug metabolism', *Annu. Rev. Pharmacol. Toxicol.* **39**: 1–17.

Guengerich, F. P., Martin, M. V., Beaune, P. H., Kremers, P., Wolff, T. and Waxman, D. J. (1986) 'Characterization of rat and human liver microsomal cytochrome P-450 forms involved in nifedipine oxidation, a prototype for genetic polymorphism in oxidative drug metabolism', *J. Biol. Chem.* **261**: 5051–60.

Guengerich, F. P., Parikh, A., Turesky, R. J. and Josephy, P. D. (1999) Inter-individual differences in the metabolism of environmental toxicants: cytochrome P450 1A2 as a prototype', *Mutat. Res.* **428**: 115–24.

Guillouzo, A. (1998) 'Liver cell models in in vitro toxicology', *Environ. Health Perspect.* **106**: 511–32.

Guo, Z., Raeissi, S., White, R. B. and Stevens, J. C. (1997) 'Orphenadrine and methimazole inhibit multiple cytochrome P450 enzymes in human liver microsomes', *Drug Metab. Dispos.* **25**: 390–3.

Gut, J., Catin, T., Dayer, P., Kronbach, T., Zanger, U. and Meyer, U. A. (1986) 'Debrisoquine/sparteine-type polymorphism of drug oxidation. Purification and characterization of two functionally different human liver cytochrome P-450 isozymes involved in impaired hydroxylation of the prototype substrate bufuralol', *J. Biol. Chem.* **261**: 11734–43.

Haehner, B. D., Gorski, J. C., Vandenbranden, M., Wrighton, S. A., Janardan, S. K., Watkins, P. B. and Hall, S. D. (1996) 'Bimodal distribution of renal cytochrome P450 3A activity in humans', *Mol. Pharmacol.* **50**: 52–9.

Hakkola, J., Pasanen, M., Pelkonen, O., Hukkanen, J., Evisalmi, S., Anttila, S., Rane, A., Mäntylä, M., Purkunen, R., Saarikoski, S., Tooming, M. and Raunio, H. (1997) 'Expression of CYP1B1 in human adult and fetal tissues and differential inducibility of CYP1B1 and CYP1A1 by Ah receptor ligands in human placenta and cultured cells', *Carcinogenesis* **18**: 391–7.

Hakkola, J., Pasanen, M., Purkunen, R., Saarikoski, S., Pelkonen, O., Mäenpää, J., Rane, A. and Raunio, H. (1994) Expression of xenobiotic-metabolizing cytochrome P450 forms in human adult and fetal liver', *Biochem. Pharmacol.* **48**: 59–64.

Hakkola, J., Raunio, H., Purkunen, R., Pelkonen, O., Saarikoski, S., Cresteil, T. and Pasanen, M. (1996) 'Detection of cytochrome P450 gene expression in human placenta in first trimester of pregnancy', *Biochem. Pharmacol.* **52**: 379–83.

Hakkola, J., Tanaka, E. and Pelkonen, O. (1998) 'Developmental expression of cytochrome P450 enzymes in the human liver', *Pharmacol. Toxicol.* **82**: 209–17.

Harlow, G. R. and Halpert, J. R. (1998) 'Analysis of human cytochrome P450 3A4 cooperativity: construction and characterization of a site-directed mutant that displays hyperbolic steroid hydroxylation kinetics', *Proc. Natl. Acad. Sci. USA* **95**: 6636–41.

Hashimoto, H., Nakagawa, T., Yokoi, T., Sawada, M., Itoh, S. and Kamataki, T. (1995a) 'Fetus-specific CYP3A7 and adult-specific CYP3A4 expressed in Chinese hamster CHL cells have similar capacity to activate carcinogenic mycotoxins', *Cancer Res.* **55**: 787–91.

Hashimoto, H., Toide, K., Kitamura, R., Fujita, M., Tagawa, S., Itoh, S. and Kamataki, T. (1993) 'Gene structure of CYP3A4, an adult-specific form of cytochrome P450 in human livers, and its transcriptional control', *Eur. J. Biochem.* **218**: 585–95.

Hashimoto, H., Yanagawa, Y., Sawada, M., Itoh, S., Deguchi, T. and Kamataki, T. (1995b) 'Simultaneous expression of human CYP3A7 and N-acetyltransferase in Chinese hamster CHL cells results in high cytotoxicity for carcinogenic heterocyclic amines', *Arch. Biochem. Biophys.* **320**: 323–9.

Hayashi, S.I., Watanabe, J., Nakachi, K. and Kawajiri, K. (1991) 'Genetic linkage of lung cancer-associated MspI polymorphisms with amino acid replacement in the heme binding region of the human cytochrome P450IA1 gene', *J. Biochem.* **110**: 407–11.

Heim, M. and Meyer, U. A. (1990) 'Genotyping of poor metabolisers of debrisoquine by allele-specific PCR amplification', *Lancet* **336**: 529–32.

Hemeryck, A., De Vriendt, C. and Belpaire, F. M. (1999) 'Inhibition of CYP2C9 by selective serotonin reuptake inhibitors: in vitro studies with tolbutalide and S-warfarin using human liver microsomes', *Eur. J. Clin. Pharmacol.* **54**: 947–51.

Hickman, D., Wang, J. P. and Unadkat, J. D. (1998) 'Evaluation of the selectivity of in vitro probes and suitability of organic solvents for the measurement of human cytochrome P450 monooxygenase activities', *Drug Metab. Dispos.* **26**: 207–15.

Hirvonen, A. (1999) 'Polymorphisms of xenobiotic-metabolizing enzymes and susceptibility to cancer', *Environ. Health Perspect.* **107** (Suppl. 1): 37–47.

Högstedt, S., Lindberg, B. and Rane, A. (1983) 'Increased oral clearance of metoprolol in pregnancy', *Eur. J. Clin. Pharmacol.* **24**: 217–20.

Högstedt, S., Lindberg, B., Peng, D., Regårdh, C.-G. and Rane, A. (1985) 'Pregnancy-induced increase in metoprolol metabolism', *Clin. Pharmacol. Ther.* **37**: 688–92.

Honkakoski, P. and Negishi, M. (2000) 'Regulation of cytochrome P450 (CYP) genes by nuclear receptors', *Biochem. J.* **347**: 321–37.

Hosea, N. A. and Guengerich, F. P. (1998) 'Oxidation of nonionic detergents by cytochrome P450 enzymes', *Arch. Biochem. Biophys.* **353**: 365–73.

Hu, Y., Hakkola, J., Oscarson, M. and Ingelman-Sundberg, M. (1999) 'Structural and functional characterization of the 5′-flanking region of the rat and human cytochrome P450 2E1 genes: identification of a polymorphic repeat in the human gene', *Biochem. Biophys. Res. Commun.* 263: 286–93.

Hu, Y., Oscarson, M., Johansson, I., Yue, Q. Y., Dahl, M. L., Tabone, M., Arinco, S., Albano, E. and Ingelman-Sundberg, M. (1997) 'Genetic polymorphism of human CYP2E1: characterization of two variant alleles', *Mol. Pharmacol.* 51: 370–6.

Huang, Z., Fasco, M. J., Figge, H. L., Keyomarsi, K. and Kaminsky, L. S. (1996) 'Expression of cytochromes P450 in human breast tissue and tumors', *Drug Metab. Dispos.* 24: 899–905.

Hukkanen, J., Lassila, A., Paivarinta, K., Valanne, S., Sarpo, S., Hakkola, J., Pelkonen, O. and Raunio, H. (2000) 'Induction and regulation of xenobiotic-metabolizing cytochrome P450s in the human A549 lung adenocarcinoma cell line', *Am. J. Respir. Cell. Mol. Biol.* 22: 360–6.

Imaoka, S., Yamada, T., Hiroi, T., Hayashi, K., Sakaki, T., Yabusaki, Y. and Funae, Y. (1996) 'Multiple forms of human P450 expressed in Saccharomyces cerevisiae, systematic characterization and comparison with those of the rat', *Biochem. Pharmacol.* 51: 1041–50.

Ingelman-Sundberg, M., Johansson, I., Penttila, K. E., Glaumann, H. and Lindros, K. O. (1988) 'Centrilobular expression of ethanol-inducible cytochrome P-450 (IIE1) in rat liver', *Biochem. Biophys. Res. Commun.* 157: 55–60.

Ingelman-Sundberg, M., Oscarson, M. and McLellan, R. A. (1999) 'Polymorphic human cytochrome P450 enzymes: an opportunity for individualized drug treatment', *Trends Pharmacol. Sci.* 20: 342–9.

Inoue, K., Yamazaki, H., Imiya, K., Akasaka, S., Guengerich, F. P. and Shimada, T. (1997) 'Relationship between CYP2C9 and 22C19 genotype and tolbutamide methyl hydroxylation and S-mephenytoin 4′-hydroxylation activities in livers from Japanese and Caucasian populations', *Pharmacogenetics* 7: 103–13.

Iyer, K. R. and Sinz, M. W. (1999) 'Characterization of Phase I and Phase II hepatic drug metabolism activities in a panel of human liver preparations', *Chem. Biol. Interact.* 118: 151–69.

Jacquet, M., Lambert, V., Baudoux, E., Muller, M., Kremers, P. and Gielen, J. (1996) 'Correlation between P450 CYP1A1 inducibility, MspI genotype and lung cancer incidence', *Eur. J. Cancer* 32: 1701–6.

Jacquet, M., Lambert, V., Todaro, A. and Kremers, P. (1997) 'Mitogen-activated lymphocytes: a good model for characterising lung CYP1A1 inducibility', *Eur. J. Epidemiology* 13: 177–83.

Janardan, S. K., Lown, K. S., Schmiedlin-Ren, P., Thummel, K. E. and Watkins, P. B. (1996) 'Selective expression of CYP3A5 and not CYP3A4 in human blood', *Pharmacogenetics* 6: 379–85.

Jeppesen, U., Gram, L. F., Vistisen, K., Loft, S., Poulsen, H. E. and Brosen, K. (1996) 'Dose-dependent inhibition of CYP1A2, CYP2C19 and CYP2D6 by citalopram, fluoxetine, fluvoxamine and paroxetine', *Eur. J. Clin. Pharmacol.* 51: 73–8.

Johansson, I., Lindros, K. O., Eriksson, H. and Ingelman-Sundberg, M. (1990) 'Transcriptional control of CYP2E1 in the perivenous liver region and during starvation', *Biochem. Biophys. Res. Commun.* 173: 331–8.

Johansson, I., Lundqvist, E., Bertilsson, L., Dahl, M. L., Sjoqvist, F. and Ingelman-Sundberg, M. (1993) 'Inherited amplification of an active gene in the cytochrome P450 CYP2D locus as a cause of ultrarapid metabolism of debrisoquine', *Proc. Natl. Acad. Sci. USA* **90**: 11825–9.

Jounaidi, Y., Hyrailles, V., Gervot, L. and Maurel, P. (1996) 'Detection of CYP3A5 allelic variant: a candidate for the polymorphic expression of the protein', *Biochem. Biophys. Res. Commun.* **221**: 466–70.

Juchau, M. R., Boutelet-Bochan, H. and Huang, Y. (1998) 'Cytochrome-P450-dependent biotransformation of xenobiotics in human and rodent embryonic tissues', *Drug Metab. Rev.* **30**: 541–68.

Kahn, G. C., Boobis, A. R., Brodie, M. J., Toverud, E. L., Murray, S. and Davies, D. S. (1985) 'Phenacetin O-deethylase: an activity of a cytochrome P-450 showing genetic linkage with that catalysing the 4-hydroxylation of debrisoquine', *Br. J. Clin. Pharmacol.* **20**: 67–76.

Kalow, W. and Tang, B. K. (1991) 'Caffeine as a metabolic probe: exploration of the enzyme-inducing effect of cigarette smoking', *Clin. Pharmacol. Ther.* **49**: 44–8.

Kenworthy, K. E., Bloomer, J. C., Clarke, S. E. and Houston, J. B. (1999) 'CYP3A4 drug interactions: correlation of 10 in vitro probe substrates', *Br. J. Clin Pharmacol.* **48**: 716–27.

Kerr, B. M., Thummel, K. E., Wurden, C. J., Klein, S. M., Kroetz, D. L., Gonzalez, F. J. and Levy, R. H. (1994) 'Human liver carbamazepine metabolism. Role of CYP3A4 and CYP2C8 in 10,11-epoxide formation', *Biochem. Pharmacol.* **47**: 1969–79.

Kim, H., Wang, R. S., Elovaara, E., Raunio, H., Pelkonen, O., Aoyama, T., Vainio, H. and Nakajima, T. (1997) 'Cytochrome P450 isozymes responsible for the metabolism of toluene and styrene in human liver microsomes', *Xenobiotica* **27**: 657–65.

Kinirons, M. T., O'Shea, D., Kim, R. B., Groopman, J. D., Thummel, K. E., Wood, A. J. and Wilkinson, G. R. (1999) 'Failure of erythromycin breath test to correlate with midazolam clearance as a probe of cytochrome P4503A', *Clin. Pharmacol. Ther.* **66**: 224–31.

Kitada, M., Kamataki, T., Itahashi, K., Rikihisa, T., Kato, R. and Kanakubo, Y. (1985a) 'Purification and properties of cytochrome P-450 from homogenates of human fetal livers', *Arch. Biochem. Biophys.* **241**: 275–80.

Kitada, M., Kamataki, T., Itahashi, K., Rikihisa, T., Kato, R. and Kanakubo, Y. (1985b) 'Immunochemical examinations of cytochrome P-450 in various tissues of human fetuses using antibodies to human fetal cytochrome P-450, P-450 HFLa', *Biochem. Biophys. Res. Commun.* **131**: 1154–9.

Kivistö, K. T., Bookjans, G., Fromm, M. F., Griese, E. U., Munzel, P. and Kroemer, H. K. (1996) 'Expression of CYP3A4, CYP3A5 and CYP3A7 in human duodenal tissue', *Br. J. Clin. Pharmacol.* **42**: 387–9.

Kivistö, K. T., Lilja, J. J., Backman, J. T. and Neuvonen, P. J. (1999) 'Repeated consumption of grapefruit juice considerably increases plasma concentrations of cisapride', *Clin. Pharmacol. Ther.* **66**: 448–53.

Kliewer, S. A., Lehmann, J. M., Milburn, M. V. and Willson, T. M. (1999) 'The PPARs and PXRs: nuclear xenobiotic receptors that define novel hormone signaling pathways', *Recent Prog. Horm. Res.* **54**: 345–67.

Kolars, J. C., Lown, K. S., Schmiedlin-Ren, P., Ghosh, M., Fang, C., Wrighton, S.

A., Merion, R. M. and Watkins, P. B. (1994) 'CYP3A gene expression in human gut epithelium', *Pharmacogenetics* 4: 247–59.

Kolars, J. C., Schmiedlin-Ren, P., Schuetz, J. D., Fang, C. and Watkins, P. B. (1992) 'Identification of rifampin-inducible P450IIIA4 (CYP3A4) in human small bowel enterocytes', *J. Clin. Invest.* 90: 1871–8.

Kondoh, N., Wakatsuki, T., Ryo, A., Hada, A., Aihara, T., Horiuchi, S., Goseki, N., Matsubara, O., Takenaka, K., Shichita, M., Tanaka, K., Shuda, M. and Yamamoto, M. (1999) 'Identification and characterization of genes associated with human hepatocellular carcinogenesis', *Cancer Res.* 59: 4990–6.

Koskela, S., Hakkola, J., Hukkanen, J., Pelkonen, O., Sorri, M., Saranen, A., Anttila, S., Fernandez-Salguero, P., Gonzalez, F. J. and Raunio, H. (1999) 'Expression of CYP2A gene in human liver and extrahepatic tissues', *Biochem. Pharmacol.* 57: 1407–13.

Koudriakova, T., Iatsimirskaia, E., Utkin, I., Gangl, E., Vouros, P., Storozhuk, E., Orza, D., Marinina, J. and Gerber, N. (1998) 'Metabolism of the human immunodeficiency virus protease inhibitors indinavir and ritonavir by human intestinal microsomes and expressed cytochrome P4503A4/3A5: mechanism-based inactivation of cytochrome P4503A by ritonavir', *Drug Metab. Dispos.* 26: 552–61.

Kremers, P. (1999) 'Liver microsomes: a convenient tool for metabolism studies but . . .', in, A. R. Boobis, P. Kremers, O. Pelkonen and K. Pithan (eds) *Drug Metabolism in Man*, Luxembourg, EUR 18569, pp. 39–52.

Kress, S., Reichert, J. and Schwarz, M. (1998) 'Functional analysis of the human cytochrome P4501A1 (CYP1A1) gene enhancer', *Eur. J. Biochem.* 258: 803–12.

Kronbach, T., Mathys, D., Umeno, M., Gonzalez, F. J. and Meyer, U. A. (1989) 'Oxidation of midazolam and triazolam by human liver cytochrome P450IIIA4', *Mol. Pharmacol.* 36: 89–96.

Kumar, G. N., Rodrigues, A. D., Buko, A. M. and Denissen, J. F. (1996) 'Cytochrome P450-mediated metabolism of the HIV-1 protease inhibitor ritonavir (ABT-538) in human liver microsomes', *J. Pharmacol. Exp. Ther.* 277: 423–31.

Lacroix, D., Sonnier, M., Moncion, A., Cheron, G. and Cresteil, T. (1997) 'Expression of CYP3A in the human liver – evidence that the shift between CYP3A7 and CYP3A4 occurs immediately after birth', *Eur. J. Biochem.* 247: 625–34.

Ladona, M. G., Park, S. S., Gelboin, H. V., Hammar, L. and Rane, A. (1988) 'Monoclonal anti-body directed detection of cytochrome P-450 (PCN) in human fetal liver', *Biochem. Pharmacol.* 37: 4735–41.

Lake, B. G., Charzat, C., Tredger, J. M., Renwick, A. B., Beamand, J. A. and Price, R. J. (1996) 'Induction of cytochrome P450 isoenzymes in cultured precision-cut rat and human liver slices', *Xenobiotica* 26: 297–306.

Lakehal, F., Wendum, D., Barbu, V., Becquemont, L., Poupon, R., Balladur, P., Hannoun, L., Ballet, F., Beaune, P. H. and Housset, C. (1999) 'Phase I and phase II drug-metabolizing enzymes are expressed and heterogeneously distributed in the biliary epithelium', *Hepatology* 30: 1498–506.

Landi, M. T., Bertazzi, P. A., Shields, P. G., Clark, G., Lucier, G. W., Garte, S. J., Cosma, G. and Caporaso, N. E. (1994) 'Association between CYP1A1 genotype, mRNA expression and enzymatic activity in humans', *Pharmacogenetics* 4: 242–6.

Landi, M. T., Sinha, R., Lang, N. P. and Kadlubar, F. F. (1999) 'Human cytochrome P4501A2', *IARC Sci. Publ.* **148**: 173–95.

Lasker, J. M., Wester, M. R., Aramsombatdee, E. and Raucy, J. L. (1998) 'Characterization of CYP2C19 and CYP2C9 from human liver: respective roles in microsomal tolbutamide, S-mephenytoin and omeprazole hydroxylations', *Arch. Biochem. Biophys.* **353**: 16–28.

Lechevrel, M., Casson, A. G., Wolf, C. R., Hardie, L. J., Flinterman, M. B., Montesano, R. and Wild, C. P. (1999) 'Characterization of cytochrome P450 expression in human oesophageal mucosa', *Carcinogenesis* **20**: 243–8.

Lehmann, J. M., McKee, D. D., Watson, M. A., Willson, T. M., Moore, J. T. and Kliewer, S. A. (1998) 'The human orphan nuclear receptor PXR is activated by compounds that regulate CYP3A4 gene expression and cause drug interactions', *J. Clin. Invest.* **102**: 1016–23.

Li, A. P., Kaminski, D. L. and Rasmussen, A. (1995) 'Substrates of human hepatic cytochrome P450 3A4', *Toxicology* **104**: 1–8.

Li, A. P., Maurel, P., Gomez-Lechon, M. J., Cheng, L. C. and Jurima-Romet, M. (1997) 'Preclinical evaluation of drug–drug interaction potential: present status of the application of primary human hepatocytes in the evaluation of cytochrome P450 induction', *Chem. Biol. Interact.* **107**: 5–16.

Li, W., Harper, P. A., Tang, B. K. and Okey, A. B. (1998) 'Regulation of cytochrome P450 enzymes by aryl hydrocarbon receptor in human cells: CYP1A2 expression in the LS180 colon carcinoma cell line, after treatment with 2,3,7,8-tetrachlorodibenzo-p-dioxin or 3-methylcholanthrene', *Biochem. Pharmacol.* **56**: 599–612.

Liang, H. C., Li, H., McKinnon, R. A., Duffy, J. J., Potter, S. S., Puga, A. and Nebert, D. W. (1996) 'Cyp1a2(-/-) null mutant mice develop normally but show deficient drug metabolism', *Proc. Natl. Acad. Sci. USA* **93**: 1671–6.

Liehr, J. G., Ricci, M. J., Jefcoate, C. R., Hannigan, E. V., Hokanson, J. A. and Zhu, B. T. (1995) '4-hydroxylation of estradiol by human utering myometrium and myoma microsomes: implications for the mechanism of uterine tumorigenesis', *Proc. Natl. Acad. Sci. USA* **92**: 9220–4.

Liu, G., Gelboin, H. V. and Myers, M. J. (1991) 'Role of cytochrome P450 IA2 in acetanilide 4-hydroxylation as determined with cDNA expression and monoclonal antibodies', *Arch. Biochem. Biophys.* **284**: 400–6.

Lown, K. S., Kolars, J. C., Thummel, K. E., Barnett, J. L., Kunze, K. L., Wrighton, S. A. and Watkins, P. B. (1994) 'Interpatient heterogeneity in expression of CYP3A4 and CYP3A5 in small bowel. Lack of prediction by the erythromycin breath test', *Drug Metab. Dispos.* **22**: 947–55.

Lukkari, E., Taavitsainen, P., Juhakoski, A. and Pelkonen, O. (1998) 'Cytochrome P450 specificity of metabolism and interactions of oxybutynin in human liver microsomes', *Pharmacol. Toxicol.* **82**: 161–6.

McCarver, D. G., Byun, R., Hines, R. N., Hichme, M. and Wegenek, W. (1998) 'A genetic polymorphism in the regulatory sequences of human CYP2E1: association with increased chlorzoxazone hydroxylation in the presence of obesity and ethanol intake', *Toxicol. Appl. Pharmacol.* **152**: 276–81.

McKinnon, R. A., Burgess, W. M., Hall, P. M., Roberts-Thomson, S. J., Gonzalez, F. J. and McManus, M. E. (1990) 'Characterisation of CYP3A gene subfamily expression in human gastrointestinal tissues', *Gut* **36**: 259–67.

McManus, M. E., Burgess, W. M., Veronese, M. E., Huggett, A., Quattrochi, L. C. and Tukey, R. H. (1990) 'Metabolism of 2-acetylaminofluorene and benzo(a) pyrene and activation of food-derived heterocyclic amine mutagens by human cytochromes P-450', *Cancer Res.* 50: 3367–76.

Manyike, P. T., Kharasch, E. D., Kalhorn, T. F. and Slattery, J. T. (2000) 'Contribution of CYP2E1 and CYP3A to acetaminophen reactive metabolite formation', *Clin. Pharmacol. Ther.* 67: 275–82.

Marre, F., de Sousa, G., Orloff, A. M. and Rahmani, R. (1993) 'In vitro interaction between cyclosporin A and macrolide antibiotics', *Br. J. Clin. Pharmacol.* 35: 447–8.

Masubuchi, Y., Hosokawa, S., Horie, T., Suzuki, T., Ohmori, S., Kitada, M. and Narimatsu, S. (1994) 'Cytochrome P450 isozymes involved in propranolol metabolism in human liver microsomes. The role of CYP2D6 as ring-hydroxylase and CYP1A2 as N-desisopropylase', *Drug Metab. Dispos.* 22: 909–15.

Mattes, W. B. and Li, A. P. (1997) 'Quantitative reverse transcriptase/PCR assay for the measurement of induction in cultured hepatocytes', *Chem. Biol. Interact.* 107: 47–61.

Maurel, P. (1996) 'The use of adult human hepatocytes in primary culture and other in vitro systems to investigate drug metabolism in man', *Adv. Drug Del. Rev.* 22: 105–32.

Maurel, P. (1996) 'The CYP3A family', in, C. Ioannides (ed.) *Cytochromes P450: Metabolic and Toxicological Aspects*, Boca Raton: CRC, pp. 241–70.

Miners, J. O. and Birkett, D. J. (1996) 'The use of caffeine as a metabolic probe for human drug metabolizing enzymes', *Gen. Pharmacol.* 27: 245–9.

Miners, J. O. and Birkett, D. J. (1998) 'Cytochrome P4502C9: an enzyme of major importance in human drug metabolism', *Br. J. Clin. Pharmacol.* 45: 525–38.

Moore, L. B., Goodwin, B., Jones, S. A., Wisely, G. B., Serabjit-Singh, C. J., Willson, T. M., Collins, J. L. and Kliewer, S. A. (2000) 'St. John's wort induces hepatic drug metabolism through activation of the pregnane X receptor', *Proc. Natl. Acad. Sci. USA* 97: 7500–2.

Morel, F., Beaune, P. H., Ratanasavanh, D., Flinois, J. P., Yang, C. S., Guengerich, F. P. and Guillouzo, A. (1990) 'Expression of cytochrome P450 enzymes in cultured human hepatocytes', *Eur. J. Biochem.* 191: 437–44.

Mortimer, O., Persson, K., Ladona, M. G., Spalding, D., Zanger, U. M., Meyer, U. A. and Rane, A. (1990) 'Polymorphic formation of morphine from codeine in poor and extensive metabolizers of dextromethorphan: relationship to the presence of immunoidentified cytochrome P-450IID1', *Clin. Pharmacol. Ther.* 47: 27–35.

Murray, G. I., McFayden, M. C., Mitchell, R. T., Cheung, Y. L., Kerr, A. C. and Melvin, W. T. (1999) 'Cytochrome P450 CYP3A in human renal cell cancer', *Br. J. Cancer* 79: 1836–42.

Murray, G. I., Pritchard, S., Melvin, W. T. and Burke, M. D. (1995) 'Cytochrome P450 CYP3A5 in the human anterior pituitary gland', *FEBS Lett* 364: 79–82.

Nakajima, M., Kobayashi, K., Shimada, N., Tokudome, S., Yamamoto, T. and Kuroiwa, Y. (1998) 'Involvement of CYP1A2 in mexiletine metabolism', *Br. J. Clin. Pharmacol.* 46: 55–62.

Nakajima, M., Yamamoto, T., Nunoya, K.-I., Yokoi, T., Nagashima, K., Inoue, K., Funae, Y., Shimada, N., Kamataki, T. and Kuroiwa, Y. (1996a) 'Characterization of CYP2A6 involved in 3′-hydroxylation of cotinine in human liver microsomes', *J. Pharmacol. Exp. Ther.* **277**: 1010–5.

Nakajima, M., Yamamoto, T., Nunoya, K.-I., Yokoi, T., Nagashima, K., Inoue, K., Funae, Y., Shimada, N. and Kuroiwa, Y. (1996b) 'Role of human cytochrome P4502A6 in C-oxidation of nicotine', *Drug Metab. Dispos.* **24**: 1212–7.

Nakajima, M., Yokoi, T., Mizutani, M., Kinoshita, M., Funayama, M. and Kamataki, T. (1999) 'Genetic polymorphism in the 5′-flanking region of human CYP1A2 gene: effect on the CYP1A2 inducibility in humans', *J. Biochem. (Tokyo)* **125**: 803–8.

Nakajima, M., Yokoi, T., Mizutani, M., Shin, S., Kadlubar, F. E. and Kamataki, T. (1994) 'Phenotyping of CYP1A2 in Japanese population by analysis of caffeine urinary metabolites: absence of mutation prescribing the phenotype in the CYP1A2 gene', *Cancer Epidemiol. Biomarkers Prev.* **3**: 413–21.

Nelson, D. R. (2000) 'Bioinformatics and mining the human genome', Abstracts of 13th International Symposium on Microsomes and Drug Oxidations, Stresa, Italy, Abstr. PL1-1: 24.

Nordmark, A., Lundgren, S., Cnattingius, S. and Rane, A. (1999) 'Dietary caffeine as a probe agent for assessment of cytochrome P4501A2 activity in random urine samples', *Br. J. Clin. Pharmacol.* **47**: 397–402.

Notarianni, L. J., Oliver, S. E., Dobrocky, P., Bennett, P. N. and Silverman, B. W. (1995) 'Caffeine as a metabolic probe: a comparison of the metabolic ratios used to assess CYP1A2 activity', *Br. J. Clin. Pharmacol.* **39**: 65–9.

Ogg, M. S., Williams, J. M., Tarbit, M., Goldfarb, P. S., Gray, T. I. and Gibson, G. G. (1999) 'A reporter gene assay to assess the molecular mechanisms of xenobiotic-dependent induction of the human CYP3A4 gene in vitro', *Xenobiotica* **29**: 269–79.

Ohmori, S., Fujiki, N., Nakasa, H., Nakamura, H., Ishii, I., Itahashi, K. and Kitada, M. (1998a) 'Steroid hydroxylation by human fetal CYP3A7 and human NADPH-cytochrome P450 reductase coexpressed in insect cells using baculovirus', *Res. Commun. Mol. Pathol. Pharmacol.* **100**: 15–28.

Ohmori, S., Nakasa, H., Asanome, K., Kurose, Y., Ishii, I., Hosokawa, M. and Kitada, M. (1998b) 'Differential catalytic properties in metabolism of endogenous and exogenous substrates among CYP3A enzymes expressed in COS-7 cells', *Biochem. Biophys. Acta.* **1380**: 297–304.

Ong, S., Hatanaka, T., Hotta, H., Satoh, T., Gonzalez, F. J. and Tsutsui, M. (1996) 'Specificity of substrate and inhibitor probes for cytochrome P450s: evaluation of in vitro metabolism using cDNA-expressed human P450s and human liver microsomes', *Xenobiotica* **26**: 681–93.

Ono, S., Hatanaka, T., Hotta, H., Tsutsui, M., Satoh, T. and Gonzalez, F. J. (1995) 'Chlorzoxazone is metabolized by human CYP1A2 as well as by human CYP2E1', *Pharmacogenetics* **5**: 143–50.

Oscarson, M., Gullstén, H., Rautio, A., Bernal, M. L., Sinues, B., Dahl, M.-L., Stengård, J. H., Pelkonen, O., Raunio, H. and Ingelman-Sundberg, M. (1998) 'Genotyping of human cytochrome P450 2A6 (CYP2A6), a nicotine C-oxidase', *FEBS Lett.* **438**: 201–5.

Oscarson, M., McLellan, R. A., Gullstén, H., Yue, Q.-Y., Lang, M. A., Bernal, M. L., Sinues, B., Hirvonen, A., Raunio, H., Pelkonen, O. and Ingelman-Sundberg, M. (1999a) 'Characterisation and PCR-based detection of a CYP2A6 gene deletion found at high frequency in a Chinese population', *FEBS Lett.* **448**: 105–10.

Oscarson, M., McLellan, R. A., Gullstén, H., Agundez, J. A. G., Benitez, J., Rautio, A., Raunio, H., Pelkonen, O. and Ingelman-Sundberg, M. (1999b) 'Identification and characterisation of novel polymorphisms in the CYP2A6 locus: implications for nicotine metabolism', *FEBS Lett.* **460**: 321–7.

Otto, S., Bhattacharyya, K. K. and Jefcoate, C. R. (1992) 'Polycyclic aromatic hydrocarbon in rat adrenal, ovary, and testis microsomes is catalyzed by the same novel cytochrome P450 (P450RAP)', *Endocrinology* **131**: 3067–76.

Pantuck, E. J., Hsaiao, K. C., Conney, A. H., Garland, W. A., Kappas, A., Anderson, K. E. and Alvares A. P. (1976) 'Effect of charcoal-broiled beef on phenacetin metabolism in man', *Science* **194**: 1055–7.

Paris, P. L., Kupelian, P. A., Hall, J. M., Williams, T. L., Levin, H., Klein, E. A., Casey, G. and Witte, J. S. (1999) 'Association between a CYP3A4 genetic variant and clinical presentation in African–American prostate cancer patients', *Cancer Epidemiol. Biomarkers Prev.* **8**: 901–5.

Pascussi, J. M., Jounaidi, Y., Drocourt, L., Domergue, J., Balabaud, C., Maurel, P. and Vilarem, M. J. (1999) 'Evidence for the presence of a functional pregnane X receptor response element in the CYP3A7 promoter gene', *Biochem. Biophys. Res. Commun.* **260**: 377–81.

Paulussen, A., Lavrijsen, K., Bohets, H., Hendrickx, J., Verhasselt, P., Luyten, W., Konings, F. and Armstrong, M. (2000) 'Two linked mutations in transcriptional regulatory elements of the CYP3A5 gene constitute the major genetic determinant of polymorphic activity in humans', *Pharmacogenetics* **10**: 415–24.

Pearce, R. E., McIntyre, C. J., Madan, A., Sanzgiri, U., Draper, A. J., Bullock, P. L., Cook, D. C., Burton, L. A., Latham, J., Nevins, C. and Parkinson, A. (1996b) Effects of freezing, thawing, and storing human liver microsomes on cytochrome P450 activity', *Arch. Biochem. Biophys.* **331**: 145–69.

Pearce, R. E., Rodrigues, A. D., Goldstein, J. A. and Parkinson, A. (1996a) Identification of the human P450 enzymes involved in lansoprazole metabolism', *J. Pharmacol. Exp. Ther.* **277**: 805–16.

Pelkonen, O., Mäenpää, J., Taavitsainen, P., Rautio, A. and Raunio, H. (1998) 'Inhibition and induction of human cytochrome P450 (CYP) enzymes', *Xenobiotica* **28**: 1203–53.

Pelkonen, O. and Raunio, H. (1995) 'Individual expression of carcinogen-metabolizing enzymes: cytochrome P4502A', *J. Occup. Environ. Med.* **37**: 19–24.

Pelkonen, O., Raunio, H., Pasanen, M., Rautio, A. and Lang, M. A. (1997) 'The metabolism of coumarin', in, R. O'Kennedy and R. D. Thornes (eds) *Coumarins: Biology, Applications and Mode of Action*, Chichester: Wiley, pp. 67–92.

Pelkonen, O., Rautio, A. and Raunio, H. (1995) 'Specificity and applicability of probes for drug metabolizing enzymes', in, G. Alvan, L. P. Balant, P. R. Bechtel, A. R. Boobis, L. F. Gram, G. Paintaud and K. Pithan (eds) European cooperation in the field of scientific and technical research – COST B1 conference on the variability and specificity in drug metabolism. Luxembourg: European Commission, 1995, pp. 147–58.

Pelkonen, O., Raunio, H., Rautio, A., Mäenpää, J. and Lang, M. A. (1993) 'Coumarin 7-hydroxylase: characteristics and regulation in mouse and man', *J. Irish Coll. Phys. Surg.* **22**: 24–8.

Pelkonen, O., Rautio, A., Raunio, H. and Pasanen, M. (2000) 'CYP2A6: a human coumarin 7-hydroxylase', *Toxicology* 144: 139–47.

Peter, R., Böcker, R. G., Beaune, P. H., Iwasaki, M., Guengerich, F. P. and Yang, C.-S. (1990) 'Hydroxylation of chlorzoxazone as a specific probe for human liver cytochrome P-450 IIE1', *Chem. Res. Toxicol.* 3: 566–73.

Pichard, L., Fabre, I., Fabre, G., Domergue, J., Saint Aubert, B., Mourad, G. and Maurel, P. (1990) 'Cyclosporin A drug interactions. Screening for inducers and inhibitors of cytochrome P-450 (cyclosporin A oxidase) in primary cultures of human hepatocytes and in liver microsomes', *Drug Metab. Dispos.* 18: 595–606.

Poli-Scaife, S., Attias, R., Dansette, P. and Mansuy, D. (1997) 'The substrate binding site of human liver cytochrome P450 2C9: an NMR study', *Biochemistry* 36: 12672–82.

Prueksaritanont, T., Ma, B., Tang, C., Meng, Y., Assang, C., Lu, P., Reider, P. J., Lin, J. H. and Baillie, T. A. (1999) 'Metabolic interactions between mibefradil and HMG-CoA reductase inhibitors: an in vitro investigation with human liver preparations', *Br. J. Clin. Pharmacol.* 47: 291–8.

Quattrochi, L. C. and Tukey, R. H. (1989) 'The human cytochrome Cyp1A2 gene contains regulatory elements responsive to 3-methylcholanthrene', *Mol. Pharmacol.* 36: 66–71.

Quattrochi, L. C., Vu, T. and Tukey, R. H. (1994) 'The human CYP1A2 gene and induction by 3-methylcholanthrene. A region of DNA that supports AH-receptor binding and promoter-specific induction', *J. Biol. Chem.* 269: 6949–54.

Rane, A., Wilkinson, G. R. and Shand, D. G. (1977) 'Prediction of hepatic extraction ratio from in vitro measurement of intrinsic clearance', *J. Pharmacol. Exp. Ther.* 200: 420–4.

Rannug, A., Alexandrie, A. K., Persson, I. and Ingelman-Sundberg, M. (1995) 'Genetic polymorphism of cytochromes P450 1A1, 2D6 and 2E1: regulation and toxicological significance, *J. Occup. Environ. Med.* 37: 25–36.

Rao, Y., Hoffmann, E., Zia, M., Bodin, L., Zeman, M., Sellers, E. M. and Tyndale, R. F. (2000) 'Duplications and defects in the *CYP2A6* gene: identification, genotyping, and *in vivo* effects on smoking', *Mol. Pharmacol.* 58: 747–55.

Raunio, H., Pasanen, M., Mäenpää, J., Hakkola, J. and Pelkonen, O. (1995) 'Expression of extrahepatic cytochrome P450 in humans', in G. M. Pacifici and G. N. Fracchia (eds) *Advances in Drug Metabolism in Man*, Luxembourg: European Commission, Office for Official Publications of the European Communities, pp. 234–87.

Raunio, H., Rautio, A., Gullstén, H. and Pelkonen, O. (2001) 'Polymorphisms of CYP2A6 and its practical consequences', *Br. J. Clin. Pharmacol.* (in press)

Raunio, H., Rautio, A. and Pelkonen, O. (1999) 'The CYP2A subfamily: function, expression and genetic polymorphism, in, P. Vineis, N. Malats, M. Lang, A. d'Errico, N. Caporaso, J. Cuzick and P. Boffetta (eds) *Metabolic Polymorphisms and Susceptibility to Cancer*, IARC Scientific Publications No 148, International Agency for Research on Cancer, Lyon, 1999, pp. 197–207.

Rebbeck, T. R., Jaffe, J. M., Walker, A. H., Wein, A. J. and Malkowicz, S. B. (1998) 'Modification of clinical presentation of prostate tumors by a novel genetic variant in CYP3A4', *J. Natl. Cancer Inst.* 90: 1225–9.

Rendic, S. and Di Carlo, F. J. (1997) 'Human cytochrome P450 enzymes: a status report summarizing their reactions, substrates, inducers and inhibitors', *Drug Metab. Rev.* **29**: 413–580.

Ring, B. J., Binkley, S. N., Roskos, L. and Wrighton, S. A. (1995) 'Effect of fluoxetine, norfluoxetine, sertraline and desmethyl sertraline on human CYP3A catalyzed 1´-hydroxy midazolam formation in vitro', *J. Pharmacol. Exp. Ther.* **275**: 1131–5.

Rodrigues, A. D. (1994) 'Use of in vitro human metabolism studies in drug development. An industrial perspective', *Biochem. Pharmacol.* **48**: 2147–56.

Ronis, M. J. J., Lindros, K. O. and Ingelman-Sundberg, M. (1996) 'The cytochrome P4502E subfamily', in, I. Ioannides (ed.) *Cytochromes P450, Pharmacological and Toxicological Aspects*, Boca Raton: CRC Press, pp. 211–39.

Roots, I., Holbe, R., Hovermann, W., Nigam, S., Heinemeyer, G. and Hildebrandt, A. G. (1979) 'Quantitative determination by HPLC of urinary 6beta-hydroxy-cortisol, an indicator of enzyme induction by rifampicin and antiepileptic drugs', *Eur. J. Clin. Pharmacol.* **16**: 63–71.

Rost, K. L., Brosicke, H., Brockmoller, J., Scheffler, M., Helge, H. and Roots, I. (1992) 'Increase of cytochrome P450IA2 activity by omeprazole: evidence by the 13C-[N-3-methyl]-caffeine breath test in poor and extensive metabolizers of S-mephenytoin', *Clin. Pharmacol. Ther.* **52**: 170–80.

Rostami-Hodjegan, A., Nurminen, S., Jackdon, P. R. and Tucker, G. T. (1996) 'Caffeine urinary metabolite ratios as markers of enzyme activity: a theoretical assessment', *Pharmacogenetics* **6**: 121–49.

Rowland, M., Benet, L. Z. and Graham, G. (1973) 'Clearance concepts in pharmacokinetics', *J. Pharmacokin. Biopharm.* **1**: 123–36.

Roy, P., Yu, L. J., Crespi, C. L. and Waxman, D. J. (1999) 'Development of a substrate-activity based approach to identify the major human liver P-450 catalysts of cyclophosphamide and ifosfamide activation based on cDNA-expressed activities and liver microsomal P-450 profiles', *Drug Metab. Dispos.* **27**: 655–66.

Sachse, C., Brockmoller, J., Bauer, S. and Roots, I. (1999) 'Functional significance of a C→A polymorphism in intron 1 of the cytochrome P450 CYP1A2 gene tested with caffeine', *Br. J. Clin. Pharmacol.* **47**: 445–9.

Sadek, C. M. and Allen-Hoffmann, B. (1994) 'Cytochrome P450IA1 is rapidly induced in normal human keratinocytes in the absence of xenobiotics', *J. Biol. Chem.* **269**: 16067–74.

Santos, A., Zanetta, S., Cresteil, T., Deroussent, A., Pein, F., Raymond, E., Vernillet, L., Risse, M. L., Boige, V., Gouyette, A. and Vassal, G. (2000) 'Metabolism of irinotecan (CPT-11) by CYP3A4 and CYP3A5 in humans', *Clin. Cancer Res.* **6**: 2012–20.

Sata, F., Sapone, A., Elizondo, G., Stocker, P., Miller, V. P., Zheng, W., Raunio, H., Crespi, C. L. and Gonzalez, F. J. (2000) 'CYP3A4 allelic variants with amino acid substitutions in exons 7 and 12: evidence for an allelic variant with altered catalytic activity', *Clin. Pharmacol. Ther.* **67**: 48–56.

Satarug, S., Lang, M. A., Yongvanit, P., Sithithaworn, P., Mairiang, E., Mairiang, P., Pelkonen, P., Bartsch, H. and Haswell-Elkins, M. R. (1996) 'Induction of cytochrome P450 2A6 expression in humans by the carcinogenic parasite infection, Opisthorchiasis viverrini', *Cancer Epidemiol. Biomarkers Prev.* **5**: 795–800.

Säwe, J., Kager, I., Svensson, J.-O. and Rane, A. (1985) 'Oral morphine in cancer patients: in vivo kinetics and in vitro hepatic glucuronidation', *Br. J. Clin. Pharmacol.* 19: 495–501.

Schellens, J. H., Soons, P. A., Breimer, D. D. (1988) 'Lack of bimodality in nifedipine plasma kinetics in a large population of healthy subjects', *Biochem. Pharmacol.* 37: 2507–10.

Schmiedlin-Ren, P., Edwards, D. J., Fitzsimmons, M. E., He, K., Lown, K. S., Woster, P. M., Rahman, A., Thummel, K. E., Fisher, J. M., Hollenberg, P. F. and Watkins, P. B. (1997) 'Mechanisms of enhanced oral availability of CYP3A4 substrates by grapefruit constituents. Decreased enterocyte CYP3A4 concentration and mechanism-based inactivation by furanocoumarins', *Drug Metab. Dispos.* 25: 1228–33.

Schrenk, D., Brockmeier, D., Morike, K., Bock, K. W. and Eichelbaum, M. (1998) 'A distribution study of CYP1A2 phenotypes among smokers and non-smokers in a cohort of healthy Caucasian volunteers', *Eur. J. Clin. Pharmacol.* 53: 361–7.

Schuetz, E. G., Schuetz, J. D., Grogan, W. M., Naray-Fejes-Toth, A., Fejes-Toth, G., Raucy, J., Guzelian, P., Gionela, K. and Watlington, C. O. (1992) 'Expression of cytochrome P450 3A in amphibian, rat, and human kidney', *Arch. Biochem. Biophys.* 294: 206–14.

Schuetz, E. G., Schuetz, J. D., Strom, S. C., Thompson, M. T., Fisher, R. A., Molowa, D. T., Li, D. and Guzelian, P. S. (1993b) 'Regulation of human liver cytochromes P-450 in family 3A in primary and continuous culture of human hepatocytes', *Hepatology* 18: 1254–62.

Schuetz, J. D., Beach, D. L. and Guzelian, P. S. (1994) 'Selective expression of cytochrome P450 CYP3A mRNAs in embryonic and adult human liver', *Pharmacogenetics* 4: 11–20.

Schuetz, J. D., Kauma, S. and Guzelian, P. S. (1993a) 'Identification of the fetal liver cytochrome CYP3A7 in human endometrium and placenta', *J. Clin. Invest.* 92: 1018–24.

Schuetz, J. D., Molowa, D. T. and Guzelian, P. S. (1989) 'Characterization of a cDNA encoding a new member of the glucocorticoid-responsive cytochromes P450 in human liver', *Arch. Biochem. Biophys.* 274: 355–65.

Schuetz, J. D., Schuetz, E. G., Thottassery, J. V., Guzelian, P. S., Strom, S. and Sun, D. (1996) 'Identification of a novel dexamethasone responsive enhancer in the human CYP3A5 gene and its activation in human and rat liver cells', *Mol. Pharmacol.* 49: 63–72.

Schweikl, H., Taylor, J. A., Kitareewan, S., Linko, P., Nagorney, D. and Goldstein, J. A. (1993) 'Expression of CYP1A1 and CYP1A2 genes in human liver', *Pharmacogenetics* 3: 239–49.

Sesardic, D., Boobis, A. R., Edwards, R. J. and Davies, D. S. (1988) 'A form of cytochrome P450 in man, orthologous to form d in the rat, catalyses the O-deethylation of phenacetin and is inducible by cigarette smoking', *Br. J. Clin. Pharmacol.* 26: 363–72.

Sesardic, D., Boobis, A. R., Murray, B. P., Murray, S., Segura, J., de la Torre, R. and Davies, D. S. (1990a) 'Furafylline is a potent and selective inhibitor of cytochrome P450IA2 in man', *Br. J. Clin. Pharmacol.* 29: 651–63.

Sesardic, D., Pasanen, M., Pelkonen, O. and Boobis, A. R. (1990b) 'Differential expression and regulation of members of the cytochrome P450IA gene subfamily in human tissues', *Carcinogenesis* **11**: 1183–8.

Shimada, T. and Guengerich, F. P. (1989) 'Evidence for cytochrome P-450NF, the nifedipine oxidase, being the principal enzyme involved in the bioactivation of aflatoxins in human liver', *Proc. Natl, Acad. Sci. USA* **86**: 462–5.

Shimada, T., Hayes, C. L., Yamazaki, H., Amin, S., Hecht, S. S., Guengerich, F. P. and Sutter, T. R. (1996) 'Activation of chemically diverse procarcinogens by human cytochrome P-450 1B1', *Cancer Res.* **56**: 2979–84.

Shimada, T., Yamazaki, H. and Guengerich, F. P. (1996) 'Ethnic-related differences in coumarin 7-hydroxylation activity catalyzed by cytochrome P2402A6 in liver microsomes of Japanese and Caucasian populations', *Xenobiotica* **26**: 395–403.

Shimada, T., Yamazaki, H., Mimura, M., Inui, Y. and Guengerich, F. P. (1994) 'Interindividual variations in human liver cytochrome P-450 enzymes involved in the oxidation of drugs, carcinogens and toxic chemicals: studies with liver microsomes of 30 Japanese and 30 Caucasians', *J. Pharmacol. Exp. Ther.* **270**: 414–23.

Shimizu, M., Lasker, J. M., Tsutsumi, M. and Lieber, C. S. (1990) 'Immunohistochemical localization of ethanol-inducible P450IIE1 in the rat alimentary tract', *Gastroenterology* **99**: 1044–53.

Shou, M., Grogan, J., Mancewicz, J. A., Krausz, K. W., Gonzalez, F. J., Gelboin, H. V. and Korzekwa, K. R. (1994) 'Activation of CYP2A4: evidence for the simultaneous binding of two substrates in a cytochrome P450 active site', *Biochemistry* **33**: 6450–5.

Silva, J. M., Morin, P. E., Day, S. H., Kennedy, B. P., Payette, P., Rushmore, T., Yergey, J. A. and Nicoll-Griffith, D. A. (1998) 'Refinement of an in vitro cell model for cytochrome P450 induction', *Drug Metab. Dispos.* **26**: 490–6.

Skoda, R. C., Gonzalez, F. J., Demierre, A. and Meyer, U. A. (1988) 'Two mutant alleles of the human cytochrome P-450dbl gene (P450C2D1) associated with genetically deficient metabolism of debrisoquine and other drugs', *Proc. Natl. Acad. Sci. USA* **85**: 5240–3.

Song, B. J., Veech, R. L., Park, S. S., Gelboin, H. V. and Gonzalez, F. J. (1989) 'Induction of rat hepatic N-nitrosodimethylamine demethylase by acetone due to protein stabilization', *J. Biol. Chem.* **264**: 3568–72.

Sotaniemi, E. A., Rautio, A., Bäckström, M., Arvela, P. and Pelkonen, O. (1995) Hepatic cytochrome P450 isoenzyme (CYP2A6 and CYP3A4) activities and fibrotic process in liver', *Br. J. Clin. Pharmacol.* **39**: 71–6.

Spaldin, V., Madden, S., Adams, D. A., Edwards, R. J., Davies, D. S. and Park, B. K. (1995) 'Determination of human hepatic cytochrome P4501A2 activity in vitro use of tacrine as an isoenzyme-specific probe', *Drug Metab. Dispos.* **23**: 929–34.

Spink, D. C., Hayes, C. L., Young, N. R., Christou, M., Sutter, T. R., Jefcoate, C. R. and Gierthy, J. F. (1994) 'The effect of 2,3,7,8-tetrachloro-dibenzo-p-dioxin on estrogen metabolism in MCF-7 breast cancer cells: evidence for induction of a novel 17b-estradiol-4-hydroxylase', *J. Steroid Biochem. Mol. Biol.* **51**: 251–8.

Steward, D. J., Haining, R. L. and Henne, K. R. (1997) 'Genetic association between sensitivity to warfarin and expression of CYP2C9*3', *Pharmacogenetics* **7**: 361–7.

Stoilov, I., Akarsu, A. N. and Sarfarazi, M. (1997) 'Identification of three different truncating mutations in cytochrome P4501B1 (CYP1B1) as the principal cause of primary congenital glaucoma (Buphthalmos) in families linked to the GLC3A locus on chromosome 2p21', *Human Mol. Genet.* 6: 641–7.

Streetman, D. S., Bertino, J. S. and Nafziger, A. N. (2000) 'Phenotyping of drug-metabolizing enzymes in adults: a review of in vivo cytochrome P450 phenotyping probes', *Pharmacogenetics* 10: 187–216.

Strom, S., Pisarov, L. A., Dorko, K., Thompson, M. T., Schuetz, J. D. and Schuetz, E. G. (1996) 'Use of human hepatocytes to study P450 gene induction', *Methods in Enzymology* 272: 388–401.

Stubbins, M. J., Harries, L. W., Smith, G., Tarbit, M. H. and Wolf, C. R. (1996) 'Genetic analysis of the human cytochrome P450 CYP2C9', *Pharmacogenetics* 6: 429–39.

Sumida, A., Kinoshita, K., Fukuda, T., Matsuda, H., Yamamoto, I., Inaba, T. and Azuma, J. (1999) 'Relationship between mRNA levels quantified by reverse transcription-competitive PCR and metabolic activity of CYP3A4 and CYP2E1 in human liver', *Biochem. Biophys. Res. Commun.* 262: 499–503.

Sutter, T. R., Guzman, K., Dold, K. M. and Greenlee, W. F. (1991) 'Targets for dioxin: genes for plasminogen activator inhibitor-2 and interleukin-1 beta', *Science* 254: 415–8.

Sutter, T. R., Tang, Y. M., Hayes, C. L., Wo, Y. Y., Jabs, E. W., Li, X., Yin, H., Cody, C. W. and Greenlee, W. F. (1994) 'Complete cDNA sequence of a human dioxin-inducible mRNA identifies a new gene subfamily of cytochrome P450 that maps to chromosome 2', *J. Biol. Chem.* 269: 13092–9.

Tang, B. K., Zhou, Y., Kadar, D. and Kalow, W. (1994) 'Caffeine as a probe for CYP1A2 activity: potential influence of renal factors on urinary phenotypic trait measurements', *Pharmacogenetics* 4: 117–24.

Tang, Y. M., Wo, Y. Y. P., Stewart, J., Hawkins, A. L., Griffin, C. A., Sutter, T. R. and Greenlee, W. F. (1996) 'Isolation and characterization of the human cytochrome P450 CYP1B1 gene', *J. Biol. Chem.* 271: 28324–30.

Tassaneeyakul, W., Birkett, D. J., Veronese, M. E., McManus, M. E., Tukey, R. H., Quattrochi, L. C., Gelboin, H. V. and Miners, J. O. (1993) 'Specificity of substrate and inhibitor probes for human cytochromes P450 1A1 and 1A2', *J. Pharmacol. Exp. Ther.* 265: 401–7.

Tateishi, T., Watanabe, M., Moriya, H., Yamaguchi, S., Sato, T. and Kobayashi, S. (1999) 'No ethnic difference between Caucasian and Japanese hepatic samples in the expression frequency of CYP3A5 and CYP3A7 proteins', *Biochem. Pharmacol.* 57: 935–9.

Thummel, K. E. and Wilkinson, G. R. (1998) 'In vitro and in vivo drug interactions involving human CYP3A', *Annu. Rev. Pharmacol. Toxicol.* 38: 389–430.

Transon, C., Lecoeur, S., Leemann, T., Beaune, P. and Dayer, P. (1996) 'Interindividual variability in catalytic activity and immunoreactivity of three major human liver cytochrome P450 isozymes', *Eur. J. Clin. Pharmacol.* 51: 79–85.

Turesky, R. J., Constable, A., Richoz, J., Varga, N., Markovic, J., Martin, M. V. and Guengerich, F. P. (1998) 'Activation of heterocyclic aromatic amines by rat and human liver microsomes and by purified rat and human cytochrome P450 1A2', *Chem. Res. Toxicol.* 11: 925–36.

Umeno, M., Song, B. J., Kozak, C., Gelboin, H. V. and Gonzalez, F. J. (1988) 'The rat P450IIE1 gene: complete intron and exon sequence, chromosome mapping, and correlation of developmental expression with specific 5′ cytosine demethylation', *J. Biol. Chem.* **263**: 4956–62.

Vanden Heuvel, J. P., Clark, G. C., Thompson, C. L., McCoy, Z., Miller, C. R., Lucier, G. W. and Bell, D. A. (1993). 'CYP1A1 mRNA levels as a human exposure biomarker: use of quantitative polymerase chain reaction to measure CYP1A1 expression in human peripheral blood lymphocytes', *Carcinogenesis* **14**: 2003–6.

Villikka, K., Kivisto, K. T. and Neuvonen, P. J. (1998) 'The effect of dexamethasone on the pharmacokinetics of triazolam', *Pharmacol. Toxicol.* **83**: 135–8.

von Moltke, L. L., Greenblatt, D. J., Schmider, J., Duan, S. X., Wright, C. E., Harmatz, J. S. and Shader, R. I. (1996) 'Midazolam hydroxylation by human liver microsomes in vitro: inhibition by fluoxetine, norfluoxetine, and by azole antifungal agents', *J. Clin. Pharmacol.* **36**: 783–91.

Wacher, V. J., Wu, C. Y. and Benet, L. Z. (1995) 'Overlapping substrate specificities and tissue distribution of cytochrome P450 3A and P-glycoprotein: implications for drug delivery and activity in cancer chemotherapy', *Mol. Carcinog.* **13**: 129–34.

Wadelius, M., Darj, E., Frenne, G. and Rane, A. (1997) 'Induction of CYP2D6 in pregnancy', *Clin. Pharmacol. Ther.* **62**: 400–7.

Walker, A. H., Jaffe, J. M., Gunasegaram, S., Cummings, S. A., Huang, C. S., Chern, H. D., Olopade, O. I., Weber, B. L. and Rebbeck, T. R. (1998) 'Characterization of an allelic variant in the nifedipine-specific element of CYP3A4: ethnic distribution and implications for prostate cancer risk. Mutations in brief No. 191', *Hum. Mutat.* **12**: 289.

Watkins, P. B., Wrighton, S. A., Maurel, P., Schuetz, E. G., Mendez-Picon, G., Parker, G. A. and Guzelian, P. S. (1985) 'Identification of an inducible form of cytochrome P-450 in human liver', *Proc. Natl. Acad. Sci. USA* **82**: 6310–4.

Waxman, D. J., Attisano, C., Guengerich, F. P. and Lapenson, D. P. (1988) 'Human liver microsomal steroid metabolism: identification of the major microsomal steroid hormone 6 beta-hydroxylase cytochrome P-450 enzyme', *Arch. Biochem. Biophys.* **263**: 424–36.

Waxman, D. J., Lapenson, D. P., Aoyama, T., Gelboin, H. V., Gonzalez, F. J. and Korzekwa, K. (1991) 'Steroid hormone hydroxylase specificities of eleven cDNA-expressed human cytochrome P450s', *Arch. Biochem. Biophys.* **290**: 160–6.

Welfare, M. R., Aitkin, M., Bassendine, M. F. and Daly, A. K. (1999) 'Detailed modelling of caffeine metabolism and examination of the CYP1A2 gene: lack of a polymorphism in CYP1A2 in Caucasians', *Pharmacogenetics* **9**: 367–75.

Werlinder, V., Zhukov, A. and Ingelman-Sundberg, M. (2000) 'Posttranslational regulation of cytochrome P4501A2', Abstracts of 13th International Symposium on Microsomes and Drug Oxidations, Stresa, Italy, Abstr. 160: 149.

Westlind, A., Lofberg, L., Tindberg, N., Andersson, T. B. and Ingelman-Sundberg, M. (1999) 'Interindividual differences in hepatic expression of CYP3A4: relationship to genetic polymorphism in the 5′-upstream regulatory region', *Biochem. Biophys. Res. Commun.* **259**: 201–5.

Wilkinson, G. R. and Shand, D. G. (1975) 'Commentary: a physiological approach to hepatic drug clearance', *Clin. Pharmacol. Ther.* **18**: 377–90.

Willey, J. C., Coy, E. L., Frampton, M. W., Torres, A., Apostolakos, M. J., Hoehn, G., Schuermann, W. H., Thilly, W. G., Olson, D. E., Hammersley, J. R., Crespi,

C. L. and Utell, M. J. (1997) 'Quantitative RT-PCR measurement of cytochromes p450 1A1, 1B1, and 2B7, microsomal epoxide hydrolase, and NADPH oxidoreductase expression in lung cells of smokers and nonsmokers', *Am. J. Respir. Cell. Mol. Biol.* **17**: 114–24.

Windmill, K. F., McKinnon, R. A., Zhu, X., Gaedigk, A., Grant, D. M. and McManus, M. E. (1997) 'The role of xenobiotic metabolizing enzymes in arylamine toxicity and carcinogenesis: functional and localization studies', *Mutat. Res.* **376**: 153–60.

Wolbold, R., Burk, O., Eichelbaum, M., Fischer, J., Klein, K., Neuhaus, P., Nüssler, A. K. and Zanger, U. M. (2000) 'Expression variability of CYP3A4 and pregnane X-receptor (PXR) in human livers', Abstracts of 13th International Symposium on Microsomes and Drug Oxidations, Stresa, Italy, Abstr. 159: 149.

Woosley, R. L. (1996) 'Cardiac actions of antihistamines', *Annu. Rev. Pharmacol. Toxicol.* **36**: 233–52.

Wrighton, S. A., Brian, W. R., Sari, M. A., Iwasaki, M., Guengerich, F. P., Raucy, J. L., Molowa, D. T. and Vandenbranden, M. (1990) 'Studies on the expression and metabolic capabilities of human liver cytochrome P450IIIA5 (HLp3)', *Mol. Pharmacol.* **38**: 207–13.

Wrighton, S. A., Ring, B. J., Watkins, P. B. and Vandenbranden, M. (1989) 'Identification of a polymorphically expressed member of the human cytochrome P-450III family', *Mol. Pharmacol.* **36**: 97–105.

Wrighton, S. A. and Vandenbranden, M. (1989) 'Isolation and characterization of human fetal liver cytochrome P450HLp2: a third member of the P450III gene family', *Arch. Biochem. Biophys.* **268**: 144–51.

Wrighton, S. A., Vandenbranden, M. and Ring, B. J. (1996) 'The human drug metabolizing cytochromes P450', *J. Pharmacokin. Biopharm.* **24**: 461–73.

Xu, L., Li, A. P., Kaminski, D. L. and Ruh, M. (2000) '2,3,7,8 Tetrachlorodibenzo-p-dioxin induction of cytochrome P4501A in cultured rat and human hepatocytes', *Chem. Biol. Interact.* **124**: 173–89.

Yamakoshi, Y., Kishimoto, T., Sugimura, K. and Kawashima, H. (1999) 'Human prostate CYP3A5: identification of a unique 5´-untranslated sequence and characterization of purified recombinant protein', *Biochem. Biophys. Res. Commun.* **260**: 676–81.

Yamano, S., Tatsuno, J. and Gonzalez, F. J. (1990) 'The CYP2A3 gene product catalyzes coumarin 7-hydroxylation in human liver microsomes', *Biochemistry* **29**: 1322–9.

Yamazaki, H., Inoue, K., Hashimoto, M. and Shimada, T. (1999) 'Roles of CYP2A6 and CYP2B6 in nicotine C-oxidation by human liver microsomes', *Arch. Toxicol.* **73**: 65–70.

Yamazaki, H., Inoue, K., Turvy, G. C., Guengerich, F. P. and Shimada, T. (1997) 'Effect of freezing, thawing, and storage of human liver samples on the microsomal contents and activities of cytochrome P450 enzymes', *Drug Metab. Dispos.* **25**: 168–74.

Yamazaki, H., Shaw, P. M., Guengerich, F. P. and Shimada, T. (1998) 'Roles of cytochromes P450 1A2 and 3A4 in the oxidation of estradiol and estrone in human liver microsomes', *Chem. Res. Toxicol.* **11**: 659–65.

Yang, H. Y., Lee, Q. P., Rettie, A. E. and Juchau, M. R. (1994) 'Functional cytochrome P4503A isoforms in human embryonic tissues: expression during organo-genesis', *Mol. Pharmacol.* **46**: 922–8.

Yokose, T., Doy, M., Kakiki, M., Horie, T., Matsuzaki, Y. and Mukai, K. (1998) 'Expression of cytochrome P450 3A4 in foveolar epithelium with intestinal metaplasia of the human stomach', *Jpn. J. Cancer Res.* **89**: 1028–32.

Yun, C.-H., Shimada, T., Guengerich, F. P. (1991) 'Purification and characterization of human liver microsomal cytochrome P-450 2A6', *Mol. Pharmacol.* **40**: 679–85.

Zhai, S., Dai, R., Friedman, F. K. and Vestal, R. E. (1998) 'Comparative inhibition of human cytochromes P450 1A1 and 1A2 by flavonoids', *Drug Metab. Dispos.* **26**: 989–92.

Zhang, Q. Y., Dunbar, D., Ostrowska, A., Zeisloft, S., Yang, J. and Kaminsky, L. S. (1999) 'Characterization of human small intestinal cytochromes P-450', *Drug Metab. Dispos.* **27**: 804–9.

Zhao, K., Murray, S., Davies, D. S., Boobis, A. R. and Gooderham, N. J. (1994) 'Metabolism of the food derived mutagen and carcinogen 2-amino-1-methyl-6-phenylimidazo(4,5-b)pyridine (PhIP) by human liver microsomes', *Carcinogenesis* **15**: 1285–8.

Zhukov, A. and Ingelman-Sundberg, M. (1999) 'Relationship between cytochrome P450 catalytic cycling and stability: fast degradation of ethanol-inducible cytochrome P450 2E1 (CYP2E1) in hepatoma cells is abolished by inactivation of its electron donor NADPH-cytochrome P450 reducatase', *Biochem. J.* **340**: 453–8.

Chapter 11

Interindividual variability of arylamine N-acetyltransferases

G. N. Levy and W. W. Weber

Introduction

This chapter will consider the molecular mechanisms and the consequences of interindividual variability of human N-acetyltransferase (E.C. 2.3.1.5). The two known isoforms of the human enzyme (NAT1 and NAT2) catalyze transfer of an acetyl group, primarily from AcCoA, to the amino nitrogen of an acceptor amine producing an acetamide. Certain hydrazines can also serve as substrates for acetylation and the acetylation of the anti-tubercular hydrazine isoniazid has been instrumental in the discovery and understanding of variability in human acetylation activity.

Clinical trials and widespread use of isoniazid to combat tuberculosis beginning in 1952, brought N-acetyltransferase into the spotlight of drug metabolism research. NAT is a conjugation enzyme catalyzing phase II of drug metabolism leading to the formation and excretion of water soluble non-toxic metabolites of active drugs. In the case of isoniazid, acetylation produces a non-bacteriocidal metabolite identified as acetylisoniazid. The amount of this metabolite produced varied between individuals, but was quite constant in each individual over time (Bönicke and Reif, 1953). The rates of isoniazid elimination in patients, as well as in healthy controls, fell into two distinct groups, known as good and poor eliminators. As the relation of acetylation and inactivation of isoniazid became known, the division of the population became known as rapid and slow acetylators. Being a rapid or slow acetylator has consequences beyond the simple elimination of isoniazid. Rapid acetylators needed to receive more frequent doses of isoniazid to maintain serum concentrations in the therapeutic range, while slow acetylators were more prone to peripheral neuritis and central nervous system toxicities caused by isoniazid therapy (Devadatta et al., 1960).

N-acetylation of pharmacological and environmental compounds

As the understanding of N-acetylation in drug metabolism grew, the list of drugs known to be substrates for NAT also grew. Arylamines and hydrazines are substrates and so are compounds which do not have a free amino group initially, but are converted by metabolism to amino-containing metabolites. Important examples of this are caffeine which is the most widely used drug in many cultures, sulfasalazine, nitrazepam, and acebutolol. In addition to isoniazid, hydrazine drugs subject to acetylation include hydralazine, phenelzine, and acetylhydrazine. The list of arylamine drugs that are acetylated includes sulfamethazine and many other sulfa drugs, aminoglutethimide, procainamide, promizole, dapsone, p-amino-benzoic acid, and p-aminosalicylic acid (Weber 1987: 52). The possibility that a new drug or its metabolic product is a substrate for acetylation should always be considered as rapid, and slow acetylators may be affected differently in regard to efficacy and/or toxicity. An example of this point is the experimental anticancer drug amonafide which, because of increased toxicity among rapid acetylators, requires NAT2 phenotyping of patients and adjustment of dosage for use (Ratain et al., 1996).

In addition to their important role in metabolism of arylamine and hydrazine drugs, N-acetyltransferases are key enzymes in the metabolic disposition of arylamine carcinogens. Carcinogenic compounds previously used in various industrial processes such as benzidine, β-naphthylamine, and methylene-bis-(2-chloroaniline) are substrates for NAT. Arylamines found in environmental hazards such as 4-aminobiphenyl in tobacco smoke and the (never released for use) insecticide 2-aminofluorene are substrates which are now often used as model compounds to study NAT activity and DNA damage. Recently, attention has been focused on the role of NAT in activation of heterocyclic arylamines formed in cooking meats and other foods. More than a score of these compounds have been isolated and the mutagenicity and carcinogenicity of several have been demonstrated (de Meester, 1989). As in the case of therapeutic drugs, there is interindividual variability in the acetylation of arylamine carcinogens, and this leads to differences in risk of carcinogenesis in those exposed to the carcinogen. Identification of the high-risk subpopulations and their protection from carcinogen exposure is an important goal in NAT research.

From the discovery of interindividual variation in the acetylation of isoniazid to the present, there have been numerous studies of variation in metabolism of NAT substrates and the effects of these variations on occurrence of drug toxicities, cancers, and other maladies. In some instances the mechanisms of such associations are clear, in some the mechanisms are hypothetical, and in others the mechanisms are unknown. In addition to the example of increased toxicity of isoniazid among slow acetylators, procainamide, a widely used anti-arrhythmic agent, is differentially acetylated and has differential toxic and therapeutic activity among rapid and slow acetylators (Reidenberg et al., 1975, 1980). Studies have shown that the major pathway for metabolism and elimination of procainamide involves N-acetylation. In individuals with impaired acetylation ability, competing pathways, primarily involving *N*-oxidation of the free amino group lead to toxicity. Administration of *N*-acetylprocainamide, also possessing anti-arrhythmic activity, avoids the toxicity seen in slow acetylators. Thus the more frequent occurrence or more rapid onset of drug-induced lupus erythematosus in slow acetylators taking procainamide or hydralazine may be understood (Strandberg *et al.*, 1976; Woosley *et al.*, 1978).

The association of acetylator status with several cancers has been examined in humans by epidemiological methods and by experimental methods in several animal models. The classical study of Cartwright *et al.* (1982) showed an excess of slow acetylators amongst bladder cancer patients with previous occupational exposure to arylamine carcinogens compared with population controls. The mechanisms by which slow acetylators could be more at risk for arylamine-induced bladder cancer have been postulated to involve a decrease in hepatic *N*-acetylation of the parent amine allowing for microsomal activation by *N*-oxidation to form *N*-hydroxyamines followed by *N*-glucuronidation. The *N*-glucuronide is then transported from the liver through blood to the kidneys and filtered into the urine. The normal acidic urine of humans causes hydrolysis of the glucuronide, leaving the active hydroxylamine which forms an arylnitrenium ion that reacts with cellular macromolecules including the guanosine residue of DNA, initiating the mutagenic and carcinogenic process (Lang and Kadlubar, 1991).

There are a number of other disorders for which an association with acetylator status has been reported. For most of these, the association has not gone unchallenged, and the mechanism for the role of acetylation is unknown. Diabetes and its complications (Bodansky *et al.*, 1981), spontaneous lupus erythematosus (Reidenberg *et al.*, 1980), leprosy (Evans, 1986), and Parkinson's disease (Bandmann *et al.*, 1997) among other disorders have all been claimed to be associated with rapid or slow acetylation, at least in some ethnic groups. It may be worthwhile to re-investigate some of these associations using NAT isozyme specific methods for phenotyping and molecular techniques for genotyping. Confirmation of a role for acetylation in some of these disorders may lead to new understanding of the etiology and mechanism of the disease.

Fundamental to our current understanding of variability of NAT activity in man is the finding that there are two isozymes of NAT (Grant *et al.*, 1991). Both isozymes can catalyze the *N*-acetylation, *O*-acetylation, and *N,O*-acetyltransfer reactions. Both isozymes are expressed in human liver, but differ in extrahepatic expression. The isozymes differ in substrate selectivity making certain substrates useful in determining which isozyme is present in a tissue by *N*-acetyltransferase activity assays. The isozyme known as NAT2 is active with sulfamethazine, procainamide, and isoniazid, while NAT1 is active with *p*-aminosalicylic and *p*-aminobenzoic acids (reviewed in Vatsis and Weber, 1997). Thus, NAT2 corresponds to "polymorphic NAT" in older papers while NAT1 is the "monomorphic NAT" of the older literature. It is important to understand that both enzymes are indeed polymorphic, having numerous alleles, as will be discussed later.

NAT phenotypes

The differing substrate selectivity of the NAT isozymes must be considered in attempts to relate acetylator status to risk of cancers and other conditions. Before the discovery of the isozymic nature of NAT, human phenotyping was carried out *in vivo* with sulfamethazine or another sulfa drug, dapsone, procainamide, hydralazine, or isoniazid (Weber, 1987: 154). These drugs showed significant interindividual differences in acetylation and are primarily NAT2 substrates. Determination of acetylator status *in vitro* was elusive and, for NAT2 at least, still is. In a healthy population, the only readily obtainable tissue is blood. However, in human leukocytes NAT1 but not NAT2 is expressed in the mononuclear cells and NAT1 is expressed to a much greater extent than NAT2 in the polymorphonuclear cells (Cribb *et al.*, 1991). This makes human leukocytes unsatisfactory for determining NAT2 phenotype.

Currently most studies involving human NAT2 phenotyping use a ratio of certain caffeine metabolites in urine (Grant *et al.*, 1984). The advantage of caffeine as a test drug is that most individuals include caffeine as a component of the normal diet so that introduction of an additional drug, perhaps with undesirable side-effects, is avoided. Metabolites are analyzed in urine, thus avoiding a blood draw. The actual determination of acetylator phenotype with caffeine is based on a ratio of the substance produced by acetylation, 5-acetylamino-6-formylamino-3-methyluracil (AFMU), to metabolites produced by cytochrome P-450 demethylation of a common precursor. The simple ratio of AFMU/1X (1-methylxanthine) is commonly determined by HPLC and the value of the antimode of the distribution is found. Thus individuals with AFMU/1X values greater than the antimode are rapid acetylators and those below are slow. A slightly more complex ratio which accounts for possible variation in xanthine oxidase activity as well includes 1-methyluracil (1U) in the denominator (Kashuba *et al.*, 1998). The ratio AFMU/(AFMU+1U+1X) distinguishes rapid and slow acetylators. The actual values of the antimodes using either ratio may shift for populations of different ethnicities.

An important and so far unanswered question concerning caffeine phenotyping is whether NAT1 is involved in caffeine metabolism. Excellent correlation has been found between caffeine and sulfamethazine phenotype determination, which argues for the validity of caffeine for NAT2 activity determinations, but specific studies of caffeine metabolites as substrates for NAT1 are lacking (Cribb *et al.*, 1994).

Interindividual variability in NAT2

Variability in NAT2, the basis of the classical (isoniazid/sulfamethazine) acetylation polymorphism, is due to mutation of the *NAT2** gene. Located on chromosome 8 (8p22) (Matas *et al.*, 1997), *NAT2** has an 870 base pair intronless coding region. Numerous (more than 20) alleles have been described for this locus. Nomenclature for and a description of the alleles identified up to 1994 are given in Vatsis *et al.* (1995). Additional alleles of *NAT2** continue to be reported as additional individuals are genotyped. The *NAT2*4* allele is taken as the "wild-type" as it is found in individuals phenotyped as rapid acetylators. The other alleles are all associated with reduced acetylation when any two of them are paired in an individual. Thus, homozygosity in a mutant allele or compound heterozygosity of two different mutant alleles produces a slow acetylator. The mechanism of slow acetylation may involve reduced catalytic activity of the mutant allele, reduced protein production or stability, or decreased mRNA production or stability by the mutant allele.

The following nucleotide changes have been found in the coding region of *NAT2* alleles: G191A, C282T, T341C, A434C, C481T, G590A, A803G, A845C, and G857A (Table 11.1). The large number of *NAT2** alleles results from these mutations occurring singly or in combinations of two or three. Not all possible combinations of mutations have been found and there is the possibility of nucleotide changes at other sites yet to be discovered. Seven of the nine nucleotide changes listed result in changes in the deduced amino acid, C282T and C481T being the exceptions. Some of these amino acid substitutions result in significant changes in charge and local hydrophobicity which may strongly affect peptide folding and stability (Martell *et al.*, 1991) as well as altering substrate (AcCoA or

Table 11.1 Mutations of NAT2* coding region

Base No.	Base change	Amino acid No.	Amino acid change	Restriction site	Activity[a]	Allele name[b]
191	G→A	64	Arg→Gln	*Msp*I deleted	decreased	14 family
282	C→T	994	–	*Fok*I deleted	normal	13
341	T→C	114	Ile→Thr	–	decreased	5 family
434	A→C	145	Glu→Pro	*Msp*I added	?	17
481	C→T	161	–	*Kpn*I deleted	decreased	5A and 5B
590	G→A	197	Arg→Gln	*Taq*I deleted	decreased	6 family
803	A→G	268	Lys→Arg	*Dde*I added	normal	12 family
845	A→C	282	Lys→Thr	*Dra*III added	?	18
857	G→A	286	Gly→Arg	*Bam*HI deleted	decreased	7 family

Notes
[a]Activity for allele expressed in heterologous system relative to NAT2*4 (compiled by Vatsis *et al.*, 1995).
[b]See http://athena.louisville.edu/medschool/pharmacology/NAT.html for latest information on NAT nomenclature.

arylamine) binding. For genotyping purposes, all the known nucleotide changes except T341C add or delete an endonuclease restriction site (Doll *et al.*, 1995).

It is apparent from the NAT2* alleles reported, that the coding region of the gene has been the site of multiple mutations. Most studies of the NAT2* alleles have examined only the coding region and very little analysis has been done with the regions upstream or downstream from it. Thus, it is possible that additional mutations exist in several of the alleles described. The methodology used to genotype NAT2* in individuals is usually PCR amplification of the coding region and restriction endonuclease digestion, or nested PCR followed by endonuclease digestion, or allele-specific PCR. These methods, when properly used can detect all known NAT2* alleles, but may be unable to detect previously undescribed alleles. Greater use of sequencing and other confirmatory techniques would make allele identification more certain (Cascorbi and Roots, 1999).

Ethnic variation in NAT2*

The distribution of NAT2* alleles is neither uniformly nor randomly distributed across humans, but varies with racial, ethnic, and geographic origin. Ignoring the population genetics of allele frequencies can lead to major errors in the interpretation of the association of genetic polymorphisms and disease risk (Garte, 1998). The pattern of distribution of alleles probably is due to the origination of NAT2* mutations in different populations and either the isolation of or the subsequent migration and mixing of peoples who were originally separated by geography, custom, etc. As we do not know the natural or endogenous substrate for NAT, we can not determine the role of natural selection on the preservation or spread of NAT gene mutations.

Among American and European Caucasians, the frequency of the NAT2*4 allele is about 20–25%. The frequency of this rapid allele is higher in African-Americans (36%), Hispanic Americans (42%), and still higher in Asiatics. Hong Kong Chinese have about a 48% NAT2*4 frequency, Koreans living in the U.S. about 66%, and a native population of Japanese over 70% frequency of NAT2*4 (Vatsis and Weber, 1997).

Available data for the distribution of mutant NAT2* alleles give some interesting results. American and European Caucasians have NAT2*5B as the most frequent mutant allele (40%), followed closely by NAT2*6A with a 30% frequency. Thus for Caucasians, the alleles 4, 5B, and 6A account for approximately 95% of all NAT2* alleles. Among African-Americans, the frequencies of both 5B (30%) and 6A (23%) are decreased with part of the deficit made up by the 14A and 14B alleles (10%) which are very rare in non-African populations. In the Hispanic American population, 5B (23%) and 6A (17%) are further reduced and 7A and 7B become significant with a frequency of (17%). In Oriental populations, the 5B allele becomes rare (5% in Hong Kong Chinese to <1% in Japanese) and the 6A (20–30%) and 7A/7B (7–16%) alleles are the most frequent mutant alleles (Vatsis and Weber, 1997).

As a practical matter, one may not need to use methods to distinguish every known NAT2* mutation in studies of the correlation of NAT2 and cancer or other diseases. Where the frequency of alleles is known for a population, genotyping diagnostic for three or four major alleles in that population may be sufficient. Further, the low frequency of some alleles means that the number of individuals with the rare alleles will be so small that statistically meaningful results related to the rare alleles will be very unlikely. More useful than exhaustive analysis of every known allele would be a determination of the major alleles in the population being studied. If three or four alleles account for 95% or more of all alleles in the population, it may not be necessary or useful to consider other alleles.

As is obvious from the differences in distribution of rapid and slow alleles in different populations, the NAT2 acetylator phenotype frequencies vary in different populations. The phenotype frequency of rapid acetylators (homozygous and heterozygous individuals) is about 45% in Caucasian populations and nearly 90% in Japanese. Obviously such differences in phenotype are important in determining the safety and efficacy profile of therapeutic agents which may be or may become substrates for acetylation.

Human variability in NAT2 and drug toxicity

Detrimental effects of acetylation may occur when an NAT substrate is encountered by the individual. A decreased ability to *N*-acetylate compounds does not appear to be disadvantageous by itself, but when the deficit in *N*-acetylation and the occurrence of an environmental factor coincide, undesirable consequences may follow. As previously described, no unusual problems were encountered by slow acetylators with tuberculosis until they were exposed to isoniazid, when the increased occurrence of neural toxicities became apparent. Similarly with procainamide, hydralazine, sulfa drugs, and so on, the interaction of decreased acetylation capacity and an environmental factor produced increased incidence or severity of toxicity.

The effect of polymorphic expression of NAT2 on the pharmacokinetics of NAT2 substrate drugs varies from drug to drug but usually produces a three- to six-fold difference in metabolism and elimination. For procainamide the plasma ratio of *N*-acetylprocainamide to procainamide is 3-fold greater in rapid acetylators than in slow, yet the renal clearance of procainamide does not differ between phenotypes (Reidenberg *et al.*, 1975). Variation in renal function of the patient population studied probably obliterated any NAT phenotype-related differences in clearance.

Sulfamethazine (sulphadimidine), a sulfa drug that is a substrate for NAT2, is polymorphically acetylated at a rate three to eight times greater in rapid than slow acetylators (Van Oudtshoorn and Potgieter, 1972). For isoniazid both the first-order rate constant for elimination and the urinary ratio of acetylisoniazid to non-acetylated isoniazid are three- to six-fold higher in rapid acetylators than slow (Ellard and Gammon, 1976). A significant number of examples can be cited where the NAT2 phenotype is an important determinant of differences in pharmacokinetics. Similarly, the role of NAT2 phenotype in frequency and severity of many drug toxicities has been definitely established in a multitude of reports over the past several decades.

An interesting practical problem has arisen as to whether decreased acetylation capacity can occur by non-genetic mechanisms. Can the slow acetylator phenotype be acquired? One way that alteration of phenotype can occur is via liver transplantation. *In vivo* acetylator phenotyping is based on the N-acetylation capacity of the liver while genotyping based on DNA from peripheral blood cells (or any other extrahepatic source) indicates the inherited genetic information of the individual. This has been shown in a study of fifty-eight liver transplant patients where the genotype of the grafted liver determined the phenotype of the recipient following transplantation (Bendriss *et al.*, 1998).

Clinical experience with HIV/AIDS patients has also provided some evidence of altered acetylation capacity and its consequences. Many case reports and studies have shown an increase in adverse reactions to a multitude of drugs among AIDS patients as compared with non-HIV positive patients (Harb and Jacobson, 1993). Although many different drugs show this increase, sulfamethoxazole, sulfadiazine, and isoniazid stand out because of the importance of acetylation in their metabolism. To examine the effect of HIV infection (or treatment of HIV infection) on drug metabolism, patients were phenotyped and compared with matched, non-HIV controls. The patients were grouped as AIDS-acutely ill, AIDS-stable, and HIV+ but non-symptomatic. The control group was 62% slow acetylator (18 of 29). The acutely ill AIDS group was 93% slow acetylator (27 of 29). The stable AIDS patients and the asymptomatic HIV individuals did not differ from controls (66% and 56% slow acetylators, respectively) (Lee *et al.*, 1993). Other results indicated increased 8-hydroxylation and decreased demethylation activity in the acute patients, but no differences from the controls for the other categories and no difference from controls for xanthine oxidase activity in any group. Liver enzymes (ALT and AST) were two- to four-fold higher in acutely ill patients than in the other groups (Lee *et al.*, 1993). A separate study by Kaufmann *et al.* (1996) found no difference in distribution of acetylator phenotype between control and patients with various stages of HIV infection. This study also genotyped the subjects and found 96% concordance of phenotype and genotype, verifying the accuracy of the caffeine results. These authors suggest that the combination of other drugs that undergo acetylation act as competitive inhibitors of caffeine acetylation and thus cause an erroneous phenotyping result. If the patients in Lee's study were receiving large doses of drugs metabolized by acetylation, it would be competition for available enzyme rather than liver damage, nutritional status, degree of immuno-suppression, or HIV infection itself that decreased apparent NAT2 activity as measured by caffeine (Kaufmann *et al.*, 1996).

Quite different results and conclusions have been presented by O'Neil *et al.* (1997). They found a discordance of 36% (18/50) between genotype and phenotype among HIV positive and AIDS patients. Although twelve had a fast genotype and a slow phenotype, six had the opposite, a slow genotype and a fast phenotype. The authors suggest that disease progression is the strongest candidate for altering acetylator phenotype, however a mechanism for this, beyond a small effect of wasting, is not elaborated. A decrease in the observed rate of acetylation could possibly be explained by exposure to a drug that inhibits or competes for NAT. An example of this is acetaminophen which has been reported to bind to NAT2 and prevent arylamine substrate from becoming acetylated (Rothen *et al.*, 1998). Plausible explanations for increased NAT2 activity are not known.

Human variability in NAT2 and cancer

The interaction of environment and genetics is extremely important in risk of cancer. Many studies of the interaction of arylamine carcinogens and polymorphic N-acetylation have been performed. It had been suggested that differences in the metabolism of arylamine carcinogens, such as by NAT, might lead to differences in risk of cancer (Weber, 1978). This possibility was strengthened by evidence that carcinogenic arylamines were polymorphically acetylated in the same manner as isoniazid and sulfa-methazine in rabbit and human liver (Glowinski *et al.*, 1978). Examples of studies of NAT2 polymorphism and human cancer are presented in Table 11.2. The principal cancers investigated have been bladder, colon, and breast. The strongest evidence of an effect of NAT2 polymorphism on cancer risk is for bladder cancer. For bladder cancer, the environmental element has often been identified as cigarette smoke or occupational exposure to arylamines.

The relation of acetylation to colon or colorectal cancer is somewhat different than for bladder cancer. First, the association of increased risk is with the rapid instead of the slow phenotype, and second, the environmental component is not identified. The increased risk for rapid acetylators has been explained as due to hepatic N-oxidation of arylamines, formation of the glucuronide which is transported via bile to the colon where bacterial glucuronidases release the N-hydroxyarylamine, and subsequent O-acetylation by NAT to the reactive N-acetoxyarylamine (Lang and

Table 11.2 Variability in NAT2 and cancer susceptibility

Cancer	Higher risk	Comment	Reference
Bladder	Slow[a]	occupational	Cartwright et al., 1982
	Neither	benzidine - Chinese	Hayes et al., 1993
	Slow	all, smokers, occup.	Risch et al., 1995
	Slow	Taiwanese	Su et al., 1998
	Slow	31 studies compiled	Vineis and Martone, 1998
Colorectal	Rapid[a]		Lang et al., 1986
	Rapid[a]		Ilett et al., 1987
	Rapid[a]	includes Lang et al.	Wohlleb et al., 1990
	Neither	Japanese	Shibuta et al., 1994
	Neither		Probst-Hensch et al., 1995
	Rapid[a]		Roberts-Thompson et al., 1996
	Slow	NAT2*7A in Chinese	Lee et al., 1998
Breast	Rapid[a]		Bulovskaya et al., 1978
	Rapid[a]	benign & malignant	Cartwright 1984
	Slow	smokers, postmeno	Ambrosone et cl., 1996
	Neither	smoking not a factor	Hunter et al., 1997
	Neither	meat intake	Ambrosone et cl., 1998
	Rapid	smokers, postmeno	Millikan et al.,1998
Lung	Rapid		Cascorbi et al., 1996
Mesothelioma	Slow	asbestos exposure	Hirvonen et al., 1995
Larynx	Slow[a]	especially smokers	Drózdz et al., 1987
Head and Neck	Slow	smokers - Spanish	González et al., 1998
Glioma	Rapid		Trizna et al., 1998

Notes
[a]Subjects phenotyped with a test drug, all other studies involved genotyping.
occup.=occupational exposure; postmeno=postmenopausal women.

Kadlubar, 1991). In this model the environmental arylamine is not identified, but could be food-borne heterocyclic amines or arylamine reduction
products of airborne nitroaromatic hydrocarbons. However, it has been
reported that the NAT activity of human intestine is due predominantly to
NAT1 rather than NAT2 (Hickman et al., 1998), which might invalidate
increased activity of NAT2 in the colon as an explanation for any increased risk of colorectal cancer among rapid acetylators.

A study of a Chinese population has shown an association of the
NAT2*7A allele with colorectal cancer. The combination of NAT2*7A
with the rapid NAT2*4 allele resulted in a slight increase in colorectal
cancer risk compared with homozygous rapid or other heterozygous
intermediate acetylators, but the combination of NAT2*7A with another
slow allele increased risk approximately three-fold (Lee et al., 1998). Any
effect of NAT2 activity on colon cancer risk probably involves carcinogen
metabolism at a site other than the colon as NAT2 is not the predominant
isozyme in colon (Hickman et al., 1998).

As the metabolism and disposition of arylamine and other carcinogens is complex and involves several enzymes, the association of genetic differences in drug metabolizing enzymes and cancer risk is multifactorial. Differences in activity of many enzymes involved in carcinogen metabolism need to be considered. In addition to NATs, cytochrome P450s, prostaglandin H synthases, glutathione S-transferases, glucuronosyl transferases, and sulfotransferases are among the activities that may modify cancer risk from chemical carcinogens. Ideally, these genetic factors should be studied in combination, but this is very difficult to carry out as the number of individuals in a study must be large because the individuals with the desired combination of genotypes will be only a fraction of the total. Thus, if NAT2 polymorphism together with glutathione S-transferase and a single CYP enzyme are considered, a 50% frequency of the slow phenotype combined with a 50% frequency of the GSTμ null genotype and say a 10% frequency of deficient CYP activity will leave only 2.5% of the original study population matching the characteristics to be studied.

The environmental factors encountered by the population also confound the problem (Ambrosone *et al.*, 1996, 1998). Should smokers be analyzed separately from non-smokers? What adjustments are required for occupational exposures? Should menopausal status be considered for female subjects? It is also possible that heavy environmental exposure to carcinogens can overcome and block out the significance of genetic risk factors. An interesting example of this was reported from Taiwan, where a significant increase in risk of bladder cancer was found among slow acetylators. However, in areas with high levels of arsenic in the drinking water, the risk of bladder cancer was similar between rapid and slow acetylators (Su *et al.*, 1998).

Interindividual variability in NAT I

One of the most troubling questions concerning the biology of NAT has been the existence of substrates such as isoniazid and sulfamethazine that are clearly polymorphically acetylated and substrates such as PABA and PAS which are apparently monomorphically acetylated. Individuals who are clearly rapid or slow acetylators based on isoniazid, SMZ, and similar compounds do not show polymorphic differences in acetylation of PABA or PAS. A number of possible models to answer this paradox have been proposed (Weber, 1987: 136–9). After almost three decades of various investigations, the answer was found by Grant *et al.* (1991) who isolated 2 distinct NAT isozymes from human liver. One of the isozymes, NAT1, acetylated "monomorphic" substrates, while the other isozyme, NAT2, acetylated the "polymorphic" substrates. Unfortunately the term "monomorphic" came to be applied to NAT1 because, although significant interindividual variation was found in acetylation of its substrates (Glowinski *et al.*, 1978; McQueen and Weber, 1980), bimodality in activity had not been reported. Although structural mutations in the coding region of *NAT2** were found quite readily (Ohsako and Deguchi, 1990, Ebisawa and Deguchi, 1991, Vatsis *et al.*, 1991), and these structural mutations correlated with decreased functionality of the variants (Blum *et al.*, 1991), a survey of possible *NAT1** mutations did not follow immediately.

In 1993, Vatsis and Weber (1993) clearly demonstrated structural heterogeneity of *NAT1**. The wild-type (*NAT1*4*) and two variant alleles (*NAT1*10* and *NAT1*11*) were identified. Further, Mendelian inheritance of the variants was demonstrated, as was independent expression of NAT1 and NAT2 (Vatsis and Weber, 1993) although *NAT1**, like *NAT2** is located at 8p22 (Matas *et al.*, 1997). Mutant *NAT1** alleles have continued to be found so that currently about twenty human *NAT1** alleles are known. Initially it was believed that *NAT1** mutations occurred mainly in the 3′-UTR and caused an altered polyadenylation signal which might be reflected in changed NAT1 mRNA stability and subsequent alteration in NAT1 protein levels (Vatsis and Weber, 1993). While this mechanism is still tenable, more recent work (Lin *et al.*, 1998; Hughes *et al.*, 1998; Butcher *et al.*, 1998) has demonstrated the occurrence and importance of mutations in the 870 base pair intronless coding region of *NAT1** leading to changes in *in vitro*, *in vivo*, and in heterologously expressed enzyme activity. Currently recognised mutations of *NAT1** are shown in Tables 11.3 and 11.4.

Ethnic variation in *NAT1**

Unlike the situation for *NAT2**, very little is known about the distribution of *NAT1** alleles. This lack of information is most likely due to the many years when NAT2 phenotyping was carried out under the presumption of "NAT" phenotyping as well as the assumption that NAT1, once discovered, was monomorphic. The information concerning mutant frequencies that is available is incomplete and somewhat contradictory. The original report of mutant *NAT1** alleles showed 42% of alleles of unrelated individuals to be variant (Vatsis and Weber, 1993). Hughes *et al.* (1998) reported 28.5% of 288 *NAT1** alleles genotyped were mutant. In the largest study to date, Lin *et al.* (1998) reported an identical mutation frequency of 5% among 976 alleles from controls and 888 alleles from colorectal cancer patients. However Lin's numbers do not include *NAT1*10*. Lin's study does not show any significant differences in mutation frequency between Asian, Black, Hispanic, and White subjects. In a small study of Japanese, Chinese, and Koreans (five subjects each), 47% of the *NAT1** alleles were mutant (Vatsis and Weber, unpublished). A recent report by Zhao *et al.* (1998) of 140 Indians, 122 Malay, and 181 Chinese living in Singapore showed an *NAT1** allele distribution of 30–33% *NAT1*3*,

Table 11.3 Mutations of NAT1* coding region

Base No.	Base change	Amino acid No.	Amino acid change	Acitivity[a]	Allele name
97	C→T	33	Arg→STOP	none	19
190	C→T	64	Arg→Trp	low/none	17
350,351	G→C	117	Arg→Thr	?	5
402	T→C	134	–	normal	20
445	G→A	149	Val→Ile	normal	11
459	G→A	153	–	normal	11
497,498	G→C	166	Arg→Thr	?	5
499	G→C	167	Glu→Gln ,	?	5
559	C→T	187	Arg→STOP	none	15
560	G→A	187	Arg→Gln	low	14
613	A→G	205	Met→Val	high	21
640	T→G	214	Ser→Ala	normal	11
752	A→T	251	Asp→Val	none	22
777	T→C	259	–	normal	23
781	G→A	261	Glu→Lys	high	24
787	A→G	263	Ile→Val	high	25

Notes
[a]Activity determined with PAS for NAT1 variants expressed in E. coli compared with wild-type NAT1*4 (Lin et al., 1998).

Table 11.4 Mutations of NAT1* untranslated regions

Region	Base No.	Base change	Activity[a]	Allele name
5′-UTR	−344	C→T	normal	11
	−40	A→T	normal	11
3′-UTR	884	A→G	?	5
	976	deleted	?	5
	1066–1090	9 bases deleted	normal	11
	1088	T→A	10 high, 14 low	10, 14
	1089–1091	AAA inserted	?	16
	1095	C→A	varies	3, 10, 11, 14, 16
	1105	deleted	?	5

Notes
[a]Activity determined as in Table 11.3. It is not known if the altered activity of certain NAT1 alleles is due to coding or non-coding region mutations.

30–35% *NAT1*4*, and 30–39% *NAT1*10* among the Malay and Chinese. The Indian population was similar except that *NAT1*4* was increased to 51% and *NAT1*10* decreased to 17%. All three ethnic groups had only 2% *NAT1*11* alleles. It is important to note that in this study only the four alleles *3, *4, *10, and *11 were considered.

At present, the actual frequencies of *NAT1** mutations is only beginning to be established, as is the importance of ethnicity in the distribution of *NAT1** alleles. The *NAT1*4* allele is referred to as the "wild-type" allele among Caucasians while *NAT1*3* is considered the "wild type" among

Asians (Vatsis *et al.*, 1995). It seems likely that something similar to the situation for *NAT2** will be found; certain alleles will be more prevalent in particular racial or ethnic populations while other alleles will be found to have a more nearly universal distribution.

Human variability in NAT1 and drug metabolism

After the original discovery of structural heterogeneity in human *NAT1** involving base changes in the 3′-UTR (*NAT1*10, NAT1*11*), alteration in enzyme amount due to decreased formation and stability of mRNA was hypothesised (Vatsis and Weber, 1993). Additional alleles have since been found that have coding mutations that introduce a premature stop codon (*NAT1*15, NAT1*19*), and as expected these mutations produce no active NAT1. Other coding region changes have been found which produce high, low, or normal NAT1 activity when expressed in *E. coli* expression systems (see Table 11.3).

It would be expected that if mutant alleles of *NAT1** occur with a significant frequency, and have altered acetylation activity, acetylation of NAT1 substrates should show variation. Such results have been observed for some time. An 80-fold variation in PAS acetylation by 131 human blood samples (Motulsky and Steinman, 1962; Evans 1963), a four-fold variation in PABA acetylation by seven human liver biopsy samples (Glowinski *et al.*, 1978), a 90-fold variation in V_{max} values for PABA acetylation by thirty-nine (Grant *et al.*, 1991) and eight (Cribb *et al.*, 1993) liver samples, and several other examples of variability in NAT1 activity have been described (Weber and Vatsis, 1993).

The lack of a clearly bimodal (or trimodal) distribution of activities for NAT1 substrates in the early studies and the lack of knowledge of the existence of a separate NAT1, led to the thinking that the acetylation of PAS and PABA was monomorphic even though large variability was shown. Recent studies have provided evidence for bimodal distribution of NAT1 activity. Whole blood lysates from 200 individuals displayed PABA acetylation that had a six-fold variation and a tendency toward bimodality (Weber and Vatsis, 1993). In another study, 130 subjects were given caffeine and PAS and the urine analysed for AFMU/1X ratio and N-Ac-PAS to PAS ratio. The two urinary ratios were not correlated, demonstrating independent expression of NAT1 and NAT2. NAT1 activity was highly variable with a tendency towards bimodality (Grant *et al.*, 1992). Using lysed human white cells from eighty-five individuals, Butcher *et al.* (1998) found a bimodal distribution of PABA acetylation activity with about 8% of the individuals being slow (NAT1) acetylators. Genotyping of the subjects showed the seven slow subjects to have either $G^{560}A$ (*NAT1*14*) or $C^{190}T$ (*NAT1*17*) in conjunction with an allele lacking these mutations. Both mutations caused a V_{max} that was roughly half that of the wild type.

The large variation and bimodal distribution of NAT1 activities defines a second N-acetylation polymorphism, the significance of which is only beginning to be explored. In a small sample of frozen tissue (twenty-six bladder, nineteen colorectal mucosa) a statistical but not an individual correlation was found between increased PABA acetylation activity and the occurrence of the NAT1*10 allele. Samples that were NAT1*4/*10 heterozygotes averaged about twice the activity of NAT1*4 homozygotes, the difference being statistically significant in bladder, but not in colon due to large variations. However, a single NAT1*10 homozygous colon sample had activity that was little different from the mean of all samples (Bell et al., 1995a). Another laboratory's analysis of NAT1 activity in human colon specimens failed to show differences between genotypes NAT1*4/4, 3/4, 10/10, and 4/10, providing evidence that the NAT1*10 allele does not produce higher activity than the NAT1*4 allele (Feng et al., 1998).

Human variability in NAT1 and cancer

The interest in the NAT1*10 allele is based on a presumed change in the polyadenylation signal caused by mutation $T^{1088}A$ which changes the AAT sequence to AAA at bases 1086–1088. This mutation may decrease the destabilising effect of the AT-rich segment and prolong the half-life of allele NAT1*10 mRNA, or conversely, the mutation in this polyadenylation signal may prevent cleavage and polyadenylation which would lead to rapid destruction of the mRNA (Vatsis and Weber, 1993). However there are eight other AAT sequences immediately preceding the lost AAT and these may be well-suited to carry out the function of the mutated triplet without significant alteration in the stability of the mRNA. Another reason for the heightened interest in NAT1*10 is that it appears to be the second most common allele after NAT1*4 (Bell et al., 1995a; Probst-Hensch et al., 1996). An unresolved problem, however, is whether the N-acetylation activity of the allele is different from that of NAT1*4. Expression of NAT1* alleles in bacterial or mammalian cell systems often result in unsatisfactory comparisons because activity is determined per unit of total protein rather than per unit of NAT1 protein. In one limited example where production of NAT1 immunoreactive protein in COS-1 cells transfected with NAT1*4, *10, *11, or *16 was determined, NAT1 16 protein was produced at only 50% of the level of the other three alleles. However, NAT1 activity, normalized to NAT1 protein, did not differ significantly for PABA, PAS, 5-ASA, or 2-AF (de León, 1996). Also the specific activity of NAT1 from leukocytes for PABA, PAS, 2-AF, p-phenetidine, and p-anisidine did not differ between individuals homozygous for NAT1*4 and NAT1*10 (de León, 1996). At this time, there is insufficient evidence to call NAT1*10 rapid or slow relative to NAT1*4. There are, however, other alleles which actually are "slow". These include mutated alleles that produce truncated protein (*NAT1*15, *19*) and two alleles reported to cause slow PABA acetylation by peripheral blood mononuclear cells of heteozygous individuals (*NAT1*14, *17*) (Butcher *et al.*, 1998).

In spite of the lack of convincing evidence that *NAT1*10* confers altered NAT1 activity either *in vivo* or *in vitro*, there is continued interest in exploring the association of this allele with colorectal and other cancers. However, because of a number of contradictory study results, lack of precision or completeness of some studies, and mainly lack of sufficient numbers of studies, the relation of NAT1 phenotype or genotype to risk of human cancer can not be simply stated. As the following examples (listed in Table 11.5) show, no strong conclusion about NAT1 and cancer risk can be made at present.

A study of 202 English colorectal adenocarcinoma patients showed an excess of the *NAT1*10* allele relative to matched controls (OR=1.9) (Bell *et al.* 1995b). In contrast, rapid acetylator genotypes of *NAT2** were not risk factors. However, there was significant gene-gene interaction as the increased risk associated with *NAT1*10* was most apparent among *NAT2** rapid genotypes (OR=2.8). In another study of NAT1 and colorectal cancer, Chen *et al.* (1998) found evidence for a gene–environment interaction between the *NAT1*10* allele and red meat consumption in men. A rapid NAT2 phenotype also interacted to increase risk of cancer. No genotype/phenotype of NAT1 or NAT2 nor their combination significantly influenced risk until red meat consumption was included in the analysis. Red meat consumption by itself was a factor only in men over 60 years of age. For all men, the risk of colorectal cancer was increased with the combination of higher red meat consumption, the *NAT1*10* allele, and

Table 11.5 Variability in *NAT1** and cancer susceptibility

Cancer	Association	Comment	Reference
Colorectal adenoma	None with *Nat1*10* None with any allele	NAT2 not a factor NAT2 not a factor	Probst-Hensch *et al.*, 1996 Lin *et al.*, 1998
Colorectal cancer	Higher risk *Nat1*10* Higher risk *Nat1*10*	rapid NAT2 a factor rapid NAT2, red meat older age are factors	Bell *et al.*, 1995b Chen *et al.*, 1998
Bladder	Higher risk *Nat1*10* Higher risk *Nat1*10*	slow NAT2 a factor smokers, slow NAT2 a factor	Badawi *et al.*, 1995 Taylor *et al.*, 1998
Breast	Higher for *Nat1*10*	postmenopausal smokers	Millikan *et al.*, 1998
Lung	Higher for "slow" *NAT1** alleles	smokers, NAT activity not measured	Bouchardy *et al.*, 1998

the NAT2*4 allele. Among men of 60 years and older, consuming more than one serving of red meat per day, the relative risk was 3.7 for NAT1*10, 4.1 for NAT2*4, and 5.8 for NAT1*10/NAT2*4 compared with consumption of 0–0.5 servings per day.

In contrast to the above studies, Probst-Hensch et al. (1996) found no association between the NAT1*10 allele and the prevalence of adenomas in sigmoidoscopy specimens from 441 adenoma cases compared with 484 controls. In addition, no interaction between NAT1* and NAT2* was found. Another study by the same laboratory (Lin et al., 1998) found no significant correlation between any high, low, or normal activity NAT1* allele and colorectal adenoma.

An examination of O-acetylation of N-OH-4-aminobiphenyl, DNA adduct formation, and NAT1* genotype of the twenty-six bladder samples examined previously by Bell et al. (1995a) showed a correlation of the NAT1*10 allele, increased PABA acetylation activity, and increased formation of N-OH-4-aminobiphenyl DNA adducts (Badawi et al., 1995). The increased formation of bladder DNA adducts was greatest in the samples (n=4) having the NAT1*10 allele and a slow NAT2* genotype.

A three-way gene–gene–exposure interaction of the NAT polymorphisms and smoking in risk of bladder cancer was described by Taylor et al. (1998). They found no effect of the NAT2 polymorphism on bladder cancer in smokers or non-smokers. Smoking tripled the risk of bladder cancer independent of NAT2 phenotype. NAT1*10 did not influence bladder cancer risk among non-smokers, but the presence of the allele slightly increased risk among smokers, the effect being greater with longer duration of smoking. They also found a gene dose effect among the smokers such that the OR was 2.4 for no NAT1*10 alleles, 3.6 for one allele, and 5.9 for two alleles (homozygotes). When NAT2 was included in the analysis, little change in risk was seen except for slow NAT2 (no NAT2*4 alleles) in combination with NAT1*10 and smoking which increased OR from 3.8 to 5.7.

Millikan et al. (1998) examined the relationship of smoking, menopausal status, and NAT1* and NAT2* genotype to breast cancer among 473 control individuals and 498 cases of invasive breast cancer in North Carolina. Among their findings was an increased risk for postmenopausal women who smoked within the previous 3 years and had the NAT1* 10 allele (OR=9.0) compared with those not having the NAT1*10 allele (OR=2.5). In the same subgroup, those with an NAT2* rapid genotype had an OR of 7.4 and those with a slow NAT2* genotype had an OR of 2.8.

Bouchardy et al. (1998) have examined lung cancer risk in a population of French Caucasian smokers. They found no association between NAT2* genotype and lung cancer. To examine any association with NAT1*, they genotyped for NAT1*3, *4, *10, *11, *14, and *15. Alleles *10 and *11 were assumed to be rapid alleles, *3 and *4 "normal" alleles, and *14 and

*15 slow alleles. No examples of *15 were found. "Homozygous rapid" acetylators were considered individuals with NAT1*10/*10 or NAT1* 10/*11 genotypes, "heterozygous rapid" acetylators had either NAT1*3 or *4 with NAT1*10 or *11, "normal" acetylators were those with NAT1*3 or *4 combined with *3 or *4, as well as the combination of NAT1*10 or *11 with NAT1*14, and "heterozygous slow" acetylators were those with NAT1*3 or *4 with NAT1*14. No "homozygous slow" acetylators were found.

In this study, the "homozygous rapid" group was used as the reference category, although only two individuals of the 150 lung cancer cases had this assumed phenotype. The OR for "heterozygous rapid" was 4.0, for the "normal" group it was 6.4, and for the "heterozygous slow" it was 11.7. In no instance was the acetylation activity measured. As the classification of the individuals or their alleles as rapid, slow, or otherwise has not been confirmed, the results of Bouchardy et al. (1998) can not be considered conclusive.

As the initial studies of NAT1 as a risk factor for various cancers (summarized in Table 11.5) demonstrate, much more work needs to be done to understand the role of the isozyme in risk. In the case of NAT2, knowledge of phenotype as rapid or slow acetylator was in hand well before genotyping was possible. For NAT1 the opposite situation prevails; genotyping is widely carried out, but knowledge of the expression of a genotype as a phenotype lags far behind. In any event, most of the epidemiological studies seem to link NAT1*10 with altered risk of cancers. As NAT1 appears to be the isozyme that is highly expressed in most tissues, the association of NAT1 phenotype/genotype with risk of cancer and other diseases deserves and requires further exploration.

Future considerations

Further investigations of the importance of variation of N-acetyltransferases in humans need to include a comprehensive survey of NAT isozyme expression in various tissues. Knowledge of the relative contribution of each isozyme to tissue-specific, as well as total metabolism of drugs and environmental carcinogens should lead to a better understanding of the role of differences in NAT1 and NAT2 activities caused by mutations of the NAT genes. A more thorough determination of the distribution and activity of NAT1* alleles in particular seems to be required to find any correlation between NAT1* genotype and risk of cancer and other diseases or drug toxicities.

An area that has not yet been addressed in man is control of NAT expression. In mice, androgenic control of NAT2 (the functional homolog of human NAT1 (Estrada-Rodgers et al., 1998a)) has been shown in the kidney (Smolen et al., 1993, Estrada-Rodgers et al., 1998b). Glucocorticoid enhancement of *in vivo* acetylation of sulfamethazine in the rabbit (Reeves *et al.,* 1989) and induction of hepatic NAT activity in the rat (Zaher and Svensson, 1994) have been reported. Reported differences between pre- and postmenopausal women in the role of NAT as a risk factor in breast cancer (Ambrosone *et al.,* 1996; Millikan *et al.,* 1998) also suggest a potential effect for steroids in NAT expression. A study of regulation of NAT expression in the various target tissues of arylamine carcinogens in humans would be helpful in understanding the roles of high and low activity of NATs in carcinogen activation. Cell culture and molecular techniques now make such studies possible.

Summary

The isozymes of human NAT catalyse identical reactions but differ in substrate selectivity and tissue distribution. Both NAT1 and NAT2 are polymorphic in structure and in function, multiple alleles of both *NAT1** and *NAT2** having been identified. There is conclusive evidence from epidemiologic, clinical, and biochemical studies that certain NAT2 phenotypes are at increased risk of adverse drug reactions and there is strong evidence of increased susceptibility to environmentally induced cancers. Further information is needed concerning specific *NAT2** genotypes and increased risk. Preliminary evidence suggests an involvement of certain *NAT1** genotypes in increased risk of cancer, but the identification of NAT1 phenotype is presently unresolved. Overall, the evidence suggests that NATs must be considered along with several other xenobiotic metabolising enzymes as susceptibility factors for human cancers.

References

Ambrosone, C. B., Freudenheim, J. L., Graham, S. and Marshall, J. R. *et al.* (1996) 'Cigarette smoking, N-acetyltransferase 2 genetic polymorphisms, and breast cancer risk', *J. Amer. Med. Assoc.* 276: 1494–501.

Ambrosone, C. B., Freudenheim, J. L., Sinha, R. and Graham, S. *et al.* (1998) 'Breast cancer risk, meat consumption and N-acetyltransferase (*NAT2*) genetic polymorphisms', *Int. J. Cancer* 75: 825–30.

Badawi, A. F., Hirvonen, A., Bell, D. A., Lang, N. P. and Kadlubar, F. F. (1995) 'Role of aromatic amine acetyltransferases, NAT1 and NAT2, in carcinogen-DNA adduct formation in the human urinary bladder', *Cancer Res.* 55: 5230–7.

Bandmann, O., Vaughn, J., Holmans, P., Marsden, C. D. and Wood, N. W. (1997) 'Association of slow acetylator genotype for N-acetyltransferase 2 with familial Parkinson's disease', *Lancet* 350: 1136–9.

Bell, D. A., Badawi, A. F., Lang, N. P., Ilett, K. F., Kadlubar, F. F. and Hirvonen, A. (1995a) 'Polymorphism in the N-acetyltransferase 1 (*NAT1*) polyadenylation signal: association of *NAT1*10* allele with higher N-acetylation activity in bladder and colon tissue', *Cancer Res.* 55: 5226–9.

Bell, D. A., Stephens, E. A., Castranio, T. and Umbach, D. M. *et al.* (1995b) 'Polyadenylation polymorphism in the acetyltransferase 1 gene (*NAT1*) increases risk of colon cancer', *Cancer Res.* **55**: 3537–42.

Bendriss, E. K., Bechtel, Y. C., Paintaud, G., Brientini, M. P., Mantion, G., Miguet, J. P., Bennani A. and Bechtel, P. R. (1998) 'Acetylation polymorphism expression in patients before and after liver transplantation: influence of host/graft genotypes', *Pharmacogenetics* **8**: 201–9.

Blum, M., Demierre, A., Grant, D. M., Heim, M. and Meyer, U. A. (1991) 'Molecular mechanism of slow acetylation of drugs and carcinogens in humans', *Proc. Nat. Acad. Sci. USA* **88**: 5237–41.

Bodansky, H. J., Drury, P. L., Cudworth, A. G. and Evans, D. A. P. (1981) 'Acetylator phenotypes and type I (insulin-dependent) diabetes with microvascular disease', *Diabetes* **30**: 907–10.

Bönicke, R. and Reif, W. (1953) 'Enzymatische Inaktivierung von Isonicotinsaure hydrazide im menschlichen und tierschen Organismus', *Arch. Exp. Pathol. Pharmakol.* **220**: 321–33.

Bouchardy, C., Mitrunene, K., Wikman, H., Husgavfel-Pursianen, K., Dayer, P., Benhamou, S. and Hirvonen, A. (1998) 'N-acetyltransferase *NAT1* and *NAT2* genotypes and lung cancer risk', *Pharmacogenetics* **8**: 291–8.

Bulovskaya, L. N., Krupkin, R. G., Bochina, T. A., Shipkova, A. A. and Pavlova, M. V. (1978) 'Acetylator phenotype in patients with breast cancer', *Oncology* **35**: 185–8.

Butcher, N. J., Ilett, K. F. and Minchin, R. F. (1998) 'Functional polymorphism of the human arylamine N-acetyltransferase type 1 gene caused by $C^{190}T$ and $G^{560}A$ mutations', *Pharmacogenetics* **8**: 67–72.

Cartwright, R. A. (1984) 'Epidemiological studies of N-acetylation and C-center ring oxidation in neoplasia', in G. S. Omenn and H. V. Gelboin (eds) *Genetic Variability in Responses to Chemical Exposure.* Banbury Report No. 16. Cold Spring Harbor: Cold Spring Harbor Laboratory, pp. 359–68.

Cartwright, R. A., Glasham, R. W., Roger, H. J., Ahmad, R. A., Hall, D. B., Higgins, E. and Kahn, M. A. (1982) "The role of N-acetyltransferase phenotypes in bladder carcinogenesis. A pharmacogenetics epidemiological approach to bladder cancer', *Lancet* **2**: 842–6.

Cascorbi, I., Brockmoller, J., Mrozikiewicz, P. M., Bauer, S., Loddenkemper, R. and Roots, I. (1996) 'Homozygous rapid arylamine N-acetyltransferase (*NAT2*) genotype as a susceptibility factor for lung cancer', *Cancer Res.* **56**: 3961–6.

Cascorbi, I. and Roots, I. (1999) 'Pitfalls of *NAT2* genotyping', *Pharmacogenetics* **9**: 123–7.

Chen, J., Stamfer, M. J., Hough, H. L., Garcia-Closas, M., Willett, W. C., Hennekens, C. H., Kelsey, K. T. and Hunter, D. J. (1998) 'A prospective study of N-acetyltransferase genotype, red meat intake, and risk of colorectal cancer', *Cancer Res.* **58**: 3307–11.

Cribb, A. E., Grant, D. M., Miller, M. A. and Spielberg, S. P. (1991) 'Expression of monmorphic arylamine N-acetyltransferase (NAT1) in human leukocytes', *J. Pharmacol. Exp. Ther.* **259**: 1241–6.

Cribb, A. E., Isbrucker, R., Levatte, T., Tsui, B., Gillespie, C. T., Renton, K. W. (1994) 'Acetylator phenotyping: the urinary caffeine metabolite ratio in slow acetylators correlates with a marker of systemic NAT1 activity', *Pharmaco-genetics* **4**: 166–70.

Cribb, A. E., Nakamura, H., Grant, D. M., Miller, M. A. and Spielberg, S. P. (1993) 'Role of polymorphic and monomorphic human arylamine N-acetyl-transferases in determining sulfamethoxazole metabolism', *Biochem. Pharmacol.* **45**: 1277–82.

de León, J. H. (1996) 'Characterization of congenic mouse (*Nat2**) and human (*NAT1**) N-acetyltransferases', Ph.D. thesis, University of Michigan, Ann Arbor.

de Meester, C. (1989) 'Bacterial mutagenicity of heterocyclic amines found in heat-processed food', *Mutat. Res.* **221**: 235–62.

Devadatta, S., Gangadharam, P. R. J., Andrews, R. H., Fox, W., Ramakrishnan, C. V., Selkon, J. B., and Velu, S. (1960) 'Peripheral neuritis due to isoniazid', *Bull World Hlt. Org.* **23**: 587–98.

Doll, M. A., Fretland, A. J., Dietz, A. C. and Hein, D. W. (1995) 'Determination of human *NAT2* acetylator genotype by restriction fragment-length polymophism and allele-specific amplification', *Anal. Biochem.* **231**: 413–20.

Drózdz, M., Gierek, T., Jendryczko, A., Pilch, J. and Piekarska, J. (1987) 'N-acetyltransferase phenotype of patients with cancer of the larynx', *Neoplasma* **34**: 481–4.

Ebisawa, T. and Deguchi, T. (1991) 'Structure and restriction fragment length polymorphism of genes for human liver arylamine N-acetyltransferases', *Biochem. Biophys. Res. Comm.* **177**: 1252–7.

Ellard, G. A. and Gammon, P. T. (1976) 'Pharmacokinetics of isoniazid metabolism in man', *J. Pharmacokinet. Biopharm.* **4**: 83–113.

Estrada-Rodgers, L., Levy, G. N. and Weber, W. W. (1998a) 'Substrate selectivity of mouse N-acetyltransferases 1, 2, and 3 expressed in COS-1 cells', *Drug Metab. Disp.* **26**: 502–5.

Estrada-Rodgers, L., Levy, G. N. and Weber, W. W. (1998b) 'Characterization of a hormone response element in the mouse N-acetyltransferase 2 (*Nat2**) promoter', *Gene Expression* **7**: 13–24.

Evans, D. A. P. (1963) 'Pharmacogenetics', *Am. J. Med.* **34**: 639–62.

Evans, D. A. P. (1986) 'Acetylation', in: W. Kalow, H. W. Goedde and D. P. Agarwal (eds) *Ethnic Differences in Reactions to Drugs and Xenobiotics*. New York: Alan R. Liss Inc., pp. 209–42.

Feng, Y., Rustan, T. D., Doll, M. A., *et al.* (1998) 'Human N-acetyltransferase-1 (NAT1) and -2 (NAT2) genotype/phenotype determination in cytosolic pre-parations from surgical human colon specimens', Abst. No. 21 First Inter-national Workshop on the Arylamine N-Acetyltransferases, Cairns, Queensland, Australia.

Garte, S. (1998) 'The role of ethnicity in cancer susceptibility gene polymorphisms: the example of *CYP1A1*', *Carcinogenesis* **19**: 1329–32.

Glowinski, I. B., Radtke, H. E. and Weber, W. W. (1978) 'Genetic variation in N-acetylation of carcinogenic arylamines by human and rabbit liver', *Mol. Pharmacol.* **14**: 940–9.

González, M. V., Alvarez, V., Pello, M. F., Menéndez, M. J., Suárez, C. and Coto, E. (1998) 'Genetic polymorphism of N-acetyltransferase-2, glutatione S-transferase-M1, and cytochromes P450IIE1 and P450IID6 in the susceptibility to head and neck cancer', *J. Clin. Pathol.* **51**: 294–8.

Grant, D. M., Blum, M., Beer, M. and Meyer, U. A. (1991) 'Monomorphic and polymorphic human arylamine N-acetyltransferases: a comparison of liver isozymes and expressed products of two cloned genes', *Mol. Pharmacol.* **39**: 184–91.

Grant, D. M., Tang, B. K. and Kalow, W. (1984) 'A simple test for acetylator phenotype using caffeine', *Br. J. Clin. Pharmacol.* **17**: 459–64.

Grant, D. M., Vohra, P., Avis, Y. and Ima, A. (1992) 'Detection of a new polymorphism of human arylamine N-acetyltransferase NAT1 using *p*-aminosalicylic acid as an *in vivo* probe', *J. Basic. Clin. Physiol. Pharmacol.* **3** (Suppl): 244.

Harb, G. E. and Jacobson, M. A. (1993) 'Human immunodeficiency virus (HIV) infection: does it increase susceptibility to adverse drug reactions?', *Drug Safety* **9**: 1–8.

Hayes, R. B., Bi, W., Rothman, N., Broly, F. *et al.* (1993) 'N-Acetylation phenotype and genotype and risk of bladder cancer in benzidine-exposed workers', *Carcinogenesis* **14**: 675–8.

Hickman, D., Pope, J., Patil, S. D., Fakis, G. *et al.* (1998) 'Expression of arylamine N-acetyltransferase in human intestine', *Gut* **42**: 402–9.

Hirvonen, A., Pelin, K., Tammilehto, L., Karjalainen, A., Mattson, K. and Linnainmaa, K. (1995) 'Inherited *GSTM1* and *NAT2* defects as concurrent risk modifiers in asbestos-related human malignant mesothelioma', *Cancer Res.* **55**: 2981–3.

Hughes, N. C., Janezic, S. A., McQueen, K. L., Jewett, M. A. S., Castranio, T., Bell, D. A. and Grant D. M. (1998) 'Identification and characterization of variant alleles of human acetyltransferase NAT1 with defective function using *p*-aminosalicylate as an in-vivo and in-vitro probe', *Pharmacogenetics* **8**: 55–66.

Hunter, D. J., Hankinson, S. E., Hough, H., Getig, D. M. *et al.* (1997) 'A prospective study of *NAT2* acetylation genotype, cigarette smoking, and risk of breast cancer', *Carcinogenesis* **18**: 2127–32.

Ilett, K. F., David, B. M., Detchon, P., Castleden, W. M. and Kwa, R. (1987) 'Acetylation phenotype in colorectal carcinoma', *Cancer Res.* **47**: 1466–9.

Kashuba, A. D. M., Bertino, J. S., Kearns, G. L., Leeder, J. S., James, A. W., Gotschall, R. and Nafziger, A. N. (1998) 'Quantitation of three-month intraindividual variability and influence of sex and menstrual cycle phase on CYP1A2, N-acetyltransferase-2, and xanthine oxidase activity determined with caffeine phenotyping', *Clin. Pharmacol. Ther.* **63**: 540–51.

Kaufman, G. R., Wenk, M., Taeschner, W., Peterli, B., Gyr, K., Meyer, U. A. and Haefeli, W. E. (1996) 'N-acetyltransferase 2 polymorphism in patients infected with human immunodeficiency virus', *Clin. Pharmacol. Ther.* **60**: 62–7.

Lang, N. P., Chu, D. Z. J., Hunter, C. F., Kendall, D. C., Flammang, T. J. and Kadlubar, FF (1986) 'Role of aromatic amine acetyltransferase in human colorectal cancer', *Arch. Surg.* **121**: 1259–61.

Lang, N. P. and Kadlubar, F. F. (1991) 'Aromatic and heterocyclic amine metabolism and phenotyping in humans', in B. L. Gledhill and F. Mauro (eds) *New Horizons in Biological Dosimetry*. New York: Wiley-Liss, pp 33–47.

Lee, B. L., Wong, D., Benowitz, M. D. and Sullam, P. M. (1993) 'Altered patterns of drug metabolism in patients with acquired immunodeficiency syndrome', *Clin. Pharmacol. Ther.* **53**: 529–35.

Lee, E. J. D, Zhao, B. and Seow-Chen, F. (1998) 'Relationship between poly-morphism of *N*-acetyltransferase gene and susceptibility to colorectal carcinoma in a Chinese population', *Pharmacogenetics* **8**: 513–7.

Lin, H. J., Probst-Hensch, N. M., Hughes, N. C., Sakamoto, G. T. *et al.* (1998) 'Variants of N-acetyltransferase NAT1 and a case-control study of colorectal adenomas', *Pharmacogenetics* **8**: 269–81.

McQueen, C. A. and Weber, W. W. (1980) 'Characterization of human lymphocyte *N*-acetyltransferase and its relationship to the isoniazid acetylator poly-morphism', *Biochem. Genet.* **18**: 889–904.

Martell, K. J., Vatsis, K. P. and Weber, W. W. (1991) 'Molecular genetic basis of rapid and slow acetylation in mice', *Mol. Pharmacol.* **40**: 218–27.

Matas, N., Thygesen, P., Stacey, M., Risch, A. and Sim, E. (1997) 'Mapping AAC1, AAC2 and AACP, the genes for arylamine N-acetyltransferases, carcinogen metabolizing enzymes on human chromosome 8p22, a region frequently deleted in tumors', *Cytogen. Cell. Genet.* **77**: 290–5.

Millikan, R. C., Pittman, G. S., Newman, B., Tse, C. J. *et al.* (1998) 'Cigarette smoking, N-acetyltransferases 1 and 2, and breast cancer risk', *Cancer Epidemiol. Biomark. Prev.* **7**: 371–8.

Motulsky, A. G. and Steinman, L. (1962) 'Aryl amine acetylation in human red cells', *J. Clin. Invest.* **41**: 1387.

Ohsako, S. and Deguchi, T. (1990) 'Cloning and expression of cDNAs for poly-morphic and monomorphic arylamine N-acetyltransferases from human liver', *J. Biol. Chem.* **265**: 4630–4.

O'Neil, W. M., Gilfix, B. M., DiGirolamo, A., Tsoukas, C. M. and Wainer, I. W. (1997) 'N-acetylation among HIV-positive patients and patients with AIDS: when is fast, fast and slow, slow?', *Clin. Pharmacol. Ther.* **62**: 261–71.

Probst-Hensch, N. M., Haile, R. W., Ingles, S. A., Longnecker, M. P. *et al.* (1995) 'Acetylation polymorphism and prevalence of colorectal adenomas', *Cancer Res.* **55**: 2017–20.

Probst-Hensch, N. M., Haile, R. W., Li, D. S., Sakamoto, G. T. *et al.* (1996) 'Lack of association between the polyadenylation polymorphism in the *NAT1* (acetyl-transferase 1) gene and colorectal adenomas', *Carcinogenesis* **17**: 2125–9.

Ratain, M. J., Mick, R., Janisch, L., Berezin, F., Schilsky, R., Vogelzang, N. J. and Kut, M. (1996) 'Individualized dosing of amonafide based on a pharmaco-dynamic model incorporating acetylator phenotype and gender', *Pharmaco-genetics* **6**: 93–101.

Reeves, P. T., Minchin, R. F. and Ilett, K. F. (1989) '*In vivo* mechanisms for the enhanced acetylation of sulfamethazine in the rabbit after hydrocortisone treat-ment', *J. Pharmacol. Exp. Ther.* **248**: 348–52.

Reidenberg, M. M., Drayer, D. E., Levy, M. and Warner, E. (1975) 'Polymorphic acetylation of procainamide in man', *Clin. Pharmacol. Ther.* **17**: 722–30.

Reidenberg, M. M., Levy, M., Drayer, D. E., Zylber-Katz, E. and Robbins, W. C. (1980) 'Acetylator phenotype in idiopathic systemic lupus erythematosus', *Arthritis. Rheum.* **23**: 569–73.

Risch, A., Wallace, D. M. A., Bathers, S. and Sim, E. (1995) 'Slow N-acetylation genotype is a susceptibility factor in occupational and smoking related bladder cancer', *Human Mol. Genetics.* **4**: 231–6.

Roberts-Thomson, J. C., Ryan, P., Khoo, K. K., Hart, W. J., McMichael, A. J. and

Butler, R. N. (1996) 'Diet, acetylator phenotype, and risk of colorectal neoplasia', *Lancet* **347**: 1372–4.

Rothen, J.-P., Haefeli, W. E., Meyer, U. A., Todesco, L. and Wenk, M. (1998) 'Acetaminophen is an inhibitor of hepatic N-acetyltransferase 2 *in vitro* and *in vivo*', *Pharmacogenetics* **8**: 553–9.

Shibuta, K., Nakashima, T., Abe, M., Mashimo, M. *et al.* (1994) 'Molecular genotyping for N-acetylation polymorphism in Japanese patients with colorectal cancer', *Cancer* **74**: 3108–12.

Smolen, T. N., Brewer, J. A. and Weber, W. W. (1993) 'Testosterone modulation of N-acetylation in mouse kidney', *J. Pharmacol. Exp. The.* **264**: 854–8.

Strandberg, I., Boman, G., Hassler, I. and Sjoqvist, F. (1976) 'Acetylator phenotype in patients with hydralzine-induced lupoid syndrome', *Acta. Med. Scand.* **1**: 269–74.

Su, H. J., Guo, Y. L., Lai, M.-D., Huang, J., Cheng, Y. and Chritiani, D. C. (1998) 'The NAT2* slow acetylator genotype is associated with bladder cancer in Taiwanese, but not in the Black Foot disease endemic area population', *Pharmacogenetics* **8**: 187–90.

Taylor, J. A., Umbach, D. M., Stephens, E., Castranio, T., Paulson, D., Robertson, C., Mohler, J. L. and Bell, D. A. (1998) 'The role of N-acetylation polymorphisms in smoking-associated bladder cancer: evidence of a gene–gene–exposure three-way interaction', *Cancer Res.* **58**: 3603–10.

Trizna, Z., de Andrade, M., Kyritis, A. P., Briggs, K. *et al.* (1998) 'Genetic polymorphisms in glutathione S-transferase μ and, θ N-acetyltransferase, and CYP1A1 and risk of gliomas', *Cancer Epidemiol. Biomar. Prevent.* **7**: 553–5.

Van Oudtshoorn, M. C. B. and Potgieter, F. J. (1972) 'Determination of pharmacokinetic parameters for rapid and slow acetylators of sulphadimidine', *J. Pharm. Pharmacol.* **24**: 357–60.

Vatsis, K. P., Martell, K. J. and Weber, W. W. (1991) 'Diverse point mutations in the human gene for polymorphic N-acetyltransferase', *Proc. Nat. Acad. Sci. USA* **88**: 6333–7.

Vatsis, K. P. and Weber, W. W. (1993) 'Structural heterogeneity of Caucasian N-acetyltransferase at the NAT1 gene locus', *Arch. Biochem. Biophys.* **301**: 71–6.

Vatsis, K. P. and Weber, W. W. (1997) 'Acetyltransferases', in I. G. Sipes, C. A. McQueen and A. J. Gandolfi (eds) *Comprehensive Toxicology*, New York: Elsevier Science, pp. 385–99.

Vatsis, K. P., Weber, W. W., Bell, D. A., Dupret, J. M., Evans, D. A. P., Grant, D. M. *et al.* (1995) 'Nomenclature for N-acetyltransferases', *Pharmacogenetics* **5**: 1–9.

Vineis, P. and Martone, T. (1998) 'The role of genetically-based metabolic polymorphisms in human cancer: an ecological study of bladder cancer and N-acetyltransferase in 23 populations', *Biotherapy* **11**: 201–4.

Weber, W. W. (1978) 'Genetic variability and extrapolation from animals to man: some perspectives on susceptibility to chemical carcinogenesis from aromatic amines', *Envir. Hlth. Persp.* **22**: 141–4.

Weber, W. W. (1987) *The Acetylator Genes and Drug Response.* New York: Oxford University Press.

Weber, W. W. and Vatsis, K. P. (1993) 'Individual variability in *p*-aminobenzoic acid N-acetylation by human N-acetyltransferase (NAT1) of peripheral blood', *Pharmacogenetics* **3**: 209–12.

Wohlleb, J. C., Hunter, C. F., Blass, B., Kadlubar, F. F., Chu, D. Z. J. and Lang, N. P. (1990) 'Aromatic amine acetyltransferase as a marker for colorectal cancer: environmental and demographic associations', *Int. J. Cancer* **46**: 22–30.

Woosley, R. L., Drayer, D. E., Reidenberg, M. M., Nies, A. S., Carr, K. and Oates, J. A. (1978) 'Effect of acetylator phenotype on the rate at which procainamide induces antinuclear antibodies and the lupus syndrome', *N. Engl. J. Med.* **298**: 1157–9.

Zaher, H. and Svensson, C. K. (1994) 'Glucocorticoid induction of hepatic acetyl CoA:arylamine *N*-acetyltransferase activity in the rat', *Res. Commun. Chem. Pathol. Pharmacol.* **83**: 195–208.

Zhao, B., Lee, E. J. D., Yeoh, P. N. and Gong, N. H. (1998) 'Detection of mutations and polymorphisms of N-acetyltransferase 1 gene in Indian, Malay and Chinese populations', *Pharmacogenetics* **8**: 299–304.

Chapter 12

Interindividual variation of UDP-glucuronosyltransferases and drug glucuronidation

B. Burchell, B. Ethell, M. J. Coffey, K. Findlay,
G. Jedlitschky, M. Soars, D. Smith and R. Hume

Introduction

Glucuronidation of pharmacologically active xenobiotic compounds and endogenous substances by a major phase 2 detoxication system in human has profound effects on the disposition, metabolism and excretion of many drugs (Dutton, 1980; Clarke and Burchell, 1994).

Glucuronide formation is catalysed by a family of UDP-glucurono-syltransferases (UGTs) using thousands of endobiotic and xenobiotic compounds as substrates (Figure 12.1) (Burchell *et al.*, 1997). The xeno-biotic substrate range of an individual UGT isoform may be dictated by the evolved structure of an individual UGT to accept endobiotic substrates, such as bilirubin or a steroid (Brierley and Burchell, 1993). A thorough understanding of the evolved endobiotic UGT substrate range is essential. Although an extensive list of drugs are glucuronidated by humans (Clarke and Burchell, 1994), it remains difficult to determine and predict UGT specificity. The fallibility of the evolved detoxication systems has been revealed by the implication of drug glucuronides in adverse drug reactions

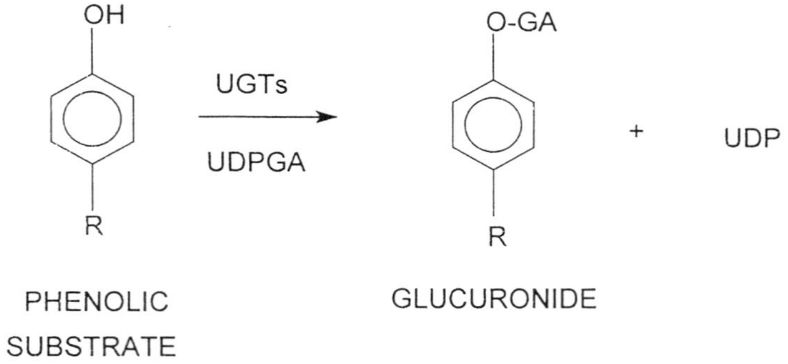

Figure 12.1 The reaction catalysed by UDP-glucuronosyltransferases is illustrated using a phenolic compound involved in the formation of an ether glucuronide.

that resulted in hypersensitivity of immune response (Sphann-Langguth and Benet, 1992).

Many xenobiotics are substrates for both UGTs and sulphotransferases (SULTs), and the different subcellular location and kinetic properties of the enzymes and the availability of co-substrate influence the relative contribution of each system. Similarly, variation of drug oxidation pathways may affect rates of drug glucuronidation. The availability of cloned human UGT cDNAs and genes has allowed significant progress to be made (Burchell *et al.*, 1995), although our excitement needs to be tempered by our lack of knowledge of the contribution of each isoform to xenobiotic conjugation *in vivo* (Remmel and Burchell, 1993). Moreover, the use of 'rate' data obtained using recombinant cell lines may lead to prediction of *in vivo* pharmacokinetics, although there are a number of limitations to those predictions that have to be circumvented.

This review will assess recent work on the inter-individual variation of glucuronidation in human caused by genetic differences in expression of UGTs. Further, we shall briefly examine the bioactivation of xenobiotics following conjugation with glucuronic acid as a mechanism of potential toxicity in man. The literature reviewed for this article was up to October 1998.

Biologically active glucuronides

Glucuronidation has been described as a safe detoxication process and glucuronides were never considered to be biologically active intermediates. However, in recent years the potential toxicity and biological activity of certain glucuronides have been well recognised. There is one notable example reported where such metabolites have been found to be pharmacologically active. (−)-Morphine is glucuronidated in a stereoselective manner to (−)-morphine-3-glucuronide and (−)-morphine-6-glucuronide in the liver (Paul *et al.*, 1989). Detailed pharmacological characterisation of the glucuronides has established that (−)-morphine-6-glucuronide is 650 times more potent that the parent drug as an analgesic, whereas morphine-3-glucuronide is a potent antagonist of morphine and has no analgesic activity (Paul *et al.*, 1989). This discovery has led to (−)-morphine-6-glucuronide being commercially marketed by Ultra Fine Chemicals, Manchester, UK.

Acyl glucuronidation in drug immune hypersensitivity

Acyl glucuronides are formed when conjugation with glucuronic acid occurs via a carboxyl group, resulting in an ester-type linkage. Ester-type glucuronides are much more unstable than ether-linked glucuronides and can easily undergo nucleophilic substitution. The chemical properties of acyl-linked glucuronides are extensively reviewed (Sphann-Langguth and Benet, 1992).

One important reaction that acyl glucuronides undergo is acyl migration, a process whereby the aglycone moves from the 1-hydroxyl group of the glucuronic acid sugar to the 2, 3 or 4 hydroxyl groups. This rearrangement of the glucuronide leads to β-glucuronidase-resistant isomers and is completely reversible with one exception: the C1-glucuronide does not appear to reform from the C1-isomer (Sphann-Langguth and Benet, 1992). The extent of acyl migration may only become detectable when the excretion of conjugates is impaired and their plasma concentrations are raised (Sphann-Langguth and Benet, 1992).

The rate of acyl migration differs from compound to compound and their stability is also highly variable (Sphann-Langguth and Benet, 1992). At physiological or slightly alkaline pH, acyl migration and hydrolysis of acyl glucuronides are extensive (Sphann-Langguth and Benet, 1992).

A number of acyl glucuronides have been shown to bind irreversibly to proteins *in vitro* and *in vivo* (Boelsterli, 1993). Evidence exists for two principal mechanisms of this reversible (covalent) binding; however, it is not known which of these is principally responsible (Ding *et al.*, 1993).

The *UGT* gene superfamily

More than fifteen human liver *UGT* cDNAs have been cloned and classified into two subfamilies based on sequence analysis (see Figure 12.2). The *UGT1* subfamily of enzymes glucuronidate xenobiotic phenols and bilirubin, whilst *UGT2* enzymes glucuronidate steroids and bile acids. An early observation was that *UGT1* cDNA clones shared an identical C-terminal coding sequence whereas the N-terminal 246 amino acids show a striking lack of identity (24–49%) (Burchell *et al.*, 1991).

Southern blot analysis indicated that the region encoding the conserved 3′ half of four separate human *UGT1* cDNAs (the common domain) was a single copy in the human genome, suggesting a role for alternative splicing in the synthesis of different isoforms. In support of this, the common domain and the isoform specific 5′ half of the four *UGT1* cDNAs co-localised to chromosome 2 at 2q.37 (Brierley and Burchell, 1993). Owens and Ritter (1992) described the existence of a gene complex by the isolation of overlapping cosmid clones containing six alternative substrate-determining first exons upstream of the four exons which make up the common domain. The human liver cDNA clone HP4 isolated by Wooster *et al.* (1991) had the same common domain sequence as other *UGT1* cDNAs, but contained a novel substrate determining exon that was eventually named *UGT1A9* and was not among those already genomically cloned. This suggested that the *UGT1* gene locus was larger than had previously been described, presumably extending further upstream. Human genomic Southern blotting indicated the presence of multiple sequences homologous to the 5′ portion of HP4 (Moghrabi *et al.*, 1992). Further work has shown that the human *UGT1* gene is a single copy gene consisting of four common exons and more than 13 variable exons that span more than 350 kb of the human genome (Mackenzie *et al.*, 1997) (see Figure 12.2).

In contrast, comparison of members of the *UGT2* gene family, the steroid metabolising isoforms, indicates that amino acid differences between different isoforms of this family occur throughout the length of the protein. The outline structure of the *UGT2B4* gene has been determined to consist of six exons and five introns thereby providing evidence for the existence of independent *UGT* genes rather than a single gene complex (Monaghan *et al.*, 1996). Three *UGT2B* genes were mapped to chromosome 4 using somatic cell hybrid cell lines and PCR. A YAC library

(a)

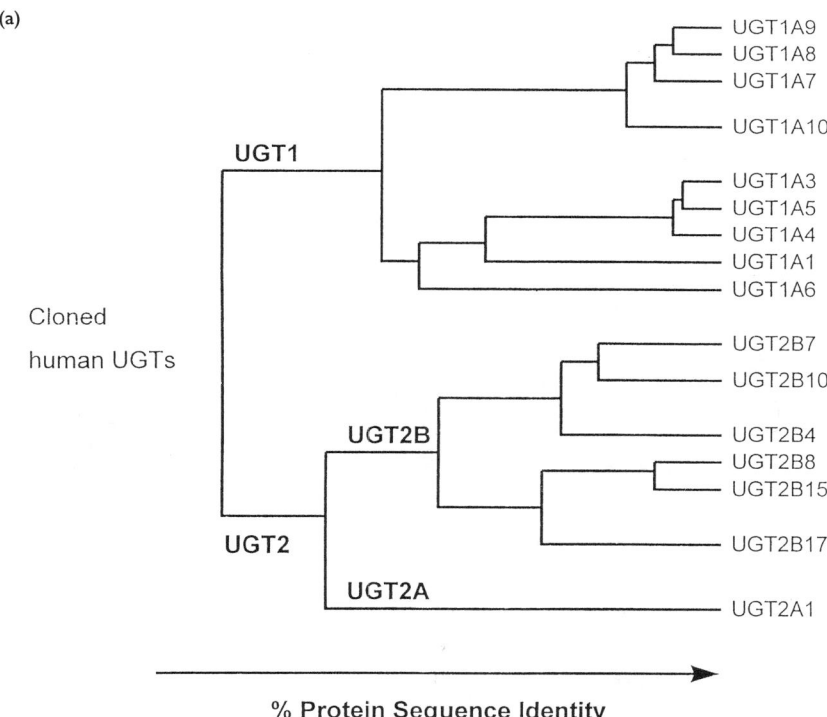

% Protein Sequence Identity

Figure 12.2 A dendogram comparing the sequence identity of human UGTs: (a) The figure indicates the separation of UGTs into two subfamilies and the identities of each isoform within each subfamily. (b) The structural organisation of the UGT-1 gene locus and the nomenclature dependent on the physical location is shown. The figure further indicates the possible mechanism of message splicing to form mature mRNA for synthesis of an individual UGT.

Figure 12.2 (continued)

(b)

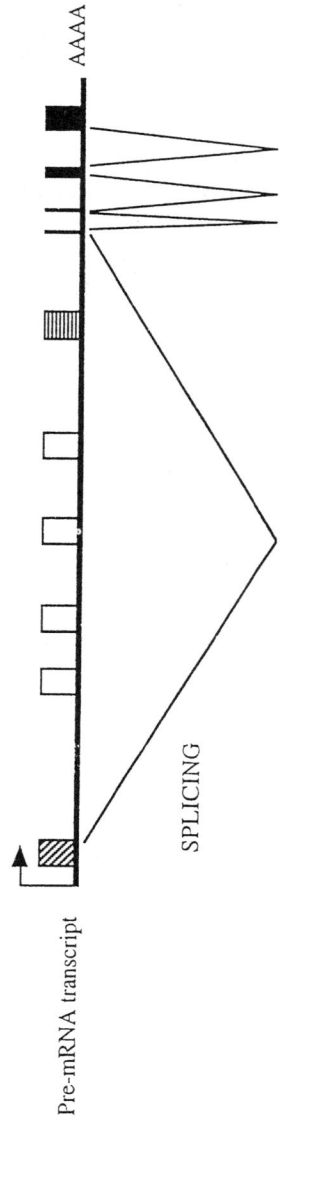

was screened to determine whether they were clustered we screened a YAC library and isolated a five YAC contig. One of these YACs was found to contain at least three *UGT2B* genes in 195 kb. FISH analysis indicated that the *UGT2B* gene cluster was localised at 4q13 (Monaghan *et al.*, 1994). Recently, an olfactory UGT2A1 has been cloned and this gene is also chromosomally located at 4q13 (Jedlitschky *et al.*, 1999).

Nomenclature for UGTs

A nomenclature for UDP-glucuronosyltransferases has been proposed based on the divergent evolution of gene sequences (Burchell *et al.*, 1991). In naming each gene the root symbol *UGT1* for humans (Ugt for mouse) followed by an Arabic number denoting the family, a letter designating the subfamily, and an Arabic numeral representing the individual gene within the family or subfamily (e.g. human *UGT2B1* and mouse *Ugt2b-1*).

Comparison of amino acid sequences leads to a definition of families and subfamilies. Gene products in the UGT-1 family are 38–48% identical with the gene products in the UGT-2 family. Therefore, a convenient value to choose for family divergence is less than 50%. Deduced protein sequences of members of the UGT-1 family are 62–80% identical; the UGT-2 family are 57–93% identical. Therefore, within a single family there is greater than 50% identity; within a subfamily the identity is increased to more than 60%. The result of the application of this nomenclature has produced the dendogram observed in Figure 12.2. The actual numbering of the family members is the result of the chronological order of discovery of new UGT cDNAs of various species, except in the *UGT-1* gene complex for which numbering is based on structural order of the variable exons within the genome (see Figure 12.2a) (Mackenzie *et al.*, 1997).

Specificity of cloned/expressed human UGTs

Fifteen human UGT isoforms have been identified by gene sequencing and cDNA cloning (Burchell *et al.*, 1991), most of these are known to be expressed *in vivo* (see tissue specific expression). However one sequence is known to contain stop codons that would prevent functional enzyme expression (Burchell *et al.*, 1991). Thirteen human UGTs have been substantially characterised (see Table 12.1).

All of the UGT enzymes exhibit similar molecular weights between 50 and 57 kDa on analysis of SDS gel electrophoresis. The variation in the size of the proteins may be the result of different folding or post-translation modification by glycosylation (Tephly and Burchell, 1990) or other unknown covalently attached ligands, because all the amino acid coding sequences are very similar in length, i.e., approximately 527–530 residues (Mackenzie *et al.*, 1997).

Table 12.1 Possible probe substrates for human UGTs

UGT-1 subfamily		UGT-2 subfamily	
Isoenzyme	Substrate	Isoenzyme	Substrate
UGT1A1	Bilirubin	UGT2A1	S(-)-B-citronellol
		UGT2B4	Hyodeoxycholic acid
	Buprenorphine	(UGT2B11)	
UGT1A3	?		
UGT1A4	Imipramine	UGT2B7	Morphine
UGT1A6	1-Naphthol	UGT2B8	Androstanediol (17β only)
		(UGT2B15)	8-hydroxyquinoline
			Dihydrotestosterone
UGT1A7	?		
UGT1A8	?		
UGT1A9	Propofol	UGT2B17	Androstanediol (3α and 17β)
UGT1A10	?		

Glucuronidation of drugs containing a wide range of acceptor groups has been reported including phenols (e.g. propofol, paracetamol, naloxone), alcohols (e.g. chloramphenicol, codeine, oxazepam), aliphatic amines (e.g. ciclopiroxalamine, lamorigine, amitriptyline), acidic carbon atoms (e.g. feprazone, phenylbutazone, sulphinpyrazone) and carboxylic acids (e.g. naproxen, zomepirac, ketoprofen). This indicates the variability of acceptor groups that can be conjugated to glucuronic acid in humans (Clarke *et al.*, 1994).

Thirteen cloned human hepatic UDP-glucuronosyltransferase cDNAs have been stably expressed in tissue culture cell lines. More than 100 drug xenobiotics and endobiotics were used as substrates for glucuronidation catalysed by the cloned human transferases to determine the chemical structure accepted as substrates (e.g. see Senafi *et al.*, 1994).

UGT1A1

A cloned human bilirubin UDP-glucuronosyltransferase (UGT1A1) accepted wide diversity of compounds such as phenols, anthraquinones, flavones, and steroids were glucuronidated by the isoform (Senafi *et al.*, 1994). Seven substrates were glucuronidated at a comparable or higher rate than bilirubin. Octyl gallate was glucuronidated at the highest rate among all substrates tested. The UGT-1A1 isoform exhibited stereospecificity towards simple non-planar phenols and estriols. The increasing number of carbon atoms in the alkyl side chain of gallate analogues improved the specific activity from no glucuronide formed in gallic acid to 0.72 and 1.90 mmol/min/mg protein in propyl and octyl gallate, respectively (Senafi *et al.*, 1994). Seventeen steroids were tested and only four that had both 17β-

and 3β-hydroxy substituents were glucuronidated (Senafi *et al.*, 1994). UGT1A1 also effectively catalysed ethinyl estradiol specifically forming the 3-β-glucuronide but not the 17-β-glucuronide (Ebner *et al.*, 1993). Site-specific mutation analysis of UGT1A1 has suggested that ethinylestradiol and bilirubin are bound in overlapping sites (Ciotti and Owens, 1996).

UGT1A1 is also the major contributor to glucuronidation of buprenorphine (King *et al.*, 1996) and the SN38 metabolite of irinotecan (Iyer *et al.*, 1998).

UGT1A3

UGT1A3 has been extensively studied by three groups. Initially, the enzyme was shown to catalyse the glucuronidation of a series of benzo(a)pyrene and α-acetyaminofluorene metabolites indicating an active role in the formation of planar phenols (Mojarrabi *et al.*, 1996). UGT1A3 also catalysed the glucuronidation of a wide range of coumarins, flavanoids, anthraquinones, phenols (but not propofol), carboxylic acids, opioids, primary and tertiary amines (Green *et al.*, 1998). Albert *et al.*, (1998) has shown that UGT1A3 is active in catalysing estrogen and bile acid glucuronidation including hyodeoxycholic acid. Coumarins, in particular scopoletin, flavanoids and anthraquinones appear to be the best substrates for this isoform.

UGT1A4

Tertiary and primary amine glucuronidation is efficiently catalysed by UGT1A4, napthylamines and 4-aminobiphenyl are good substrates (Green *et al.*, 1994). Indeed, UGT1A4 appears to be catalytically more effective in N-glucuronidation than UGT1A3. However, the existence of two isoforms capable of catalysing these glucuronidation reactions may explain the biphasic kinetics of quateriary ammonium glucuronide formation of amitryptyline and diphenylhydramine in human liver microsomes (Breyer-Pfaff *et al.*, 1997).

UGT1A6, UGT1A7, UGT1A8, UGT1A9

UGT1A6 exhibited a limited substrate specificity for planar phenolic compounds, whereas UGT1A7, UGT1A8, UGT1A9 were more promiscuous in acceptance of non-planar phenols, anthraquinones, flavones, aiphatic alcohols, aromatic carboxylic acids, steroids and many drugs of varied structure (Ebner and Burchell, 1993; Strassburg *et al.*, 1998; Cheng *et al.*, 1998). Propofol is a good probe substrate for UGT1A9. UGT1A9 is also an effective catalyst of tolcapone and entacapone drugs used to treat Parkinson's disease (Lautala *et al.*, 2000).

UGT1A8, UGT1A9 and possibly UGT1A10 may catalyse the glucuronidation of many similar compounds including mycophenolic acid

(Cheng *et al.*, 1998; Mojarrabi and Mackenzie, 1997; Ethell *et al.*, 1998) although differential tissue localisation of the different isoforms UGT1A8 in intestine, UGT1A9 in kidney and UGT1A10 in intestine, may explain the overlapping versatility.

Subfamily 2 contains at least five UGTs catalysing steroid or bile acid glucuronidation. All of these isoforms also catalysed the glucuronidation of some xenobiotics (Burchell *et al.*, 1995). It is difficult to assess the number of different forms in this family accurately, because possible sequence differences between laboratories may account for some isoforms such that UGT2B4 and UGT2B11 are possibly identical (Mackenzie *et al.*, 1997) and similarly for UGT2B8 and UGT2B15 (see Figure 12.1 and Table 12.1).

UGT2B4

UGT2B4 was observed to catalyse glucuronidation of hyodeoxycholic acid and estriol (Fournel-Gigleux *et al.*, 1989a).

UGT2B7

UGT2B7 is also involved in synthesis of these glucuronides (Jin *et al.*, 1993). UGT2B7 catalysed glucuronidation in a wide range of substrates including 50 hydroxylated androgens and pregnanes (Ritter *et al.*, 1992, Jin *et al.*, 1997) and importantly carboxylic acids, opioids, morphinan derivatives and other drugs (Jin *et al.*, 1993, Coffman *et al.*, 1997).

UGT2B8 (UGT2B15)

UGT2B8 (UGT2B15) catalysed the glucuronidation of androgens, some flavanoids and anthraquinones. Phenophthalein and 8-hydroxyquinoline are useful probe substrates (Green *et al.*, 1994).

UGT2B17

UGT2B17 has been demonstrated to glucuronidate C19 steroids and some phenols (Beaulieu *et al.*, 1996), but was differentiated from UGT2B8 (UGT2B15) by catalysing the glucuronidation of dihydrotestosterone and 5α-androstane-3α, 17β diol of both the 3α and 17β positions, whereas UGT2B15 is restricted to the 17β position. Indeed, serine residue 121 appears to be important for 3α glucuronidation of androgens by UGT2B17 (Dubois *et al.*, 1998).

Screening of catechol substrates using five different UGTs allows comparison with human liver microsomes and identification of the most effective enzyme in catechol drug/xenobiotic glucuronidation, and UGT1A9 was a more efficient catalyst than UGT1A1, 1A6, 2B7 and 2B15 (Ethell *et al.*, 1998).

Levels of UGT activity of cloned/expressed enzymes were sufficient to allow determination of kinetic parameters for the enzyme reaction. Further, metabolism and toxicity of drugs could be studied by addition to the recombinant cell lines in culture and extraction of the media allowed further analysis of glucuronide formation. Suggested probe substrates for individual UGT isoforms are listed in Table 12.1.

Additional methods to assess specificity of tissue microsomal UGTs

The use of specific antibodies

Some problems in the use of expressed human drug metabolising enzymes in the analysis of drug metabolism and drug–drug interactions have been discussed in a recent commentary (Remmel and Burchell, 1993). The value of these *in vitro* systems is their relevance to human drug metabolism *in vivo*.

Recently, attempts have been made to assess the contribution of a specific UGT to the microsomal glucuronidation of an endobiotic or xenobiotic in a specific tissue by using inhibitory antibodies. Monospecific polyclonal antibodies raised against the N-terminal portion (14–150 residues) of human liver UGT2B4 protein expressed in *E. coli* were used to immuno-inhibit and immunoprecipitate this transferase from human liver and kidney microsomes (Pillot *et al.*, 1993). These experiments demonstrated that UGT2B4 activity was responsible for more than 90% of the hyodeoxycholate 6-0-glucuronidation activity in human liver microsomes, but did not contribute significantly towards the glucuronidation of estriol, 4-hydroxy-esterone, 1-naphthol or hyocholic acid (Pillot *et al.*, 1993).

Similarly, antibodies were raised against the N-terminal half of UGT1A6 expressed in *E. coli*, and immuno-inhibition analysis of human liver and kidney microsomes demonstrated that this isoenzyme represented up to 50% of the total microsomal 1-naphthol glucuronidation (Ouzzine *et al.*, 1994). UGT activities towards hyodeoxycholic acid, 4-hydroxybiphenyl, 4-t-butylphenol and bilirubin were not inhibited by these specific anti-UGT1A6-antibody.

Additional studies are needed to produce a "glucuronidation pie" and an assessment of the contribution of each isoform to glucuronidation of a single drug, such that a significant variation of this metabolic event can be predicted *in vivo*.

Specific inhibition of UGT

The studies of inhibition of UGTs are difficult and confused by the micro-somal membrane location of transferases. Many compounds that have been considered inhibitors of glucuronidation may cause membrane disruption or reduce cellular UDPGA concentrations (Mulder *et al.*, 1990).

Specific analysis is perhaps more easily achieved by measurement of the endogenous compound glucuronidation, such as the inhibition of bilirubin UDP-glucuronosyltransferase activity. Gentamycin was shown to be a weak inhibitor of bilirubin UGT *in vitro*, but also inhibited salicylamide glucuronidation *in vivo* (Malaka-Zafiriu *et al.*, 1973). Bilirubin has been shown to specifically inhibit the 3α hydroxyestradiol glucuronide formation, but not 17β hydroxyestradiol glucuronide formation by human liver microsomes indicating a stereospecific role of bilirubin UGT in formation of this endogenous glucuronide (Senafi *et al.*, 1994). Novobiocin, which caused unconjugated hyperbilirubinemia in animals and human (Duvaldstein *et al.*, 1976), was shown to exert non-competitive inhibition of rat microsomal UDP-glucuronosyltransferase in digitonin-activated preparations with either bilirubin or UDPGA. Human microsomal bilirubin UGT activity was also inhibited by novobiocin, whereas 1-naphthol UDP-glucuronosyltransferase was unaffected (Burchell *et al.*, 1987). Further studies with purified rat liver bilirubin UGT suggested that novobiocin competitively inhibited bilirubin binding to the enzyme, but the drug did not appear to be a substrate for the purified enzyme.

D-ring glucuronidation of estriol, testosterone and dihydrotestosterone have been shown to possess pharmacological activity and mediate cholestasis (Meyers *et al.*, 1981). In contrast, A-ring conjugates of these steroids are inactive (Slikker *et al.*, 1983). Human bilirubin UGT has been shown to be the major enzyme responsible for E_2-3-glucuronide (Vore *et al.*, 1985).

Androsterone glucuronide is the predominant C-19 steroid glucuronide in plasma (Thompson *et al.*, 1990). The marked rise in testosterone during puberty was strongly correlated with increases of androsterone glucuronide and androstane-3α, 17β-diol glucuronide. Both steroid glucuronides are plasma biochemical markers of adrenal hyperandrogenism in hirsuitism in women (Salman *et al.*, 1992) and virilising congenital adrenal hyperplasia (Pang *et al.*, 1991). Direct inhibition of UGTs by competitive xenobiotics could significantly affect the production of steroid glucuronides and in turn the physiological function responsive tissues, such as ovary.

Tertiary amine drugs, chlorpromazine, amitriptyline, imipramine, promethazine and cyproheptadine were potent inhibitors of the glucuronidation of testosterone, androsterone and estriol. Structural features required for inhibition of a rigid tricyclic ring and either a dimethylaminopropyl or a methylpiperidine side chain (Sharp *et al.*, 1992).

Ketoprofen and other substrates of human UGT2B7 have been shown to be competitive inhibitors of (S) oxazepam glucuronidation in human liver microsomes, but not an effective inhibitor of (R) oxazepam glucuronidation indicating a stereoselective competitive inhibition of oxazepam glucuronidation which may be catalysed by two different UGTs (Patel *et al.*, 1995a).

Oxazepam inhibits morphine UGT activity in human fetal liver microsomes (Pacifici and Rane, 1981) which may again involve UGT2B7. Chloramphenicol and 1-naphthol were poor competitive inhibitors of a low-affinity morphine UGT in adult human liver microsomes (Miners et al., 1988). Tricyclic anti-depressants also inhibited human hepatic morphine glucuronidation (Wahlstrom et al., 1994).

Competitive substrates

Triphenylacetic acid and related compounds have been shown to competitively inhibit rat and human liver microsomal bilirubin UGT (Fournel et al., 1986). Among twenty compounds tested, 7,7,7-triphenyl-heptanoic acid most strongly inhibited rat liver mirosomal bilirubin UGT and had a weaker effect on 1-naphthol, androsterone, and testosterone glucuronidation (Fournel et al., 1986, Fournel-Gigleux et al., 1989). This arylalkanoic acid showed competitive inhibition with rat liver microsomal and purified bilirubin UGT activities, with respective K_I values of 12 μM and 16 μM. The inhibitory potency on bilirubin UGT was a function of presence of the hydrophobic triphenyl moiety, the length of the aliphatic chain, and presence of the carboxylic acid group. The glucuronidation of these compounds was also studied. 7,7,7-Triphenylheptanoic acid was actively glucuronidated by purified bilirubin UGT, in contrast to its analogues having decreased alkyl chain length (Fournel-Gigleux et al., 1988, 1989). Further studies of purified UGTs also suggested that triphenylheptanoic acid was also glucuronidated by another member of the rat UGT1 subfamily (Fournel-Gigleux et al., 1989b).

The next step in the development of UGT inhibitors was the synthesis of transition state analogues (Noort et al., 1991). W,w,w-triphenyl alkyl UDPs were more potent inhibitors than their parent compounds (Noort et al., 1990). Addition to UDP to triphenyl-heptanoic acid yielded a good inhibitor of 1-naphthol and testosterone glucuronidation without effecting bilirubin UGT activity (Said et al., 1992).

A recent further attempt to develop a specific inhibitor of human UGTs was by synthesis of a steroid transition state analogue (TSA). Two epimers were obtained from the synthesis (Timmers et al., 1997). There was a distinct difference in the inhibition of four individual UGTs by the two epimers. Epimer (2) exhibited a consistent competitive effect on UGT1A1 and UGT2B15. Both of these UGTs are capable of metabolising steroids (see Specificity section), suggesting that the active sites afford a good fit for the conformation of the transition state analogue. However, the noncompetitive inhibition of UGT1A9 suggests the TSA binds excluding UDPGA from the active site. Preferential inhibition of individual UGTs was observed, but the TSA is not sufficiently specific to be routinely useful (Timmers et al., 1997).

Brequinar is glucuronidated in human and has been suggested as a preferential inhibitor of UGT-1 family isoenzymes from studies using rat liver microsomes (Diamond and Christ, 1996). This suggestion was further investigated using human UGTs. Brequinar was shown to potently inhibit UGT-1 activities towards bilirubin and 1-naphthol in human liver microsomes (Ethell, 1998). Brequinar was also shown to competitively inhibit UGT1A1, UGT1A9 and UGT2B15, i.e. members of both UGT enzyme families; UGT-1A6 appeared to be non-competitively inhibited by Brequinar. K_1 values for inhibition of individual UGTs are between 80 and 250 μM. The hope of a specific inhibitor of individual human UGTs has again proved elusive (Ethell, 1998).

Discrimination of individual UGT isoform catalysing substrate glucuronidation using competitive inhibition

The glucuronidation of the anticancer drug 5,6-dimethylxanthenone-4-acetic acid (DXAA) was screened using individually expressed human UGT enzymes and human liver microsomes. UGT1A9 and UGT2B7 were shown to catalyse the glucuronidation DXAA (Miners et al., 1997). Microsomal glucuronidation of DXAA was significantly inhibited by diclofenac at 100 μM compared to the other twenty drug substrates tested. Diclofenac was then demonstrated to more efficiently inhibit DXAA glucuronidation catalysed by UGT2B7 and therefore this UGT isoform was deemed the most likely candidate for this role in vivo (Miners et al., 1997).

Tissue specific variation in expression of UGTs

Recently, several research teams have investigated the tissue distribution of individual UGTs using functional assay with specific substrates such as bilirubin (Peters and Jansen, 1988) with specific antibodies (Coughtrie et al., 1987; Peters and Jansen, 1988; Radominska-Pandya et al., 1998), isoform specific cDNA probes (Sutherland et al., 1993) or specific RT/PCR analysis (Strassburg et al., 1998; Radominska-Pandya et al., 1998, Beaulieu et al., 1996). A survey of this literature allows tissue localisation of different UGT isoforms to be recorded. Table 12.2 shows the location of different UGTs in liver, kidney and intestine. Only certain isoforms are present in individual tissues, e.g. UGT1A1 is absent from kidney, but present in liver and intestine, UGT1A6 appears to be present in all tissues, whereas expression of UGT1A8 is apparently only present in kidney (Table 12.2).

UGT2A1 was only observed in brain and olfactory tissue (Jedlitschky et al., 1999). This variable tissue distribution is useful in determination of the involvement of a specific enzyme in glucuronidation of a particular substrate. Table 12.3 illustrates the value of using different tissue microsomes to determine the role of certain UGTs in thyroid hormone glucuronidation (Findlay et al., 2000).

Table 12.2 Location of human UGTs

Isoform	Liver	Kidney	Intestine		
			Gastric	Biliary	Colonic
UGTIAI	+	−	+	+	+
UGTIA3	+	+	+	+	+
UGTIA4	+	−	+	+	+
UGTIA5	−		−	−	−
UGTIA6	+	+	+	+	+
UGTIA7	−		+	−	−
UGTIA8	−	+	−	−	+
UGTIA9	+	+	−	−	+
UGTIA10	−	+	+	+	+
UGTIAII					
UGTIA12					
UGT2AI					
UGT2B4	+	+			−
UGT2B7	+	+	+		+
UGT2B8	+				
UGT2B10	+		+		+
UGT2B15	+	+	+		+
UGT2B17	+	(+)			

Notes
References for this work are Strassburg et al., 1998; Sutherland et al., 1993; Radominska-Pandya et al.,1998 and Levesque et al., 1998.

Table 12.3 Comparison of UGT activity in human liver and kidney microsomes

Substrate	Bilirubin	UGT activity	
		Propofol (nmol/min/mg protein)	T4 (pmol/min/mg protein)
Liver	0.5	0.3	0.43
Kidney	0	1.8	0.08

Certainly for steroid glucuronidation specific UGTs may be prominently expressed in steroidogenic tissues such as UGT2B17 in testis, prostate, mammary gland and ovary (Beaulieu et al., 1996). Tissue microsomes from these sources may help to determine the specificity of endobiotic or xenobiotic glucuronidation.

Inter-individual variation of drug glucuronidation

Large interindividual variations of human hepatic microsomal drug glucuronidation has been detected in vitro, but even ten-fold differences in extremes might be expected as a normal distribution within the population. Bilirubin UGT activity was demonstrated to vary 28-fold in the liver bank of twenty-one samples (see Figure 12.3, Coffey et al., unpublished). This variation in UGT activities may well be related to gender, age, disease

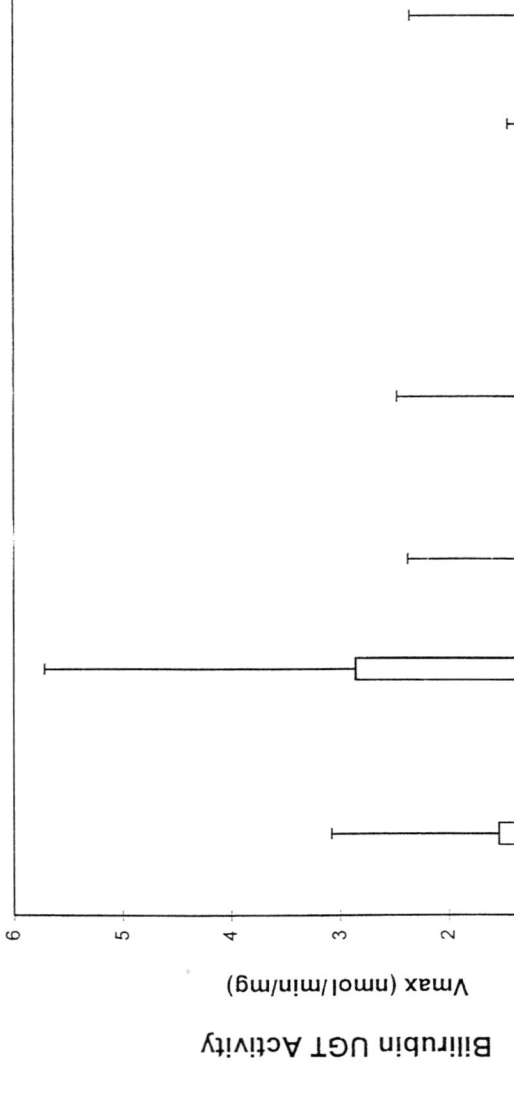

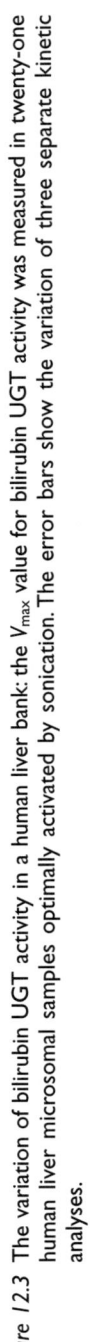

Figure 12.3 The variation of bilirubin UGT activity in a human liver bank: the V_{max} value for bilirubin UGT activity was measured in twenty-one human liver microsomal samples optimally activated by sonication. The error bars show the variation of three separate kinetic analyses.

state, or exposure to xenobiotics, as well as genetic background (Burchell and Coughtrie, 1989).

1-Hydroxypyrene UGT activity varies up to 200-fold in lung microsomes isolated from a population of 101 individual smokers and ex-smokers, but this is not due to induction of the enzyme activity in smokers (Vainio *et al.*, 1995). Urine, nicotine and cotinine N-glucuronide was almost two-fold lower in African smokers compared with Caucasian smokers, whereas 3-hydroxycotinine-o-glucuronide was two-fold higher in Africans (Benowitz *et al.*, 1998). Glucuronidation of clomipramine metabolites showed a pronounced 28-fold interindividual difference in a Japanese psychiatric population (Shimoda *et al.*, 1995). Histograms and probit plots suggest a normal distribution, although there are obviously slow and fast glucuronidators within this group of patients. It would be interesting to look for variation in the genetics of UGT expression in the slow glucuronidators. Glucuronidation was also clearly affected by gender, use of oral contraceptives and other steroids, and smoking, further indicating the problems in determination of genetic polymorphism (Shimoda *et al.*, 1995; Bock *et al.*, 1994).

Liu *et al.* (1991) reported that the glucuronide excretion of one hypolipidemic drug, clofibrate, in a healthy White population followed a normal distribution, whereas that of fenofibrate appeared to be distributed into the distinct normal groups. However, a follow-up familial study has shown a lack of a genetic polymorphism in the glucuronidation of fenofibrate (Vincent-Viry *et al.*, 1995).

Another study of the French population examined variation of dextrorphan glucuronidation (Duche *et al.*, 1993). Again, a normal distribution was observed.

A number of recent studies demonstrate extensive variation *in vivo* in man. Diphenhydramine N-glucuronide excreted in urine from a single dose of the parent drug ranged between 2.7% and 14.8% of the dose within 8 h (Fischer and Breyer-Pfaff, 1997). Zidovudine glucuronide peak levels in serum varied seven-fold in a patient population (Sherwood *et al.*, 1997). The ratio of urinary concentration of glucuronides of benzo(a) pyrene 7,10/8,9 tetrol and 1-hydroxy pyrene was shown to vary 6000-fold in coal tar treated psoriasis patients (Bowman *et al.*, 1997). Thus, there are many new examples of interindividual variation of glucuronidation being recognised in recent studies.

UDP glucuronic acid concentration

Variation in drug glucuronidation may be caused by changes of UDPGA availability, although no specific examples of extreme changes of UDPGA concentration have been reported in humans, they have been observed in rats. For example, Ericksson and Sträth (1981) reported that UDPGA concentrations are reduced after ether narcosis. Interference with liver redox state by adenosine reduced levels of UDPGA by approximately 60% and subsequently caused a 60% decrease in glucuronide formation (Shipley and Weiner, 1987).

UDPGA concentration has been determined to vary five-fold between fetal and adult stages of hepatic development and such variations in UDPGA level were suggested as the potential cause of variation in drug glucuronidation in humans (Capiello *et al.*, 1998).

Problems of drug selection for studies of polymorphism of drug glucuronidation

Phase I metabolism

Drugs which are largely excreted as glucuronides in humans may well be oxidised to their active metabolite prior to glucuronidation. Propranolol is metabolised by side chain oxidation to naphthoxylactic acid (NLA) as major metabolite, and by direct glucuronidation and ring hydroxylation to 4-hydroxypropranolol (4-OH-P), which is then conjugated to glucuronide or sulphate (Walle *et al.*, 1985). The formation of NLA was 55% less in poor metabolisers of mephenytoin and formation of 4-OH-P was 75% less in poor metabolisers of debrisoquine (Ward *et al.*, 1989). Therefore apparent polymorphic variation in formation of propranolol glucuronides would be considerably influenced by polymorphism of drug oxidation. Thus drugs, which are almost entirely eliminated by phase 2 metabolism in humans, should be studied.

Sulphation

Many hydroxylated drug metabolites are potential substrates for sulpho-transferases and UGTs. Sulphation is classically considered the high affinity, low capacity system, whereas glucuronidation is believed to be a low affinity high capacity system (Mulder *et al.*, 1990). Obviously, this generalisation is rather naive, due to the existence of several isoenzymes within each family capable of catalysing the conjugation of phenols. The structure of the substrate will to a large extent determine the affinity of the interaction with the isoenzyme, although a high capacity, low affinity glucuronidation system with its demonstrable multiplicity of isoenzymes with identified overlapping capacities, may compensate for a defect in an individual enzyme. The dose of drug administered may determine whether variation of sulphation or glucuronidation is the primary system studied. Thus a drug which is a preferred substrate for one isoenzyme within a family would be a useful tool for investigation of polymorphism of drug glucuronidation.

Caldwell *et al.*, (1982) have studied the variation of paracetamol and salicylamide conjugation in a cohort of normal human volunteers. The glucuronide:sulphate ratio for conjugation with paracetamol and salicylamide can vary up to sixteen-fold in the population studied. Four of the volunteers were remarkable for their relative inability to form paracetamol sulphate and therefore the measurement of the G:S ratio may merely reflect variation of sulphate conjugation.

Variation of drug glucuronidation in humans has not been extensively studied due to problems in the selection of suitable drugs for screening. The identification and measurement of metabolites, including the interaction between pathways of glucuronidation and sulphation, complicates the interpretation of the data. Indeed, measured variations of acetaminophen glucuronidation in healthy individuals *in vivo* are not more than three-fold (Osborne *et al.*, 1991) although there may not be great variability in enzyme activity levels. There may be compensation by competing metabolic pathways.

Temellini *et al.* (1991) have reported a nineteen-fold variation of ethinylestradiol glucuronidation and seven-fold variation of ethinylestradiol sulphation in human liver. Analysis of the polymorphic variation of diflunisal phenol and its acyl glucuronide showed a unimodal population distribution, especially when excluding females using oral contraceptives (Herman *et al.*, 1994), although metabolism in via phenol sulphation is an added complication. Readers are referred to the reviews of polymorphic variation of drug sulphation in humans by Weinshilboum *et al.* (1997).

Criteria for candidate drugs in the study of polymorphism of glucuronidation

- Mainly directly eliminated by glucuronidation
- Simple metabolism
- Relatively non-toxic
- Excretion in urine not via bile and feces.

Obviously many candidate drugs for such a study, e.g. tamoxifen, chloramphenicol, propranolol and frusemide are rapidly eliminated by these four criteria. Paracetamol and salicylamide have been studied and the results were generally inconclusive except to demonstrate possible variation of conjugation with sulphate.

Menthol and diflunisal would appear to be good candidates for further study, although their elimination still involves conjugation with sulphate, as well as glucuronide. Several other drugs such as chlorpromazine, valproate, lorazepam, codeine, morphine, ketophen, naproxen, lamotrigine, labetralol, gemfibrozil, cyproheptadine, propofol, tamezepam and probenacid are under consideration for further study.

Genetic variation of human *UGT* genes and enzymes

Recently, the existence of polymorphisms in *UGT*s has been established and a more intensive investigation of *UGT*s has revealed the predictable genetic variations.

A summary of the mutations/polymorphisms in *UGT* genes and the resultant possible enzymological effects are shown in Table 12.4. Each genetic mutation will be discussed in a little more detail.

Genetic variation of *UGTIAI*

The known defects of glucuronidation in humans are best illustrated within the group of hereditary hyperbilirubinemias (Clarke *et al.*, 1997) where molecular genetic studies have revealed the association between genetic defects and loss of function.

Crigler–Najjar syndrome: *UGTIAI* mutations

Crigler–Najjar syndrome is a familial form of severe unconjugated hyper-bilirubinemia caused by a dysfunction in bilirubin glucuronidation in humans. The molecular basis of these syndromes has recently been charac-

Table 12.4 Genetic variation of human *UGT* genes and enzymes

Gene	Mutation	Substrate/Function	References
UGTIAI	Mutations in exons 1A,2,3,4,5 G71R and Y486D	Bilirubin glucuronidation Reduced 0–32%	Clarke *et al.*, 1997 Yamamoto *et al.*, 1998
UGTIAI	TA mutations in promoter	Bilirubin glucuronidation Reduced to 30% SN-38 glucuronidation reduced	Bosma *et al.*, 1995 Monaghan *et al.*, 1996 Iyer *et al.*, 1998
UGTIA3	G284R	Scopoletin ?	Smith, Cassidy and Burchell (unpublished work) Green *et al.*, 1998
UGTIA6	T181A	Planar phenols Up to 70% reduction in glucuronidation	Ciotti *et al.*, 1997
UGTIA9	M269X	Propofol	Cassidy, Brierley and Burchell (unpublished work)
UGT2B4	D458E	Hyodeoxycholic acid D-reduced glucuronidation	Levesque *et al.*, 1998
UGT2B7	Y268H	S-oxazepam, morphine	Patel *et al.*, 1995b Coffman *et al.*, 1998
UGT2B15	D85Y	Androstanediol (17β only)	Levesque et al., 1998

terised by enzymological, immunochemical and molecular genetic analysis. *In vitro* analysis of Crigler–Najjar type 1 liver samples has revealed that, as well as complete absence of bilirubin UGT activity, these patients also poorly glucuronidate phenols, 5-hydroxytryptamine and the drugs ethinyl-estradiol and propofol depending on the molecular basis of the defect (Clarke *et al.*, 1994, 1997).

Recently, as a result of the elucidation of the *UGT1* gene complex, several groups have determined some of the genetic lesions that cause Crigler–Najjar syndrome (Clarke *et al.*, 1997). These mutations that result in Crigler–Najjar syndrome have been found in exons 1, 2, 3, and 5 encoding the constant region of all UGT1 proteins thus explaining the decreased activity towards other aglycones, as well as bilirubin (see Clarke *et al.*, 1997). More than thirty-five different genetic lesions have been demonstrated to be associated with the severe hyperbilirubinemia of Crigler–Najjar syndrome (Mackenzie *et al.*, 1997; Clarke *et al.*, 1997). Menthol glucuronidation is considerably reduced in many patients with Crigler–Najjar syndrome, such that the menthol excretion test is often used as a confirmatory diagnosis of the disorder and as a study of the genetic inheritance of the disease (Arias, 1962; Szabo and Ebrey, 1963). In a study of a family in which two Crigler–Najjar children were born from the same marriage, only five of sixteen members of the family showed a normal menthol glucuronide output. This menthol test demonstrated likely hetero-zygotes in the family members who were not revealed by serum bilirubin analyses (Arias, 1962). In other hands, the tests failed to discriminate between icteric patients and anicteric family members suspected to be heterozygotes. Indeed jaundiced patients may show normal menthol glucuronide excretion (Arias *et al.*, 1969). Bloomer *et al.* (1971) also detected normal menthol conjugation in the parents of a Crigler–Najjar child. These accumulated data suggest that menthol glucuronidation is independently variable within the population.

Menthol is conjugated with glucuronic acid prior to excretion in bile and urine (Szabo and Ebrey, 1963) and is therefore an interesting, relatively harmless test compound for study of polymorphism of drug glucuronidation in humans. However, glucuronidation of menthol was only reduced to about 20% of controls in some of the Crigler–Najjar type 1 patients, which suggests that menthol may be a substrate for more than one UGT isoenzyme, which may complicate studies of menthol glucuro-nidation in the normal population.

Liver tissue may be removed from Crigler–Najjar type I patients during liver transplantation for treatment of this lethal disorder, although with orthotopic partial transplant supplementation this tissue is becoming rare. However, some ageing tissue samples are still resident in $-80°C$ freezers around the world. Table 12.5 illustrates the value of this rare tissue in the investigation of glucuronidation.

Table 12.5 UGT activities towards various substrates in Crigler–Najjar liver microsomes

Substrate	UGT activity (nmol/min/mg protein)		References
	Normal	CN	
Bilirubin	0.5	0	Findlay et al., 2000
T4[a]	0.38	0.05	Findlay et al., 2000
Propofol	0.3	0.21	Findlay et al., 2000
Buprenorphine	2.1	0.57	King et al., 1996
Ethinylestradiol	1.03	0.10	Ebner et al., 1993
Naltrexane	0.23	0.22	King et al., 1996
SN38	++	0	Iyer et al., 1998
Propofol[b]	0.3	0	Moghrabi et al., 1993
1-Naphthol[b]	0.47	0.19	Moghrabi et al., 1993

Notes
[a] pmol/min/mg protein of T4 glucuronide.
[b] Crigler–Najjar patient with stop codon in exon 3 leads to loss of all UGT-1 family of enzymes.

There are mutations in Crigler–Najjar patients specifically in the UGT1A1 exon which may affect only the expression of bilirubin UGT activity (see Table 12.5) and mutations in the UGT1A common exons, which may cause the loss of several members or even all of the UGT1A family (see Clarke et al., 1997 and Table 12.5). Loss of the whole family of UGT1 enzymes, will provide an indication of which sub-family will catalyse glucuronidation of compound X. Specific loss of UGT1A1 (bilirubin UGT) may implicate this isoform in glucuronidation of a xenobiotic such as ethinylestradiol (Ebner et al., 1993) or SN38 (Iyer et al., 1998) (Table 12.5).

Gilbert's disease: UGT1A1 promoter polymorphism

Gilbert's disease, a familial hyperbilirubinemia previously estimated to be present in up to 5% of the population in 1980, is characterised by a mild unconjugated hyperbilirubinemia (Fevery, 1981). Decreased formation of bilirubin diglucuronide and increased levels of bilirubin monoglucuronide were found in bile in parallel with decreased hepatic UGT activity (Fevery et al., 1977). This disease provides an opportunity to study variation in drug glucuronidation due to the prevalence of the familial disorder within the population. There is no obvious indication of impaired drug oxidation, acetylation or sulphation (Ullrich et al., 1987). Decreased clearance of several drugs such as tolbutamide, rifamycin, josamycin and paracetamol has been observed (Macklon et al., 1979), although decreased clearance was not apparently associated with a decreased rate of glucuronidation measured in overnight urine samples (Ullrich et al., 1987).

De Morais et al. (1989) have reported that paracetamol glucuronide formation, measured in six Gilbert's patients by clearance from plasma within 2 h, was 31% lower than normal controls. The timing of measurements may be critical in determination of these significant differences and on overnight urine may be a better measurement (Ulrich *et al.*, 1987) since UGT1A1 is not considered to be a key enzyme in paracetamol glucuronidation (Bock *et al.*, 1993).

A paper by Bosma *et al.* (1995) suggested a correlation between homozygosity for a 2 bp insertion in the TATA box upstream of *UGT1A1* exon 1 and GS (no mutations were found in the coding sequence of the *UGT1A1* gene). The primary genetic factor contributing to the variation in the serum and total bilirubin concentration in the Eastern Scottish population was demonstrated to be the sequence variation reported by Bosma *et al.* (1995) and a direct correlation is only revealed by a controlled study of a drug-free, alcohol-free, non-smoking population (Monaghan *et al.*, 1996). Drugs, alcohol and smoking induce human bilirubin UGT (Monaghan *et al.*, 1996) and thereby interfere with the phenotype in the general population, creating 'latent' Gilbert's patients.

GS is strongly associated with homozygosity for allele 7 (7/7 genotype) (Monaghan *et al.*, 1996) and is present in 11–13% and 17–19% of the Eastern Scottish and Canadian Inuit populations, respectively (Monaghan *et al.*, 1996, 1997). Several very recent studies have examined the world populations for TA dinucleotide polymorphisms in the *UGT1A1* promoter. These results are summarised in Table 12.6. These data show that the 7/7 allele associated with GS is present in up to 23% of the Africans, but is very infrequent in Japanese and Asians (<3%). A recent Italian study has determined that 90% of individuals classified as GS exhibited the 7/7 genotype (Sampietro *et al.*, 1998).

Recent work has shown that the mildly affected members of families in which CN type 2 occurs are heterozygous for mutations in the UDP-glucuronosyltransferase *UGT1A1* (G71R and Y486D) may be classified as Gilbert's patients (Koiwai *et al.*, 1995; Sato *et al.*, 1996). A Japanese and Asian population study has revealed a high frequency of the G71R allele

Table 12.6 Frequency of *UGT1A1* promoter mutation (Gilbert's) in different populations

Population (n)		Genotypes			References
		6/6 %	6/7 %	7/7 %	
African[a]	(82)	32 (26)	45 (37)	23 (19)	Beutler *et al.*, 1998
Asian	(47)	70 (33)	27 (13)	3 (1)	Beutler *et al.*, 1998
European	(71)	34 (24)	55 (39)	11 (8)	Beutler *et al.*, 1998
Inuit (Canadian)	(88)	34 (30)	49 (43)	17 (15)	Monaghan *et al.*, 1997
Japanese	(58)	76 (44)	21 (12)	3 (2)	Ando *et al.*, 1998a
Scottish	(77)	40 (31)	38 (37)	12 (9)	Monaghan *et al.*, 1996

Note
[a]The frequency of all promoter mutations including rarer alleles 5 and 8 in this population is 36% (Beutler *et al.*, 1998).

especially in jaundiced Japanese neonates (Akaba *et al.*, 1998, see Table 12.7).

The frequency of the G71R allele is zero in a European population analysed (Akaba *et al.*, 1998). The heterozygous and homozygous G71R mutation causes an approximate 40% and 70% reduction in expression of bilirubin UGT (Yamamoto *et al.*, 1998). Obviously both of these genotypes can lead to clinically defined phenotype in the different population. Compound genetic defects which lead to a more severe hyperbilirubinemia may be termed Crigler–Najjar type 2 patients in some Japanese, because each polymorphic genotype is fairly frequent in Japanese (Aono *et al.*, 1995).

Variation in drug glucuronidation associated with the Gilbert's phenotype

It is now recognised that there are better xenobiotic substrates of UGT1A1 (the major bilirubin-metabolising form) than bilirubin itself, examples including octyl gallate and emodin (Senafi *et al.*, 1994; King *et al.*, 1996) which obviously have the potential to cause jaundice by competitive inhibition of UGT1A1, especially in Gilbert's patients whose hepatic activity is reduced to 35% of normal levels.

Importantly, polymorphic variation in Gilbert's patients has been shown to be associated with reduced glucuronidation of the anticancer drug, irinotecan (CPT-11). Wasserman *et al.* (1997) observed toxicity with this drug in two Gilbert's patients. A study of forty patients showed there was no difference in the incidence and severity of toxicity based on race and sex. The interpatient variability suggests pharmacogenetic variation (Gupta *et al.*, 1997). The topoisomerase 1 inhibitor induced delayed-onset diarrhea in patients with colorectal cancer (Saliba *et al.*, 1998). Bilirubin UGT1A1 has been demonstrated to glucuronidate the CPT-11 metabolite SN-38 (Iyer *et al.*, 1998).

The metabolic ratios (SN-38/SN-38 glucuronide) in the patient with 7/7 genotype were uncharacteristically higher than those in the patients with

Table 12.7 Allele frequency of genetic mutations causing the Gilbert's phenotype

Genotype	(n)	Population	Allele frequency (%)
TA 6	(77)	European	64
TA 7		European	36
TA 6	(58)	Japanese	86
TA 7		Japanese	14
G71R		Japanese (controls)	13
G71R	(42)	Japanese (jaundiced neonates)	32
G71R		Chinese and Korean (controls)	23
G71R	(50)	European (German)	0

other genotypes (6/6 and 6/7). Biliary index was 6980 versus 2180±1110 (range 840–3730) in patients with 7/7 versus 6/6 genotypes, respectively (Ando *et al.*, 1998b).

Other *UGT1* family polymorphisms

Polymorphic variation of UGT1A6

Ciotti *et al.* (1997) have identified two missense mutations T181A and R184S. Approximately 32% (33/98) DNA samples in the population studied were heterozygous with both mutations on one allele. *In vitro* analysis of wild-type and mutant transferases showed that the catalysis of salicylates, β-blockers and 3-o-methyl dopa glucuronidation by the mutant UGT1A6 were reduced by 30–70%. The functional effect of this mutation in humans *in vivo* remains to be examined. UGT1A6 is thought to be a key enzyme in paracetamol (acetamenophen) glucuronidation (Bock *et al.*, 1993). Paracetamol glucuronidation in small Chinese and Caucasian groups has been compared, but no interethnic differences were observed (Osborne *et al.*, 1991). In a more recent study of paracetamol glucuronidation the distribution in a random population appeared to be unimodel although skewed (Bock *et al.*, 1994). Glucuronidation was also clearly affected by gender, oral contraceptive, steroids and smoking, further indicating the problems in determination of genetic polymorphism (Bock *et al.*, 1994).

UGT2 family polymorphisms

UGT2B4

UGT2B4 was identified to catalyse the glucuronidation of hyodeoxycholic acid (Fournel-Gigleux *et al.*, 1989) and this isoform appears to be the major isoform catalysing this reaction (Pillot *et al.*, 1993). Very recently, a polymorphism D458E, was identified with an allele frequency of 38.5% in a small Caucasian population (Levesque *et al.*, 1998). E458 was more active in glucuronidation of hyodeoxycholic acid, and may lead to interindividual variation in glucuronidation.

UGT2B7 (H268Y)

Recently, oxazepam administered as a racemic mixture was shown to be preferentially excreted as the (S) glucuronide and a low S/R glucuronide ratio was used to assess poor glucuronidation of oxazepam (Patel *et al.*, 1995b). A group of 10% of the whole population was determined to be poor glucuronidators of (S) oxazepam and suggested a genetic relationship to the UGT2B7 isoform (Patel *et al.*, 1995a). However, oxazepam may not be solely glucuronidated by UGT2B7 *in vivo* and this relationship requires additional investigation. A *UGT2B7* variant H268Y was originally identified by Jin *et al.* (1993). Miners *et al.* (1998) have determined that the frequencies of the H268/Y268 alleles was 52/48%, respectively, in a Caucasian population whereas the ratio was H88/Y12 in Japanese subjects. Expression of the two polymorphic variants *in vitro* has indicated that UGT2B7 activity towards morphine and many other drugs may be slightly reduced but may not be significantly different (Coffman *et al.*, 1998). Miners *et al.* (1998) did not see any functional difference between menthol and androsterone glucuronidation. These substrates may be glucuronidated by other UGTs and a more specific substrate may be more revealing. Interethnic differences in codeine glucuronidation, reduced in Han Chinese men when compared with a Swedish population are known to exist (Yue *et al.*, 1989, 1995).

UGT2B15 (D85Y)

Characterisation of the UGT2B15(Y-85) cDNA, which was isolated from human prostate and LNCaP cell cDNA libraries, revealed twenty nucleotide differences between UGT2B15(Y-85) and the previously characterized UGT2B15 protein UGT2B15(D-85). However, only one of the two variations in the coding region leads to an amino acid change from aspartic acid to a tyrosine residue at position 85. The genomic DNA of 27 subjects was analysed by direct sequencing of polymerase chain reaction (PCR) products and demonstrated that UGT2B15(D-85) and UGT2B15(Y-85) are encoded by variant alleles with a frequency D85 48% and Y85 52% prevalent in the Caucasian population (Levesque *et al.*, 1997). Expression of UGT2B15(D-85) and UGT2B15(Y-85) in HK293 cells demonstrated similar substrate specificities. Both proteins displayed similar K_m values of 2.2 and 2.4 μM for androstane-3 alpha, 17 beta-diol and dihydrotestosterone, respectively. However, results suggest that UGT2B15(Y-85) has a two-fold higher V_{max} than UGT2B15(D-85) (Levesque *et al.*, 1997).

A 50% reduction in androgen glucuronidation may be very important in steroidogenic or androgen-responsive tissues, such as prostate. Steroids may act as tumor promoters and conjugation of steroids may also be an important restriction mechanism controlling androgen levels. Therefore, it would be logical to assess the role of UGT2B15 polymorphism in association with prostate cancer and those studies are underway in Lang's group (MacLeod *et al.*, 1998).

Xenobiotic and hormonal regulation of UGTs

Environmental chemicals including drugs and changes in endobiotic concentrations during physiological changes can lead to altered expression of

UGTs and hence interindividual variation. Induction of glucuronidation reactions has been reported in man (Clarke and Burchell, 1994). The Indoles present in cruciferous vegetables (brussel sprouts and cabbage) appear to enhance oxazepam and paracetamol glucuronidation modestly (Pantuck et al., 1984). The anticonvulsant agents phenobarbitone, phenytoin and carbamazepine either separately or in combination, induce the glucuronidation of paracetamol (Bock and Bock-Hennig, 1987) and possibly norcodeine (Bock et al., 1994). Carbamazepine also induces valproic acid glucuronidation (Panesar et al., 1989). Co-administration of phenobarbitone and phenytoin induces chloramphenicol glucuronidation (Bloxham et al., 1979). Several oral contraceptive drugs have been demonstrated to increase the glucuronidation of paracetamol (Bock et al., 1994), clofibric acid (Miners et al., 1984) and temazepam (Stoehr et al., 1984). Cimetidine has been shown to specifically increase the urinary excretion of naproxen acyl glucuronide, in contrast to other naproxen glucuronide metabolites (Vree et al., 1993). There are many other examples where glucuronidation of drugs has been shown to be enhanced by other drugs inducing UGTs. Dexamethasone and phenobarbital have been shown to cause up to a two-fold induction of digitoxigenin monodigitoxoside UGT in human liver (Schuetz et al., 1986).

Ethanol treatment of a Gilbert's patient led to a three-fold decrease in serum bilirubin associated with a corresponding 2.5-fold increase in hepatic bilirubin UGT activity (Ideo et al., 1971) and bilirubin UGT mRNA encoded by the UGT1A1 gene, was reported to be selectively induced in human livers from patients treated with phenytoin and phenobarbital (Sutherland et al., 1993). Indeed, widespread consumption of therapeutic and social drugs, e.g. ethanol, and exposure to environmental chemicals induce UGTs and may mask genetic variation for example in Gilbert's patients (see above).

Thyroid hyperplasia

Plasma thyroxine (T4) concentrations are monitored by the pituitary gland and, if thyroxine levels decrease, the pituitary secretes thyroid stimulating hormone that increases the production of thyroxine by the thyroid follicular cells. TSH synthesis is under negative feedback regulation by thyroxine, hence, when plasma thyroxine concentrations return to normal, TSH secretion stops. However, continuous depression of plasma thyroxine results in sustained increases of plasma TSH leading to follicular cell proliferation hyperplasia and ultimately neoplasia (Saito et al., 1991).

Plasma thyroxine levels may be decreased by either direct inhibition of its synthesis or by increased metabolism and excretion. A major route of thyroxine metabolism is conjugation with glucuronic acid in the liver followed by biliary excretion.

Rats given four different microsomal enzyme inducers had elevated UGT activity towards T3 and T4 of up to 66%, and the circulating T3 and T4 concentrations fell to 70–75% of control levels. Furthermore, this reduction in hormone levels was not mediated by the thyroid (Barter and Klaassen, 1994). This effect results in continuous TSH synthesis of thyroid hyperplasia.

The hyperplastic mechanism is one that is potentially operative in many species including humans. Glucuronidation of thyroxine is catalysed by bilirubin UGT and other transferases in human liver (Visser *et al.*, 1993). Therefore chemical induction of bilirubin UGT by alcohol and other drugs could increase risk of hypothyroidism and subsequent thyroid hyperplasia.

Steroid regulation of UGTs in target tissues

Glucuronidation of androgens was observed in prostate, breast cyst fluid and ovary follicular fluid (Bélanger *et al.*, 1998). Two key UGTs involved in androgen glucuronidation, UGT2B15 and UGT2B17 are present in a prostate-derived cell line, LNCaP cells. Treatment of LNCaP cells with dihydrotestosterone decreased UGT2B levels. Glucuronidation of androgens also led to a reduced androgen response (Bélanger *et al.*, 1998). Therefore, glucuronidation, as well as sulphation, has a key role in regulation of androgen action in target tissues such as prostate.

Genetic variation of β-glucuronidase

Variation in the expression of β-glucuronidase especially in relevant tissues such as intestine, may lead to longer half-life of drugs due to enterohepatic circulation. This interindividual difference may be interpreted as a variation in glucuronidation.

Severe genetic mutation of the β-glucuronidase gene in mice and humans can lead to mucopolysaccharidoses (Kyle *et al.*, 1990). Minor defects or heterozygous mutations may affect glucuronide hydrolysis, as well as glycosaminoglycan synthesis. Indeed, a wide range of activities for β-glucuronidase activity towards 4-methylumbelliforme glucuronide has been recorded in human liver and kidney (Sperker *et al.*, 1997). A log normal distribution of enzyme activity was observed, which closely correlated with enzyme protein levels in the human tissue libraries (Sperker *et al.*, 1997). These data indicate the possibility of wide interindividual variability in β-glucuronide mediated hydrolysis of drug glucuronides, which may be interpreted as variation of UGT activity.

Acknowledgements

We thank the Wellcome Trust and the Commission of the European Communities (contract number BMH4-97-2621) for their support of the research work in our laboratories.

References

Akaba, K., Kimura, T., Sasaki, A., Tanabe, S., Ikogami, T., Hashimoto, M., Umeda, H., Yoshida, H., Umetsu, K., Chiba, H., Yuasa, I. and Hayasaka, K. (1998) 'Neonatal hyperbilirubinaemia and mutation of bilirubin UDP-glucuronosyltransferase gene: a common missense mutation among Japanese, Koreans and Chinese', *Biochem. Mol. Biol. Int.* **46**: 21–6.

Albert, C., Vallee, M., Belanger, A. and Hum, D. W. (1998) 'Characterisation of human UDP-glucuronosyltransferase UGT1A3 on active estrogens and bile acids', paper presented at 12th Microsomes and Drug Oxidations Meeting, Montpelier, France.

Ando, Y., Chida, M., Nakayama, K., Saka, H. and Kamataki, T. (1998a) 'The UGT1A1*28 allele is relatively rare in a Japanese population', *Pharmacogenet* **8**: 357–60.

Ando, Y., Saka, H., Asai, G., Suriura, S., Shimokata, K. and Kamataki, T. (1998b) 'UGT1A1 genotypes and glucuronidation of SN38, the active metabolite of irinotecan', *Ann. Oncol.* **9**: 845–7.

Aono, S., Adachi, Y., Uyama, E., Yamada, Y., Keino, H., Nanno, T., Koiwai, O. and Sato, H. (1995) 'Analysis of genes for bilirubin UDP-glucuronosyltransferase in Gilbert's syndrome', *Lancet* **345**: 958–9.

Arias, I. M. (1962) 'Chronic unconjugated hyperbilirubinaemia without overt signs of hemolysis in adolescents and adults', *J. Clin. Invest.* **41**: 2233–45.

Arias, I. M., Gartner, L. M., Cohen, M., Ezzer, J. B. and Levi, A. J. (1969) 'Chronic nonhemolytic unconjugated hyperbilirubinemia with glucuronyltransferase deficiency: clinical, biochemical, pharmacologic and genetic evidence for heterogeneity', *Am. J. Med.* **47**: 395–409.

Barter, R. A. and Klaassen, C. D. (1994) 'Reduction of thyroid hormone levels and alteration of thyroid function by four representative UDP-glucuronosyltransferase inducers in rats', *Toxicol. Appl. Pharmacol.* **128**: 9–17.

Beaulieu, M., Levesque, E., Hum, D.W. and Bélanger, A. (1996) 'Isolation and characterisation of a novel cDNA encoding a human UDP-glucuronosyltransferase active on C19 steroids', *J. Biol. Chem.* **271**: 22855–62.

Bélanger, A., Hum, D. W., Beaulieu, M., Levesque, E, Guillemette, C., Tehernot, A., Bélanger, G., Turgeon, D. and Dubois, S. (1998) 'Characterisation and regulation of UDP-glucuronosyltransferase in steroid target tissues', *J. Ster. Biochem. and Mol. Biol.* **65**: 301–10.

Benowitz, N. L., Perez-Stable, E., Fong, I. and Jacob, P. (1998) 'Differences in N- and O-glucuronide formation in African-American vs Caucasian smokers', *Clin. Pharmacol. Therap.* **63**: 148.

Beutler, E., Gelbert, T. and Demina, A. (1998) 'Racial variability in the UDP-glucuronosyltransferase 1 (UGT1A1) promoter: a balanced polymorphism for regulation of bilirubin metabolism', *Proc. Natl. Acad. Sci. USA* **95**: 8170–4.

Bloomer, J. R., Berk, P. D., Howe, R. B. and Berlin, N. I. (1971) 'Bilirubin metabolism in congenital nonhemolytic jaundice', *Pediat. Res.* **5**: 256–64.

Bloxham, R. A., Durbin, G. M., Johnson, T. and Winterborn, M. H. (1979) 'Chloramphenicol and phenobarbitone – a drug interaction', *Arch. Dis. Child.* **54**: 76–7.

Bock, K. W. and Bock-Hennig, B. S. (1987) 'Differential Induction of human liver UDP-glucuronosyltransferase activities by phenobarbital-type inducers', *Biochem. Pharmacol.* **36**: 4137–43.

Bock, K. W., Forster, A., Gschaidmeier, H., Bruck, M., Munzel, P., Scharek, W., Fournel-Gigleux, S. and Burchell, B. (1993) 'Paracetamol glucuronidation by recombinant rat and human phenol UDP-glucuronosyltransferase', *Biochem. Pharmacol.* **45**: 1809–14.

Bock, K. W., Schrenk, D., Forster, A., Griese, E., Morike, K., Brockmeier, D. and Eichelbaum, M. (1994) 'The influence of environmental and genetic factors on CYP2D6, CYP1A2 and UDP-glucuronosyltransferases in man using sparteine, caffeine, and paracetamol as probes', *Pharmacogenetics* **4**: 209–18.

Boelsterli, U. A. (1993) 'Specific targets of covalent drug-protein interactions in hepatocytes and their toxicological significance in drug-induced liver-injury', *Drug Metab. Rev.* **25**: 395–451.

Bosma, P. J., Roy Chowdhury, J., Bakker, C., Gantla, S., De Boer, A., Oostra, B. A., Lindhout, D., Tytgat, G. N. J., Jansen, P. L. M., Oude Elferink, R. P. J. and Roy Chowdhury, N. (1995) 'The genetic basis of the reduced expression of bilirubin UDP-glucuronosyltransferase 1 in Gilbert's syndrome', *New Eng. J. Med.* **333**: 1171–218.

Bowman, E. D., Rothman, N., Hackl, C., Santella, R. M. and Weston, A. (1997) 'Interindividual variation in the levels of certain urinary polycyclic aromatic hydrocarbon metabolites following medicinal exposure to coal tar ointment', *Biomarkers* **2**: 321–7.

Breyer-Pfaff, U., Fischer, D. and Winne, D. (1997) 'Biphasic kinetics of quaternary ammonium glucuronide formation from anitryptyline and diphenhydramine', *Drug Metab. Disp.* **25**: 340–5.

Brierley, C. H. and Burchell, B. (1993) 'Human UDP-glucuronosyltransferases: chemical defence, jaundice and gene therapy', *Bioessays* **15**: 749–54.

Burchell, B., Coughtrie, M. W. H., Jackson, M. R., Shepherd, S. R. P. and Harding, D. (1987) 'Genetic deficiency of bilirubin glucuronidation in rats and humans', *Mol. Asp. Med.* **9**: 429–55.

Burchell, B. and Coughtrie, M. W. H. (1989) 'UDP-glucuronyltransferases in genetic factors influencing the metabolism of foreign compounds', *Pharmacol. Therap.* **43**: 261–89.

Burchell, B., Brierley, C. H. and Rance, D. (1995) 'Specificity of human UDP-glucuronosyltransferases and xenobiotic glucuronidation', *Life. Sci.* **57**: 1819–31.

Burchell, B., Nebert, D. W., Nelson, D. R., Bock, K. W., Iyanagi, T. and Jansen, P. L. M. (1991) 'The UDP glucuronosyltransferase gene superfamily: suggested nomenclature based on evolutionary divergence', *DNA Cell. Biol.* **10**: 487–94.

Burchell, B., McGurk, K., Brierley, C. H. and Clarke, D. J. (1997) UDP-'Glucuronosyltransferases', in I. G. Sipes, A. J. Gandolfi and C. A. Mcqueen (eds) *Comprehensive Toxicology*, Amsterdam: Pergamon Elsevier Science, pp. 401–35.

Caldwell, J., Davies, S., Boote, D. J. and O'Gorman, J. (1982) 'Interindividual variation in the sulfation and glucuronidation of paracetamol and salicylamide in human volunteers', in G. J. Mulder, J. Caldwell, G. M. J. Van Kempen and R. J. Vonk (eds) *Sulphate Metabolism and Sulphate*, London: Taylor and Francis, pp. 251–61.

Capiello, M., Giuliani, L., Rane, A. and Pacifici, G. M. (1998) '5′ Diphosphos-phoglucuronic acid (UDPGA) in the human fetal liver, kidney and placenta', *Biol. Neonate.*

Cheng, Z., Radominska-Paydya, A. and Tephly, T. R. (1998) 'Cloning and expression of human UDP-glucuronosyltransferase 1A8', *Arch. Biophys. Biochem.* **356**: 301–5.

Ciotti, M., Marrone, A., Potter, C. and Owen, I. S. (1997) 'Genetic polymorphism in the human UGT1A6 (planar phenol) UDP-glucuronosyltransferase: pharmacological implications', *Pharmacogenet* **7**: 485–95.

Ciotti, M. and Owens, I. S. (1996) 'Evidence for overlapping active sites for 17a-ethinylestradiol and bilirubin in the human major bilirubin UDPglucuronosyltransferase', *Biochem.* **35**: 10119–24.

Clarke, D. J. and Burchell, B. (1994) 'The uridine diphosphate glucuronosyltransferase multigene family: function and regulation', *Handb. Exper. Pharmcol.* **112**: 3–43.

Clarke, D. J., Moghrabi, N., Monaghan, G., Cassidy, A., Boxer, M., Hume, R. and Burchell, B. (1997) 'Genetic defects of the UDP-glucuronosyltransferase-1 (UGT1) gene that cause familial non-haemolytic unconjugated hyperbilirubinaemias', *Clin. Chim. Acta.* **266**: 63–74.

Coffman, B. L., King, C. D., Rios, G. R. and Tephly, T. R. (1998) 'The glucuronidation of opiods, other xenobiotics and androgens by human UGT2B7Y(2b8) and UGT2B7H(2b8)', *Drug Metab. Disp.* **26**: 73–7.

Coffman, B. L., Rios, G. R., King, C. D. and Tephly, T. R. (1997) 'Human UGT2B7 catalyses morphine glucuronidation', *Drug Metab. Dispos.* **25**: 1–4.

Coughtrie, M. W. H., Burchell, B., Shepherd, I. M. and Bend, J. R. (1987) 'Defective induction of phenol glucuronidation by 3-methylcholanthrene in Gunn rats is due to the absence of a specific UDP-glucuronosyltransferase isoenzyme', *Mol. Pharmacol.* **31**: 585–91.

De Morais, S. M. F., Uetricht, J. P. and Wells, P. G. (1992) 'Decreased glucaronidation and increased bioactivation of acetaminophen in Gilbert's Syndrome', *Gastroenterology* **102**: 577–86.

Diamond, S. and Christ, D. D. (1996) 'Effects of the novel immunosuppresent brequinar on hepatic UDP-glucuronic acid levels and UDP-glucuronosyltransferase activities in the rat', *Drug Metab. Dispos.* **24**: 375–6.

Ding, A., Ojingwa, J. C., McDonagh, A. F., Burlingame, A. L. and Benet, L. Z. (1993) 'Evidence for covalent binding of acyl glucuronides to serum-albumin via an imine mechanism as revealed by tandem mass-spectrometry', *Proc. Nat. Acad. Sci. USA* **90**: 3797–801.

Dubois, S., Beaulieu, M., Levesque, E., Albert, C., Hum, D. W. and Bélanger, A. (1998) 'Residue 121 is involved in the specificity of the UGT2B17 steroid metabolising enzyme', paper presented at the 12th Microsomes and Drug Oxidations Meeting, Montpellier, France.

Duche, J. C., Querol-Ferrer, V., Barre, J., Mesangeau, M. and Tillement, J. P. (1993) 'Dextromethorphan O-demethylation and dextrorphan glucuronidation in a French population', *Int. J. Clin. Pharmacol. Ther. Toxicol.* **31**: 392–8.

Dutton, G. J. (ed.) (1980) *Glucuronidation of Drugs and Other Compounds,* Boca Raton: CRC Press.

Duvaldestin, P., Mahu, J.-L., Preaux, A.-M. and Berthelot, P. (1976) 'Novobiocin-inhibition and magnesium-interaction of rat liver microsomal bilirubin UDP-glucuronosyltransferase', *Biochem. Pharmacol.* **25**: 2587–92.

Ebner, T. and Burchell, B. (1993) 'Substrate specificities of two stably expressed human liver UDP-glucuronosyltransferases of the UGT1 gene family', *Drug Metab. Dispos.* **21**: 50–5.

Ebner, T., Burchell, B. and Remmel, R. P. (1993) 'Human bilirubin UDP-glucuronosyltransferase catalyses the glucuronidation of ethinylestradiol', *Mol. Pharmacol.* **43**: 649–54.

Eriksson, G. and Strath, D. (1981) 'Decreased UDP-glucuronic acid in rat liver after ether narcosis', *FEBS Letts.* **124**: 39–42.

Ethell, B. (1998) 'Structure/activity relationships for cloned and expressed human UDP-glucuronosyltransferases', PhD thesis, University of Dundee.

Ethell, B., Lautala, P., Taskinen, J. and Burchell, B. (1998) 'Screening of catechol substrates for the development of predictive models of catechol drug glucuronidation', proceedings of the 5th International ISSX Meeting, Cairns, Australia.

Fevery, J. (1981) 'Pathogenesis of Gilbert's syndrome', *Eur. J. Clin. Invest.* **11**: 417–8.

Fevery, J., Blanckaert, N., Heirwegh, K. P., Preaux, A. M. and Berthelot, P. (1977) 'Unconjugated bilirubin and an increased proportion of bilirubin monoconjugates in the bile of patients with Gilbert's syndrome and Crigler–Najjar disease', *J. Clin. Invest.* **60**: 970–9.

Findlay, K. (2000) 'Characterization of the UGTs catalysing thyroid hormone glucuronidation in man', *J. Clin. Endocrinology and Metab.* **85**: 2879–83.

Fischer, D. and Breyer-Pfaff, U. (1997) 'Variability of diphenhydramine N-glucuronidation in healthy subjects', *Europ. J. Drug. Metab. Pharmacokinet.* **22**: 151–4.

Fournel, S., Gregoire, B., Magdalou, J., Carre, M.-C., Lafaurie, C., Siest, G. and Caubere, P. (1986) 'Inhibition of bilirubin UDPglucuronosyltransferase activity by triphenylacetic and related compounds', *Biochim. Biophys. Acta.* **883**: 190–6.

Fournel-Gigleux, S., Jackson, M. R., Wooster, R. and Burchell, B. (1989a) 'Expression of a human liver cDNA encoding hydeoxycholic acid UDP-glucuronosyltransferase in cell culture', *FEBS Letts.* **243**: 119–22.

Fournel-Gigleux, S., Magdalou, J., Siest, G., Carre, M.C., Shepherd, S. R. P., Jackson, M.R., Harding, D. and Burchell, B. (1988) 'Carboxylic acids as inhibitors and substrates of UDP-glucuronosyltransferases', in G. Siest, J. Magdalou and B. Burchell (eds) *Cellular and Molecular Aspects of Glucuronidation*, London–Paris: Colloque INSERM/John Libbey Eurotext Ltd, pp. 43–50.

Fournel-Gigleux, S., Shepherd, S. R. P., Carre, M.-C., Burchell, B., Siest, G. and Caubere, P. (1989b) 'Novel inhibitors and substrates of bilirubin UDP-glucuronyltransferase (arylalkylcarboxylic acids)', *Eur. J. Biochem.* **183**: 653–9.

Green, M. D., King, C. D., Mojarrabi, B., Mackenzie, P. I. and Tephly, T. R. (1998). 'Glucuronidation of amines and other xenobiotics catalysed by expressed human UDP-glucuronosyltransferase 1A3', *Drug Metab. Disp.* **26**: 507–12.

Green, M. D., Oturu, E. M. and Tephly, T. R. (1994) 'Stable expression of a human liver UDP-glucuronosyltransferase (UGT2B15) with activity toward steroid and xenobiotic substrates', *Drug Metabolism and Disposition* **22**: 799–805.

Gupta, E., Mick, R., Ramirez, J., Wang, X. L., Lestingi, T. M., Vokes, E. E. and Ratain, M. J. (1997) 'Pharmacokinetic and pharmacodynamic evaluation of the topoisomerase inhibitor irinotecan in cancer patients', *J. Clin. Oncol.* **15**: 1502–10.

Herman, R. J., Loewen, G. R., Antosh, D. M., Taillon, M. R., Hussein, S. and Verbeeck, R. K. (1994) 'Analysis of polymorphic variation in drug metabolism:

III. Glucuronidation and sulfation of diflunisal in man', *Clin. Invest. Med.* **17**: 297–307.

Ideo, G., De Franchis, R., Del Ninno, E. and Dioguardi, N. (1971) 'Ethanol increases liver uridine-diphosphate-glucuronosyltransferase', *Experientia* **27**: 24–5.

Iyer, L., King, C. D., Whitington, P. F., Green, M. D., Roy, S.K., Tephly, T. R., Coffman, B. L. and Ratain, M. J. (1998) 'Genetic predisposition to the metabolism of irinotecan (CPT11)', *J. Clin. Invest.* **101**: 847–54.

Jedlitschky, G., Cassidy, A. J., Sales, M., Pratt, N. and Burchell, B. (1999) 'Cloning and characterization of a novel human olfactory UGT', *Biochem. J.* **340**: 837-43.

Jin, C. J., Mackenzie, P. I. and Miners, J. O. (1997) 'The regio- and stereoselectivity of C19 and C21 hydroxysteroid glucuronidation by UGT2B7 and UGT2B11', *Arch. Biochem. Biophys.* **341**: 207–11.

Jin, C.J., Miners, J. O., Lillywhite, K. J. and MacKenzie, P. I. (1993) 'Complementary deoxyribonucleic acid cloning and expression of a human liver uridine diphosphate-glucuronosyltranferase glucuronidating carboxylic acid-containing drugs', *J. Pharmacol. Exp. Ther.* **264**: 475–9.

King, C. D., Green, M. D., Rios, G. R., Coffman, B. L., Owens, I. S., Bishop, W. P. and Tephly, T. R. (1996) 'The glucuronidation of exogenous and endogenous compounds by stably expressed rat and human UDP-glucuronosyltransferase 1.1', *Arch. Biochem. Biophys.* **332**: 92–100.

Koiwai, O., Nishizawa, M., Hasada, K., Aono, S., Adachi, Y., Mamiya, N. and Sato, H. (1995) 'Gilbert's syndrome is caused by heterozygous missense mutation in the gene for bilirubin UDP-glucuronosyltransferase', *Human Molecular Genetics* **4**: 1183–6.

Kyle, J. W., Birkenmeier, E. H., Gwynn, B., Vogler, C., Hoppe, P. C., Hoffmann, J. W. and Sly, W. S. (1990) 'Correction of murine mucopolysaccharidosis VII by a human β-glucuronidase transgene', *Proc. Natl. Acad. Sci. USA* **87**: 3914–8.

Lautala, P., Ethell, B., Burchell, B. and Taskinen, J. (2000) 'The COMT inhibitors and entacapone and tolcapone are good substrates for UGT1A4 and UGT1A9', *Drug Metab. Disp.* **28**: 1385–9.

Levesque, E., Beaulieu, M., Green, M. D., Tephly, T. R., Bélanger, A. and Hum, D. W. (1997) 'T1: isolation and characterization of UGT2B15(Y-85): a UDP-glucuronosyltransferase encoded by a polymorphic gene', *Pharmacogenet* **7**: 317–25.

Levesque, E., Beaulieu, M., Vallée, M. and Bélanger, A. (1998) 'UGT2B4 (E^{458}), a UDP-glucuronosyltransferase encoded by a polymorphic gene with differential substrate specificity', paper abstract presented at the 12th meeting of Microsomes and Drug Oxidations in Montpellier.

Liu, H. F., Vincentviry, M., Galteau, M. M., Gueguen, R., Magdalou, J., Nicolas, A., Leroy, P. and Siest, G. (1991) 'Urinary glucuronide excretion of fenofibric and clofibric acid glucuronides in man – is it polymorphic', *Europ. J. Clin. Pharmacol.* **41**: 153–9.

Mackenzie, P., Owens, I. S., Burchell, B., Bock, K. W., Bairoch, A., Bélanger, A., Fournel-Gigleux, S., Green, M., Hum, D. W., Iyanagi, T., Lancet, D., Louisot, P., Magdalou, J., Roy Chowdhury, J., Ritter, J. K., Schachter, H., Tephly, T. R., Tipton, K. E. and Nebert, D. W. (1997) 'The UDP glycosyltransferase gene superfamily: recommended nomenclature update based on evolutionary divergence', *Pharmacogen.* **7**: 255–69.

Macklon, A. F., Savage, R. L. and Rawlins, M. D. (1979) 'Gilbert's syndrome and drug metabolism', *Clin. Pharmacokinet.* **4**: 223–32.

MacLeod, S. L., Nowell, S. A. and Lang, N. P. (1998) 'Determination of genetic polymorphisms in UGT2B15 by allele-specific PCR.', paper abstract presented at the 5th International ISSX Meeting in Cairns, Australia.

Malaka-Zafiriu, K., Tsiouris, I. and Cassimos, C. (1973) 'The effect of gentamicin on liver glucuronosyltransferase', *J. Paediat.* **82**: 118–20.

Meyers, M., Slikker, W. and Vore, M. (1981) 'Steroid D-ring glucuronides: characterisation of a new class of cholestatic agents in the rat', *J. Pharmacol. Exp. Ther.* **218**: 63–73.

Miners, J. O., Attwood, J. and Birkett, D. J. (1984) 'Determinants of acetaminophen metabolism: inhibitors of drug metabolism on acetaminophen's metabolic pathways', *Clin. Pharmacol. Therap.* **35**: 480–86.

Miners, J. O., Lillywhite, K. J. and Birkett, D. J. (1988) 'In vitro evidence for the involvement of at least two forms of human liver UDP-glucuronosyltransferase in morphine 3-glucuronidation', *Biochem. Pharmacol.* **37**: 2839–45.

Miners, J. O., McKinnon, W. M., Angus, C. T., Lo, A. C. T., Kubota, T., Ishizaki, T. and Bhasker, C. R. (1998) 'Polymorphism in the UGT2B7 gene', paper abstract presented at the International Glucuronidation Workshop, Brisbane, Australia.

Miners, J. O., Volete, L., Lilleywhite, K., Mackenzie, P. I., Burchell, B., Baguley, B. C. and Kestell, P. (1997) 'Preclinical prediction of factors influencing the elimination of 5,6 dimethyl xenthenone-4-acetic acid, a new anticancer drug', *Cancer Res.* **57**: 284–9.

Moghrabi, N., Sutherland, L., Wooster, R., Povey, S., Boxer, M. and Burchell, B. (1992) 'Chromosomal assignment of human phenol and bilirubin UDP-glucuronosyltransferase genes (UGT1A subfamily)', *Ann. Hum. Genet.* **56**: 83–93.

Moghrabi, N., Clarke, D. J., Burchell, B. and Boxer, M. (1993) 'Cosegration of intragenic markers with a novel mutation that causes Crigler–Najjar syndrome type 1: implications for carrier detection and prenatal diagnosis', *Am. J. Hum. Genet.* **53**: 722–9.

Mojarrabi, B., Butler, R. and Mackenzie, P. I. (1996) 'cDNA cloning and characterization of the human UDP glucuronosyltransferase, UGT1A3', *Biochem. Biophys. Res. Commun.* **225**: 785–90.

Mojarrabi, B. and Mackenzie, P. I. (1997). 'The human UDP-glucuronosyltransferase, UGT1A10 glucuronidates mycophenolic acid', *Biochem. Biophys. Res. Commun.* **238**: 775–8.

Monaghan, G., Clarke, D. J., Povey, S., Gee See, C., Boxer, M. and Burchell, B. (1994) 'Isolation of a human YAC contig encompassing a cluster of UGT2 genes and its regional localization to chromosome 4q13', *Genomics* **23**: 496–9.

Monaghan, G., Foster, B., Jurima-Romet, M., Hume, R. and Burchell, B. (1997) 'UGT1*1 genotyping in a Canadian inuit population', *Pharmacogenetics* **7**: 153–6.

Monaghan, G., Ryan, M. F., Seddon, R., Hume, R. and Burchell, B. (1996) 'Genetic variation in bilirubin UDP-glucuronosyltransferase gene promoter and Gilbert's syndrome', *Lancet* **347**: 578–81.

Mulder, G. J., Coughtrie, M. W. H. and Burchell, B. (1990) 'Glucuronidation', in G. J. Mulder (ed.) *Conjugation Reactions in Drug Metabolism: An Integrated Approach*', London: Taylor & Francis, pp. 51–105.

Noort, D., Coughtrie, M. W. H., Burchell, B., van der Morel, G. A., van Boom, J. H., van der Gen, A. and Mulder, G. J. (1990) 'Inhibition of UDP-glucurono-syltransferase activity by possible transition state analogues in rat liver microsomes', *Eur. J. Biochem.* 281: 170–5.

Noort, D., Vandermarel, G. A., Vandergen, A., Mulder, G. J. and Vanboom, J. H. (1991) 'Synthesis of potential UDP-glucuronosyltransferase inhibitors containing a diphosphate function', *Royal Netherlands Chem.* 110: 53–6.

Osborne, N. J., Tonkin, A. L. and Miners, J. O. (1991) 'Interethnic differences in drug glucuronidation: a comparison of paracetamol metabolism in Caucasians and Chinese', *Br. J. Clin. Pharmac.* 32: 765–7.

Ouzzine, M., Pillot, T., Fournelgigleux, S., Magdalou, J., Burchell, B. and Siest, G. (1994) 'Expression and role of the human liver UDP- glucurono-syltransferase UGT1*6 analyzed by specific antibodies raised against a hybrid protein produced in Escherichia-coli', *Arch. Biochem. Biophys.* 310: 196–204.

Owens, I. S. and Ritter, J. K. (1992) 'The novel bilirubin/phenol UDP-glucurono-syltransferase UGT 1 gene locus: implications for multiple nonhemolytic familial hyperbilirubinaemia phenotypes', *Pharmacogenetics* 2: 93–108.

Pacifici, G. M. and Rane, A. (1981) 'Inhibition of morphine glucuronidation by oxazepam in human fetal liver microsomes', *Drug Metab. and Disp.* 9: 569–72.

Panesar, S. K., Orr, J. M., Farrell, K., Burton, R. W., Kassahun, K. and Abbott, F. S. (1989) 'The effect of carbamazepine on valproic acid disposition in adult volunteers', *Brit. J. Clin. Pharmacol.* 27: 323–8.

Pang, S., Macgillivary, M., Wang, M., Jeffries, S., Clark, A., Rosenthal, I., Weigensberg, M. and Riddick, L. (1991) '3a-androstanediol glucuronide in virilizing congenital adrenal hyperplasia: a useful serum metabolic marker of integrated adrenal androgen secretion', *J. Clin. Endocrinol. Metab.* 73: 166–74.

Pantuck, E. J., Pantuck, C. B., Anderson, K. E., Wattenberg, L. W., Conney, A. H. and Kappas, A. (1984) 'Effect of brussels-sprouts and cabbage on drug conjugation', *Clin. Pharmacol. Therap.* 35: 161–9.

Patel, M., Tang, B. K., Grant, D. M. and Kalow, W. (1995b) 'Interindividual variability in the glucuronidation of (S) oxazepam contrasted with that of (R) oxazepam', *Pharmacogenetics* 5: 287–97.

Patel, M., Tang, B. K. and Kalow, W. (1995a) (S) 'Oxazepam glucuronidation is inhibited by ketoprofen and other substrates of UGT 2B7', *Pharmacogentics* 5: 43–9.

Paul, D., Standifer, K. M., Inturrisi, C. E. and Pasternak, G. W. (1989) 'Pharmacological characterization of morphine-6-b-glucuronide, a very potent morphine metabolite', *Pharmacol. Exp. Therap.* 251: 477–83.

Peters, W. H. M. and Jansen, P. L. M. (1988) 'Immunocharacterization of UDP-glucuronyltransferase isoenzymes in human liver, intestine and kidney', *Biochem. Pharmacol.* 37: 564–7.

Pillot, T., Ouzzine, M., Fournel-Gigleux, S., Lafaurie, C., Radominska, A., Burchell, B., Siest, G. and Magdalou, J. (1993) 'Glucuronidation of hyodeoxy-choic acid in human liver – evidence for a selective role for UDP-glucurono-syltransferase-2B4', *J. Biol. Chem.* 268: 25636–42.

Radominska-Pandya, A., Little, J. M., Pandya, J. T., Tephly T. R., King, C. D.,

Barone, G. W. and Raufman, J. P. (1998) 'UDP-glucuronosyltransferases in human intestinal mucosa', *Biochem. Biophys. Acta.* **1394**: 199–208.

Remmel, R. P. and Burchell, B. (1993) 'Validation and use of cloned, expressed human drug metabolising enzymes in heterologous cells for analysis of drug metabolism and drug–drug interactions', *Biochem. Pharmacol.* **46**: 559–66.

Ritter, J. K., Chen, F., Sheen, Y. Y., Lubet, R. A. and Owens, I. S. (1992) 'Two human liver cDNAs encode UDP-glucuronosyltransferase with 2 log differences in activity toward parallel substrates including hyodeoxycholic acid and certain estrogen derivatives', *Biochem.* **31**: 3409–14.

Said, M., Noort, D., Magdalou, J., Ziegler, J. C., van der Marel, G. A., van Boom, J. H., Mulder, G. J. and Siest, G. (1992) 'Selective and potent inhibition of differnt hepatic UDP-glucuronosyltransferase activities by w,w,w-triphenyl-alcohols and UDP derivatives. *Biochem. Biophys. Res. Commun.* **187**: 140–5.

Saito, K., Kaneko, H., Sato, K., Yoshitake, A. and Yamada, H. (1991) 'Hepatic UDP-glucuronsyltransferase(s) activity toward thyroid hormones in rats: induction and effects on serum thyroid hormone levels following treatment with various enzyme inducers', *Toxicology* **111**: 99–106.

Saliba, F., Higipantelli, R., Misset, J. L., Bastian, G., Vassal, G., Ronnay, M., Herait, P., Cote, C., Mahjoubi, M., Mignard, D. and Critkovic, E. (1998) 'Pathophysiology and therapy of irinotecan-induced onset diarrhea in patients with advanced colorectal cancer', *J. Clin. Oncol.* **16**: 2745–51.

Salman, K., Spielvogel, R. L., Shulman, L. H., Miller, J. L., Vanderlinde, R. E. and Rose, L. I. (1992) 'Serum androstanediol glucuronide in women with facial hirsutism', *J. Am. Acad. Dermatol.* **26**: 411–4.

Sampietro, M., Lupica, L., Perrero, L., Romano, R., Molteni, V and Fionelli, G. (1998) 'TATA-box promoter mutant in the promoter of UDP-glucuronosyltransferase gene in Italian patients with Gilbert's syndrome', *Ital. J. Gastroenterol. Hepatol.* **30**: 194–8.

Sato, H., Adachi, Y. and Koiwai, O. (1996) 'The genetic basis of Gilbert's syndrome', *Lancet* **347**: 557–8.

Schuetz, E. G., Hazelton, G. A., Hall, J., Watkins, P. B., Klaassen, C. D. and Guzelian, P. S. (1986) 'Induction of digitoxigenin monodigitoxoside UDP-glucuronosyltransferase activity by glucocorticoids and other inducers of cytochrome-P-450 in primary monolayer-cultures of adult-rat hepatocytes and in human-liver', *J. Biol. Chem.* **261**: 8270–5.

Senafi, S. B., Clarke, D. J. and Burchell, B. (1994) 'Investigation of the substrate-specificity of a cloned expressed human bilirubin UDP-glucuronosyltransferase - UDP-sugar specificity and involvement in steroid and xenobictic glucuronidation', *Biochem. J.* **303**: 233–40.

Sharp, S., Mak, L. Y., Smith, D. J. and Coughtrie, M. W. H. (1992) 'Inhibition of human and rabbit liver steroid and xenobiotic UDP-glucuronosyltransferases by tertiary amine drugs-implications for adverse drug reactions', *Xenobiotica* **22**: 13–25.

Sherwood, R. A, Marsden, J. T., Stein, C. A., Somasundaram, S., Aitken, C., Oxford, J. S., Menzies, I. S. and Bjarnason, I. (1997) 'Intra-individual variation in serum AZT is not related to intestinal absorption or small intestinal inflammatory changes in human HIV-infected subjects', *Antiviral Chem. & Chemotherap.* **8**: 327–32.

Shimoda, K., Noguchi, T., Ozeki, Y., Morita, S., Shibasaki, M., Someya, T. and Takahashi, S. (1995) 'Metabolism of clomipramine in a Japanese psychiatric population: hydroxylation, desmethylation, and glucuronidation', *Neuropsychopharmacology* **12**: 323–33.

Shipley, L. A. and Weiner, M. (1987) 'Effects of adenosine on glucuronidation and uridine diphosphate glucuronic acid (UDPGA) synthesis in isolated rat hepatocytes', *Biochem. Pharmacol.* **36**: 2993–3000.

Slikker, W., Vore, M., Bailey, J. R., Meyers, M. and Montgomery, C. (1983) 'Hepatotoxic effects of estradiol-17-b-D-glucuronide in the rat and monkey', *J. Pharmacol. Exp. Ther.* **225**: 138–43.

Spahn-Langguth, H. and Benet, L. Z. (1992) 'Acyl glucuronides revisited: is the glucuronidation process a toxification as well as detoxification mechanism?', *Drug. Metab. Rev.* **24**: 5–48.

Sperker, B., Backman, J. T. and Kroemer, H. K. (1997) 'The role of beta-glucuronidase in drug disposition and drug targeting in humans', *Clin. Pharmacokin.* **331**: 18–31.

Stoehr, G. P., Kroboth, P. D., Juhl, R. P., Wender, D. B., Phillips, J. P. and Smith, R. B. (1984) 'Effect of oral contraceptives on triazolam, temazepam, alprazolam and lorazepam kinetics', *Clin. Pharmacol. Ther.* **36**: 683–90.

Strassburg, C. P., Mann, M. P. and Tukey, R. H. (1998) 'Expression of the UDP-glucuronosyltransferase 1A locus in human colon', *J. Biol. Chem.* **273**: 8719–26.

Sutherland, L., Ebner, T. and Burchell, B. (1993) 'The expression of UDP-glucuronosyltransferase of the UGT1 family in human liver and kidney and in response to drugs', *Biochem. Pharmacol.* **45**: 295–301.

Szabo, L. and Ebrey, P. (1963) 'Studies on the inheritance of Crigler-Najjar syndrome by the menthol test', *Acta. Paediatr. Scand.* **4**: 153–8.

Temellini, A., Giuliani, L. and Pacifici, G. M. (1991) 'Interindividual variability in the glucuronidation and sulphation of ethinyloestradiol in human liver', *Br. J. Clin. Pharmac.* **31**: 661–4.

Tephly, T. R. and Burchell, B. (1990) 'The UDP-glucuronosyltransferases: a family of detoxifying enzymes', *Trends Pharmacol. Sci.* **11**: 276–9.

Thompson, D. L., Horton, N. and Rittmaster, R. S. (1990) 'Androsterone glucuronide is a marker of adrenal hyperandrogenism in hirsute women', *Clinical Endocrinology* **32**: 283–92.

Timmers, C. M., Dekker, M., Buijsman, R. C., Van der Marel, G. A., Ethell, B., Anderson, G., Burchell, B., Mulder, G. J. and van Boom, J. H. (1997) 'Synthesis and inhibitory effect of a trisubstrate transition state analogue for UDP-glucuronosyltransferases', *Bioorg. Med. Chem. Lett.* **7**: 1501–6.

Ullrich, D., Sieg, A., Blume, R., Bock, K. W., Schrotter, W. and Bircher, J. (1987) 'Normal pathways for glucuronidation, sulphation and oxidation of paracetamol in Gilbert's syndrome', *Eur. J. Clin. Investig.* **17**: 237–40.

Vainio, H., Elovaara, E., Luukkanen, L., Anttila, S., Ulmanen, I., Fournel-Gigleux, S., Ouzzine, M., Pillot, T. and Magdalou, J. (1995) 'Expression and co-induction of CYP1A1 and UGT1*6 in human lungs', *Europ. J. Drug. Metab. Pharmacokinet.* (Special Issue): 47–8.

Vincent-Viry, M., Cossy, C., Galteau, M. M., Gueguen, R., Magdalou, J., Nicolas, A., Leroy, P. and Siest, G. (1995) 'Lack of a genetic polymorphism in the glucuronidation of fenofibric acid', *Pharmacogenetics* **5**: 50–2.

Visser, T. J., Kaptein, E., Gijzel, A. L., de Herder, W. W., Ebner, T. and Burchell, B. (1993) 'Glucuronidation of thyroid hormone by humanbilirubin and phenol UDP-glucuronosyltransferase isoenzymes', *FEBS Lett.* **324**: 358–60.

Vore, M. and Slikker, W. (1985) 'Steroid D-ring glucuronides: a new class of cholestatic agents', *TIPS* **6**: 256–9.

Vree, T. B., Van der biggelaar-Martea, M., Verwey Van Wissen, C. P. W. G. M., Vree, M. L. and Guelen, P. J. M. (1993) 'The pharmacokinetics of naproxen, its metabolite o-desmethylnaproxen, and their acyl glucuronides in humans – effect of cimetidine', *Brit. J. Clin. Pharmacol.* **35**: 467–72.

Wahlstrom, A., Lenhammar, B., Ask, B. and Rane, A. (1994) 'Tricyclic antidepressants inhibit opioid receptor binding in human brain and hepatic morphine glucuronidation', *Pharmacol. Toxicol.* **75**: 23–7.

Walle, T., Walle, U. K., and Olanoff, L. S. (1985) 'Quantitative account of propranolol metabolism in urine of normal man', *Drug Metab. Dispos.* **13**: 204–9.

Ward, S. A., Walle, T., Walle, U. K., Wilkinson, G. R. and Branch, R. A. (1989) 'Propanolol's metabolism is determined by both mephenytoin and debrisoquine hydroxylase activities', *Clinical Pharmacology and Therapeutics* **45**: 72–9.

Wasserman, E., Myara, A., Lokiec, F., Goldwasser, F., Trivin, F., Mahjoubi, M., Misset, J. L. and Cvitkovic, E. (1997) 'Severe CPT-11 toxicity in patients with Gilbert's syndrome: two case reports', *Ann. Oncol.* **810**: 1049–51.

Weinshilboum, R. M., Otterness, D. M., Aksoy, I. A., Wood, T. C., Her, C. and Raffogianis, R. B. (1997) 'Sulfotransferase molecular biology', *FASEB J.* **11**: 3–14.

Wooster, R., Sutherland, L., Ebner, T., Clarke, D. J., Da Cruz e Silva, O. and Burchell, B. (1991) 'Cloning and stable expression of a new member of the human liver phenol/bilirubin UDP-glucuronosyltransferase cDNA family', *Biochem. J.* **278**: 465–9.

Yamamoto, K., Sato, H., Fujiyama, Y., Doida, Y. and Bamba, T. (1998) 'Contribution of two missense mutation (G71R and Y486D) of the bilirubin UDP-glucuronosyltransferase (UGT1A1) gene to phenotypes of Gilbert's syndrome and Crigler–Najjar syndrome type II', *Biochim. Biophys. Acta.* **1406**: 267–73.

Yue, Q. Y., Svensson, J. O., Alm, C., Sioqvist, F. and Sawe, J. (1989) 'Interindividual and interethnic differences in the demethylation and glucuronidation of codeine', *Br. J. Clin. Pharmacol.* **28**: 629–37.

Yue, Q.-Y., Svensson, J.-O., Sawe, J. and Bertilsson, L. (1995) 'Codeine metabolism in three Oriental populations: a pilot study in Chinese, Japanese and Koreans', *Pharmacogenet* **5**: 173–7.

Chapter 13

Interindividual variability of methyltransferases

L. Yan and R. Weinshilboum

Introduction

Methylation of an exogenous compound was first described by Wilhelm His over one hundred years ago when he observed the excretion of N-methylpyridine in the urine of dogs after the oral administration of pyridine (His, 1887). Methyl conjugation was subsequently shown to be an important pathway in the biotransformation of many drugs and other xenobiotics, as well as endogenous compounds such as neurotransmitters (Weinshilboum, 1989b; Weinshilboum and Raftogianis, 2000). Today we know that methyltransferase enzymes can catalyze the methyl conjugation not only of small molecules such as drugs, hormones and neurotransmitters, but also macromolecules such as proteins, RNA and DNA (Tollervey, 1996; Klein and Costa, 1997; Aletta *et al.*, 1998). Over 100 methyltransferase enzymes have already been identified (Enzyme Nomenclature, 1992), and many more will be identified after completion of ongoing "genome projects" for humans and other organisms. The methyl conjugating enzymes described in this chapter are all "small molecule" methyltransferases that participate in the biotransformation of drugs, xenobiotics and endogenous compounds. Although a great deal is known about the biochemistry, molecular biology and regulation of methyltransferase enzymes in experimental animals, this chapter will focus on human enzymes selected from each major methyltransferase functional class. The biochemical and molecular properties of selected members of each of these groups of enzymes will be outlined briefly, followed by a description of their variation in humans – with a focus on pharmacogenetics. Although variations in methyltransferase activities related to age, gender and exposure to drugs or other chemicals have been described, the quantitatively most important and best-studied examples of variation for this family of drug-metabolising enzymes are pharmacogenetic in nature. The clinical implications of those variations in activity will also be discussed. However, before turning to the properties and regulation of methyltransferase enzymes, it might be helpful to briefly discuss the synthesis of

S-adenosyl-L-methionine (AdoMet), the high energy methyl donor cosubstrate for the majority of methyltransferase enzymes.

AdoMet biosynthesis

AdoMet, also abbreviated "SAM", is the methyl donor for most methyltransferase enzymes. AdoMet was discovered by Cantoni in 1953 and is synthesized *in vivo* from adenosine triphosphate (ATP) and L-methionine by methionine adenosyltransferase (MAT, EC 2.5.1.6) (Figure 13.1). Conserved amino acid sequence motifs present in MAT from several different species are thought to be critical for the enzyme's catalytic activity (Markham and Satishchandran, 1988; Pajares *et al.*, 1991). An example of such a sequence is the ATP-binding motif Gly-X-Gly-X-X-Gly, in which X indicates any amino acid. During the reaction catalysed by MAT the adenosyl group of ATP is transferred to the sulfur atom of methionine. The triphosphate group of ATP remains bound to the enzyme after the first step in the reaction, but MAT subsequently hydrolyses the triphosphate to form pyrophosphate and phosphate (Figure 13.1; Cantoni and Durell, 1957). After donating its methyl group during a methyltransferase reaction, AdoMet is converted to S-adenosyl-L-homocysteine (AdoHcy) – a potent inhibitor of AdoMet-dependent reactions (Borchardt, 1977).

In mammals, MAT exists in three different forms, MAT I, II and III (Kotb and Geller, 1993). MAT I is composed of four α_1 subunits, while MAT III is a dimer of α_1 subunits. Both of these isoforms are constitutively expressed in liver. MAT I has a K_m value for methionine of 23 μM, while MAT III has a much higher K_m of 200–600 μM. Therefore, MAT III is also referred to as the "high K_m" form. MAT II is widely distributed in extrahepatic tissues and is composed of an α_2 catalytic subunit and a

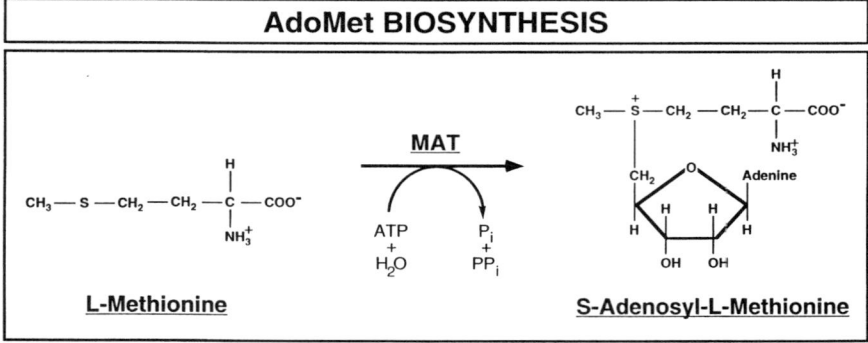

Figure 13.1 Methionine adenosyltransferase (MAT) catalysed biosynthesis of S-adenosyl-L-methionine (AdoMet).

catalytically inactive regulatory β subunit. MAT II has the lowest K_m value (4–10 μM) for methionine of the three MAT isoforms and is also referred to as the "low K_m" form of the enzyme. In mammals, two different genes, *MAT1A* and *MAT2A*, encode the MAT α_1 and α_2 catalytic subunits, respectively (Horikawa and Tsukada, 1991, 1992; Kotb *et al.*, 1997). Amino acid sequences of the proteins encoded by these two genes in humans are approximately 85% identical (Kotb and Geller, 1993). The gene that encodes the β subunit has not yet been cloned. The methyl group of AdoMet can be transferred to a variety of heteroatoms, including oxygen, sulfur and nitrogen. The products of those methyltransferase-catalysed reactions are AdoHcy and O-, S-, or N-methylated products.

Methyltransferase biochemistry and molecular biology

Background

Most methyltransferase enzymes also share "signature" amino acid sequence motifs (Ingrosso *et al.*, 1989; Wu *et al.*, 1992; Gomi *et al.*, 1992). Ingrosso *et al.* (1989) first reported the presence of three areas of high amino acid sequence homology in many methyltransferase enzymes. They designated these sequences as regions I, II and III. Since virtually all methyltransferase enzymes utilize AdoMet as a cosubstrate, it was reasonable to suggest that those amino acid sequences might be required for binding of the methyl donor. These common sequence motifs were further characterized by Wu *et al.* (1992) and Gomi *et al.* (1992), authors who emphasized the possible functional importance of regions I and III (Figure 13.2). However, when Gomi *et al.* (1992) performed site-directed mutagenesis studies of region III with rat guanidinoacetate methyltransferase, they found that all five of the mutants studied, Lys160, Pro161, Gly162, Gly163 and Leu165, were just as catalytically active as the "wild-type" enzyme and also displayed similar kinetic constants. Hamahata *et al.* (1996) performed site-directed mutagenesis with region I of the same enzyme. They found that conversion of either of two glycine residues within region I (Gly67 and Gly69) to alanine resulted in an inactive enzyme. Those results suggested that region I might participate in substrate binding and/or catalysis, while region III did not – at least in this specific methyltransferase. The widespread presence of these signature amino acid sequences in methyltransferase enzymes was emphasised when they were used recently to identify enzymes potentially capable of catalysing methyl conjugation from among all proteins encoded by genes identified as a result of conclusion of the *S. cerevisiae* genome project (Niewmierzycka and Clarke, 1999). X-ray crystallographic analysis has also been performed with the bacterial DNA methyltransferases, *M. Hal* (Cheng *et al.*, 1993) and *M. Taq1* (Labahn *et al.*, 1994), as well as small molecule methyl-

METHYLTRANSFERASE SIGNATURE SEQUENCES				

	REGION I		REGION III	
ENZYME	SEQUENCE	POSITION	SEQUENCE	POSITION
NNMTm	I D I G S G P T	60-67	L K P G G F L	187-193
NNMTh	I D I G S G P T	60-67	L K P G G F L	187-193
INMTrab	I D I G S G P T	60-67	L K P G G H L	187-193
TEMTm	I D I G S G P T	61-68	L K P G G H L	188-194
PNMTh	I D I G S G P T	76-83	L R P G G H L	205-211
PNMTm	I D I G S G P T	87-94	L R P G G H L	216-222
PNMTr	I D I G S G P T	62-69	L R P G G H L	191-197
PNMTb	I D I G S G P T	76-83	L R P G G H L	188-194
PCMTh	L D V G S G S G	82-89	L K P G G R L	172-178
PCMTm	L D V G S G S G	82-89	L K P G G R L	170-176
PCMTr	P D V G S G S G	82-89	L K P G G R L	173-179
HNMTh	L S I G G G A G	57-64	V V S G S S G	171-177
HNMTr	L S I G G G A G	57-64	L V S G T S G	171-177
COMTh	L E L G A Y C G	113-120	L R K G T V L	210-216
COMTr	L E L G A Y C G	106-113	L R K G T V L	203-209
HIOMTh	C D L G G T R I	184-191	C K P G G G I	273-279
HIOMTb	C D L G G G S G	184-191	C R T G G G I	301-307
GAMTr	L E V G F G M A	65-72	L K P G G I L	160-166
GMTr	L D V A C G T G	62-69	V R P G G L L	165-171

CONS	L D o G s G s G
	  I T
			L R P G G x L
			  K	

Figure 13.2 Methyltransferase signature sequence regions I and III as described by Ingrosso et al. (1989). When identical residues or two residues belonging to the same group of amino acids were present in the aligned sequences of at least fourteen of the nineteen enzymes listed, that amino acid or those two amino acids have been included in the consensus sequence (CONS). The symbols "o" and "s" in the consensus sequence line represent hydrophobic and small-neutral amino acids, respectively, while "x" represents any amino acid. The enzymes for which sequences are compared include: mouse liver NNMT (NNMTm) (Yan et al., 1997); human liver NNMT (NNMTh) (Aksoy et al., 1994); rabbit lung INMT (INMTrab) (Thompson and Weinshilboum, 1998); mouse lung thioether methyltransferase (TEMTm) (Warner et al., 1995); human pheochromocytoma (Kaneda et al., 1988), mouse (Morita et al., 1992), rat (Weisberg et al., 1989) and bovine adrenal medullary (Baetge et al., 1986) phenylethanolamine N-methyltransferase (PNMTh, PNMTm, PNMTr and PNMTb, respectively); human brain (MacLaren et al., 1992), mouse testis (Romanik et al., 1992), and rat brain (Sato et al., 1989) protein carboxyl methyltransferase (PCMTh, PCMTm and PCMTr), respectively; human kidney (Girard et al., 1994) and rat kidney (Takemura et al., 1992) histamine N-methyltransferase (HNMTh and HNMTr); human placental (Lundström et al., 1991) and rat liver (Salminen et al., 1990) catechol O-methyltransferase (COMTh and COMTr); human (Donohue et al., 1993) and bovine pineal (Donohue et al., 1992) hydroxyindole O-methyltransferase (HIOMTh and HIOMTb); rat liver guanidinoacetate methyltransferase (GAMTr) (Ogawa et al., 1988); and rat liver glycine methyltransferase (GMTr) (Ogawa et al., 1987).

transferases such as rat liver catechol O-methyltransferase (Vidgren *et al.*, 1994) and rat liver glycine N-methyltransferase (Fu and Takusagawa, 1994). Those analyses provided three-dimensional structural evidence that a glycine within region I forms a hydrogen bond with the carboxyl oxygen of the methionine moiety in AdoMet.

A comprehensive classification of methyltransferase enzymes based on amino acid sequence identity like that which has been used to classify the cytochromes P450 (Nelson *et al.*, 1996) has not yet been developed. That is true in part because fewer of these genes have been cloned than have those for the cytochromes P450 and in part because, with the exception of the signature sequence motifs described previously, these enzymes do not show as high a degree of overall amino acid sequence homology as do the cytochromes P450. Therefore, one of the most commonly used classifications for drug-metabolising small molecule methyltransferase enzymes continues to be based on the type of heteroatom methylated. That functional approach to classification will be used in the subsequent discussion and three large functional classes of these enzymes; O-, S- and N-methyltransferases will each be described in turn, with an emphasis on enzymes for which pharmacogenetic studies have been performed in humans. Because abbreviations of the names for these enzymes can easily become a jumble of "MTs", Table 13.1 is provided to help the reader keep track of the enzymes that will be discussed subsequently.

O-Methyltransferases

Catechol O-methyltransferase (COMT, EC 2.1.1.6) is a Mg^{2+}-dependent enzyme that catalyses the O-methylation of catechols, but not phenols (Axelrod and Tomchick, 1958). The O-methylation of norepinephrine catalyzed by COMT is shown in Figure 13.3. COMT plays an important role in the metabolism of catecholamine neurotransmitters such as dopamine, norepinephrine and epinephrine (Guldberg and Marsden, 1975), as well as the anti-Parkinson's disease drug levodopa (Martinez-Martin and O'Brien, 1998) and the antihypertensive agent methyldopa (Campbell *et al.*, 1984). Recently, several non-toxic COMT inhibitors such as nitecapone and tolcapone have entered clinical practice as adjuncts to the levodopa therapy of patients with Parkinson's disease (De Santi *et al.*, 1998). COMT is widely distributed in many tissues and cells, with highest levels of activity in liver and kidney (Axelrod and Tomchick, 1958; Guldberg and Marsden, 1975; Inoue and Creveling, 1991). Two forms of COMT are present in most tissues, a "soluble" form localised to the cytosol (S-COMT) and a "membrane-bound" form (M-COMT). S-COMT predominates in the liver, while M-COMT is highly expressed in the central nervous system (Tenhunen *et al.*, 1994) and in pheochromocytoma tissue (Eisenhofer *et al.*, 1998).

Table 13.1 Small molecule methyltransferase enzymes

Enzyme	Abbreviation	EC number	Substrates	Example
Catechol O-methyltransferase	COMT	EC 2.1.1.6	Catechols	Dopamine
Thiopurine methyltransferase	TPMT	EC 2.1.1.67	Aromatic and Heterocyclic Sulfhydryls	6-Mercaptopurine
Thiol methyltransferase	TMT	EC 2.1.1.9	Aliphatic Sulfhydryls	2-Mercaptoethanol
Phenylethanolamine N-methyltransferase	PNMT	EC 2.1.1.28	Phenylethanolamines	Norepinephrine
Histamine N-methyltransferase	HNMT	EC 2.1.1.8	Imidazolethylamines	Histamine
Nicotinamide N-methyltransferase	NNMT	EC 2.1.1.1	Pyridines	Nicotinamide

Note
The table lists the most common abbreviation for each enzyme, its EC number, the general class of compound methylated and a common or "prototypic" substrate for each enzyme.

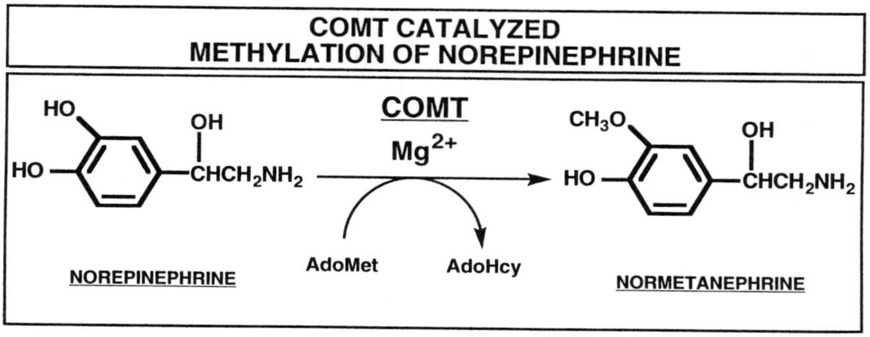

**COMT CATALYZED
METHYLATION OF NOREPINEPHRINE**

Figure 13.3 COMT reaction with norepinephrine as the methyl acceptor substrate.

cDNAs for COMT have been cloned from both human (Bertocci *et al.*, 1991; Lundström *et al.*, 1991) and rat tissues (Salminen *et al.*, 1990). The amino acid sequences of S- and M-COMT within a given species are identical except that the N-terminus of M-COMT is longer than is that of S-COMT. For example, there is an additional, highly hydrophobic 50 amino acid N-terminal segment for M-COMT in humans that is thought to anchor the enzyme to the membrane (Bertocci *et al.*, 1991; Lundström *et al.*, 1991). Human and rat COMT genes have also been cloned (Tenhunen *et al.*, 1993, 1994). The genes in both species have two separate promoters that direct the transcription of two different mRNAs which encode S- and M-COMT. The human gene has six exons, the first two of which are noncoding. Two separate ATG codons are located within exon 3 that are responsible for translation initiation for the membrane-bound and soluble forms of the enzyme (Tenhunen *et al.*, 1994). The COMT gene maps to human chromosome 22 between bands q11.1 and q11.2 (Winqvist *et al.*, 1992; Grossman *et al.*, 1992). As mentioned previously, the X-ray crystallographic structure of rat COMT at a resolution of 2 Å has been reported by Vidgren *et al.* (1994). The AdoMet binding site in COMT as defined by X-ray crystallography was similar to that of DNA methylases (Cheng *et al.*, 1993; Labahn *et al.*, 1994). In addition to being the first small molecule methyltransferase for which a crystal structure was solved, COMT was also the first methyltransferase for which pharmacogenetic studies were performed, as will be described subsequently.

S-Methyltransferases

Thiopurine methyltransferase (TPMT, EC 2.1.1.67) and thiol methyltransferase (TMT, EC 2.1.1.9) are two S-methyltransferases that, like COMT, have been studied in humans from a pharmacogenetic perspective. Both of these enzymes catalyse the S-methylation of sulfhydryl groups, but they differ in subcellular location, substrate specificity, inhibitor sensitivity and regulation (Weinshilboum, 1989a, 1989b). TPMT is a cytosolic enzyme that preferentially catalyses the S-methylation of aromatic and heterocyclic sulfhydryl compounds, including thiopurine drugs such as 6-mercaptopurine (6-MP) (Figure 13.4; Remy, 1963; Woodson and Weinshilboum, 1983). Thiopurines are used to treat childhood leukemia, autoimmune diseases and organ transplant recipients (Paterson and Tidd, 1975; Lennard, 1992). No endogenous substrates for TPMT are known, although the plasma of patients with chronic renal failure contains unidentified TPMT substrate(s) (Pazmiño *et al.*, 1980). TPMT is inhibited by benzoic acid derivatives, including the aminosalicylates that are used to treat inflammatory bowel disease (Woodson *et al.*, 1983; Szumlanski and Weinshilboum, 1995). However, it is not inhibited by SKF-525A or the arylalkylamines that have been shown to be potent inhibitors of TMT (Weinshilboum *et al.*, 1979; Woodson *et al.*, 1983; Glauser *et al.*, 1993). TPMT cDNAs were cloned and characterised from a T84 human colon carcinoma cell cDNA library (Honchel *et al.*, 1993) and, subsequently, from a human liver cDNA library (Lee *et al.*, 1995). TPMT mRNA is expressed in most human tissues, including kidney, liver and gut (Lee *et al.*, 1995). Most tissues express three different transcripts that are approximately 1.4, 2.0 and 3.6 kb in length (Lee *et al.*, 1995). These different TPMT mRNAs all encode the same protein, but they differ in 3′-untranslated region (3′-UTR) length (Lee *et al.*, 1995). A processed pseudogene for TPMT is located on the long arm of human chromosome 18 (Lee *et al.*, 1995), and the active gene maps to the short arm of chromosome 6 at band 6p22.3 (Szumlanski *et al.*, 1996). The human TPMT gene is approximately 34 kb in length and consists of ten exons, eight of which encode protein (Szumlanski *et al.*, 1996). The encoded protein consists of 245 amino acids and has a calculated M_r value of 28.2 kDa (Honchel *et al.*, 1993).

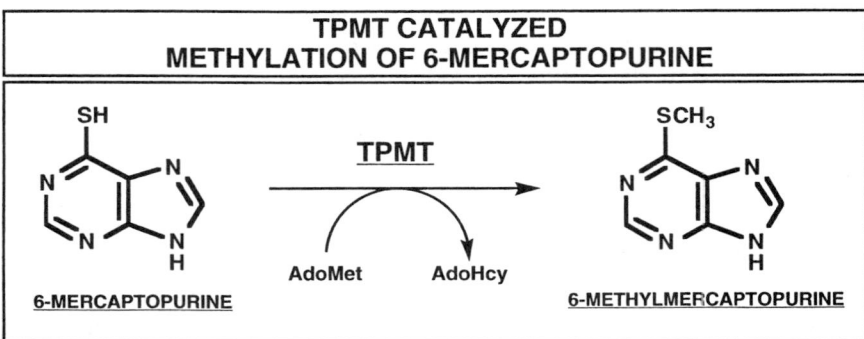

Figure 13.4 TPMT reaction with 6-mercaptopurine as the methyl acceptor substrate.

TMT is a membrane-bound enzyme that preferentially catalyses the S-methylation of aliphatic sulfhydryl compounds such as 2-mercaptoethanol, captopril, D-penicillamine and N-acetylcysteine (Bremer and Greenberg, 1961; Weinshilboum *et al.*, 1979; Keith *et al.*, 1983, 1984, 1985). TMT, unlike TPMT, is inhibited by SKF-525A and arylalkylamines such as 2,3-dichloro-α-methylbenzylamine (Weinshilboum *et al.*, 1979; Glauser *et al.*, 1993). However, it is not inhibited by the benzoic acid derivatives that inhibit TPMT (Weinshilboum, 1989a). TMT has not been purified, and neither cDNAs nor genes for TMT have been reported for any species.

N-Methyltransferases

N-Methyltransferases catalyze the conjugation of amines and nitrogen-containing heterocyclic compounds, including many endogenous compounds. One example of an N-methyltransferase that conjugates endogenous compounds is phenylethanolamine N-methyltransferase (PNMT, EC 2.1.1.28). Even though PNMT does not play a role in drug metabolism, it is included in this chapter because it is an N-methyltransferase and because the structure of its gene is similar to that of the gene for nicotinamide N-methyltransferase (NNMT, EC 2.1.1.1), an enzyme that catalyses the methylation of exogenous compounds (Aksoy *et al.*, 1995; Yan *et al.*, 1997). PNMT catalyses the N-methylation of norepinephrine, the final step in the biosynthesis of epinephrine, as well as that of other β-hydroxylated phenylethylamines (Axelrod, 1962). PNMT is expressed in the cytosol of adrenal medullary cells and is also present in the heart and in certain nuclei in the central nervous system (Saavedra and Axelrod, 1973). The human enzyme consists of 282 amino acids and has an M_r value of 31 kDa (Kaneda *et al.*, 1988). Structures have been reported for the human (Baetge *et al.*, 1988), bovine (Batter *et al.*, 1988), rat (Suh *et al.*, 1994) and mouse (Morita *et al.*, 1992) PNMT genes. Each of these genes consists of three exons; in each case the central exon is 208 bp in length; and the structures of all these genes are similar to those of the human and mouse NNMT genes (Aksoy *et al.*, 1995; Yan *et al.*, 1997). The human gene for PNMT has been mapped to chromosome bands 17q21–22 (Kaneda *et al.*, 1988; Hoehe *et al.*, 1992).

Histamine N-methyltransferase (HNMT, EC 2.1.1.8) is another example of an enzyme that catalyses the N-methylation of an endogenous substance, histamine, as well as that of structurally related compounds (Brown *et al.*, 1959). The N-methylation of histamine to form N^τ-methylhistamine catalyzed by HNMT is shown in Figure 13.5. α-Methylhistamine is also a substrate for HNMT, but the K_m value of the enzyme for histamine is approximately ten–fold lower than is that for α-methylhistamine (Hough *et al.*, 1981). Included among HNMT inhibitors are both H1 and H2 histamine receptor antagonists (Taylor and Snyder, 1972; Barth and Lorenz,

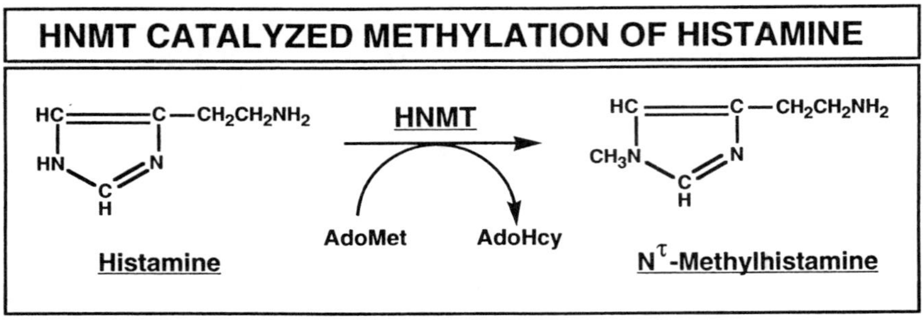

HNMT CATALYZED METHYLATION OF HISTAMINE

Figure 13.5 HNMT reaction with histamine as the methyl acceptor substrate.

1978) as well as antimalarial drugs such as amodiaquine and chloroquine (Thithapandha and Cohn, 1977). A cDNA for human kidney HNMT has been cloned (Girard et al., 1994; Yamauchi et al., 1994) and that cDNA encoded a 292 amino acid protein with a calculated M_r value of 33 kDa. The human gene for HNMT has also been cloned and is approximately 34 kb in length with six exons (Aksoy et al., 1996). The human HNMT gene mapped to chromosome 2 (Aksoy et al., 1996).

NNMT is another small molecule N-methyltransferase. NNMT is of historical significance because it is almost certainly the enzyme that catalysed the N-methylation of pyridine in the dog when Wilhelm His first demonstrated that methylation is a pathway for the biotransformation of exogenous compounds (His, 1887). NNMT also catalyses the N-methylation of nicotinamide and structurally related compounds (D'Souza et al., 1980). Since the lipid-lowering drug nicotinic acid is converted to nicotinamide in vivo (Lee et al., 1972), NNMT plays an important role in the biotransformation of that drug. Unlike most other methyltransferase enzymes, no highly specific NNMT inhibitors have been reported other than the products of the reaction, AdoHcy and N^1-methylnicotinamide (Rini et al., 1989). NNMT is expressed in many mammalian tissues, but it is most highly expressed in the liver (Aksoy et al., 1994). The human NNMT cDNA and gene have both been cloned and characterised (Aksoy et al., 1994; Aksoy et al., 1995). The cDNA encodes a protein with a calculated M_r value of 29.6 kDa. NNMT is a member of a growing "family" of related small molecule methyltransferase enzymes that presently also includes PNMT and mouse thioether methyltransferase (Warner et al., 1995), as well as rabbit and human indolethylamine N-methyltransferase (Thompson and Weinshilboum, 1998; Thompson et al., 1999). All of these enzymes share a high degree of identity among the amino acid sequences of their encoded proteins, as well as a striking similarity in their gene structures (Yan et al., 1998; Thompson and Weinshilboum, 1998).

Methyltransferase pharmacogenetics

Background

Methyltransferase enzymes have been studied intensively from a pharmacogenetic perspective, and several of these enzymes display functionally significant pharmacogenetic variation in humans. Historically, those pharmacogenetic studies progressed in a step-wise fashion from phenotype to genotype. The experimental strategy used in these studies frequently began with the development of an assay that could be used to measure the methyltransferase enzyme activity of interest in an easily accessible human tissue or cell, most often the red blood cell (RBC). It was then possible to determine the nature and extent of individual variation in the level of enzyme activity in the easily accessible cell – followed by an estimate of the contribution of inheritance to that variance by performing twin or family studies. It could also be determined whether inherited variation in the RBC level of the enzyme activity might reflect similar variation in organs that are involved in drug metabolism such as the liver. Finally, the possible functional consequences of that variation could be studied. Use of this experimental approach made it possible to discover and characterise pharmacogenetic variation in the activities of a series of methyltransferase enzymes including COMT (Weinshilboum and Raymond, 1977), TPMT (Weinshilboum and Sladek, 1980), HNMT (Scott *et al.*, 1988; Price *et al.*, 1993), and TMT (Keith *et al.*, 1983; Price *et al.*, 1989). During the past decade, application of the techniques of molecular biology and genomics has also made it possible to characterise molecular mechanisms responsible for this inherited variation and to develop DNA-based diagnostic tests. Human pharmacogenetic information for each of the three large functional classes of these enzymes – O-, S- and N-methyltransferases – will be discussed subsequently. Particular attention will be paid to COMT, TPMT and HNMT as "model enzymes" within each class of methyltransferase. As mentioned previously, genetic variation is currently the best characterised, but obviously not the only source of differences among individuals in these enzyme activities. Therefore, even though the subsequent discussion is focussed on pharmacogenetics, variation based on gender, age, ethnicity or the presence of drugs or other chemicals will also be addressed when appropriate.

O-Methyltransferases

COMT was the first methyltransferase enzyme studied for possible pharmacogenetic variation, and COMT pharmacogenetics offers a good example of the application of the research strategy that has been used to study these enzymes. COMT is present in the RBC (Axelrod and Cohen, 1971; Raymond and Weinshilboum, 1975), and RBC lysate COMT is biochemically and immunologically similar to the cytosolic form of the enzyme in tissues and organs in which drug metabolism occurs (Creveling *et al.*, 1973; Quiram and Weinshilboum, 1976). The first evidence that inheritance might play a role in regulating the five–fold individual variation in RBC COMT activity present in humans was provided by the discovery of a significant familial aggregation of level of the enzyme activity. Correlation coefficients for RBC COMT activities in blood samples from siblings were approximately 0.59 (Weinshilboum *et al.*, 1974), while similar values for monozygotic twins varied from 0.9 to 0.95 (Grunhaus *et al.*, 1976; Winter *et al.*, 1978). A correlation coefficient of 1.0 would be expected for monozygotic twins and a value of 0.5 for siblings in a situation in which 100% of the variance was due to the effects of additive inheritance, i.e., a situation in which heritability was 1.0 (Cavalli-Sforza and Bodmer, 1971). Therefore, estimates of heritability for levels of human RBC COMT activity ranged from 0.68 to 1.0, indicating that from 68 to 100% of the total variance was due to the effects of inheritance. However, twin studies were unable to determine whether that inheritance was Mendelian (due to a polymorphism for a major gene) or polygenic (due to the effects of many genes). The fact that the frequency distribution for level of RBC COMT activity was bimodal, with approximately 25% of subjects included in a low activity subgroup, suggested monogenic inheritance (Figure 13.6a) (Weinshilboum *et al.*, 1974). The question of the mechanism of inheritance was answered by performing family studies with 201 first-degree relatives in forty-nine nuclear families (Weinshilboum and Raymond, 1977) – studies that made it possible to determine whether levels of RBC COMT activity "segregated" across generations according to one of the patterns of monogenic inheritance (Mendel, 1865). Segregation analysis of these data showed that the trait of low activity resulted from a common genetic polymorphism (Weinshilboum and Raymond, 1977). Subsequent studies confirmed that inheritance of level of RBC COMT activity was autosomal codominant and was controlled by a single genetic locus with two alleles, with approximately equal frequencies of alleles for low and high levels of enzyme activity in Caucasian subjects (Spielman and Weinshilboum, 1981; Floderus and Wetterberg, 1981; Siervogel *et al.*, 1984).

The two alleles that regulated levels of COMT activity were also associated with differences in a physical property of the enzyme, thermal stability (Scanlon *et al.*, 1979; Weinshilboum, 1981; Boudíková *et al.*, 1990). Thermal stability is a sensitive measure of differences in amino acid sequence between two proteins, and thermal stability measurements have often been incorporated into biochemical genetic studies (Weinshilboum, 1981). The allele for low levels of COMT activity was associated with a more thermolabile enzyme – shown as a decreased "heated/control (H/C) ratio" in Figure 13.6b. Subsequent studies demonstrated that the genetic polymorphism that regulates levels of COMT activity in the RBC also

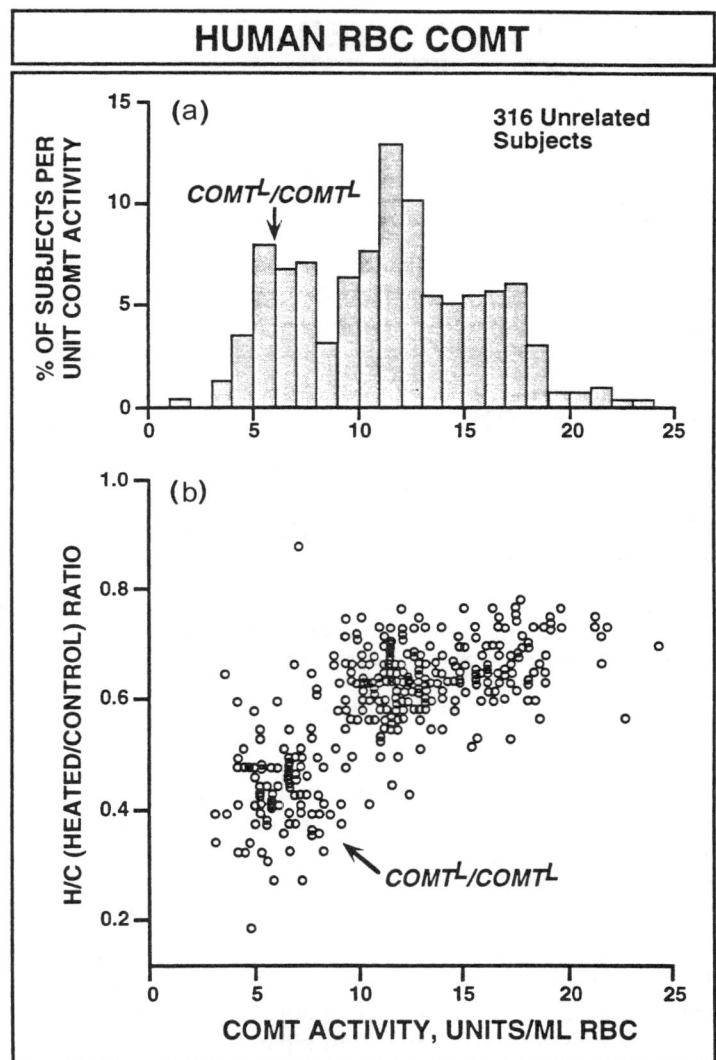

Figure 13.6 Human RBC COMT. (a) The frequency distribution of levels of RBC COMT activity in blood samples from 316 randomly selected subjects is shown. The presumed genotype for the "trait" of low COMT activity (*COMT^L*) is indicated. This allele nomenclature was used prior to the time that the molecular basis for the *COMT* genetic polymorphism was determined. (b) Correlation of RBC COMT activity and thermal stability measured as a heated/control (H/C) ratio in blood samples from the same 316 randomly selected subjects shown in (a). (Modified from Scanlon *et al.*, 1979; reproduced with permission of the American Association for the Advancement of Science.)

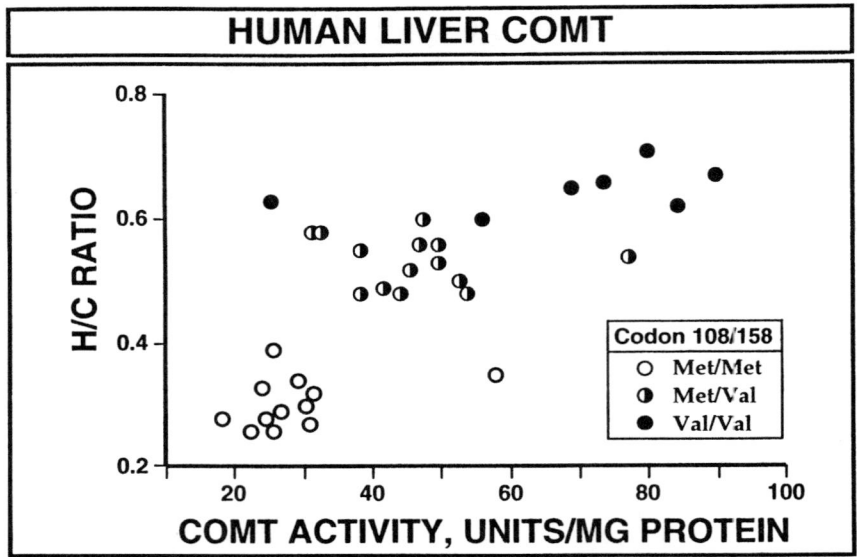

Figure 13.7 Human liver COMT activity and thermal stability measured as an H/C ratio in samples from thirty-three females who underwent clinically indicated open liver biopsies are shown. The amino acid encoded by *COMT* codon 108/158 is also indicated. (Modified from Lachman *et al.*, 1996; reproduced with permission of Lippincott-Raven Publishers.)

regulates levels of this enzyme activity in other human organs and tissues such as liver, kidney, lung and lymphocyte (Weinshilboum, 1978; Sladek-Chelgren and Weinshilboum, 1981; Boudíková *et al.*, 1990). In addition, at a functional level, genetically regulated variations in COMT activity were significantly correlated with individual differences in the methyl conjugation of orally administered catechol drugs such as levodopa and methyldopa (Reilly *et al.*, 1980; Campbell *et al.*, 1984). Therefore, as discussed subsequently, this common genetic polymorphism for a methyltransferase enzyme was functionally significant with regard to individual differences in the biotransformation of drugs.

Molecular pharmacogenetic studies performed after the cDNA and gene for COMT had been cloned (Bertocci *et al.*, 1991; Lundström *et al.*, 1991; Tenhunen *et al.*, 1994) demonstrated that the COMT genetic polymorphism resulted from a single G→A transition that caused a change in the amino acid encoded by codon 108/158 (S-COMT/M-COMT) from valine to methionine (Lachman *et al.*, 1996). The low activity, thermolabile enzyme had methionine at that position, while the high activity, thermostable enzyme had valine (Lachman *et al.*, 1996). The correlation of COMT genotype with phenotype in the human liver is depicted graphically in Figure 13.7. That Figure shows a plot of human liver COMT activity versus enzyme thermal stability measured as a heated/control (H/C) ratio (compare with Figure 13.6b which shows similar data for the RBC). The Figure also shows genotype at *COMT* codon 108/158. The genotype–phenotype correlation is striking. In addition, as anticipated on the basis of pharmacogenetic studies of other drug-metabolising enzymes (Kalow, 1992, 1997), allele frequencies for the *COMT* genetic polymorphism differed among ethnic groups. For example, Asian subjects had a significantly higher frequency of the high activity allele, approximately 0.7 to 0.8 (Kunugi *et al.*, 1997a; Li *et al.*, 1997), than did Caucasians with an average value of approximately 0.5. Although the difference between an allele frequency of 0.5 and 0.7 may not appear to be great, if Hardy–Weinberg assumptions are correct, that difference would result in a near doubling of the proportion of the population homozygous for the trait controlled by that allele, from 25% to 49%, respectively. Even though inheritance is the primary factor responsible for individual differences in COMT activity, gender can also contribute – at least in some tissues. For example, even though there are not significant differences between females and males in RBC COMT activity (Weinshilboum *et al.*, 1974; Weinshilboum and Raymond, 1977), average enzyme activity is approximately 32% higher in hepatic biopsy tissue from males than in that obtained from females (Boudíková *et al.*, 1990).

S-Methyltransferases

Pharmacogenetic studies of S-methylation catalysed by TPMT represent another example of the application of the sequential biochemical and molecular pharmacogenetic strategy that proved so successful with COMT. These studies, like those performed with COMT, began by measuring TPMT activity in RBC lysates obtained from large randomly selected population samples and family members (Weinshilboum and Sladek, 1980). The results of segregation analysis showed that approximately 89% of randomly selected Caucasian subjects were homozygous for the inherited trait of high RBC TPMT activity, approximately 11% were heterozygous and had intermediate activity, and one out of every 300 subjects was homozygous for the trait of extremely low or absent TPMT activity (Figure 13.8; Weinshilboum and Sladek, 1980; Vuchetich *et al.*, 1995). Those values fit the predictions of the Hardy–Weinberg theorem for a single genetic locus with frequencies of 0.06 and 0.94 for "low" and "high" activity alleles, respectively (Weinshilboum and Sladek, 1980; Vuchetich *et al.*, 1995). Therefore, both TPMT and COMT represent examples of "common" genetic polymorphisms, i.e., the frequency of the less common allele is 1% or greater (Cavalli-Sforza and Bodmer, 1971). Subsequent studies showed that genetically regulated levels of TPMT

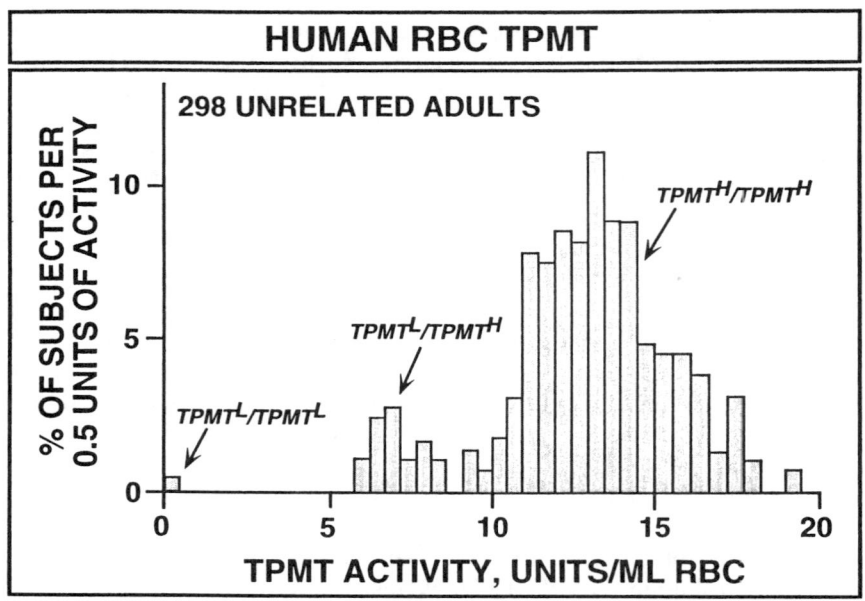

Figure 13.8 Human RBC TPMT activity. The frequency distribution of levels of RBC TPMT activity in samples from 298 randomly selected blood donors is shown. Presumed genotypes for the *TPMT* polymorphism, with *TPMT^L* and *TPMT^H* as alleles for the traits of "low" and "high" activity, are indicated. This allele nomenclature was used prior to the time that the molecular basis for the *TPMT* genetic polymorphism was determined. (Modified from Weinshilboum and Sladek, 1980; reproduced with permission of the University of Chicago Press.)

activity in the RBC reflected relative levels of this enzyme activity in other human cells and tissues such as the lymphocyte, kidney and liver (Van Loon and Weinshilboum, 1982; Woodson *et al.*, 1982; Szumlanski *et al.*, 1992).

The extension of pharmacogenetic studies of TPMT to the molecular level was made possible by cloning the cDNA and, subsequently, the gene for this enzyme in humans (Honchel *et al.*, 1993; Lee *et al.*, 1995; Szumlanski *et al.*, 1996). Those molecular cloning experiments were followed by the discovery and characterisation of a series of variant alleles that were associated with decreased levels of enzyme activity in human tissues (Szumlanski *et al.*, 1996; Otterness *et al.*, 1997, 1998). At least eight separate polymorphisms associated with very low TPMT activity have been reported (Figure 13.9). Seven of those polymorphisms alter the encoded amino acid, and one, *TPMT*4*, involves a mutation at the 3'-acceptor splice site between *TPMT* intron 9 and exon 10 (Figure 13.9).

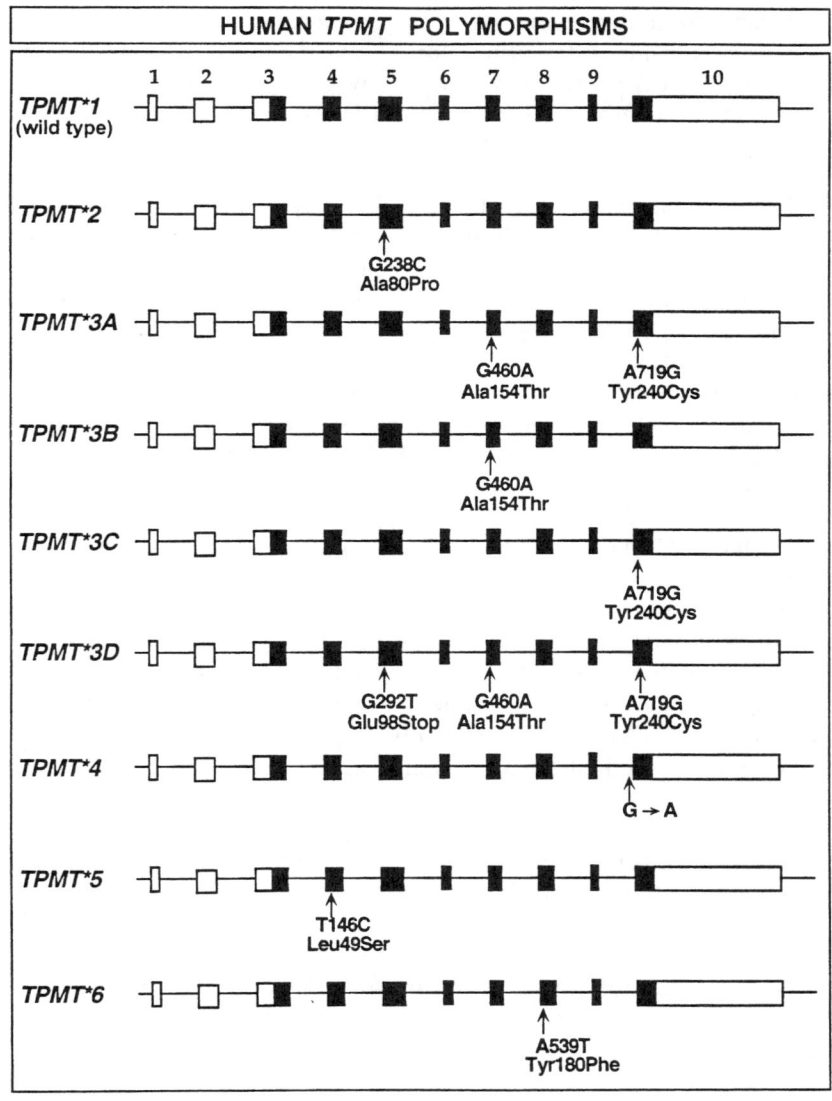

Figure 13.9 Human *TPMT* alleles. The figure depicts schematically the wild-type allele for *TPMT (TPMT*1)* as well as eight variant alleles associated with low enzyme activity. Black rectangles represent exons that encode open reading frame sequence, and white rectangles represent exons or portions of exons that encode untranslated region sequence. Arabic numerals are exon numbers. Exon sizes are proportional to their relative lengths, but introns vary greatly in length, even though they have been depicted here as equal. (Modified from Otterness *et al.*, 1997; reproduced with permission of Mosby Publishing Company.)

The most common variant allele in Caucasians, *TPMT*3A*, includes two polymorphisms, one within exon 7 that changes the amino acid at codon 154 from Ala→Thr and a second within exon 10 that results in a Try240→Cys change in encoded amino acid (Szumlanski *et al.*, 1996; Tai *et al.*, 1997; Otterness *et al.*, 1997; Yates *et al.*, 1997). The mechanism responsible for low levels of TPMT enzyme activity and immunoreactive protein in the presence of allele *TPMT*3A* appears to be an increased rate of protein degradation (Tai *et al.*, 1997, 1999). The splice junction mutation in allele *TPMT*4* results in the activation of a cryptic splice site within *TPMT* intron 9 and a striking decrease in TPMT mRNA levels (Otterness *et al.*, 1998).

Average levels of RBC TPMT activity, like those for RBC COMT activity, vary among different ethnic groups, due – at least in part – to differences in allele frequencies among those populations (Klemetsdal *et al.*, 1992; McLeod *et al.*, 1994; Park-Hah *et al.*, 1996; Jang *et al.*, 1996; Otterness *et al.*, 1997; Collie-Duguid *et al.*, 1999; McLeod *et al.*, 1999; Hon *et al.*, 1999). There are also developmental changes in levels of TPMT activity. RBC TPMT activity was approximately 50% higher in blood samples obtained from neonates than in samples from race-matched adult control subjects (McLeod *et al.*, 1995). Finally, TPMT, like COMT, displays gender-dependent differences in some tissues. Although RBC TPMT activity does not differ significantly between males and females in most large population-based studies (Weinshilboum and Sladek, 1980), average hepatic TPMT activity was approximately 13.6% higher in biopsy tissue obtained from males than in that obtained from females (Szumlanski *et al.*, 1992).

The other human S-methyltransferase that has been studied from a pharmacogenetic perspective is TMT – a membrane-bound enzyme with a preference for aliphatic sulfhydryl compounds as methyl acceptor substrates (Weinshilboum, 1989a). The development of a sensitive radio-chemical enzymatic assay for the measurement of RBC membrane TMT activity (Weinshilboum *et al.*, 1979) made it possible to perform pharmacogenetic studies of this enzyme. Those experiments demonstrated a heritability of 0.98 for the approximately five-fold individual variation in RBC TMT activity, i.e., 98% of the variance was due to the effects of inheritance (Keith *et al.*, 1983). Subsequent segregation analysis performed with data from 237 members of forty-nine nuclear families demonstrated that inherited variation for this enzyme also resulted, at least in part, from a genetic polymorphism (Price *et al.*, 1989). Future molecular pharmacogenetic studies of TMT will require cloning of its cDNA and gene to make it possible to determine the molecular basis for the TMT genetic polymorphism in a fashion similar to the approach that has been used to study COMT and TPMT.

N-Methyltransferases

Pharmacogenetic studies of N-methylation have focused on two enzymes, HNMT and NNMT. Our knowledge of HNMT pharmacogenetics is more advanced than is that of NNMT; so the subsequent discussion will begin with HNMT and then proceed to NNMT. Studies of the pharmacogenetics of HNMT, like those of COMT and TPMT, were made possible by the development of a sensitive radiochemical assay for the measurement of this enzyme activity in RBC lysates (Van Loon *et al.*, 1985). That assay was then used to measure variation of RBC HNMT activity in humans. A three-fold individual variation in RBC activity was observed (Scott *et al.*, 1988), and studies of 241 first-degree relatives in fifty-one nuclear families showed a significant familial aggregation of level of enzyme activity. The heritability of level of RBC HNMT activity was estimated to vary from 0.7 to 0.9 (i.e., from 70 to 90% of the total variance was due to the effects of inheritance) (Scott *et al.*, 1988). Furthermore, segregation analysis of data from those families demonstrated that this heritability resulted from the effects of at least one major gene (Price *et al.*, 1993).

Those biochemical pharmacogenetic observations led directly to molecular genetic experiments. As initial steps, a human HNMT cDNA was cloned (Girard *et al.*, 1994), followed by cloning of the human HNMT gene (Aksoy *et al.*, 1996). Subsequent molecular studies demonstrated the presence of at least two common *HNMT* genetic polymorphisms in Caucasians, a C→T transition at open reading frame nucleotide 314 within exon 4 of the gene that changed the amino acid encoded by codon 105 from Thr→Ile as well as an A→G transition at cDNA 3′-UTR nucleotide 939 (Preuss *et al.*, 1998). Linkage analysis demonstrated that the A939G 3′-UTR polymorphism was in linkage disequilibrium with the C314T polymorphism within the open reading frame (Preuss *et al.*, 1998). A phenotype–genotype correlation study performed with 114 human renal biopsy tissue samples showed that variations in both levels of HNMT activity and thermal stability in the kidney correlated with genotype at the exon 4 polymorphism (Figure 13.10). The data for human renal HNMT shown in Figure 13.10 should be compared with those for human hepatic COMT in Figure 13.7. Subjects homozygous or heterozygous for Ile105 had significantly lower HNMT activity and thermal stability in renal tissue than did those homozygous for the more common allele that encoded Thr105 (Figure 13.10; Preuss *et al.*, 1998). It is obvious that, although the *HNMT* codon 105 genetic polymorphism explains a portion of the variance in levels of this enzyme activity (Figure 13.10), this genotype is not as highly correlated with phenotype as is that for COMT (Figure 13.7). These observations made with tissue biopsy samples were confirmed when expression constructs that contained the cDNA sequences encoded by all four *HNMT* alleles were used to transfect COS-1 cells. Levels of HNMT

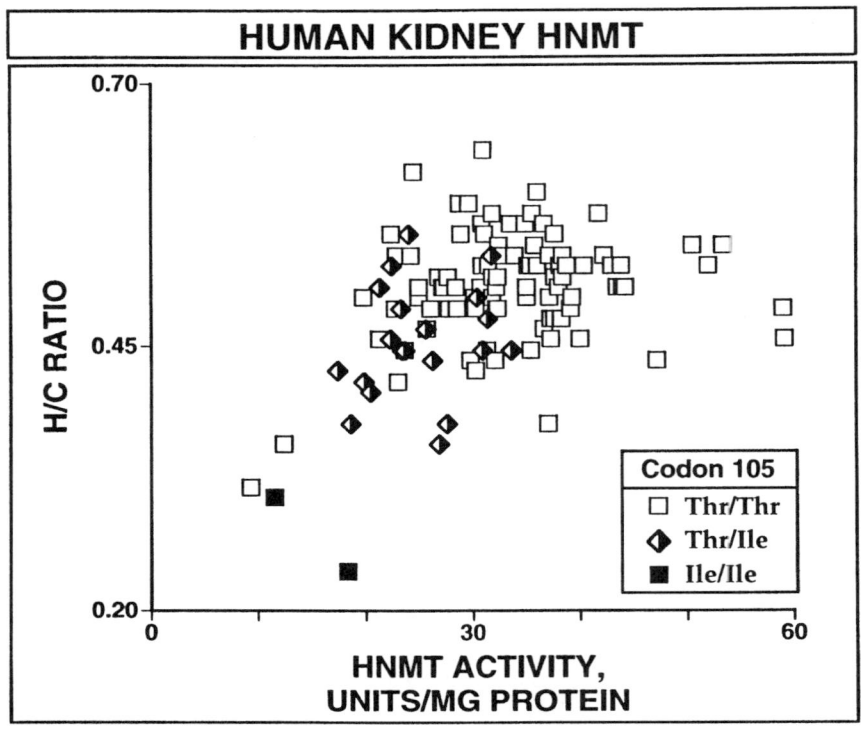

Figure 13.10 Human kidney HNMT activity and thermal stability measured as an H/C ratio in 114 human renal biopsy samples obtained during clinically indicated surgery are shown. The amino acid encoded by *HNMT* codon 105 is also indicated. (Modified from Preuss *et al.*, 1998; reproduced with permission of the American Society for Pharmacology and Experimental Therapeutics.)

activity measured under two different assay conditions (Figure 13.11a and 13.11b), as well as immunoreactive protein measured by Western blot analysis (Figure 13.11c) were reduced in cells transfected with constructs that encoded Ile105 (alleles *2A and *2B) when compared with cells transfected with constructs that encoded Thr105 (alleles *1A and *1B) (Preuss *et al.*, 1998). All of these observations indicated that the HNMT genetic polymorphism at codon 105 was of functional significance. Therefore, the biochemical and molecular pharmacogenetic research strategy that had proved successful when applied to O-methylation, COMT, and to S-methylation, TPMT, was also useful when applied to at least one N-methyltransferase, HNMT. However, application of that same strategy to NNMT has thus far failed to provide a molecular genetic explanation for the regulation of variation in that enzyme activity.

Figure 13.11 Recombinant human HNMT level of activity and immunoreactive protein. (a) Average levels of HNMT activity (mean±S.E.M., n=6) after transient expression in COS-1 cells are shown for each of the four known HNMT alleles. Alleles *1A and *1B encode Thr105, while *2A and *2B encode Ile105. Alleles *1A and *2A included 3′-UTR nucleotide A939 while alleles *1B and *2B included G939. All values were corrected for transfection efficiency. Values for the four recombinant proteins encoded by the four HNMT alleles were significantly different from each other (p<0.001 by analysis of variance). (b) The same preparations were assayed with higher histamine and AdoMet concentrations than those used in the experiments shown in (a). Values for the four alleles differed significantly from each other. (c) Western blot analysis of recombinant human HNMT performed with a rabbit polyclonal antibody to human HNMT after SDS-PAGE. (Modified from Preuss et al., 1998; reproduced with permission of the American Society for Pharmacology and Experimental Therapeutics.)

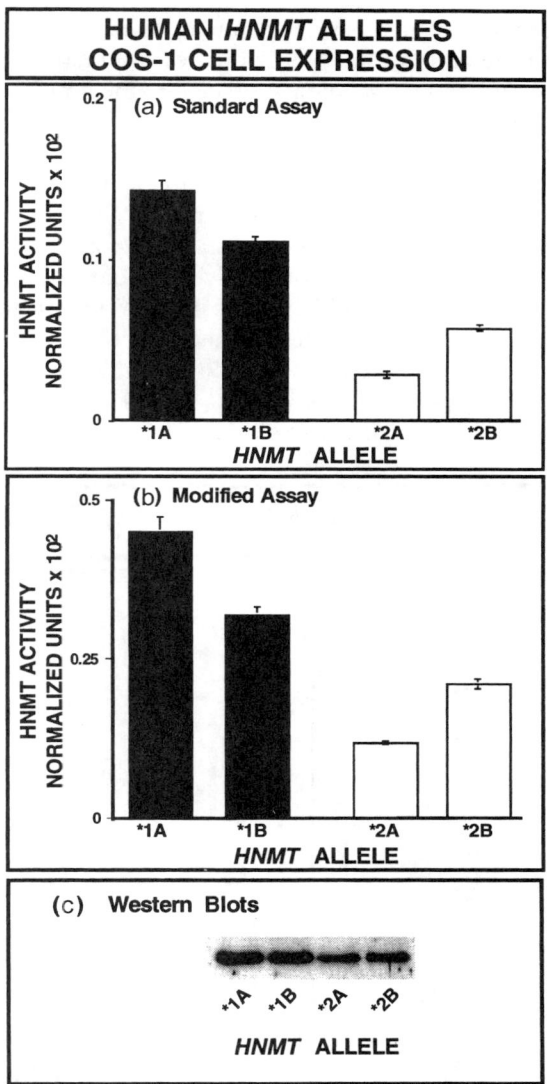

NNMT, unlike COMT, TPMT, TMT and HNMT, is not expressed in an easily accessible human cell such as the RBC. Therefore, the approach used to study human NNMT pharmacogenetics had to differ from those used to study other small molecule methyltransferases. However, the initial step, like that required to make possible similar studies of COMT, TPMT, TMT and HNMT, involved the development of a sensitive radiochemical enzymatic assay (Rini et al., 1989). That assay was then used to study the properties of NNMT in human liver preparations and to determine the nature and extent of individual variation in NNMT activity in 163 samples of human hepatic biopsy tissue obtained during clinically indicated surgery (Rini *et al.*, 1989). Levels of NNMT activity varied approximately five-fold. This fact, plus the existence of a bimodal frequency distribution (Figure 13.12), raised the possibility that a genetic polymorphism might also be involved in the regulation of human liver NNMT activity. Since NNMT was not expressed in an easily accessible tissue, it was not possible to perform segregation analysis of data obtained during family studies, because it was neither ethically nor practically possible to obtain liver biopsies from multiple members of the same family. Therefore, a direct molecular approach was adopted that involved cloning a human liver NNMT cDNA (Aksoy *et al.*, 1994), followed by cloning of the human NNMT gene (Aksoy *et al.*, 1995). However, unlike the situations found for

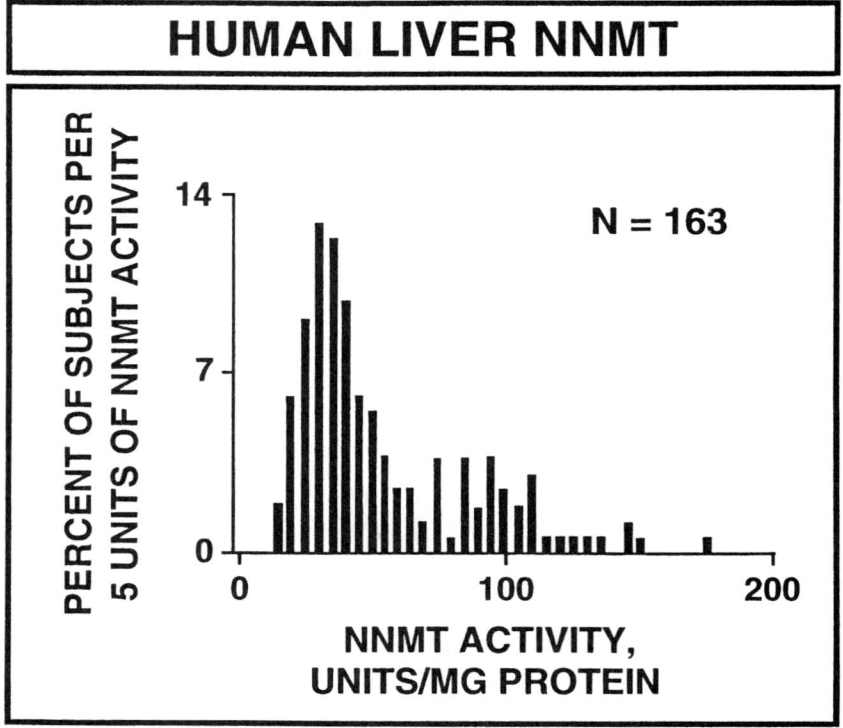

Figure 13.12 Human liver NNMT enzymatic activity. The frequency distribution histogram shows levels of NNMT activity in 163 human liver biopsy samples. Detailed descriptions of the NNMT assay and clinical data for patients from whom the biopsies were obtained have been published previously. (Modified from Rini *et al.*, 1989; reproduced with permission of Elsevier Science Publishers.)

COMT, TPMT and HNMT, use of that approach has, thus far, failed to provide a molecular explanation for the bimodal frequency distribution for NNMT activity shown in Figure 13.12 (Yan et al., 1999).

Methyltransferase variation and molecular medicine

A major goal of studies of individual variation in drug-metabolising enzymes is to enhance the diagnosis and treatment of human disease. TPMT represents a particularly striking example of the potential clinical application of this type of information. Thiopurine drugs are often used to treat life-threatening situations such as acute lymphoblastic leukemia of childhood or patients who require organ transplantation (Paterson and Tidd, 1975; Lennard, 1992). However, these drugs have relatively narrow therapeutic indices, with bone marrow suppression as a common toxicity (Lennard, 1992). Therefore, individual variations in either drug toxicity or therapeutic efficacy could potentially have profound consequences for the patient. Thiopurine drugs such as 6-mercaptopurine (6-MP) or azathioprine, which is converted to 6-MP in vivo, are metabolised by TPMT (Remy, 1963; Woodson et al., 1983). These drugs can also undergo oxidation catalysed by xanthine oxidase (Elion, 1967). Furthermore, 6-MP itself is a prodrug that undergoes bioactivation by a series of enzymes to form 6-thioguanine nucleotides (6-TGN) which can then be incorporated into DNA (Tidd and Paterson, 1974). These competing thiopurine metabolic pathways are depicted schematically in Figure 13.13. Concentrations of 6-TGN measured in the RBCs of patients being treated with 6-MP or azathioprine are directly correlated with the therapeutic efficacy and toxicity of thiopurine drugs (Lennard et al., 1983). It might be expected, based on the competing pathways shown in Figure 13.13, that an inverse relationship would exist between genetically determined levels of TPMT activity and RBC 6-TGN concentrations, and that is exactly what has been observed (Figure 13.14a; Lennard et al., 1990). As a result, patients with genetically very low or absent TPMT who are treated with 6-MP or azathioprine have consistently been shown to be at greatly increased risk for the occurrence of life-threatening thiopurine-induced myelosuppression because their RBC 6-TGN concentrations are greatly elevated (Figure 13.14b; Lennard et al., 1989; Weinshilboum et al., 1999). These patients can be treated with thiopurine drugs such as 6-MP, but the dose must be reduced to 1/10 to 1/15th of the standard dose, and even then they have to be monitored carefully for signs of toxicity (Evans et al., 1991; Lennard et al., 1997). There are also indications that patients with very high levels of TPMT activity may be at risk for undertreatment with "standard doses" of thiopurine drugs (Lennard et al., 1990). It has been suggested that such patients might be treated with higher doses of these drugs, once again with careful monitoring. Finally, a life-threatening late consequence of the

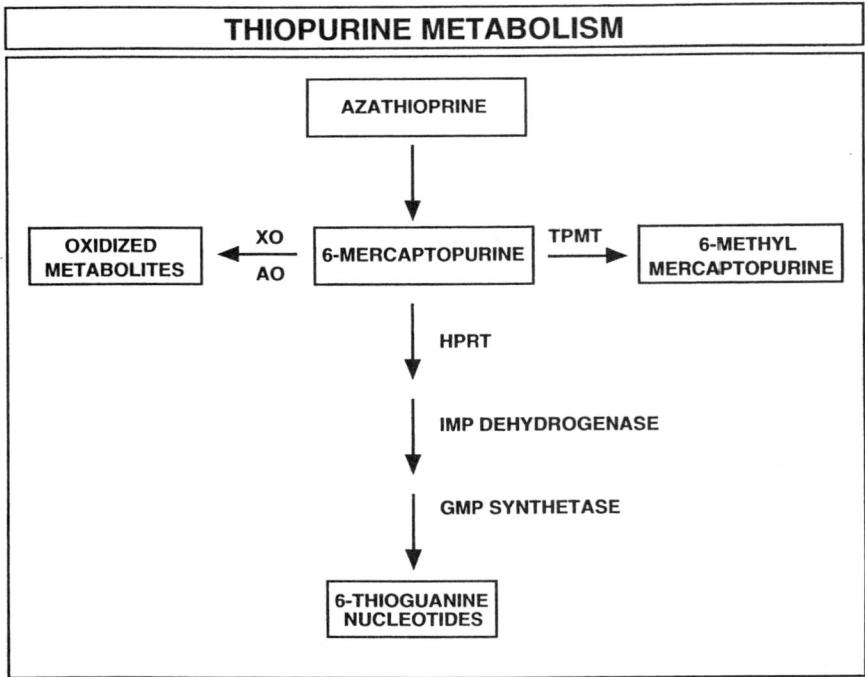

Figure 13.13 Thiopurine metabolism. Major metabolic pathways are shown for azathioprine and 6-MP. XO is xanthine oxidase, AO is aldehyde oxidase and HPRT is hypoxanthine guanine phosphoribosyltransferase.

treatment of acute lymphoblastic leukemia is the occurrence of therapy-dependent secondary acute myelogenous leukemia that appears 3–5 years after treatment of the acute lymphoblastic leukemia (Ratain and Rowley, 1992). Recent reports indicate that low TPMT activity may be a risk factor for the occurrence of secondary acute myelogenous leukemia in patients who have been exposed to thiopurines during the treatment of acute lymphoblastic leukemia (Relling *et al.*, 1998; Thomsen *et al.*, 1999). All of these clinical observations indicate that the TPMT genetic polymorphism is a major factor responsible for variations among individuals in their response to therapy with thiopurine drugs.

The observation that TPMT can be inhibited by benzoic acid derivatives (Woodson *et al.*, 1983) has also been extended into the clinic by reports that aminosalicylic acid compounds are potent inhibitors of recombinant human TPMT (Szumlanski and Weinshilboum, 1995). This observation is of potential significance because patients with inflammatory bowel disease, such as Crohn's disease, are often treated with thiopurine drugs, and those same patients may be treated with aminosalicylic acid derivatives, such as

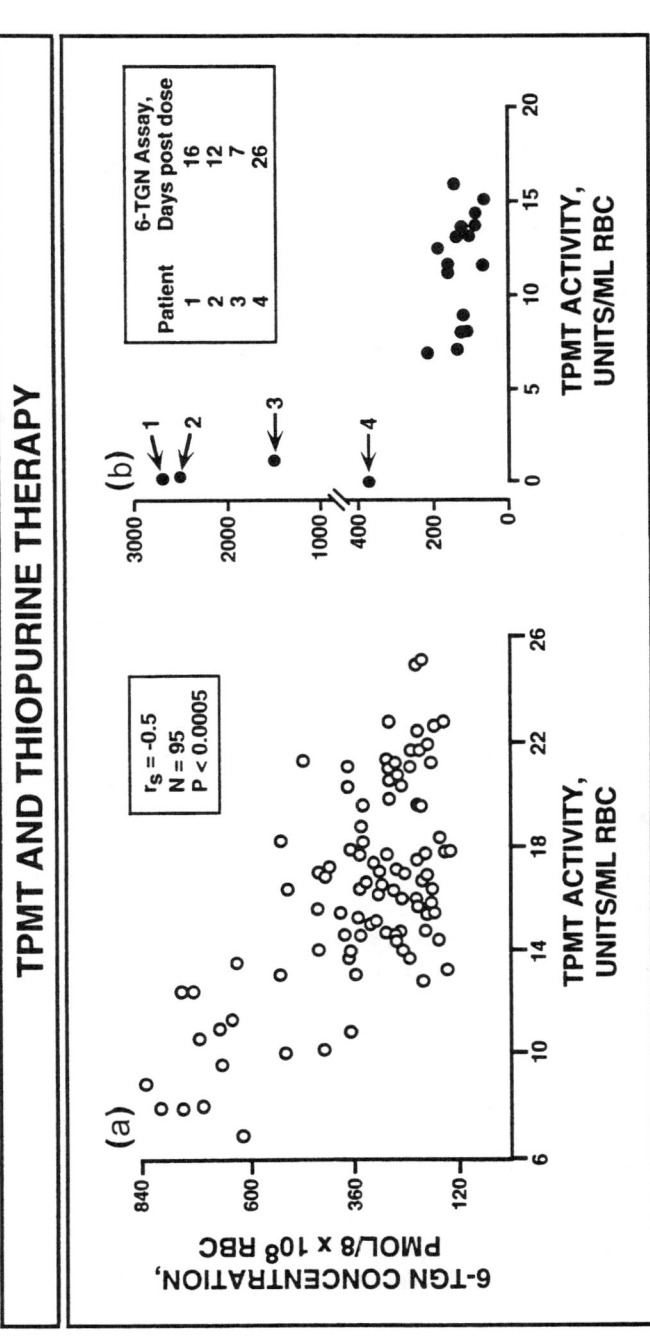

Figure 13.14 TPMT and thiopurine drug therapy. Correlations of RBC TPMT activity and RBC 6-TGN concentrations in patients treated with thiopurine drugs are shown. (a) Data for ninety-five children with acute lymphoblastic leukemia (ALL) who were on therapy with 6-MP under the protocol UK ALL VIII. (Modified from Lennard et al., 1990; reproduced with permission of the Lancet.) (b) Data for four adult dermatologic patients treated with azathioprine who developed profound myelosuppression (numbered 1–4), as well as a group of control adult dermatologic patients who were treated with comparable doses of azathioprine. (Modified from Lennard et al., 1989; reproduced with permission of Mosby Publishing Company.)

sulfasalazine and olsalazine. Both sulfasalazine and olsalazine are potent inhibitors of TPMT (Szumlanski and Weinshilboum, 1995; Lewis *et al.*, 1997). Therefore, the possibility exists that a clinically significant drug interaction might occur if patients are treated simultaneously with thiopurines and aminosalicylic acid derivatives, and at least one case report has been published which describes profound myelosuppression in such a patient (Lewis *et al.*, 1997). This situation emphasises the potential importance of drug interactions as a cause for variation in the activity of TPMT as well as other drug-metabolising enzymes. In summary, the TPMT genetic polymorphism demonstrates the potential contribution of pharmacogenetics to a medical future that could include a much greater degree of "individualisation" of drug therapy than is currently possible. Knowledge of the potential clinical implications of the pharmacogenetics of O- and N-methylation is less advanced than is our understanding of the clinical consequences of the pharmacogenetics of S-methylation, but there too, clinical consequences of inherited variation in methyltransferase activity have been described.

The COMT genetic polymorphism is of functional importance with regard to individual variations in the methylation of catechol drugs. Specifically, a significant correlation has been reported between genetically determined levels of COMT activity measured in the RBC and the ratio of the COMT metabolite 3-O-methyldopa to levodopa in patients with Parkinson's disease who were treated with that drug (Reilly *et al.*, 1980). O-Methylation is a major metabolic pathway for levodopa (Reilly *et al.*, 1980). Similar data have appeared with regard to the relationship between RBC COMT activity and methylation of the catechol antihypertensive agent methyldopa (Campbell *et al.*, 1984). In addition to its role in variation in the biotransformation of catechol drugs, the COMT genetic polymorphism is also a "candidate risk factor" for the pathophysiology of human disease. Because catecholamines are neurotransmitters, interest in the possibility that the COMT genetic polymorphism might contribute to human disease has focused primarily on neuropsychiatric illness. However, application of allele-specific assays for the *COMT* codon 108/158 genetic polymorphism has provided no convincing evidence for an association of inherited variation in COMT activity with affective disorders, schizophrenia or Parkinson's disease (Lachman *et al.*, 1998; Kunugi *et al.*, 1997b; Xie *et al.*, 1997). Therefore, it was somewhat surprising when several groups recently reported that subjects homozygous for genetically low COMT activity have an increased risk for the development of breast cancer, with odds ratios of approximately 2.0 (Lavigne *et al.*, 1997; Thompson *et al.*, 1998; Huang *et al.*, 1999). Those groups speculated that low COMT activity might increase breast cancer risk because of the role of methylation in the biotransformation of catechol estrogens that can be formed *in vivo* from estrone and 17β-estradiol (Ball *et al.*, 1972; Cavalieri *et al.*, 1997). Catechol estrogens can be "metabolically activated" to form carcinogenic DNA adducts (Cavalieri *et al.*, 1997). Therefore, COMT-catalysed O-methylation of catechol estrogens represents a possible "protective" metabolic pathway.

Histamine, the major endogenous substrate for HNMT, participates in the pathophysiology of a variety of human diseases including allergy, asthma, and peptic ulcer disease (Wasserman, 1983; Loiselle and Wollin, 1993). Therefore, individual variation in histamine metabolism could potentially represent a risk factor for the occurrence of those diseases. Cloning of the human HNMT cDNA and gene, as well as the identification of a functionally significant genetic polymorphism for this enzyme in humans (Girard *et al.*, 1994; Aksoy *et al.*, 1996; Preuss *et al.*, 1998) made it possible to study the potential clinical implications of genetic variation in HNMT activity as a risk factor for disease. The first attempt to do that involved a study of the *HNMT* codon 105 genetic polymorphism in patients with asthma. That study reported a significant increase in the frequency of the allele associated with decreased HNMT activity in patients with asthma as compared with ethnically matched control subjects (Yan *et al.*, 2000). These observations are compatible with the conclusion that lower HNMT activity might result in a decrease in histamine metabolism – leading to increased bronchospasm. Obviously, these results, like those of all molecular epidemiology association studies, require confirmation. However, all of these data – those for TPMT, COMT and HNMT – demonstrate the continuing and accelerating rate of clinical application of methylation pharmacogenetics.

Conclusions

Methylation is an important phase II pathway for the biotransformation of a large number of drugs, other xenobiotics and endogenous compounds (Weinshilboum, 1989b; Weinshilboum *et al.*, 1999). Our evolving knowledge of the regulation of enzymes that catalyse this metabolic pathway in humans provides an excellent example of the way in which decades of basic biochemical, molecular and genetic studies can ultimately have a significant impact on human health. The TPMT genetic polymorphism represents a striking example of the potential implications of pharmacogenetics for clinical medicine – and a glimpse of a future when it may be possible to individualise therapy in a way that would have seemed inconceivable only a few years ago. Pharmacogenetic studies of COMT have not only provided insight into the molecular basis for individual variation in the biotransformation of catechol drugs such as levodopa and methyldopa, but they have also provided unanticipated understanding of one factor that may be involved in the pathophysiology of a major cause of mortality in females, breast cancer. Similar pharmacogenetic studies of

HNMT may provide insight into factors involved in the etiology of asthma. As this type of knowledge expands in the near future to include not only other methyltransferase enzymes, but also other proteins responsible for individual variations in drug response, we will enter a new era in the rational use of medications to treat human disease.

Acknowledgements

We thank Luanne Wussow for her assistance with the preparation of this manuscript. The work described in this chapter was supported in part by United States National Institutes of Health grants RO1 GM28157 and RO1 GM35720.

References

Aksoy, S., Brandriff, B. F., Ward, V., Little, P. F. R. and Weinshilboum, R. M. (1995) 'Human nicotinamide N-methyltransferase gene: molecular cloning, structural characterization, and chromosomal localization', *Genomics* 29: 555–61.

Aksoy, S., Raftogianis, R. B. and Weinshilboum, R. M. (1996) 'Human histamine N-methyltransferase gene: structural characterization and chromosomal localization', *Biochem. Biophys. Res. Commun.* 219: 548–54.

Aksoy, S., Szumlanski, C. L. and Weinshilboum, R. M. (1994) 'Human liver nicotinamide N-methyltransferase: cDNA cloning, expression and biochemical characterization', *J. Biol. Chem.* 265: 14835–40.

Aletta, J. M., Cimato, R. T. and Ettinger, M. J. (1998) 'Protein methylation: a signal event in post-translational modification', *Trends Biochem Sci* 23: 89–91.

Axelrod, J. (1962) 'Purification and properties of phenylethanolamine N-methyltransferase', *J. Biol. Chem.* 237: 1657–60.

Axelrod, J. and Cohen, C. K. (1971) 'Methyltransferase enzymes in red blood cells', *J. Pharmacol. Exp. Ther.* 176: 650–4.

Axelrod, J. and Tomchick, R. (1958) 'Enzymatic O-methylation of epinephrine and other catechols', *J. Biol. Chem.* 233: 702–5.

Baetge, E. E., Behringer, R. R., Messing, A., Brinster, R. L. and Palmiter, R. D. (1988) 'Transgenic mice express the human phenylethanolamine N-methyltransferase gene in adrenal medulla and retina', *Proc. Natl. Acad. Sci. USA* 85: 3648–52.

Baetge, E. E., Suh, Y. H. and Joh, T. H. (1986) 'Complete nucleotide and deduced amino acid sequence of bovine phenylethanolamine N-methyltransferase: partial amino acid homology with rat tyrosine hydroxylase', *Proc. Natl. Acad. Sci. USA* 83: 5454–8.

Ball, P., Knuppen, R., Haupt, M. and Breuer, H. (1972) 'Interactions between estrogens and catechol amines. III. Studies on the methylation of catechol estrogens, catechol amines and other catechols by the catechol O-methyltransferase of human liver', *J. Clin. Endocrinol.* 34:736–46.

Barth, H. and Lorenz, W. (1978) 'Structural requirements of imidazol compounds to be inhibitors or activators of histamine methyltransferase: investigation of histamine analogues and H₂-receptor antagonists. *Agents and Actions* 8: 359–65.

Batter, D. K., D'Mello, S. R., Turzai, L. M., Hughes, H. B. III, Gioio, A. E. and Kaplan, B. B. (1988) 'The complete nucleotide sequence and structure of the gene encoding bovine phenylethanolamine N-methyltransferase', *J. Neurosci. Res.* 19: 367–76.

Bertocci, B., Miggiano, V., Da Prada, M., Dembic, Z., Lahm, H.-W. and Malherbe, P. (1991) 'Human catechol O-methyltransferase: cloning and expression of membrane-associated form', *Proc. Natl. Acad. Sci. USA* 88: 1416–20.

Borchardt, R. T. (1977) 'Synthesis and biological activity of analogs of adenosylhomocysteine as inhibitors of methyltransferases', in F. Salvatore, E. Borek, V. Zappia, H. G. Williams-Ashman and F. Schlenk (eds) *Biochemistry of Adenosylmethionine*, New York: Columbia University Press, pp. 151–71.

Boudíková, B., Szumlanski, C., Maidak, B. and Weinshilboum, R. (1990) 'Human liver catechol O-methyltransferase pharmacogenetics', *Clin. Pharmacol. Ther.* 48: 381–9.

Bremer, J. and Greenberg, D. M. (1961) 'Enzymatic methylation of foreign sulfhydryl compounds', *Biochim. Biophys. Acta.* 46: 217–24.

Brown, D. D., Tomchick, R. and Axelrod, J. (1959) 'The distribution and properties of a histamine-methylating enzyme', *J. Biol. Chem.* 234: 2948–50.

Campbell, N. R. C., Dunnette, J. H., Mwaluko, G., Van Loon, J. and Weinshilboum, R. M. (1984) 'Platelet phenol sulfotransferase and erythrocyte catechol-O-methyltransferase activities: correlation with methyldopa metabolism in man', *Clin. Pharmacol. Ther.* 35: 55–63.

Cantoni, G. L. (1953) 'S-Adenosylmethionine: a new intermediate formed enzymatically from L-methionine and adenosinetriphosphate', *J. Biol. Chem.* 204: 402–16.

Cantoni, G. L. and Durell, J. (1957) 'Activation of methionine for transmethylation II. The methionine-activation enzyme: studies on the mechanism of the reaction', *J. Biol. Chem.* 255: 1033–48.

Cavalieri, E. L., Stack, D. E., Devanesan, P. D., Todorovic, R., Dwivedy, I., Higginbothan, S., Johannson, S. L., Patil, K. D., Gross, M. L., Gooden, J. K., Ramanathan, R., Cerny, R. L. and Rogan, E. G. (1997) 'Molecular origin of cancer: catechol estrogen-3,4–quinones as endogenous tumor initiators', *Proc. Natl. Acad. Sci. USA* 94: 10937–42.

Cavalli-Sforza, L. L. and Bodmer, W. F. (1971) *The Genetics of Human Populations*, San Francisco: W. H. Freeman.

Cheng, X., Kumar, S., Posfai, J., Pfugrath, J. W. and Roberts, R. J. (1993) 'Crystal structure of the HhaI DNA methyltransferase complexed with S-adenosyl-L-methionine', *Cell* 74: 299–307.

Collie-Duguid, E. S. R., Pritchard, S. C., Powrie, R. H., Sludden, J., Collier, D. A., Li, T. and McLeod, H. L. (1999) 'The frequency and distribution of thiopurine methyltransferase alleles in Caucasian and Asian populations', *Pharmacogenetics* 9: 37–42.

Creveling, C. R., Borchardt, R. T. and Isersky, C. (1973) 'Immunological characterization of catechol-O-methyltransferase', in E. Usdin and S. Snyder (eds) *Frontiers in Catecholamine Research*, New York: Pergamon Press, pp. 117–119.

De Santi, C., Giulianotti, P. C., Pietrabissa, A., Mosca, F. and Pacifici, G. M. (1998) 'Catechol O-methyltransferase: variation in enzyme activity and inhibition by entacapone and tolcapone', *Eur. J. Clin. Pharmacol.* 54: 215–9.

Donohue, S. J., Roseboom, P. H., Illnerova, H., Weller, J. L. and Klein, D. C. (1993) 'Human hydroxyindole-O-methyltransferase: presence of LINE-1 fragment in a cDNA clone and pineal mRNA', *DNA Cell Biol.* 12: 715–27.

Donohue, S. J., Roseboom, P. H. and Klein, D. C. (1992) 'Bovine hydroxyindole O-methyltransferase: significant sequence revision', *J. Biol. Chem.* 267: 5184–5.

D'Souza, J., Caldwell, J. and Smith, R. L. (1980) 'Species variations in the N-methylation and quaternization of [^{14}C]pyridine', *Xenobiotica* 10: 151–7.

Eisenhofer, G., Keiser, H., Friberg, P., Mezey, E., Huynh, T. T., Hiremagalur, B., Ellingson, T., Duddempudi, S., Eijsbouts, A. and Lenders, J. W. (1998) 'Plasma metanephrines are markers of pheochromocytoma produced by catechol-O-methyltransferase within tumors', *J. Clin. Endocrinol. Met.* 83: 2175–85.

Elion, G. B. (1967) 'Biochemistry and pharmacology of purine analogues', *Fed. Proc.* 26: 898–904.

Enzyme Nomenclature (1992) 'Recommendations of the Nomenclature Committee of the International Union of Biochemistry and Molecular Biology on the nomenclature and classification of enzymes', prepared for NC-IUBMB by E. C. Webb, New York: Academic Press.

Evans, W. E., Horner, M., Chu, Y. Q., Kalwinsky, D. and Roberts, W. M. (1991) 'Altered mercaptopurine metabolism, toxic effects and dosage requirement in a thiopurine methyltransferase-deficient child with acute lymphoblastic leukemia', *J. Pediatrics* 119: 985–9.

Floderus, Y. and Wetterberg, L. (1981) 'The inheritance of human erythrocyte catechol-O-methyltransferase activity', *Clin. Genet.* 19: 392–5.

Fu, Z. and Takusagawa, F. (1994) 'Crystallization and preliminary X-ray diffraction studies of glycine methyltransferase from rat liver', *J. Struct. Biol.* 113: 247–9.

Girard, B., Otterness, D. M., Wood, T. C., Honchel, R., Wieben, E. D. and Weinshilboum, R. M. (1994) 'Human histamine N-methyltransferase pharmacogenetics: cloning and expression of kidney cDNA', *Mol. Pharmacol.* 45: 461–8.

Glauser, T. A., Nelson, A. N., Zembower, D. E., Lipsky, J. J. and Weinshilboum, R. M. (1993) 'Diethyldithiocarbamate S-methylation: evidence for catalysis by human liver thiol methyltransferase and thiopurine methyltransferase', *J. Pharmacol. Exp. Ther.* 266: 23–32.

Gomi, T., Tanihara, K., Date, T. and Fujioka, M. (1992) 'Rat guanidinoacetate methyltransferase: mutation of amino acids within a common sequence motif of mammalian methyltransferase does not affect catalytic activity but alters proteolytic susceptibility', *Intl. J. Biochem.* 24: 1639–49.

Grossman, M. H., Emanuel, B. S. and Budaf, M. L. (1992) 'Chromosomal mapping of the human catechol-O-methyltransferase gene to 22q11.1–q11.2', *Genomics* 12: 822–5.

Grunhaus, L., Ebstein, R., Belmaker, R., Sandler, S. G. and Jonas, W. (1976) 'A twin study of human red blood cell catechol-O-methyltransferase', *Br. J. Psychiat.* 128: 494–8.

Guldberg, H. C. and Marsden, C. A. (1975) 'Catechol-O-methyltransferase: pharmacological aspects and physiological role', *Pharmacol. Rev.* 27: 135–206.

Hamahata, A., Takata, Y., Gomi, T. and Fujioka, M. (1996) 'Probing the S-adenosylmethionine-binding site of rat guanidinoacetate methyltransferase', *Biochem. J.* **317**: 141–5.

His, W. (1887) 'Ueber das Stoffwechselproduct des Pyridins', *Arch. Ex. Pathol. Pharmakol.* **22**: 253–60.

Hoehe, M. R., Plaetke, R., Otterud, B., Stauffer, D., Holik, J., Byerley, W. F., Baetge, E. E., Gershon, E. S., Lalouel, J. M. and Leppert, M. (1992) 'Genetic linkage of the human gene for phenylethanolamine N-methyltransferase (PNMT), the adrenaline-synthesizing enzyme, to DNA markers on chromosome 17q21–q22', *Hum. Mol. Genet.* **1**: 175–8.

Hon, Y. Y., Fessing, M. Y., Pui, C.-H., Relling, M. V., Krynetski, E. Y. and Evans, W. E. (1999) 'Polymorphism of the thiopurine S-methyltransferase gene in African–Americans', *Human Mol. Genet.* **8**: 371–6.

Honchel, R., Aksoy, I., Szumlanski, C. L., Wood, T. C., Otterness, D. M., Wieben, E. D. and Weinshilboum, R. M. (1993) 'Human thiopurine methyltransferase: molecular cloning and expression of T84 colon carcinoma cell cDNA', *Mol. Pharmacol.* **43**: 878–87.

Horikawa, S. and Tsukada, K. (1991) 'Molecular cloning and nucleotide sequence of cDNA encoding the human liver S-adenosylmethionine synthetase', *Biochem. Int.* **25**: 81–90.

Horikawa, S. and Tsukada, K. (1992) "Molecular cloning and developmental expression of a human kidney S-adenosylmethionine synthetase', *FEBS Lett.* **312**: 37–41.

Hough, L. B., Khandelwal, J. K. and Mittag, T. W. (1981) 'Alpha-methylhistamine methylation by histamine methyltransferase', *Agents Actions* **11**: 425–8.

Huang, C.-S., Chern, H.-D., Chang, K.-J., Cheng, C.-W., Hsu, S.-M. and Shen, C.-Y. (1999) 'Breast cancer risk associated with genotype polymorphism of the estrogen-metabolising genes *CYP17*, *CYP1A1*, and *COMT*: a multigenic study on cancer susceptibility', *Cancer Res.* **59**: 4870–5.

Ingrosso, D., Fowler, A. V., Bleibaum, J. and Clarke, S. (1989) 'Sequence of the D-aspartyl/L-isoaspartyl protein methyltransferase from human erythrocytes: common sequence motifs for protein, DNA, RNA and small molecule S-adenosylmethionine-dependent methyltransferases', *J. Biol. Chem.* **264**: 20131–9.

Inoue, K. and Creveling, C. R. (1991) 'Induction of catechol-O-methyltransferase in the luminal epithelium of rat uterus by progesterone', *J. Histochem. Cytochem.* **39**: 823–8.

Jang, I. J., Shin, S. G., Lee, K. H., Yim, D. S., Lee, M. S., Koo, H. H. and Sohn, D. R. (1996) 'Erythrocyte thiopurine methyltransferase activity in a Korean population', *Br. J. Pharmacol.* **42**: 638–41.

Kalow, W. (1992) *Pharmacogenetics of Drug Metabolism*, New York: Pergamon Press.

Kalow, W. (1997) 'Pharmacogenetics in biological perspective', *Pharmacol. Rev.* **49**: 369–79.

Kaneda, N., Ichinose, H., Kobayashi, K., Oka, K., Kishi, F., Nakazawa, A., Kurosawa, Y., Fujita, K. and Nagatsu, T. (1988) 'Molecular cloning of cDNA and chromosomal assignment of the gene for human phenylethanolamine N-methyltransferase, the enzyme for epinephrine biosynthesis', *J. Biol. Chem.* **263**: 7672–7.

Keith, R. A., Jardine, I., Kerremans, A. and Weinshilboum, R. M. (1984) 'Human erythrocyte membrane thiol methyltransferase: S-methylation of captopril, N-acetylcysteine and 7-α-thio-spirolactone', *Drug Met. Dispos.* **12**: 717–24.

Keith, R. A., Otterness, D. M., Kerremans, A. L. and Weinshilboum, R. M. (1985) 'S-Methylation of D and L-penicillamine by human erythrocyte membrane thiol methyltransferase', *Drug Met. Dispos.* **13**: 669–76.

Keith, R. A., Van Loon, J., Wussow, L. F. and Weinshilboum, R. M. (1983) 'Thiol methylation pharmacogenetics: heritability of human erythrocyte thiol methyltransferase activity', *Clin. Pharmacol. Ther.* **34**: 521–8.

Klein, C. B. and Costa, M. (1997) 'DNA methylation, heterochromatin and epigenetic carcinogens', *Mutat. Res.* **386**: 163–80.

Klemetsdal, B., Tollefsen, E., Loennechen, T., Johnsen, K., Utsi, E., Gisholt, K., Wist, E. and Aarbakke, J. (1992) 'Interethnic difference in thiopurine methyltransferase activity', *Clin. Pharmacol. Ther.* **51**: 24–31.

Kotb, M. and Geller, A. M. (1993) 'Methionine adenosyltransferase: structure and function', *Pharmacol. Ther.* **59**: 125–45.

Kotb, M., Mudd, S. H., Mato, J. M., Geller, A. M., Kredich, N. M., Chou, J. Y. and Cantoni, G. L. (1997) 'Consensus nomenclature for the mammalian methionine adenosyltransferase genes and gene products', *Trends Genet.* **13**: 51–2.

Kunugi, H., Nanko, S., Ueki, A., Otsuka, E., Hattori, M., Hoda, F., Vallada, H. P., Arranz, M. J. and Collier, D. A. (1997a) 'High and low activity alleles of catechol O-methyltransferase gene: ethnic difference and possible association with Parkinson's disease', *Neurosci. Lett.* **221**: 202–4.

Kunugi, H., Vallada, H. P., Hoda, F., Kirov, G., Gill, M., Aitchison, K. J., Ball, D., Arranz, M. J., Murray, R. M. and Collier, D. A. (1997b) 'No evidence for an association of affective disorders with high- or low-activity allele of catechol-O-methyltransferase gene', *Biol. Psychiatr.* **42**: 282–5.

Labahn, J., Granzin, J., Schluckebier, G., Robinson, D. P., Jach, W. E. and Schildkraut, I. (1994) 'Three-dimensional structure of the adenine-specific DNA methyltransferase M. Taq1 in complex with the cofactor S-adenosylmethionine', *Proc. Natl. Acad. Sci. USA* **91**: 10957–61.

Lachman, H. M., Nolan, K. A., Mohr, P., Saito, T. and Volavka, J. (1998) 'Association between catechol O-methyltransferase genotype and violence in schizophrenia and schizoaffective disorder', *Am. J. Psychiatr.* **155**: 835–7.

Lachman, H. M., Papolos, D. F., Saito, T., Yu, Y.-M., Szumlanski, C. L. and Weinshilboum, R. M. (1996) 'Human catechol O-methyltransferase pharmacogenetics: description of a functional polymorphism and its potential application to neuropsychiatric disorders', *Pharmacogenetics* **6**: 243–50.

Lavigne, J. A., Helzlsouer, K. J., Huang, H.-Y., Strickland, P. T., Bell, D. A., Selmin, O., Watson, M. A., Hoffman, S., Comstock, G. W. and Yager, J. D. (1997) 'An association between the allele coding for a low activity variant of catechol O-methyltransferase and the risk for breast cancer', *Cancer Res.* **57**: 5493–7.

Lee, D., Szumlanski, C., Houtman, J., Honchel, R., Rojas, K., Overhauser, J., Wieben, E. D. and Weinshilboum, R. M. (1995) 'Thiopurine methyltransferase pharmacogenetics: cloning of human liver cDNA and presence of a processed pseudogene on human chromosome 18q21.1', *Drug Met. Dispos.* **23**: 398–405.

Lee, Y. C., McKenzie, R. M., Gholson, R. K. and Raica, N. (1972) 'A comparative study of the metabolism of nicotinamide and nicotinic acid in normal and germ-free rats', *Biochim. Biophys. Acta* **264**: 59–64.

Lennard, L. (1992) 'The clinical pharmacology of 6-mercaptopurine', *Eur. J. Clin. Pharmacol.* **43**: 329–39.

Lennard, L., Lewis, I. J., Michelagnoli, M. and Lilleyman, J. S. (1997) 'Thiopurine methyltransferase deficiency in childhood lymphoblastic leukaemia: 6-mercaptopurine dosage strategies', *Med. Pediatr. Oncol.* **29**: 252–5.

Lennard, L., Lilleyman, J. S., Van Loon, J. and Weinshilboum, R. M. (1990) 'Genetic variation in response to 6-mercaptopurine for childhood acute lymphoblastic leukaemia', *Lancet* **336**: 225–9.

Lennard, L., Rees, C. A., Lilleyman, J. S. and Maddocks, J. L. (1983) 'Childhood leukemia: a relationship between intracellular 6-mercaptopurine metabolites and neutropenia', *Br. J. Clin. Pharmacol.* **16**: 359–63.

Lennard, L., Van Loon, J. A. and Weinshilboum, R. M. (1989) 'Pharmacogenetics of acute azathioprine toxicity: relationship to thiopurine methyltransferase genetic polymorphism', *Clin. Pharmacol. Ther.* **46**: 149–54.

Lewis, L. D., Benin, A., Szumlanski, C., Otterness, D. M., Lennard, L., Weinshilboum, R. M. and Nierenberg, D. W. (1997) 'Olsalazine and 6-mercaptopurine-related hematologic suppression: a possible drug–drug interaction', *Clin. Pharmacol. Ther.* **62**: 464–75.

Li, T., Vallada, H., Curtis, D., Aaranz, M., Xu, K., Cai, G., Deng, H., Liu, J., Murray, R., Liu, X. and Collier, D. A. (1997) 'Catechol O-methyltransferase Val158Met polymorphism: frequency analysis in Han Chinese subjects and allelic association of the low activity allele with bipolar affective disorder', *Pharmacogenetics* **7**: 349–53.

Loiselle, J. and Wollin, A. (1993) 'Mucosal histamine elimination and its effect on acid secretion in rabbit gastric mucosa', *Gastroenterol.* **104**: 1013–20.

Lundström, K., Salminen, M., Jalanko, A., Savolainen, R. and Ulmanen, I. (1991) 'Cloning and characterization of human placental catechol-O-methyltransferase cDNA', *DNA Cell Biol.* **10**: 181–9.

MacLaren, D. C., Kagan, R. M. and Clarke, S. (1992) 'Alternative splicing of the human isoaspartyl protein carboxyl methyltransferase RNA leads to the generation of a C-terminal-RDEL sequence in isozyme II', *Biochem. Biophys. Res. Commun.* **185**: 277–83.

McLeod, H. L., Krynetski, E. Y., Wilimas, J. A. and Evans, W. E. (1995) 'Higher activity of polymorphic thiopurine S-methyltransferase in erythrocytes from neonates compared to adults', *Pharmacogenetics* **5**: 281–6.

McLeod, H. L., Lin, J. S., Scott, E. P., Pui, C.-H. and Evans, W. E. (1994) 'Thiopurine methyltransferase activity in American white subjects and black subjects', *Clin. Pharmacol. Ther.* **55**: 15–20.

McLeod, H. L., Pritchard, S. C., Githang, J., Indalo, A., Ameyaw, M.-M., Powrie, R. H., Both, L. and Collie-Duguid, E. S. R. (1999) 'Ethnic differences in thiopurine methyltransferase pharmacogenetics: evidence for allele specificity in Caucasian and Kenyan individual', *Pharmacogenetics* **9**: 773–6.

Markham, G. D. and Satishchandran, C. (1988) 'Identification of the reactive sulfhydryl groups of S-adenosylmethionine synthetase', *J. Biol. Chem.* **263**: 8666–70.

Martinez-Martin, P. and O'Brien, C. F. (1998) 'Extending levodopa action: COMT inhibition', *Neurology* 50 (Suppl. 6): S27–32.

Mendel, G. (1865) 'Versuche der PflanzenHybriden', *Verhandlungen des naturforschenden Vereines in Brünn* 4: 3–47.

Morita, S., Kobayashi, K., Hidaka, H. and Nagatsu, T. (1992) 'Organization and complete nucleotide sequence of the gene encoding mouse phenylethanolamine N-methyltransferase', *Mol. Brain Res.* 13: 313–9.

Nelson, D. R., Koymans, L., Kamataki, T., Stegeman, J. J., Feyereisen, R., Waxman, D. J., Waterman, M. R., Gotoh, O., Coon, M. J., Estabrook, R. W., Gunsalus, I. and Nebert, D. W. (1996) 'P450 superfamily: update on new sequences, gene mapping, accession numbers and nomenclature', *Pharmacogenetics* 6: 1–42.

Niewmierzycka, A. and Clarke, S. (1999) 'S-Adenosylmethionine-dependent methylation in *Saccharomyces cerevisiae*: identification of a novel protein arginine methyltransferase', *J. Biol. Chem.* 274: 814–24.

Ogawa, H., Date, T., Gomi, T., Konishi, K., Pitot, H. C., Cantoni, G. L. and Fujioka, M. (1988) 'Molecular cloning, sequence analysis, and expression in *Escherichia coli* of the cDNA for guanidinoacetate methyltransferase from rat liver', *Proc. Natl. Acad. Sci. USA* 85: 694–8.

Ogawa, H., Konishi, K., Takata, Y., Nakashima, H. and Fujioka, M. (1987) 'Rat glycine methyltransferase: complete amino acid sequence deduced from a cDNA clone and characterization of the genomic DNA', *Eur. J. Biochem.* 168: 141–51.

Otterness, D. M., Szumlanski, C. L., Lennard, L., Klemetsdal, B., Aarbakke, J., Park-Hah, J. O., Iven, H., Schmiegelow, K., Branum, E., O'Brien, J. and Weinshilboum, R. M. (1997) 'Human thiopurine methyltransferase pharmacogenetics: gene sequence polymorphisms', *Clin. Pharmacol. Ther.* 62: 60–73.

Otterness, D. M., Szumlanski, C. L., Wood, T. C. and Weinshilboum, R. M. (1998) 'Human thiopurine methyltransferase pharmacogenetics: kindred with a terminal exon splice junction mutation that results in loss of activity', *J. Clin. Invest.* 101: 1036–44.

Pajares, M. A., Corrales, F. J., Ochoa, P. and Mato, J. M. (1991) 'The role of cysteine-150 in the structure and activity of rat liver S-adenosyl-L-methionine synthetase', *Biochem. J.* 274: 225–9.

Park-Hah, J. O., Klemetsdal, B., Lysaa, R., Choi, K. H. and Aarbakke, J. (1996) 'Thiopurine methyltransferase activity in a Korean population sample of children', *Clin. Pharmacol. Ther.* 60: 68–74.

Paterson, A. R. P. and Tidd, D. M. (1975) '6-Thiopurines', in A. C. Sartorelli and D. G. Johns (eds) *Antineoplastic and Immunosuppressive Agents II*, New York: Springer Verlag, pp. 384–403.

Pazmiño, P. A., Sladek, S. L. and Weinshilboum, R. M. (1980) 'Thiol S-methylation in uremia: erythrocyte enzyme activities and plasma inhibitors', *Clin. Pharmacol. Ther.* 28: 356–67.

Preuss, C. V., Wood, T. C., Szumlanski, C. L., Raftogianis, R. B., Otterness, D. M., Girard, B., Scott, M. C. and Weinshilboum, R. M. (1998) 'Human histamine N-methyltransferase pharmacogenetics: common genetic polymorphisms that alter activity', *Mol. Pharmacol.* 53: 708–17.

Price, R. A., Keith, R. A., Spielman, R. S. and Weinshilboum, R. M. (1989) 'Major gene polymorphism for human erythrocyte (RBC) thiol methyltransferase (TMT)', *Genet. Epidemiol.* 6: 651–62.

Price, R. A., Scott, M. C. and Weinshilboum, R. M. (1993) 'Genetic segregation analysis of red blood cell (RBC) histamine N-methyltransferase (HNMT) activity', *Genet. Epidemiol.* **10**: 123–31.

Quiram, D. R. and Weinshilboum, R. M. (1976) 'Catechol-O-methyltransferase in rat erythrocyte and three other tissues: comparison of biochemical properties after removal of inhibitory calcium', *J. Neurochem.* **27**: 1197–203.

Ratain, M. J. and Rowley, J. D. (1992) 'Therapy-related acute myeloid leukemia secondary to inhibitors of topoisomerase II: from the bedside to the target genes', *Ann. Oncol.* **3**: 107–11.

Raymond, F. A. and Weinshilboum, R. M. (1975) 'Microassay of human erythrocyte catechol-O-methyltransferase: removal of inhibitory calcium ion with chelating resin', *Clin. Chim. Acta.* **58**: 185–94.

Reilly, D. K., Rivera-Calimlim, L. and Van Dyke, D. (1980) 'Catechol-O-methyltransferase activity: a determinant of levodopa response', *Clin. Pharmacol. Ther.* **28**: 278–86.

Relling, M. V., Yanishevski, Y., Nemec, J., Evans, W. E., Boyett, J. M., Behm, F. G. and Pui, C.-H. (1998) 'Etoposide and antimetabolite pharmacology in patients who develop secondary acute myeloid leukemia', *Leukemia* **12**: 346–52.

Remy, C. N. (1963) 'Metabolism of thiopyrimidines and thiopurines: S-methylation with S-adenosylmethionine transmethylase and catabolism in mammalian tissue', *J. Biol. Chem.* **238**: 1078–84.

Rini, J., Szumlanski, C. L., Guerciolini, R. and Weinshilboum, R. M. (1989) 'Human liver nicotinamide N-methyltransferase: ion-pairing radiochemical assay, biochemical properties and individual variation', *Clin. Chim. Acta.* **186**: 359–74.

Romanik, E. A., Ladino, C. A., Killoy, L. C., D'Ardenne, S. C. and O'Connor, C. M. (1992) 'Genomic organization and tissue expression of the murine gene encoding the protein β-aspartate methyltransferase', *Gene* **118**: 217–22.

Saavedra, J. M. and Axelrod, J. (1973) 'Demonstration and distribution of phenylethanolamine in brain and other tissues', *Proc. Natl. Acad. Sci. USA* **70**: 769–72.

Salminen, M., Lundström, K., Tilgmann, C., Savolainen, R., Kalkkinen, N. and Ulmanen, I. (1990) 'Molecular cloning and characterization of rat liver catechol O-methyltransferase', *Gene* **93**: 241–7.

Sato, M., Yoshida, T. and Tuboi, S. (1989) 'Primary structure of rat brain protein carboxyl methyltransferase deduced from cDNA sequence', *Biochem. Biophys. Res. Commun.* **161**: 342–7.

Scanlon, P. D., Raymond, F. A. and Weinshilboum, R. M. (1979) 'Catechol-O-methyltransferase: thermolabile enzyme in erythrocytes of subjects homozygous for the allele for low activity', *Science* **203**: 63–5.

Scott, M. C., Van Loon, J. A. and Weinshilboum, R. M. (1988) 'Pharmacogenetics of N-methylation: heritability of human erythrocyte histamine N-methyltransferase activity', *Clin. Pharmacol. Ther.* **43**: 256–62.

Siervogel, R. M., Weinshilboum, R., Wilson, A. F. and Elston, R. C. (1984) 'Major gene model for the inheritance of catechol-O-methyltransferase activity in five large families', *Am. J. Med. Genet.* **19**: 315–23.

Sladek-Chelgren, S. and Weinshilboum, R. M. (1981) 'Catechol-O-methyltransferase biochemical genetics: human lymphocyte enzyme', *Biochem. Genet.* **19**: 1037–53.

Spielman, R. S. and Weinshilboum, R. M. (1981) 'Genetics of red cell COMT activity: analysis of thermal stability and family data', *Am. J. Med. Genet.* **10**: 279–90.

Suh, Y.-H., Chun, Y.-S., Lee, I. S., Kim, S.-S., Choi, W., Chong, Y. H., Hong, L., Kim, S.-H., Park, C.-W. and Kim, C.-G. (1994) 'Complete nucleotide sequence and tissue-specific expression of the rat phenylethanolamine N-methyltransferase gene' *J. Neurochem.* **63**: 1603–8.

Szumlanski, C. L., Honchel, R., Scott, M. C. and Weinshilboum, R. M. (1992) 'Human liver thiopurine methyltransferase pharmacogenetics: biochemical properties, liver–erythrocyte correlation and presence of isozymes', *Pharmacogenetics* **2**: 148–59.

Szumlanski, C. L., Otterness, D. M., Her, C., Lee, D., Brandriff, B. F., Kelsell, D., Spurr, N., Lennard, L., Wieben, E. D. and Weinshilboum, R. M. (1996) 'Thiopurine methyltransferase pharmacogenetics: human gene cloning and characterization of a common polymorphism', *DNA Cell Biol.* **15**: 17–30.

Szumlanski, C. L. and Weinshilboum, R. M. (1995) 'Sulphasalazine inhibition of thiopurine methyltransferase: possible mechanism for interaction with 6-mercaptopurine and azathioprine', *Br. J. Clin. Pharmacol.* **39**: 456–9.

Tai, H.-L., Fessing, M. Y., Bonten, E. J., Yanishevsky, Y., d'Azzo, A., Krynetski, E. Y. and Evan, W. E. (1999) 'Enhanced proteasomal degradation of mutant human thiopurine methyltransferase (TPMT) in mammalian cells: mechanism for TPMT protein deficiency inherited by *TPMT*2, TPMT*3A, TPMT*3B* or *TPMT*3C*', *Pharmacogenetics* **9**: 641–50.

Tai, H.-L., Krynetski, E. Y., Schuetz, E. G., Yanishevski, Y. and Evans, W. E. (1997) 'Enhanced proteolysis of thiopurine methyltransferase (TPMT) encoded by mutant alleles in humans (TPMT*3A, TPMT*2): mechanisms for the genetic polymorphism of TPMT activity', *Proc. Natl. Acad. Sci. USA* **94**: 6444–9.

Takemura, M., Tanaka, T., Taguchi, Y., Imamura, I., Mizuguchi, H., Kuroda, M., Fukui, H., Yamatodani, A. and Wada, H. (1992) 'Histamine N-methyltransferase from rat kidney: cloning, nucleotide sequence, and expression in *Escherichia coli* cells', *J. Biol. Chem.* **267**: 15687–91.

Taylor, K. M. and Snyder, S. H. (1972) 'Histamine methyltransferase: inhibition and potentiation by antihistamines', *Mol. Pharmacol.* **8**: 300–10.

Tenhunen, J., Salminen, M., Jalanko, A., Ukkonen, S. and Ulmanen, I. (1993) 'Structure of the rat catechol-O-methyltransferase gene: separate promoters are used to produce mRNAs for soluble and membrane-bound forms of the enzyme', *DNA Cell. Biol.* **12**: 253–63.

Tenhunen, J., Salminen, M., Lundstrom, K., Kiviluoto, T., Savolainen, R. and Ulmanen, I. (1994) 'Genomic organization of the human catechol-O-methyltransferase gene and its expression from two distinct promoters', *Eur. J. Biochem.* **223**: 1049–59.

Thithapandha, A. and Cohn, V. H. (1977) 'Brain histamine N-methyltransferase purification, mechanism of action and inhibition by drugs', *Biochem. Pharmacol.* **27**: 263–71.

Thompson, M. A. and Weinshilboum, R. M. (1998) 'Rabbit lung indolethylamine N-methyltransferase: cDNA and gene cloning and characterization', *J. Biol. Chem.* **273**: 34502–10.

Thompson, M. A., Moon, E., Kim, U.-J., Xu, J., Siciliano, J. and Weinshilboum, R. M. (1999) 'Human indolethylamine N-methyltransferase: cDNA cloning and expression, gene cloning, and chromosomal localization', *Genomics* **61**: 285–97.

Thompson, P. A., Shields, P. G., Freudenheim, J. L., Stone, A., Vena, J. E., Marshall, J. R., Graham, S., Laughlin, R., Nemoto, T., Kadlubar, F. F. and Ambrosone, C. B. (1998) 'Genetic polymorphisms in catechol O-methyltransferase, menopausal status, and breast cancer risk', *Cancer Res.* **58**: 2107–10.

Thomsen, J. B., Schrøder, H., Kristinsson, J., Madsen, B., Szumlanski, C., Weinshilboum, R., Andersen, J. B. and Schmiegelow, K. (1999) 'Possible carcinogenic effect of 6-mercaptopurine on bone marrow stem cells', *Cancer* **86**: 1080–6.

Tidd, D. M. and Paterson, A. R. P. (1974) 'A biochemical mechanism for the delayed cytotoxic reaction of 6-mercaptopurine' *Cancer Res.* **34**: 738–46.

Tollervey, D. (1996) 'Small nucleolar RNAs guide ribosomal RNA methylation', *Science* **273**: 1056–7.

Van Loon, J. and Weinshilboum, R. M. (1982) 'Thiopurine methyltransferase biochemical genetics: human lymphocyte activity', *Biochem. Genet.* **20**: 637–58.

Van Loon, J. A., Pazmiño, P. A. and Weinshilboum, R. M. (1985) 'Human erythrocyte histamine N-methyltransferase: radiochemical microassay and biochemical properties', *Clin. Chim. Acta* 149, 237–51.

Vidgren, J., Svensson, L. A. and Liljas, A. (1994) 'Crystal structure of catechol O-methyltransferase', *Nature* **368**: 354–8.

Vuchetich, J. P., Weinshilboum, R. M. and Price, R. A. (1995) 'Segregation analysis of human red blood cell (RBC) thiopurine methyltransferase (TPMT) activity', *Genet. Epidemiol.* **12**: 1–11.

Warner, D. R., Mozier, N. M., Pearson, J. D. and Hoffman. J. L. (1995) 'Cloning and base sequence analysis of a cDNA encoding mouse lung thioether S-methyltransferase', *Biochim. Biophys. Acta* **1246**: 160–6.

Wasserman, S. I. (1983) 'Mediators of immediate hypersensitivity', *J. Allergy Clin. Immunol.* **72**: 101–15.

Weinshilboum, R. M. (1978) 'Human erythrocyte catechol-O-methyltransferase: correlation with lung and kidney activity', *Life Sci.* **22**: 625–30.

Weinshilboum, R. M. (1981) 'Enzyme thermal stability and population genetic studies: application to erythrocyte catechol-O-methyltransferase and plasma dopamine β-hydroxylase', in E. S. Gershon, S. Matthysse, X. O. Breakefield and R. D. Ciaranello (eds) *Genetic Strategies in Psychobiology and Psychiatry,* Pacific Grove: Boxwood Press, pp. 79–94.

Weinshilboum, R. M. (1989a) 'Thiol S-methyltransferases I. biochemistry', in L. A. Damani (ed.) *Sulphur-Containing Drugs and Related Organic Chemicals: Chemistry, Biochemistry and Toxicology* (Volume 2: Part A), Chichester: Ellis Horwood Ltd, pp. 121–42.

Weinshilboum, R. M. (1989b) 'Methyltransferase pharmacogenetics', *Pharmacol Ther.* **43**: 77–90.

Weinshilboum, R. M. and Raymond, F. A. (1977) 'Inheritance of low erythrocyte catechol-O-methyltransferase activity in man', *Am. J. Human Genet.* **29**: 125–35.

Weinshilboum, R. M. and Sladek, S. L. (1980) 'Mercaptopurine pharmacogenetics: monogenic inheritance of erythrocyte thiopurine methyltransferase activity', *Am. J. Human Genet.* **32**: 651–62.

Weinshilboum, R. M. and Raftogianis, R. B. (2000) 'Sulfotransferases and methyltransferases', in R. H. Levy, K. E. Thummel, W. F. Trager, P. D. Hansten and M. Eichelboum (eds) *Metabolic Drug Interactions*, Lippincott-Raven Publishers, pp. 191–203.

Weinshilboum, R. M., Raymond, F. A., Elveback, L. R. and Weidman, W. H. (1974) 'Correlation of erythrocyte catechol-O-methyltransferase activity between siblings', *Nature* 252: 490–1.

Weinshilboum, R. M., Sladek, S. and Klumpp, S. (1979) 'Human erythrocyte thiol methyltransferase: radiochemical microassay and biochemical properties', *Clin. Chim. Acta* 97: 59–71.

Weinshilboum, R. M., Otterness, D. M. and Szumlanski, C. L. (1999) 'Methylation pharmacogenetics: catechol O-methyltransferase, thiopurine methyltransferase and histamine N-methyltransferase', *Annu. Rev. Pharmacol. Toxicol.* 39: 19–52.

Weisberg, E. P., Baruchin, A., Stachowiak, M. K., Stricker, E. M., Zigmond, M. J. and Kaplan, B. B. (1989) 'Isolation of a rat adrenal cDNA clone encoding phenylethanolamine N-methyltransferase and cold-induced alterations in adrenal PNMT mRNA and protein', *Mol. Brain Res.* 6: 159–66.

Winqvist, R., Lundström, K., Salminen, M., Laatikainen, M. and Ulmanen, I. (1992) 'The human catechol-O-methyltransferase (COMT) gene maps to band q11.2 of chromosome 22 and shows a frequent RFLP with BglI', *Cytogenet. Cell Genet.* 59: 253–7.

Winter, H., Herschel, M., Propping, P., Friedl, W. and Vogel, F. (1978) 'A twin study on three enzymes (DBH, COMT, MAO) of catecholamine metabolism', *Psychopharmacol.* 57: 63–9.

Woodson, L. C., Ames, M. M., Selassie, C. D., Hansch, C. and Weinshilboum, R. M. (1983) 'Thiopurine methyltransferase: aromatic thiol substrates and inhibition by benzoic acid derivatives', *Mol. Pharmacol.* 24: 471–8.

Woodson, L. C. and Weinshilboum, R. M. (1983) 'Human kidney thiopurine methyltransferase: purification and biochemical properties', *Biochem. Pharmacol.* 32: 819–26.

Woodson, L. C., Dunnette, J. H. and Weinshilboum, R. M. (1982) 'Pharmacogenetics of human thiopurine methyltransferase: kidney–erythrocyte correlation and immunotitration studies', *J. Pharmacol. Exp. Ther.* 222: 174–81.

Wu, G., Williams, H. D., Zamanian, M., Gibson, F. and Poole, R. K. (1992) 'Isolation and characterization of *Escherichia coli* mutants affected in aerobic respiration: the cloning and nucleotide sequence of *ubiG*: identification of an S-adenosylmethionine-binding motif in protein, RNA and small molecule methyltransferases', *J. Gen. Microbiol.* 138: 2101–12.

Xie, T., Ho, S. L., Li, L. S. W. and Ma, O. C. K. (1997) 'G/A$_{1947}$ polymorphism in catechol O-methyltransferase (COMT) gene in Parkinson's disease', *Movement Disorders* 12: 426–7.

Yamauchi, K., Sekizawa, K., Suzuki, H., Nakazawa, H., Ohkawara, Y., Katayose, D., Ohtsu, H., Tamura, G., Shibahara, S., Takemura, M., Maeyama, K., Watanabe, T., Sasaki, H., Shirata, K. and Takishima, T. (1994) 'Structure and function of human histamine N-methyltransferase: critical enzyme in histamine metabolism in airway', *Am. J. Physiol.* 267: L342–9.

Yan, L., Otterness, D. M., Craddock, T. L. and Weinshilboum, R. M. (1997) 'Mouse liver nicotinamide N-methyltransferase: cDNA cloning, expression and nucleotide sequence polymorphisms', *Biochem. Pharmacol.* **54**: 1139–49.

Yan, L., Otterness, D. M., Kozak, C. A. and Weinshilboum, R. M. (1998) 'Mouse nicotinamide N-methyltransferase gene: molecular cloning, structural characterization and chromosomal localization', *DNA Cell. Biol.* **17**: 659–67.

Yan, L., Otterness, D. M. and Weinshilboum, R. M. (1999) 'Human nicotinamide N-methyltransferase pharmacogenetics: gene sequence analysis and promoter characterization', *Pharmacogenetics* **9**: 307–16.

Yan, L., Galinsky, R. E., Bernstein, J. A., Liggett, S. B. and Weinshilboum, R. M. (2000) 'Histamine N-methyltransferase pharmacogenetics: association of common functional polymorphism with asthma', *Pharmacogenetics* **10**: 261–6.

Yates, C. R., Krynetski, E. Y., Loennechen, T., Fessing, M. Y., Tai, H.-L., Pui, C.-H., Relling, M. V. and Evans, W. E. (1997) 'Molecular diagnosis of thiopurine S-methyltransferase deficiency: genetic basis for azathioprine and mercaptopurine intolerance', *Ann Int Med* **126**: 608–14.

Chapter 14

Interindividual variability of sulfotransferases

G. M. Pacifici and A. M. Rossi

Forms of ST

STs (EC 2.8.2) are important enzymes that catalyse the sulphation of
neurotransmitters, hormones, drugs and chemicals (Mulder and Jakoby,
1990; Falany, 1991; Pacifici and De Santi 1995; Weinshilboum, 1986).
Their subcellular localisation is mainly cytosolic, although membrane
bound STs have been found to catalyse the sulfation of glycosaminoglycans
(Inoue *et al.*, 1986; Razi and Lindahl, 1995) and tyrosyl residues within
proteins (Huttner, 1982; Lin and Roth, 1990; Rens-Domiano and Roth,
1989). However, since most of the research work on the interindividual
variability of STs has been performed on the cytosolic forms, the subsequent
discussion will deal with these ones. In human tissue, there are several forms
of ST and five forms have been characterised for their substrate specificities,
thermal stability, inhibitor sensivity and regulation. Three forms are
grouped under the expression phenol-STs (Falany, 1991; Pacifici and De
Santi 1995; Weinshilboum 1986). Two of these forms are thermostable and
their diagnostic substrate is 4-nitrophenol. They are named TS-PST
(Campbell *et al.*, 1987) or form P (Carter *et al.*, 1983), simply phenol ST
(Cappiello *et al.*, 1990; Pacifici and De Santi, 1995) or SULT1A1. The third
form is thermolabile and its diagnostic substrate is dopamine. It is then
referred to as TL-PST (Sundaram *et al.*, 1989) or form M (Carter *et al.*,
1983), simply catechol ST as the functional moiety is the catecholic group
of dopamine (Cappiello *et al.*, 1990; Pacifici and De Santi, 1995) or
SULT1A3. Furthermore, there is a form of hydroxysteroid ST named
dehydroepiandrosterone ST also referred to as DHEA-ST and its diagnostic
substrate is dehydroepiandrosterone (Falany *et al.*, 1989; Falany *et al.*,
1995). This form is believed to catalyse the sulfation of androsterone,
pregnolone, testosterone, estrone, lithocholic acid and taurolithocholic acid
(Falany, 1991; Falany *et al.*, 1989). Finally, there is a form of estrogen ST
also referred to as EST and its diagnostic substrate is estrone (Falany and
Falany, 1996) or estradiol (Song *et al.*, 1998) at nanomolar concentrations.

Variability of phenol ST activity

The variability of phenol ST activities has been studied in the human liver (Pacifici *et al.*, 1994a), duodenum (Pacifici *et al.*, 1997a) and platelets (Pacifici and Marchi 1993; Pacifici *et al.*, 1993). The distribution of phenol ST was positively skewed and the activity of this enzyme was not gender regulated. Table 14.1 summarises the results of the descriptive statistical analysis and Figure 14.1 shows the frequency distribution histograms obtained in the human liver, duodenum and adult and newborn platelets. Figure 14.2 shows the probit plots in human liver, duodenum and adult and cord platelets.

Variability of catechol ST activity

The variability of catechol ST activity has been studied in the human liver (Pacifici *et al.*, 1994a), duodenum (Pacifici *et al.*, 1997a) and platelets (Pacifici and Marchi, 1993). The frequency distribution of catechol ST did not deviate from normality in the cord platelets, whereas it was positively skewed in the other cases. The activity of this enzyme was not gender regulated and did not correlate with the age of the tissue donors (Table 14.2 and Figures 14.3 and 14.4).

Both phenol and catechol STs catalyse the sulfation of a number of compounds including drugs such as minoxidil (Anderson *et al.*, 1998; Pacifici *et al.*, 1993) and salbutamol (Pacifici *et al.*, 1997a). Minoxidil is an anti-hypertensive agent that is converted by sulfation into the active compound minoxidil sulfate (McCall *et al.*, 1983). The results of the

Table 14.1 Descriptive statistical analysis of phenol ST in the human liver, duodenum and platelets

Tissue	Liver	Duodenum	Adult platelets	Cord platelets
Number of cases	100	100	100	100
Mean[a]	1492	144	3.0	4.8
±S.D.[a]	876	56	3.2	4.3
Median[a]	1200	131	1.8	3.4
5% Percentile[a]	620	68	0.5	0.8
95% Percentile[a]	3310	252	9.1	13.4
Variation[b]	5.3	3.7	18.2	16.7
Skewness	1.570	0.758	2.350	2.239
W-statistic	0.862	0.936	0.741	0.783
p	<0.001	<0.001	<0.001	<0.001
References	A	B	C	C

Notes

[a]The enzyme activity is expressed as pmol/mg/min.

[b]The variation is calculated by dividing the 95% percentile by the 5% percentile. W-statistic is the critical value of the Shapiro and Wilk test. The distribution deviates from normality when $p < 0.05$.

A: Pacifici *et al.*, 1994a; B: Pacifici *et al.*, 1997a; C: Pacifici and Marchi, 1993.

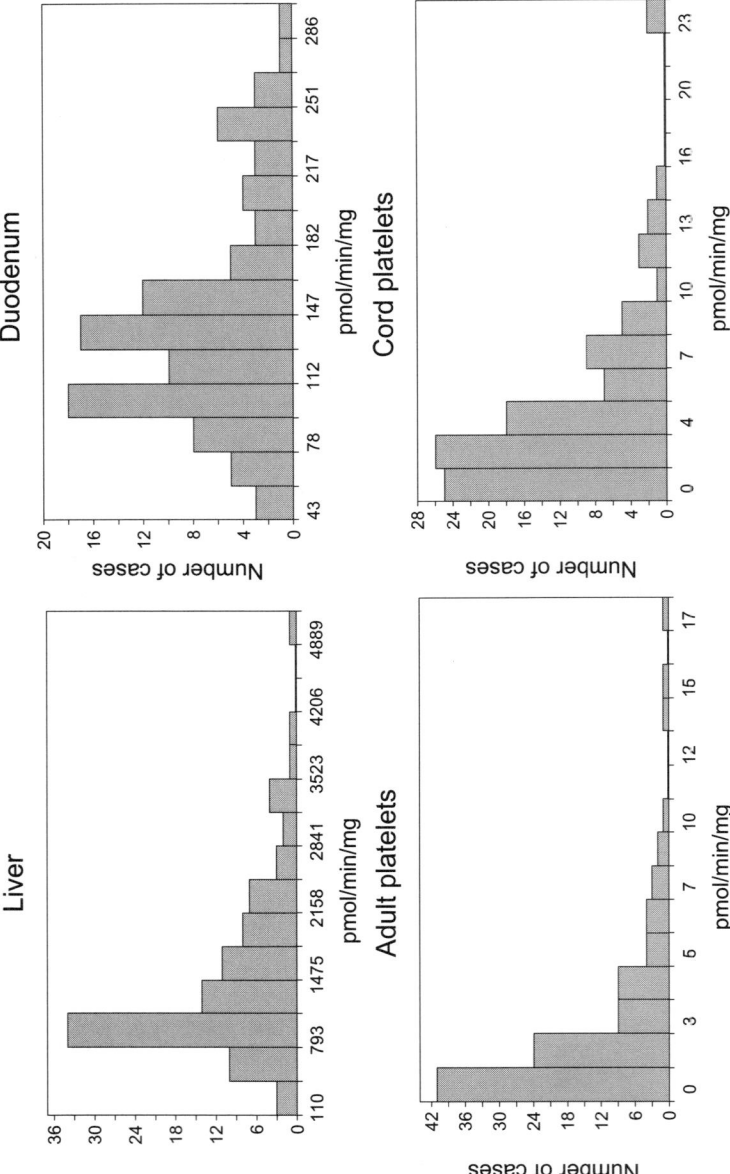

Figure 14.1 Frequency distribution histograms of phenol sulfotransferase activities in the human liver, duodenum and in the adult and cord platelets. The cord blood was obtained by full-term placentas.

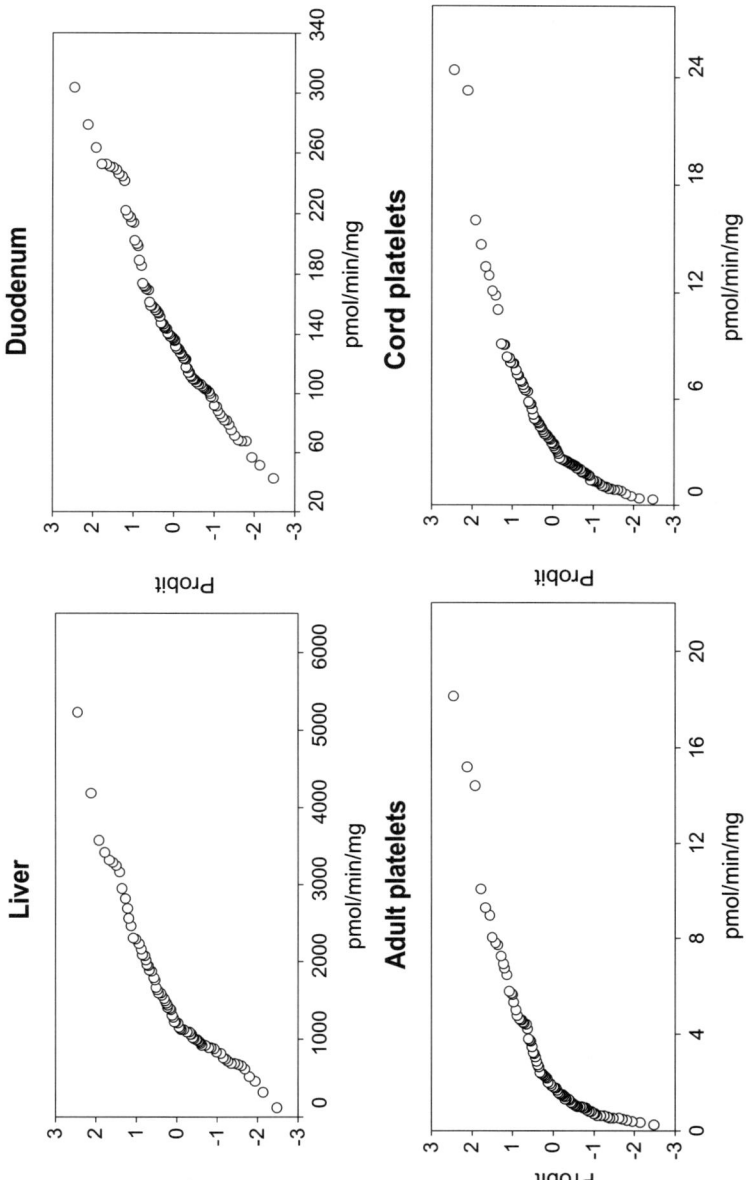

Figure 14.2 Probit plots of phenol sulfotransferase activities in the human liver, duodenum, and in the adult and cord platelets. The cord blood was obtained from full-term placentas.

Table 14.2 Descriptive statistical analysis of catechol sulfotransferase in the human liver, duodenum and platelets

Tissue	Liver	Duodenum	Adult platelets	Cord platelets
Number of cases	100	100	100	100
Mean[a]	47	631	7.7	13.3
±S.D.[a]	29	234	5.9	6.4
Median[a]	44.1	593	6.15	13.2
5% Percentile[a]	12	334	0.8	3.6
95% Percentile[a]	92	1014	21.4	24.2
Variation[b]	7.7	3.0	26.7	6.7
Skewness	1.420	0.241	1.486	0.520
W-statistic	0.886	0.910	0.863	0.970
p	<0.001	<0.001	<0.001	0.147
References	A	B	C	C

Notes
[a]The enzyme activity is expressed as pmol/mg/min.
[b]The variation is calculated by dividing the 95% percentile by the 5% percentile. W-statistic is the critical value of Shapiro and Wilk test. The distribution deviates from normality when $p < 0.05$.
A: Pacifici et al., 1994a; B: Pacifici et al., 1997a; C: Pacifici and Marchi 1993.

Table 14.3 Descriptive statistical analysis of minoxidil sulfotransferase in the human liver and (−)-salbutamol sulfotransferase in the liver and duodenum

Substrate	Minoxidil	(−)-Salbutamol	
Tissue	Liver	Liver	Duodenum
Number of cases	118	100	100
Mean[a]	631	76.2	329
±S.D.[a]	330	23.8	99
Median[a]	595	73.7	315
5% Percentile[a]	284	40.6	189
95% Percentile[a]	1270	120.4	468
Variation[b]	4.5	3.0	2.5
Skewness	0.734103	0.73400	0.75277
W-statistic	0.91117	0.95488	0.96678
p	<0.001	0.008	0.083
References	A	B	B

Notes
[a]The enzyme activity is expressed as pmol/mg/min.
[b]The variation is calculated by dividing the 95% percentile by the 5% percentile. W-statistic is the critical value of Shapiro and Wilk test. The distribution deviates from normality when $p < 0.05$.
A: Pacifici et al., 1993; B: Pacifici et al., 1997a.

descriptive statistical analysis of the hepatic minoxidil ST activity are summarised in Table 14.3. This Table also summarises the results of the descriptive statistical analysis of the hepatic and duodenal salbutamol ST activities. In the liver, the distribution of minoxidil and salbutamol ST activities is positively skewed and the range of variation is 4.5 (minoxidil) and 3 (salbutamol). In the duodenum, the activity of salbutamol ST does not deviate from normality and the range of variation is 2.5 (Table 14.3

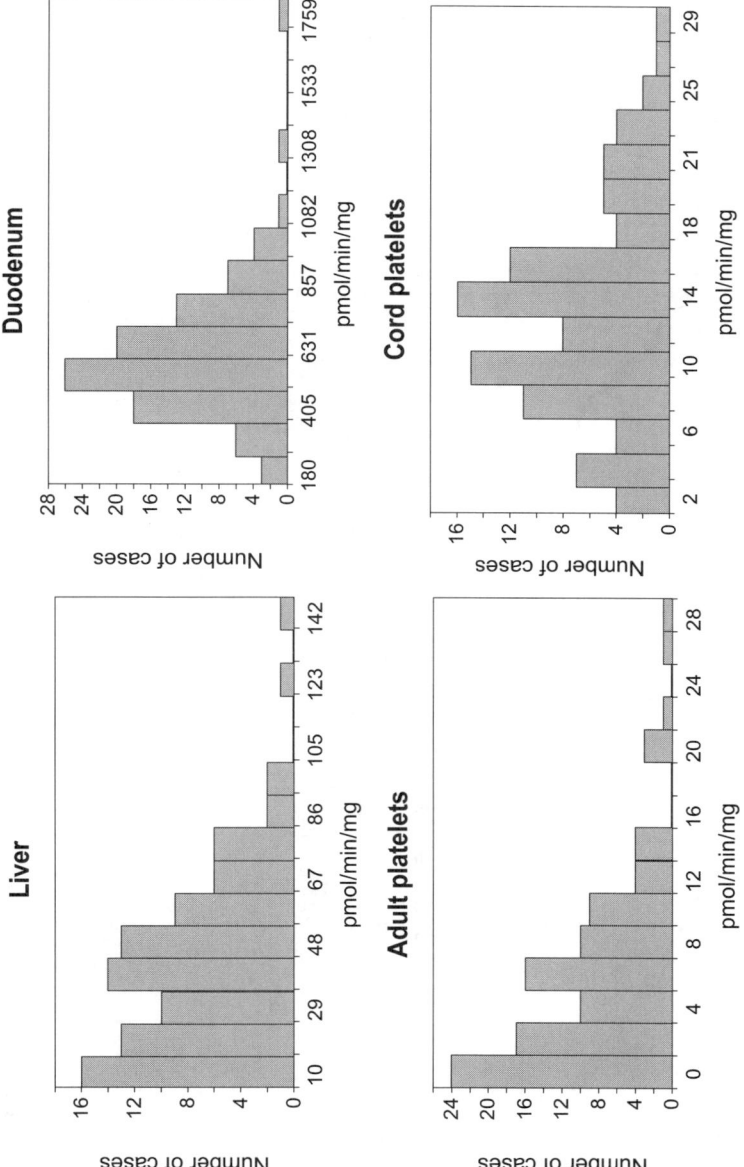

Figure 14.3 Frequency distribution histograms of the catechol sulfotransferase activity in the human liver, duodenum, adult and cord platelets. Cord blood was obtained by full-term placentas.

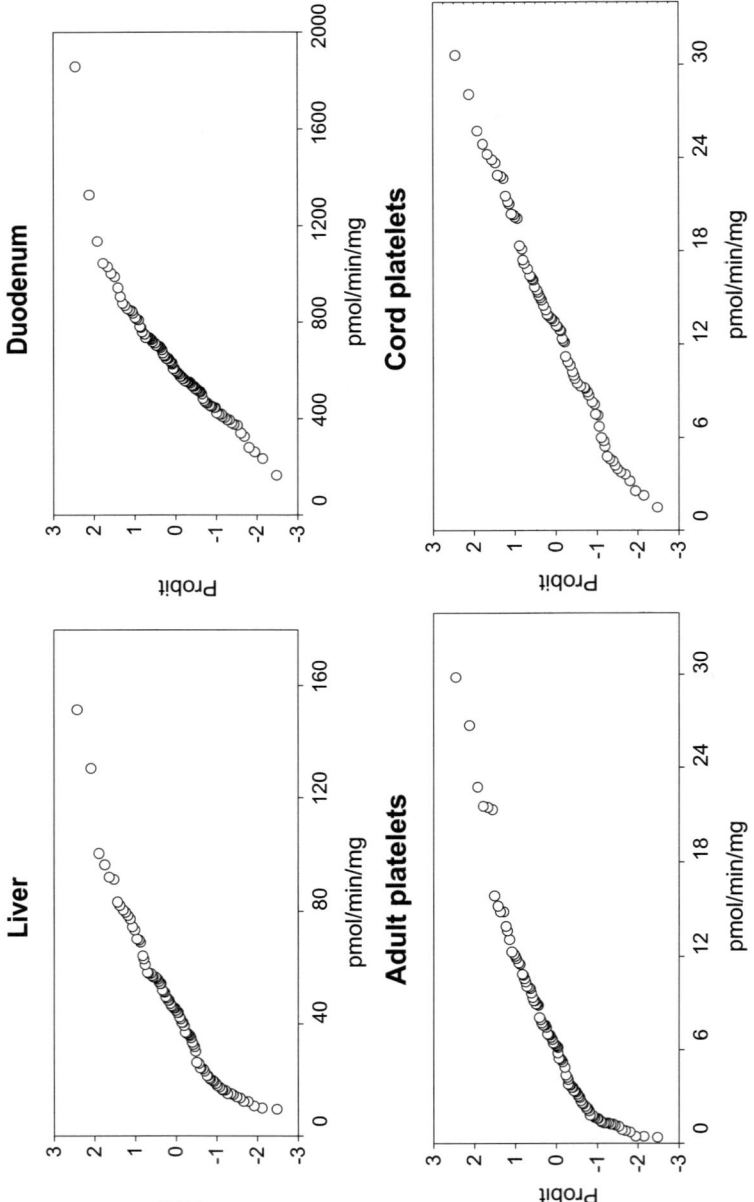

Figure 14.4 Probit plots of catechol sulfotransferase activity in the human liver, duodenum, adult and cord blood. Cord blood was obtained by full-term placentas.

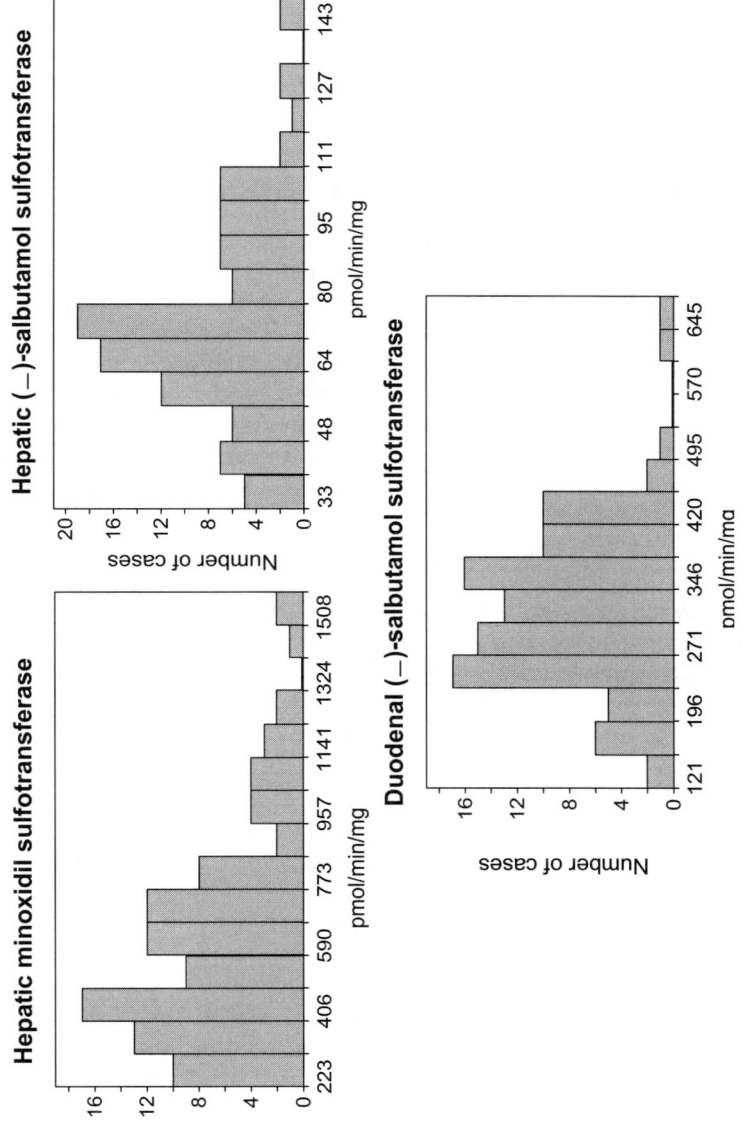

Figure 14.5 Frequency distribution histograms of sulfotransferase activities towards minoxidil and (−)-salbutamol.

and Figure 14.5). The same samples used to measure the activity of salbutamol ST were also used to measure the activities of phenol and catechol STs (results not shown). In the liver, the rate of salbutamol sulfation correlated with the activity of phenol ST ($r=0.853$; $p<0.001$), whereas in the duodenum the rate of salbutamol sulfation correlated with the activity of catechol ST ($r=0.914$; $p<0.001$), indicating that the rate of salbutamol sulfation correlated with the isoform most expressed both in liver and gut (Pacifici et al., 1997a).

Interindividual variability of dehydroepiandrosterone ST activity

The interindividual variability of dehydroepiandrosterone ST activity was described by Aksoy et al. (1993). DHEA-ST activity was assayed in 94 specimens of human liver: the authors found a lack of correlation between enzyme activity and age of the liver donors and a lack of gender regulation. The mean ($\pm$SD) was 5.3 ± 1.7 pmol/min/mg, with 4.6-fold range that varied from 2.2 to 10.2 pmol/min/mg. The frequency distribution histogram of DHEA-ST activity was bimodal with 25% included in a high activity subgroup. Consistent results were obtained with the probit analysis.

Interindividual variability of estrogen ST activity

Little is known on the interindividual variability of estrogen ST activity in man. Song et al. (1998) have observed a 25-fold variation in protein content and enzyme activity of EST in ten specimens of human liver. The enzyme activity was measured with 1.2 nM estradiol. There was no gender difference in enzyme activity. Both the content of EST and its activity were inhibited by alcohol. This finding is of particular importance as it was observed that alcohol intake increased free estrogen level in the blood by 300% in women who were given exogenous estrogen (Ginsburg et al., 1996). Likely, sulfation is quantitatively important in the metabolism of estrogens.

Interindividual variability of the ST activities is gender regulated

Dehydroepiandrosterone ST is believed to catalyse the sulfation of testosterone and other hydroxysteroids (Falany et al., 1989). The hepatic activities of ST towards testosterone (Pacifici et al., 1997b), budesonide (Pacifici et al., 1994b) and 1,2,3,4-tetrahydroisoquinoline (Pacifici et al., 1997c) were found higher in males than females. Table 14.4 and Figure 14.6 summarise the results of the ST activities gender regulated in females. The activities of ST towards testosterone and budesonide correlated

($r=0.81$; $p<0.001$). Testosterone inhibited the sulfation of budesonide and the IC_{50} of testosterone was 7 μM (Pacifici *et al.*, 1994b). The mean activities (pmol/min/mg) in males and females were 22.4 and 17.5, respectively (testosterone; $p<0.05$; Pacifici *et al.*, 1997b), 41.1 and 28.2, respectively (budesonide; $p<0.05$; Pacifici *et al.*, 1994b) and 544 and 455, respectively (1,2,3,4-tetrahydroisoquinoline; $p<0.05$; Pacifici *et al.*, 1997c). In the three studies, the number of females was greater than that of males and the results of the descriptive statistical analysis relative to females are summarised in Table 14.4 and in Figure 14.6. With the three substrates, the frequency distribution histogram was positively skewed and the fold of variation ranged from 2.2 to 4.3.

The genetic basis of ST variability

A superfamily of STs has been postulated on the basis of the considerable extent of similarity found at amino acid (aa) sequence level among sixteen different enzymes from bacterial, plant and mammalian species (Yamazoe *et al.*, 1994). More than thirty ST cDNAs have now been cloned, and they share a high degree of coding sequence homology, with conservation of the locations of most intron/exon splice junctions, further supporting the hypothesis that they arose from a common ancestor before plant–animal divergence. In particular four regions, presumably involved in the binding of PAPS, the cosubstrate for the sulfation reaction, are highly conserved throughout phylogeny (Weinshilboum *et al.*, 1997). The ST gene super-family includes phenol ST (PST), hydroxysteroid ST (HSST), and, in plants,

Table 14.4 Descriptive statistical analysis of the hepatic testosterone, budesonide and 1,2,3,4-tetrahydroisoquinoline sulfotransferase activities in females

Substrate	Testosterone	Budesonide	1,2,3,4-tetrahydro isoquinoline
Number of cases	60	65	60
Mean[a]	18.4	28.2	18.4
±S.D.[a]	8.2	12.4	8.2
Median[a]	16.8	26.0	16.8
5% Percentile[a]	9.4	11.6	294
95% Percentile[a]	20.9	50.4	872
Variation[b]	2.2	4.3	3.0
Skewness	2.770237	0.903959	0.707988
W-statistic	0.78406	0.94371	0.95129
p	<0.001	0.009	0.033
References	A	B	C

Notes
[a]The enzyme activity is expressed as pmol/mg/min.
[b]The variation is calculated by dividing the 95% percentile by the 5% percentile. W-statistic is the critical value of Shapiro and Wilk test. The distribution deviates from normality when $p<0.05$.
A: Pacifici *et al.*, 1997b; Pacifici *et al.*, 1994b; C: Pacifici *et al.*, 1997c.

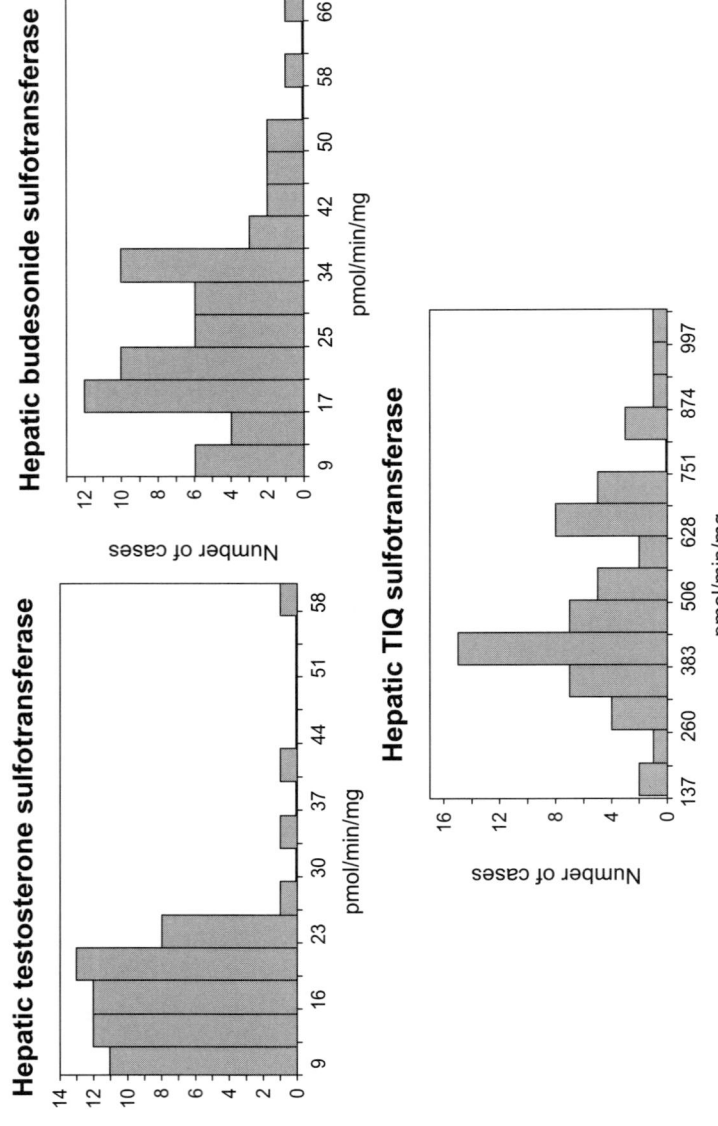

Figure 14.6 Frequency distribution histograms of sulfotransferase activities towards testosterone, budesonide and 1,2,3,4-tetrahydroisoquinoline in the liver of females.

flavonol ST (FST) families, members of which share at least 45% aa sequence identity. These families can be further subdivided into subfamilies that are at least 60% identical in aa sequence. For example, the PST family includes both PST and EST subfamilies, whereas HSST STs constitute a closely related family. Flavonol STs, showing lower degree of homology with PST-HSST families, presumably diverged earlier in the evolutionary history of STs.

Rikke and Roy (1996) conducted a phylogenetic analysis of twenty-five mammalian and four plant ST cDNA and gene sequences. This analysis supports the reliability of these family subgroupings and suggests that there are two additional groups: a thyroid hormone ST family (St1b1, also designated 1B1ST), and a N-hydroxy-2-acetylaminofluorene ST family (St1c1 or AAFST), defined so far only on the basis of their substrate specificity. A codon insertion not found in any of the other gene sequences appears to be characteristic of the St1b1 and St1c1 families.

The PST gene family

The human PST gene family presently includes three phenol ST genes (PST subfamily) and an estrogen ST gene (EST subfamily). Two additional genes, SULT1C1, the human horthologue of rat ST1C1, and a thyroid hormone preferring ST, also designated 1B1ST, have been recently identified and await better characterisation. Their divergence is comparable with that seen between PST and EST subfamilies, although it is possible that they have evolved within the PST family (Rikke and Roy, 1996).

The PST subfamily

The cloning of numerous cDNA isolates from different tissues has led to the understanding of the structural relationship between the members of the subfamily of human phenol ST genes. Three related forms of phenol-preferring STs (PST) implicated in the metabolism of catecholamines, thyroid hormones and several exogenous compounds are encoded by three genes. That is hTS-PST1 and hTS-PST2, encoding the two thermostable isoforms (TS-PST or P-PST), and hTL-PST, encoding a thermolabile or monoamine-preferring (TL-PST or MST) ST. Dooley (1998) recently reviewed the main features of this gene family.

Structure of the three PST subfamily members

The three PST genes have been finely localised to chromosome 16p12.1-p11.2, to the same region as CLN3, the gene for Batten disease (Dooley *et al.*, 1993; Dooley and Huang, 1996; Her *et al.*, 1996b). Using long PCR, Raftogianis *et al.* (1996) concluded that the hTS-PST1 is located approximately 45 kb 5′-upstream from hTS-PST2 and the two genes are aligned head to tail. They are, in turn, located about 100 kb telomeric to hTL-PST. hTS-PST1 and hTS-PST2 are 95.9% identical at the aa sequence level, whereas the TL-PST gene is only 92.9% and 90.5% identical to hTS-PST1 and hTS-PST2, respectively. Alignment of the genomic sequences indicated that all three genes have similar genomic organisation and conserved intron–exon boundaries, suggesting that all three arose by gene duplication. Further characterisation of the structural organisation of these genes better clarified the genetic mechanisms involved in the regulation of their activity in human tissues. hTS-PST1 spans approximately 4.4 kb and contains eight coding exons (Aksoy *et al.*, 1994a, b; Dooley *et al.*, 1994a, b). Bernier *et al.* (1996) compared the complete genomic sequence with the coding sequences of several cDNAs, corresponding to hTS-PST1, and confirmed that there are two mRNA species, with different 5′ UTRs. While one of the 5′ UTRs is included in the exon I, the other is located in the beginning of exon IIa. The remaining sequence in exon II that is identical to both mRNAs was termed exon IIb. Exons III to VIII, which cover the coding region and the 3′ UTR, are identical in all cDNAs. Both 5′-flanking sequences upstream from exon I and exon II, respectively, were shown to possess promoter activity, although no canonical TATA box sequences were found. These results suggested that hTS-PST1 possesses two alternative promoters that drive its expression in a tissue-specific manner. By RNA blot analysis the gene was found to be expressed in kidney, liver, lung, leukocyte, colon, small intestine and spleen.

hTS-PST2 spans approximately 5.1 kb and contains nine exons (Her *et al.*, 1996a). The two initial exons, IA and IB, are noncoding and represent two different mRNA 5′UTRs. No canonical TATA boxes, but CCAAT elements were found in the two 5′-flanking regions. hTL-PST consists of ten exons and nine introns, with a total length of approximately 8.4 kb (Aksoy and Weinshilboum, 1995). The first two exons are represented in the 5′UTR of a longer mRNA, while exon III is represented in the 5′UTR of a shorter mRNA, both being expressed in brain and liver tissues. Also in this case alternative transcription initiation and/or alternative splicing have been suggested as explanations for the existence of two mRNA species with two different 5′UTRs. The 5′-flanking region(s) contained neither canonical TATA nor CCAAT elements, but they did contain pyrimidine-rich stretches. Northern blot analyses showed that an mRNA species, approximately 1.4 kb in length, was expressed in human liver, kidney, lung, small intestine, spleen and leukocyte. Sakakibara *et al.* (1998) investigated the role of the different structure and sequence of the three loci in determining the distinct enzyme properties. They found that the internal domain spanning aa 84–148 is presumably the substrate specificity/catalytic domain of either TL-form or TS-form PST. Data on the kinetic constants (K_m, V_{max}, and V_{max}/K_m) further showed the differential roles of the two highly variable regions (region I spanning aa 84–89 and region II spanning aa 143–148) in substrate binding, catalysis and sensitivity to the inhibition by 2,6-dichloro-4-nitrophenol (DCNP).

Identification of hTS-PST1, hTS-PST2 and hTL-PST

A full length cDNA (1206 bp long) for the TS-form of phenol ST (P-PST-1) was isolated from a human liver cDNA library and characterised by Wilborn *et al.* (1993). The coding sequence predicted a 295-aa protein with a molecular mass of 34 kDa. *In vitro* expression of this cDNA generated a protein that comigrates with immunoreactive TS-PST from human liver and was endowed of ST activity toward two TS-PST-specific substrates, minoxidil and 4-nitrophenol. Northern blot analysis of human liver RNA detected a transcript of approximately 1.3 kb in length.

Other three human PST cDNAs, HAST1, HAST2 and HAST3 were isolated from liver and brain, respectively (Zhu *et al.*, 1993a, b). Liver HAST1 cDNA and brain HAST2 cDNA, respectively 1,155 bp and 1,179 bp long, had an identical coding domain but a different 5´ UTR. The coding sequence shared 80% homology to the rat aryl ST cDNA, 58% to the bovine and rat estrogen ST cDNAs, 53% to the rat hydroxysteroid ST cDNA and 51% to the human liver dehydroepiandrosterone ST cDNA. The deduced sequence was 79% homologous to that of the rat aryl ST cDNA and the putative PAPS-binding site motif GxxGxxK of the STs was strictly conserved. Brain HAST3 cDNA was 1,424 bp long and, when used as probe for Northern blot analysis, identified a 1.5 kb band in mRNA of human liver, colon, kidney and lung. The coding domains and the deduced 295-aa sequences of HAST1/2 and HAST3 were 93% identical.

COS-expressed HAST1/2 and HAST3 proteins were kinetically characterised using the model substrates for TS-PST and TL-PST, p-nitrophenol and dopamine (3,4-dihydroxyphenethylamine) respectively (Veronese *et al.*, 1994). HAST1 showed high affinity for p-nitrophenol, whereas dopamine was the preferred substrate for HAST3. Also the inhibition profiles with the ST inhibitor DCNP, thermal stabilities and electrophoretic mobilities (32 versus 34 kDa) were consistent with the differences observed for phenol preferring ST and monoamine preferring ST. Thus it was concluded that both HAST1 and HAST2 cDNAs correspond to the gene designated hTS-PST1 and HAST3 cDNA corresponds to the gene designated hTL-PST. Another cDNA for TL-PST was also isolated from human liver cDNA using a PCR-mediated strategy (Wood *et al.*, 1994). *In vitro* translation and COS-expression of this cDNA gave similar results. Two new human PST cDNAs, HAST4 and HAST4v, 1036 bp and 1060 bp long, respectively, were cloned from a liver cDNA library (Zhu *et al.*, 1996). The two COS-expressed proteins, that differed by two amino acids

(Thr7Ile and Thr235Asn), were unable to sulfonate dopamine and showed markedly different affinities for p-nitrophenol and for PAPS. HAST4v was regarded as an allelic variant of HAST4, which in turn represent a second gene encoding a thermostable phenol ST (hTS-PST2). The coding domains were 97 and 94% homologous to TS-PST1 and TL-PST, respectively.

A newly identified gene or an allelic variant (Hippocampal PST)?

Hwang *et al.* (1997) reported the characterisation of a member of the PST family, whose cDNA was isolated from human hippocampal (Hwang *et al.*, 1995). The hippocampal PST cDNA (H-PST) possesses differences in its deduced primary sequence compared with both TS and TL-PST isoforms. H-PST cDNA was expressed in bacterial expression system and the resulting protein is thermolabile, as well as TL-PST, but does not sulfate dopamine or neuropeptide substrates. In contrast with TL-PST, H-PST is sensitive to inhibition by DCNP (2,6-dichloro-4-nitrophenol) and prefers p-nitrophenol as substrate, as well as TS-PST.

The EST subfamily

The EST gene, localised to chromosome 4q13.1, spans approximately 20 kb and consists of eight exons. The locations of most exon–intron splice junctions are identical to those found in the three human PST genes. In addition, the locations of five EST introns are also conserved in the human dehydroepiandrosterone (DHEA) ST gene, HSST. The 5′-flanking region of EST gene contains one CCAAT and two TATA sequences (Her *et al.*, 1995).

Identification of EST gene

Using primers derived from the bovine placental estrogen ST (EST) sequence, Bernier *et al.* (1994a) amplified a probe to screen a human placental cDNA library in search for human placental EST. They isolated a 1.3-kb long cDNA, differing from brain PST cDNA only in the 5′ UTR. Using this cDNA as probe, Bernier *et al.* (1994b) screened a human leukocyte genomic library and isolated a clone containing almost the whole gene sequence. The chromosome location and the genomic structure were the same as those found for brain PST. They interpreted these results as indicating that brain PST and placental EST mRNA species are transcribed from a single gene by alternating two different promoters.

A distinct human estrogen ST (hEST-1) cDNA was isolated from a human liver cDNA library by Falany *et al.* (1995). The 994-bp long cDNA encodes a 294-aa protein (molecular mass of 35 kDa). Bacterial expression of the cDNA led to a purified product endowed with a significantly greater affinity for estrogen sulfation than the other human STs which also conjugate estrogens.

On the other hand, Aksoy *et al.* (1994b) had reported the cloning of a human liver EST cDNA (882-bp long) using a PCR-based strategy. They designed degenerate primers on the basis of highly conserved EST sequences in non-human species. The 294 aa deduced protein was 81%, 73%, and 72% identical to the aa sequences of guinea pig adrenocortical, bovine placental and rat liver ESTs, respectively. The transiently COS-expressed cDNA generated a protein that was characterised with regard to thermal stability, inhibition by 2,6-dichloro-4-nitrophenol (DCNP) and substrate specificity. Estrone, DHEA and 4-nitrophenol were efficiently sulfated, but not dopamine. This cDNA allowed the localisation of the estrogen ST gene (EST) to chromosome 4q13.1 by fluorescence *in situ* hybridisation (Her *et al.*, 1995).

It is possible that more than one gene encodes, ESTs and that the gene mapping to chromosome 4 by Her *et al.* (1995) and the one localised to chromosome 16 by Bernier *et al.* (1994a) are two separate EST genes. Recently, Gaedigk *et al.* (1997) reported the isolation of a genomic sequence that corresponds to TS-PST2, with a genomic structure resembling more than that of EST gene. This sequence, together with other two products, was generated from human genomic DNA or from genomic library using extra-long PCR (XL–PCR). However, the placental EST gene identified by Bernier *et al.*, (1994a) is most probably transcribed from TL-PST gene (Luu-The *et al.*, 1996).

SULT1C1, the human orthologue of rat ST1C1

Her *et al.* (1997) isolated from a fetal liver–spleen cDNA library a cDNA orthologue of a rat ST1C1 cDNA, which efficiently mediate the conversion of N-hydroxy-2-acetylaminofluorene (N-OH-AAF) into N-hydroxyary-lamine O-sulfates. The aa sequence, deduced from the 888-bp coding sequence of the cDNA designated SULT1C1, was 62% identical to that encoded by the rat ST1C1 cDNA and included signature sequences highly conserved among ST. Northern blot analyses identified a 1.4 kb mRNA, expressed in adult human stomach, kidney, and thyroid, as well as fetal kidney and liver. The gene was localised to chromosome 2q11.1-2 region by PCR-based somatic cell hybrid analysis. In spite of the structural similarity with rat ST1C1, the bacterial-expressed cDNA did not mediate PAPS-dependent DNA binding of N-OH-AAF (Yoshinari *et al.*, 1998)

Thyroid hormone-preferring ST

Human cDNAs encoding thyroid hormone ST have been isolated from liver cDNA libraries (Fujita *et al.*, 1997; Wang *et al.*, 1998). This cDNA consists of 1144 bp, contains a 888-bp coding sequence. The corresponding 296-aa sequence protein (molecular mass of 34 kDa) shares 77 and 74% homologies at nucleotidic and deduced aa levels with a rat ST1B1, but only 34% homology to DEHA-ST and 52–56% homology to TS-PST1 and 2, TL-PST and EST. These results indicate that it belongs to a new gene family of enzymes catalysing the sulfation of T3 as a typical endogenous substrate. The 5′ UTR is 127-bp long and the 3′UTR, including a 22-bp poly(A)+ tract, is 129-bp long. Northern blot and immunoblot analysis indicate that this cDNA is expressed in several human tissues. COS-expressed cDNA produced a 32.5 kDa protein, whose mobility was identical with proteins detected in human livers in Western blots using specific anti-(rat ST1B1) antibodies. The expressed protein sulfates small phenols such as 1-naphthol and p-nitrophenol and thyroid hormones, including 3,3′-diiodothyronine, triiodothyronine (T3), reverse triiodothyronine, and thyroxine. No activity was detected when several steroids, including beta-estradiol and dehydroepiandrosterone, or dopamine were tested as substrates.

The HSST family

The human gene for hydroxysteroid ST (HSST) was mapped on chromosome 19q13.3 (Otterness et al., 1995a, b). Using a biallelic polymorphism found in intron 2 and eight CEPH reference families for a refined linkage mapping, Durocher et al. (1995) confirmed the location of the HSST gene. The gene spans at least 17 kb and is composed of six exons and five introns (Otterness et al., 1995a). The 5′-flanking region was capable of promoting transcription of a reporter gene in human cells. Using primer extension analysis, Luu-The et al. (1995) located the transcription start site at nu 98 upstream from the ATG initiating codon. Putative TATA and CAAT boxes are situated at positions 72 and 96 upstream from the transcription start site, respectively. Northern blot analysis showed a strong signal in the adrenals and liver, whereas no signal was detected in the spleen, thymus, prostate, testis, ovary, small intestine, colon, peripheral blood leukocytes, heart, brain, placenta, lung, skeletal muscle, kidney, or pancreas (Luu-The et al., 1995).

Identification of HSST gene

Otterness et al. (1992), Kong et al. (1992) and Comer et al. (1993) reported the cloning of cDNAs encoding liver dehydroepiandrosterone (DHEA), or hydroxysteroid ST (STD or HSST).

Screening a human liver cDNA library, Otterness et al. (1992) isolated two cDNA clones, 1.1 kb and 1.8 kb long, respectively. Northern blot analysis confirmed the presence of 1.1 and 1.8 kb transcripts in human liver. The deduced 285-aa protein included two separate 27- and 23-aa sequences that were identical to those obtained by microsequencing of proteolytic fragments from purified human liver DHEA-ST. COS-expressed cDNAs produced enzymatically active DHEA-ST protein (molecular mass 35-kDa), which comigrated with purified human liver DHEA-ST. This translation product catalysed the sulfation of DHEA, but not the sulfation of model substrates for the two isoforms of PST. It displayed a pattern of inhibition by DCNP identical to that of human liver DHEA-ST.

Kong et al. (1992) also isolated two cDNA clones. The first consists of 1069 bp and contains an 855 bp coding sequence, beginning at nucleotide 65. A second cDNA (1563 bp long) with an identical coding region, was truncated 5′ at nucleotide 231 (lacking the first 15 amino acids). However, it had a much longer 3′ UTR. By Northern blot analysis on human liver RNA two mature mRNAs with sizes ranging from approximately 1.1 kb to 1.7 kb were detected, verifying the authenticity of the obtained cDNAs. From the sequence alignment, the coding region shares 62%/74%, 39%/59%, 35%/48%, 36%/54% identity with rSTa, rSTp (phenol), rSTe (estrogen), and bovine STe (bSTe) at the deduced amino acid and DNA levels, respectively.

Also Comer et al. (1993) isolated a 1060 bp long cDNA, designated DHEA-ST8, containing the same coding sequence. In vitro translation of DHEA-ST8 generated a protein identical in molecular size with that of DHEA-ST. The COS-expressed cDNA produced an active protein, capable of sulfating DHEA, with the same molecular mass as human liver DHEA-ST and recognised by rabbit anti-(human liver DHEA-ST) antibodies. Although Northern blot analysis of human liver RNA detected transcripts of three different sizes, Southern blot analysis of human DNA suggested that only one gene is present in the genome.

Another full-length cDNA clone, encoding human fetal adrenal HSST, was isolated by Forbes et al. (1995). The V79-expressed cDNA generated a protein identical to that isolated from adult human liver. Substrate specificity and kinetic properties of this enzyme towards various steroid hormones are very similar to the hepatic isoform.

Luu-The et al. (1996) have also cloned and sequenced the 1.8 kb DHEA-ST cDNA from human adrenal cDNA library. Except for one nucleotide difference, the human adrenal and liver DHEA-ST cDNAs were identical. Using expression vectors containing the chloramphenicol acetyl-transferase (CAT) reporter gene ligated to various fragments of the DHEA-ST gene promoter, Luu-The et al. (1996) have shown that DHEA-ST gene promoter activity is stimulated by estradiol (E2) and that E2 stimulation is inhibited by the anti-estrogen EM-139.

Genetic polymorphism and individual variation of TS and TL-PST

Evidence that there is individual variations in the activity of both TS and TL-PST in human platelets and that these variations are strongly influenced by inheritance has been known long before the PST genes were identified.

Twins and parent offspring correlation studies provided strong support for high heritability of TL-PST activity, and segregation analysis supported a major gene hypothesis or a polygenic model with high heritability (Price *et al.*, 1988). Analogously, TS-PST basal activity and thermal stability showed significant correlations among first degree relatives and segregation analysis supported a major gene hypothesis with a three-allele model. A major gene polymorphism in conjunction with a polygenic inheritance was proposed by Price *et al.* (1989). Weinshilboum (1988) suggested that a structural gene polymorphism may be one mechanism by which inheritance controls TS and TL-PST activities in humans. They suggested that the isoforms of TS-PST in the liver may represent the products of alternative alleles for this polymorphism, that is different alleles might control the structure of TS-PST in many human tissues. Later, it was clarified that TS and TL-PST activities in platelets are regulated by separate common genetic polymorphisms (Weinshilboum and Askoy, 1994). Two cDNAs, isolated from human platelets mRNA and encoding phenol and catechol sulfotransferases, contained five and two aa changes from the other two previously published sequences from human liver and brain, and they were interpreted as new allelic variants (Jones *et al.*, 1995). A *Hin*dIII RFLP polymorphism was also discovered in the hTS-PST1 (Henkel *et al.*, 1995). Common polymorphism associated with phenotypic variation in both platelets TS-PST activity and thermal stability were reported by Raftogianis *et al.* (1997). They measured platelets TS-PST activity and thermal stability on 905 human subjects. They found more than fifty-fold activity variation and over ten-fold thermal stability variation. "Extreme" TS-PST activities, that is high activity/thermal stability, were detected in thirty-three subjects. These thirty-three subjects were genotyped for TS-PST, designated SULT1A1, by PCR amplification and sequencing of the entire coding sequence, as well as approximately 1 kb of intron DNA sequence. One common allele SULT1A1*2 (Arg213His) was uniformly associated with both very low TS-PST activity and low thermal stability. The allele frequency of SULT1A1*2 in a random selected population sample of 150 Caucasian blood donors was 0.31 (31%), indicating that approximately 9% of this population would be homozygous for that allele. Two other variants (SULT1A1*3 Met223Val and SULT1A1*4 Arg37Gln) were also found. SULT1A1*2 and SULT1A1*3 alleles were also detected by Ozawa *et al.* (1998). Among fifty-two human liver samples, twenty-eight individuals were homozygous 1/1 (Arg213), fifteen individuals were heterozygous 1/2 and nine homozygous 2/2 (His213). No homozygous 3/3 and only three heterozygous (1/3) were observed, confirming that SULT1A1*3 allele is less frequent than SULT1A1*2. The SULT1A1*1 and SULT1A1*2 alleles have also been found in a Japanese population ($n=143$), with allele frequencies of 83.2 and 16.8%, respectively, whilst SULT1A1*3 allele was not found (Ozawa *et al.*, 1999).

Comparable frequencies of SULT1A1*2 allele were also found among 293 Caucasian donors and fifty-two Nigerian donors by Coughtrie *et al.* (1999). They also observed an increasing incidence of SULT1A1*1 homozygosity and decreasing incidence of SULT1A1*2 homozygosity within the Caucasian population, significantly associated with increasing age. Thus, SULT1A1*1 alleles are potentially protective against cell and/or tissue damage during ageing. Common nucleotide polymorphisms have also been found at SULT1A2 locus (Raftogianis *et al.*, 1999). Among sixty-one individuals, thirteen different alleles were detected. These ones were in linkage disequilibrium with alleles at SULT1A1 locus and were associated with individual differences in phenol SULT properties in the liver.

Genetic polymorphism and individual variation of EST and DHEA-ST

Although the pharmacogenetic strategy used to study TS and TL-PST could not be applied to EST and DHEA-ST, since these enzymes are not expressed in human blood elements, interindividual variation of both activities has been observed in liver and jejunal mucosa samples (Askoy *et al.*, 1993; Her *et al.*, 1996b; Song *et al.*, 1998). Two nucleotide changes, that is a T170C transition in exon 2, resulting in Met57Thr aa change, and a A557T transversion in exon 4, resulting in Glu186Val aa change, were detected by examining the coding region and the 5'-flanking region corresponding to the DHEA-ST gene (HSST) of three low- and three high-activity subjects (Wood *et al.*, 1996). Exon 2 and 4 were analysed in an additional 87 liver samples, that had been previously phenotyped. The allele frequency for the exon 2 polymorphism was 0.0027, whereas that for the exon 4 polymorphism was 0.038, but neither polymorphism was systematically related to the level of enzyme activity in these samples. Transient COS expression of cDNA that contained nucleotide 170 and 557 polymorphisms, either separately or together, was analysed. A decreased expression of both DHEA-ST enzyme activity and level of immuno-suppressive protein was observed only when the nucleotide 557 variant was present. It is not yet clear whether this polymorphism might affect DHEA-ST expression and/or function *in vivo* and account for the observed interindividual variation.

The variation in the hepatic expression and activity of EST observed by Song *et al.* (1998) might also be under genetic control, although no variant allele has so far been detected at the EST locus.

Although several genes encoding STs have been found to be polymorphic and the extent of these polymorphisms is currently under investigation, it is not yet clear whether the observed variability can be completely explained by the presence of various alleles in the population. The problem appears to be still bound to the separation of distinct contribution to each

ST activity by multiple enzymes with specific biochemical properties but with a largely overlapping of substrate specificity. Further studies will provide a better understanding of the regulation mechanisms underlying the expression of these enzymes, often under coordinated control, in response to either endogenous compounds and influenced by gender and age in a complex way.

References

Aksoy, I. A., Callen, D. F., Apostolou, S., Her, C. and Weinshilboum, R. M. (1994a) 'Thermolabile phenol sulfotransferase gene (STM): localisation to human chromosome 16p11.2', *Genomics* 23: 275–7.

Aksoy, I. A., Sochorova, V. and Weinshilboum, R. M. (1993) 'Human liver dehydro-epiandrosterone sulfotransferase: nature and extent of individual variation', *Clin. Pharmacol. Ther.* 54: 498–506.

Aksoy, I. A. and Weinshilboum, R. M. (1995) 'Human thermolabile phenol sulfotransferase gene (STM): molecular cloning and structural characterization', *Biochem. Biophys. Res. Commun.* 208: 786–95.

Aksoy, I. A., Wood, T. C. and Weinshilboum, R. (1994b) 'Human liver estrogen sulfotransferase: identification by cDNA cloning and expression', *Biochem. Biophys. Res. Commun.* 200: 1621–9.

Bernier, F., Leblanc, G., Labrie, F. and Luu-The, V. (1994b) 'Structure of human estrogen and aryl sulfotransferase gene. Two mRNA species issued from a single gene', *J. Biol. Chem.* 269: 28200–5.

Bernier, F., Lopez Solache, I., Labrie, F. and Luu-The, V. (1994a) 'Cloning and expression of cDNA encoding human placental estrogen sulfotransferase', *Mol. Cell. Endocrinol.* 99: R11–R15.

Bernier, F., Soucy, P. and Luu-The, V. (1996) 'Human phenol sulfotransferase gene contains two alternative promoters: structure and expression of the gene', *DNA Cell. Biol.* 15: 367–75.

Campbell, N. R. C., Van Loon, J. A. and Weinshilboum, R. M. (1987) 'Human sulphotransferase: assay conditions, biochemical properties and partial purification of isozymes of the thermostable form', *Biochem. Pharmacol.* 36: 1435–46.

Cappiello, M., Giuliani, L. and Pacifici, G. M. (1990) 'Differential distribution of phenol and catechol sulfotransferases in human liver and intestinal mucosa', *Pharmacology* 40: 69–76.

Carter, S. M. B., Rein, G., Glover, V., Sandler, M. and Caldwell, J. (1983) 'Human phenolsulfotransferase M and P: substrate specificities and correlation with in vivo sulphate conjugation of paracetamol and salicylamide', *Br. J. Clin. Pharmacol.* 15: 323–30.

Comer, K. A., Falany, J. L. and Falany, C. N. (1993) 'Cloning and expression of human liver dehydroepiandrosterone sulphotransferase', *Biochem. J.* 289: 233–40.

Coughtrie, M. W., Glissen, R. A., Shek, B., Strange, R. C., Fryer, A. A., Johes, P. W. and Bamber, D. E. (1999) 'Phenol sulfotransferase SULT1A1 polymorphism: molecular diagnosis and allele frequencies in Caucasian and African populations', *Biochem. J.* 337: 45–9.

Dooley, T. P. (1998) 'Cloning of the human phenol sulfotransferase gene family: three genes implicated in the metabolism of catecholamines, thyroid hormones and drugs', *Chem. Biol. Interact.* **109**: 29–41.

Dooley, T. P. and Huang, Z. (1996) 'Genomic organization and DNA sequences of two human phenol sulfotransferase genes (STP1 and STP2) on the short arm of chromosome 16', *Biochem. Biophys. Res. Commun.* **228**: 134–40.

Dooley, T. P., Mitchison, H. M., Munroe, P. B., Probst, P., Neal, M., Siciliano, M. J., Deng, Z., Doggett, N. A., Callen, D. F. and Gardiner, R. M., *et al.* (1994a) 'Mapping of two phenol sulphotransferase genes, STP and STM, to 16p: candidate genes for Batten disease', *Biochem. Biophys. Res. Commun.* **205**: 482–9.

Dooley, T. P., Obermoeller, R. D., Leiter, E. H., Chapman, H. D., Falany, C. N., Deng, Z. and Siciliano, M. J. (1993) 'Mapping of the phenol sulfotransferase gene (STP) to human chromosome 16p12.1-p11.2 and to mouse chromosome 7', *Genomics* **18**: 440–3.

Dooley, T. P., Probst, P., Munroe, P. B., Mole, S. E., Liu, Z. and Doggett, N. A. (1994b) 'Genomic organization and DNA sequence of the human catecholamine-sulfating phenol sulfotransferase gene (STM)', *Biochem. Biophys. Res. Commun.* **205**: 1325–32.

Durocher, F., Morissette, J., Dufort, I., Simard, J. and Luu-The, V. (1995) 'Genetic linkage mapping of the dehydroepiandrosterone sulfotransferase (STD) gene on the chromosome 19q13.3 region', *Genomics* **29**: 781–3.

Falany, C. N. (1991) 'Molecular enzymology of human liver cytosolic sulpho-transferase', *Trends. Pharmacol. Sci.* **12**: 255–9.

Falany, C. N., Krasnykh, V. and Falany, J. L. (1995) 'Bacterial expression and characterisation of a cDNA for human liver estrogen sulfotransferase', *J. Steroid. Biochem. Molec. Biol.* **52**: 529–39.

Falany, C. N., Vazquez, M. E. and Kalab, J. M. (1989) 'Purification and characterisation of human liver dehydroepiandrosterone sulphotransferase', *Biochem. J.* **260**: 641–6.

Falany, J. L. and Falany, C. N. (1996) 'Regulation of estrogen sulfotransferase in human endometrial adenocarcinoma cells by progesterone', *Endocrinology* **137**: 1395–401.

Forbes, K. J., Hagen, M., Glatt, H., Hume, R. and Coughtrie, M. W. (1995) 'Human fetal adrenal hydroxysteroid sulphotransferase: cDNA cloning, stable expression in V79 cells and functional characterisation of the expressed enzyme', *Mol. Cell. Endocrinol.* **112**: 53–60.

Fujita, K., Nagata, K., Ozawa, S., Sasano, H. and Yamazoe, Y. (1997) 'Molecular cloning and characterization of rat ST1B1 and human ST1B2 cDNAs, encoding thyroid hormone sulfotransferases', *J. Biochem. (Tokyo)* **122**: 1052–61.

Gaedigk, A., Beatty, B. G. and Grant, D. M. (1997) 'Cloning, structural organization, and chromosomal mapping of the human phenol sulfotransferase STP2 gene', *Genomics* **40**: 242–6.

Ginsburg, E. L., Mello, N. K., Mendelson, J. H., Barbieri, R. L., Teoh, S. K., Rothman, M., Gao, X. and Sholar, J. M. (1996) 'Effects of alcohol ingestion on estrogens in postmenopausal women', *JAMA* **276**: 1747–51.

Henkel, R. D., Galindo, L. V. and Dooley, T. P. (1995) 'Detection of a HindIII restriction fragment length polymorphism in the human phenol sulfotransferase (STP) locus', *Hum Genet* **95**: 245–6.

Her, C., Aksoy, I. A., Kimura, S., Brandriff, B. F., Wasmuth, J. J. and Weinshilboum, R. M. (1997) 'Human estrogen sulfotransferase gene (STE): cloning, structure, and chromosomal localization', *Genomics* 29: 16–23.

Her, C., Kaur, G. P., Athwal, R. S. and Weinshilboum, R. M. (1997) 'Human sulfotransferase SULT1C1: cDNA cloning, tissue-specific expression, and chromosomal localization', *Genomics* 41: 467–70.

Her, C., Raftogianis, R. and Weinshilboum, R. M. (1996a) 'Human phenol sulfotransferase STP2 gene: molecular cloning, structural characterization, and chromosomal localization', *Genomics* 33: 409–20.

Her, C., Szumlanski, C., Aksoy, I. A. and Weinshilboum, R. M. (1996b) 'Human jejunal estrogen sulfotransferase and dehydroepiandrosterone sulfotransferase: immunochemical characterization of individual variation', *Drug Metab. Dispos.* 24: 1328–35.

Huttner, W. B. (1982) 'Sulphation of tyrosine residues a widespread modification of proteins', *Nature* 299: 273–6.

Hwang, S. R., Kohn, A. B. and Hook, V. Y. (1995) 'Molecular cloning of an isoform of phenol sulfotransferase from human brain hippocampus', *Biochem. Biophys. Res. Commun.* 207: 701–7.

Hwang, S. R., Palkovits, M. and Hook, V. Y. (1997) 'High level expression and characterization of recombinant human hippocampus phenol sulfotransferase: a novel phenol-sulfating form of phenol sulfotransferase', *Protein. Expr. Purif.* 11: 125–34.

Inoue, H., Otsu, K., Masahiko, Y., Kimata, K., Suzuki, S. and Nakanishi, Y. (1986) 'Glycosaminoglycan sulphotransferase in human and animal sera', *J. Biol. Chem.* 261: 4460–9.

Jones, A. L., Hagen, M., Coughtrie, M. W., Roberts, R. C. and Glatt, H. (1995) 'Human platelet phenolsulfotransferases: cDNA cloning, stable expression in V79 cells and identification of a novel allelic variant of the phenol-sulfating form', *Biochem. Biophys. Res. Commun.* 208: 855–62.

Kong, A. N., Yang, L., Ma, M., Tao, D. and Bjornsson, T. D. (1992) 'Molecular cloning of the alcohol/hydroxysteroid form (hSTa) of sulfotransferase from human liver', *Biochem. Biophys. Res. Commun.* 187: 448–54.

Lin, W.-H. and Roth, J. A. (1990) 'Characterisation of a tyrosylprotein sulphotransferase in human liver', *Biochem. Pharmacol.* 40: 629–35.

Luu-The, V., Bernier, F. and Dufort, I. (1996) 'Steroid sulfotransferases', *J. Endocrinol.* 150 (Suppl.): 87–97.

Luu-The, V., Dufort, I., Paquet, N., Reimnitz, G. and Labrie, F. (1995) 'Structural characterization and expression of the human dehydroepiandrosterone sulfotransferase gene', *DNA. Cell. Biol.* 14: 511–18.

McCall, J. M., Aiken, J. W., Chigester, C. G., Ducarme, D. W. and Wendling, M. G. (1983) 'Pyrimidine and triazine 3-oxide sulfates: a new family of vasodilators', *J. Med. Chem.* 26: 1791–3.

Mulder, G. J. and Jakoby, W. B. (1990) 'Sulphation', in G. J. Mulder (ed.) *Conjugation Reactions in Drug Metabolism*, London: Taylor & Francis, 107–61.

Otterness, D. M., Her, C., Aksoy, S., Kimura, S., Wieben, E. D. and Weinshilboum, R. M. (1995a) 'Human dehydroepiandrosterone sulfotransferase gene: molecular cloning and structural characterization', *DNA Cell Biol.* 14: 331–41.

Otterness, D. M., Mohrenweiser, H. W., Brandriff, B. F. and Weinshilboum, R. M. (1995b) 'Dehydroepiandrosterone sulfotransferase gene (STD): localization to human chromosome band 19q13.3', *Cytogenet Cell Genet.* **70**: 45–7.

Otterness, D. M., Wieben, E. D., Wood, T. C., Watson, W. G., Madden, B. J., McCormick, D. J. and Weinshilboum, R. M. (1992) 'Human liver dehydroepiandrosterone sulfotransferase: molecular cloning and expression of cDNA', *Mol. Pharmacol.* **41**: 865–72.

Ozawa, S., Shimizu, M., Katoh, T., Miyajima, A., Ohno, Y., Matsumoto, Y., Fukuoka, M., Tang, Y. M., Lang, N. P. and Kadlubar, F. F. (1999) 'Sulfating-activity and stability of cDNA-expressed allozymes of human phenol sulfotransferase, ST1A3*1 ((213)Arg) and ST1A3*2 ((213)His), both of which exist in Japanese as well as Caucasians', *J. Biochem. (Tokyo)* **126**: 271–7.

Ozawa, S., Tang, Y. M., Yamazoe, Y., Kato, R., Lang, N. P. and Kadlubar, F. F. (1998) 'Genetic polymorphisms in human liver phenol sulfotransferases involved in the bioactivation of N-hydroxy derivatives of carcinogenic arylamines and heterocyclic amines', *Chem. Biol. Interact.* **109**: 237–48.

Pacifici, G. M., Bigotti, R., Marchi, G. and Giuliani, L. (1993) 'Minoxidil sulphation in human liver and platelets', *Eur. J. Clin. Pharmacol.* **45**: 337–41.

Pacifici, G. M., D'Alessandro, C., Gucci, A. and Giuliani, L. (1997c) 'Sulphation of the heterocyclic amine 1,2,3,4-tetrahydroisoquinoline in the human liver and intestinal mucosa: interindividual variability', *Arch. Toxicol.* **71**: 477–81.

Pacifici, G. M. and De Santi, C. (1995) 'Human sulphotransferase. Classification and metabolic profile of the major isoforms. The point of view of the clinical pharmacologist' in G. M. Pacifici and G. N. Fracchia (eds) *Advances in Drug Metabolism in Man*, European Commission (EUR 15439 – ISBN 92-827-3982-1) Luxembourg/Brussels: 312–49

Pacifici, G. M., Ferroni, M. A., Temellini, A., Gucci, A., Morelli, M. C. and Giuliani, L. (1994b) 'Human liver budesonide sulphotransferase is inhibited by testosterone and correlates with testosterone sulphotransferase', *Eur. J. Clin. Pharmacol.* **46**: 49–54.

Pacifici, G. M., Giulianetti, B., Quilici, M. C., Spisni, R., Nervi, M., Giuliani, L. and Gomeni, R. (1997a) '(−)-Salbutamol sulphotransferase in the human liver and duodenal mucosa: interindividual variability', *Xenobiotica* **27**: 279– 86.

Pacifici, G. M., Gucci, A. and Giuliani, L. (1997b) 'Testosterone sulphation and glucuronidation in the human liver: interindividual variability', *Eur. J. Drug. Metab. Pharmacokin.* **22**: 253–8.

Pacifici, G. M. and Marchi, G. (1993) 'Interindividual variability of phenol and catechol sulphotransferase in platelets from adult and newborn', *Br. J. Clin. Pharmacol.* **36**: 593–7.

Pacifici, G. M., Temellini, A., Castiglioni, C., D'Alessandro, C., Ducci, A. and Giuliani, L. (1994a) 'Interindividual variability of the human hepatic sulphotransferase', *Chem-Biol. Interact.* **92**: 219–31.

Price, R. A., Cox, N. J., Spielman, R. S., Van Loon, J. A., Maidak, B. L. and Weinshilboum, R. M. (1988) 'Inheritance of human platelet thermolabile phenol sulfotransferase (TL PST) activity', *Genet. Epidemiol.* **5**: 1–15.

Price, R. A., Spielman, R. S., Lucena, A. L., Van Loon, J. A., Maidak, B. L. and Weinshilboum, R. M. (1989) 'Genetic polymorphism for human platelet thermostable phenol sulfotransferase (TS PST) activity', *Genetics* **122**: 905–14.

Raftogianis, R. B., Her, C. and Weinshilboum, R. M. (1996) 'Human phenol sulfotransferase pharmacogenetics: STP1 gene cloning and structural chracterization', *Pharmacogenetics* **6**: 473–87.

Raftogianis, R. B., Wood, T. C., Otterness, D. M., Van Loon, J. A. and Weinshilboum, R. M. (1997) 'Phenol sulfotransferase pharmacogenetics in humans: association of common SULT1A1 alleles with TS PST phenotype', *Biochem. Biophys. Res. Commun.* **239**: 298–304.

Raftogianis, R. B., Wood, T. C. and Weinshilboum, R. M. (1999) 'Human phenol sulfotransferases SULT1A2 and SULT1A1: genetic polymorphisms, allozyme properties, and human liver genotype-phenotype correlations', *Biochem. Pharmacol.* **58**: 605–16.

Razi, N. and Lindahl, U. (1995) 'Biosynthesis of heparin/heparan sulphate', *J. Biol. Chem.* **270**: 11267–75.

Rens-Domiano, S. and Roth, J. A. (1989) 'Characterisation of tyrosylprotein sulphotransferase from rat liver and other tissues', *J. Biol. Chem.* **264**: 899–905.

Rikke, B. A. and Roy, A. K. (1996) 'Structural relationships among members of the mammalian sulfotransferase gene family', *Biochim. Biophys. Acta.* **1307**: 331–8.

Sakakibara, Y., Takami, Y., Nakayama, T., Suiko, M. and Liu, M. C. (1998) 'Localization and functional analysis of the substrate specificity/catalytic domains of human M-form and P-form phenol sulfotransferases', *J. Biol. Chem.* **273**: 6242–7.

Song, W.-C., Qian, Y. and Li, A. P. (1998) 'Estrogen sulphotransferase expression in the human liver: marked interindividual variation and lack of gender specificity', *J. Pharmacol. Exp. Ther.* **284**: 1197–202.

Sundaram, R. S., Szumlaski, C., Otterness, D., Van Loon, J. A. and Weinshilboum, R. M. (1989) 'Human intestinal phenol sulphotransferase: assay conditions, activity level and partial purification of the thermolabile form', *Drug Metab. Dispos.* **17**: 255–64.

Veronese, M. E., Burgess, W., Zhu, X. and McManus, M. E. (1994) 'Functional characterization of two human sulphotransferase cDNAs that encode monoamine- and phenol-sulphating forms of phenol sulphotransferase: substrate kinetics, thermal-stability and inhibitor-sensitivity studies', *Biochem. J.* **302**: 497–502.

Wang, J., Falany, J. L. and Falany, C. N. (1998) 'Expression and characterization of a novel thyroid hormone-sulfating form of cytosolic sulfotransferase from human liver', *Mol. Pharmacol.* **53**: 274–82.

Weinshilboum, R. (1988) 'Phenol sulfotransferase inheritance', *Cell. Mol. Neurobiol.* **8**: 27–34.

Weinshilboum, R. M. (1986) 'Phenol sulphotransferase in humans: properties, regulation, and function', *Federation. Proc.* **45**: 2223–8.

Weinshilboum, R. and Aksoy, I. (1994) 'Sulfation pharmacogenetics in humans', *Chem. Biol. Interact.* **92**: 233–46.

Weinshilboum, R. M., Otterness, D. M., Aksoy, I. A., Wood, T. C., Her, C. and Raftogianis, R. B. (1997) 'Sulfation and sulfotransferases 1: sulfotransferase molecular biology: cDNAs and genes', *FASEB J.* **11**: 3–14.

Wilborn, T. W., Comer, K. A., Dooley, T. P., Reardon, I. M., Heinrikson, R. L. and Falany, C. N. (1993) 'Sequence analysis and expression of the cDNA for the phenol-sulfating form of human liver phenol sulfotransferase', *Mol. Pharmacol.* **43**: 70–7.

Wood, T. C., Aksoy, I. A., Aksoy, S. and Weinshilboum, R. M. (1994) 'Human liver thermolabile phenol sulfotransferase: cDNA cloning, expression and characterization', *Biochem. Biophys. Res. Commun.* **198**: 1119–27.

Wood, T. C., Her, C., Aksoy, I., Otterness, D. M. and Weinshilboum, R. M. (1996) 'Human dehydroepiandrosterone sulfotransferase pharmacogenetics: quantitative Western analysis and gene sequence polymorphisms', *J. Steroid. Biochem. Mol. Biol.* **59**: 467–78.

Yamazoe, Y., Nagata, K., Ozawa, S. and Kato R. (1994) 'Structural similarity and diversity of sulfotransferases', *Chem. Biol. Interact.* **92**: 107–17.

Yoshinari, K., Nagata, K., Shimada, M. and Yamazoe, Y. (1998) 'Molecular characterization of ST1C1-related human sulfotransferase', *Carcinogenesis* **19**: 951–3.

Zhu, X., Veronese, M. E., Bernard, C. C., Sansom, L. N. and McManus, M. E. (1993b) 'Identification of two human brain aryl sulfotransferase cDNAs', *Biochem. Biophys. Res. Commun.* **195**: 120–7.

Zhu, X., Veronese, M. E., Iocco, P. and McManus, M. E. (1996) 'cDNA cloning and expression of a new form of human aryl sulfotransferase', *Int. J. Biochem. Cell. Biol.* **28**: 565–71.

Zhu, X., Veronese, M. E., Sansom, L. N. and McManus, M. E. (1993a) 'Molecular characterisation of a human aryl sulfotransferase cDNA', *Biochem. Biophys. Res. Commun.* **192**: 671–6.

Chapter 15

Interindividual variability of glutathione transferase expression

A.-S. Johansson and B. Mannervik

Abbreviations

ACTH, adrenocorticotropic hormone; BCNU, 1,3-bis-(2-chloroethyl)-1-nitrosourea; BHA, 2(3)-*tert*-butyl-4-hydroxyanisole; (+)-*anti*-BPDE, (+)-*anti*-benzo[*a*]pyrene-7,8-diol 9,10-epoxide; CDNB, 1-chloro-2,4-dinitrobenzene; DEB, 1,2,3,4-diepoxybutane; G-site, glutathione binding site; GST, glutathione transferase; HPLC, high performance liquid chromatography; HPV, human papilloma virus; H-site, hydrophobic substrate binding site; HSTF, heat-shock transcription factor; MGST1; microsomal glutathione transferase; NF-GMa, nuclear factor for granulocyte/macrophage colony-stimulating factor gene promoter a; PAH, polycyclic aromatic hydrocarbon; PAGE, polyacrylamide gel electrophoresis; PCR, polymerase chain reaction; RFLP, restriction fragment length polymorphism; SCE, sister chromatid exchange; SDS, sodium dodecyl sulfate

Introduction

Glutathione transferases (GSTs) function as detoxication enzymes and are generally considered to play a prominent role in cellular defense against electrophilic chemical species, of endogenous as well as xenobiotic origins. It is reasonable to assume that variabilities in the expression of these detoxication enzymes in humans would alter the biotransformation of many carcinogens and other noxious agents that may serve as etiological factors in degenerative processes. The absence of specific isoenzymes affects the tolerance of the organism to chemical challenges and may result in an increased rate of somatic mutations and higher susceptibility to disease. The following chapter describes the multiplicity of GSTs, the variability in their expression, and known genetic polymorphisms in humans. The impact on detoxication at the levels of enzymes, cells, and the organism, as well as the causes underlying the differential expression of GSTs are also reviewed. The regulation of GST gene transcription is an area subject to active research (Rushmore and Pickett, 1993; Daniel, 1993; Hayes and Pulford, 1995), but considered to be outside the scope of this chapter.

Discovery of multiple forms of glutathione transferases

GSTs were discovered in the rat liver cytosol fraction by measurement of the enzyme-catalysed conjugation of aryl halides with glutathione (Booth *et al.*, 1961; Combes and Stakelum, 1961). Crude fractionations, heat inactivation and use of alternative electrophilic substrates led to the conclusion that several enzymes with different substrate specificities exist (Boyland and Chasseaud, 1969). The introduction of purification methods with higher resolution led to the identification of "isoenzymes" in the original sense of the descriptor, i.e. enzymes catalysing the same reaction (Habig *et al.*, 1974; Askelöf *et al.*, 1975; Mannervik, 1985). The nature of the multiple forms was further clarified when it was demonstrated that GST isoenzymes occur as binary combinations of protein subunits with different substrate specificities (Mannervik and Jensson, 1982). The functional properties of a heterodimeric GST can be accurately predicted as the composite of those of the corresponding homodimers based on substrate saturation curves (Danielson and Mannervik, 1985; Gustafsson and Mannervik, 1999) as well as by titrations with inhibitors (Tahir and Mannervik, 1986). Thus, experimental tools were created for the separation and identification of the multiple forms of GST in biological tissues. Human GSTs with different isoelectric points were demonstrated in human liver (Kamisaka *et al.*, 1975). Differences in chromatographic profiles among samples from different livers were noted, but the substrates used to characterise the multiple forms did not reveal any significant differences in their catalytic properties. It was therefore believed that the multiple forms represented degraded variants of a single gene product. The existence of a true polymorphism in the occurrence of human GSTs was first demonstrated (Figure 15.1) when it was found that some, but not all, individuals expressed a major distinct GST with catalytic properties that were significantly different from those of the previously described hepatic enzyme (Warholm *et al.*, 1980). This novel form with a near-neutral isoelectric point was initially called GST μ, and is now known as GST M1-1.

Human GSTs can be divided into two main categories: membrane-bound GSTs and soluble GSTs. The latter category is often referred to as cytosolic GSTs, although it includes members that may be localised in the mitochondria and the nucleus.

Glutathione transferase nomenclature

The systematic name of GSTs is "RX: glutathione R-transferase" (EC 2.5.1.18) and the Enzyme Commission has recommended the trivial name "glutathione transferase" without a prefix. The abbreviation GST is nevertheless adequate. The commonly used "glutathione *S*-transferase" is a misnomer since the sulfur is not transferred, but the R-substituent, or the glutathionyl group (GS-) of the substrates RX and GSH, respectively.

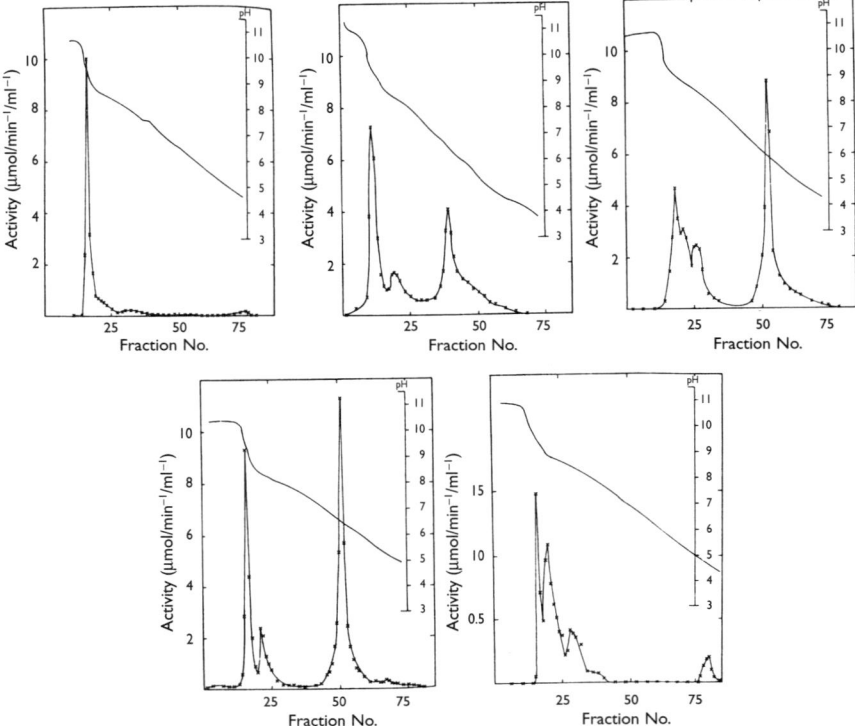

Figure 15.1 Polymorphism in the expression of glutathione transferases in human liver. The cytosol fraction of liver samples from five individuals was analysed by isoelectric focusing followed by activity measurements with 1-chloro-2,4-dinitrobenzene. The activity peaks found at high pH values (to the left in the activity profiles) correspond to Alpha class GSTs, including GST A1-1, GST A1-2, and GST A2-2. The peak found at approximately pH 6.5 in three of the samples (top middle and right, bottom left) corresponds to the polymorphic GST M1-1. Isoelectric points of human GSTs have been compiled by Mannervik and Widersten (1995). The graphs have been reproduced from Warholm et al. (1980) with permission from the publisher.

A unifying nomenclature for the mammalian GSTs and their corresponding genes has been introduced (Mannervik *et al.*, 1992). The membrane-bound GSTs, originally identified in the microsome fraction, are designated MGST followed by an Arabic numeral. The first enzyme characterised, often referred to as "microsomal GST", is thus called MGST1. The corresponding gene is designated *MGST1* (italicised). Other members in this category have not yet been incorporated into this nomenclature system.

The soluble GSTs are subdivided into classes based on sequence similarities that reflect evolutionary branches from an ancestral protein (Mannervik *et al.*, 1985). The classes are designated by the names of Greek letters: alpha, mu, pi etc., and are abbreviated A, M, P and so on. A given class may contain one or several protein sequences (i.e. subunits), and they are numbered using Arabic numerals. The gene for the Alpha class subunit 1 is accordingly written *GSTA1*. The functional form of the enzyme is a dimer of two polypeptide chains, and since both homodimers and hetero-dimers occur naturally (Mannervik and Jensson, 1982), the name of the functional enzyme should therefore reflect its subunit content. The membrane-bound GSTs appear to be homotrimeric structures (Schmidt-Krey *et al.*, 1999), and do not require further clarification of their subunit content, unless heterotrimeric structures were to be discovered. The names of the soluble GSTs explicitly specify the subunit composition. For example, the heterodimeric enzyme composed of subunits 1 and 2 of the Alpha class is designated GST A1-2. The homodimer composed of two copies of subunit 1 of the Theta class is called GST T1-1. Heterodimers of subunits from different classes are not known to occur.

Allelic variants are distinguished by letters. For example, the variant of GST M1-1 containing the amino acid residue Lys in position 173 is called GST M1a-1a, whereas the allelic variant B with Asn in position 173 is designated GST M1b-1b. The heterodimeric protein, which is present in heterozygous individuals, is called GST M1a-1b. At the level of the gene the corresponding variant alleles are designated *GSTM1*A* and *GSTM1*B*, respectively. The genotype of a heterozygous individual is indicated by specifying both alleles (Mannervik *et al.*, 1992), e.g., *GSTM1*A/GSTM1*B* in this case, and the corresponding phenotype would be referred to as GSTM1 A,B (not italicised). The null allele is denoted O (capital letter O), *GSTM1*O*. In general, human genes should be written in italicised capital letters (Shows *et al.*, 1987).

Membrane-bound glutathione transferases

The first membrane-bound GST that was characterised (Morgenstern *et al.*, 1979), MGST1, is an abundant protein in the endoplasmic reticulum and the outer mitochondrial membrane. It has been reported to represent 3–4% of the total protein content in these membranes isolated from rat liver (Morgenstern *et al.*, 1984). Like the soluble GSTs, MGST1 appears to serve as a detoxication enzyme active with both endogenous and xeno-biotic electrophiles. A particularly interesting feature of the enzyme is its ability to be activated by certain electrophiles, including sulfhydryl-mod-ifying agents, as well as by partial proteolysis (Morgenstern *et al.*, 1983).

A second member of the family of membrane-bound GSTs is leukotriene C_4 synthase, which is involved in the biosynthesis of leukotriene C_4 by catalysing the conjugation of leukotriene A_4 with glutathione (Jakschik *et al.*, 1982; Bach *et al.*, 1984; Yoshimoto *et al.*, 1985; Söderström *et al.*, 1992). The enzyme has insignificant activities with conventional GST substrates (Bach *et al.*, 1984), including those of the microsomal enzyme MGST1 (Söderström *et al.*, 1988). Additional sequences related to MGST1 have been identified, and the family of membrane-bound GSTs includes at least six members (Jakobsson *et al.*, 1999a). The functional properties of the more recently discovered proteins are in several cases linked to eicosanoid metabolism, e.g. the synthesis of prostaglandin E (Jakobsson *et al.*, 1999b). MGST1 is a trimer of three identical 17 kDa subunits (Schmidt-Krey *et al.*, 1999). However, the quaternary structure of the other members of the family has not been established.

Soluble glutathione transferases

The soluble GSTs have been divided into distinct classes, each containing one or several members. Originally the classification was based on both structural and functional properties (Mannervik *et al.*, 1985), but primary structures have subsequently been adopted as the guide for classification. Table 15.1 shows the GST classes and the human GST isoenzymes so far recognized, as well as the chromosomal location of their gene loci. The DNA sequence of human chromosome 22 has been determined, and the loci of *GSTT1* and *GSTT2* confirmed in a region, which also encodes related proteins (Dunham *et al.*, 1999).

The soluble GSTs are dimeric proteins composed of subunits from the same class (Mannervik and Jensson, 1982). The formation of both homo- and heterodimers increases the number of possible isoenzymes significantly. For example, the Mu class encompasses at least five distinct subunits, which theoretically gives the possibility of fifteen binary combinations (isoenzymes). Not all genes are expressed simultaneously or in the same cells, and it is not clear how many isoenzymes actually do occur naturally. However, both Alpha and Mu class heterodimers have been demonstrated in human tissues (Stockman *et al.*, 1985; Tsuchida *et al.*, 1990). From a functional point of view it is not obvious that the formation of hetero-dimers has any important consequences for catalytic activities.

The active site of a GST is composed of two subsites (Mannervik *et al.*, 1978), the glutathione binding site (G-site) and the hydrophobic substrate binding site (H-site). While the functional properties of the amino acid residues making up the G-site generally are well conserved among different classes, the residues forming the H-site vary considerably between GSTs. This gives the various GSTs complementary abilities to inactivate toxic substrates. Consequently, the GST family as a whole is capable of metabolising an exceedingly large number of structurally diverse substrates.

In addition to the two main categories consisting of soluble and membrane-bound enzymes, a plasmid-borne GST has been identified in clinical isolates of bacteria (Arca *et al.*, 1988; Arca *et al.*, 1990). This form of GST, which is active with the antibiotic fosfomycin, is a metalloprotein.

Table 15.1 Human glutathione transferases, classes and chromosomal locations of their genes

Enzyme[a] Designation[b]	Gene Class	Locus designation	Chromosome	Band	References
GST A1–1	Alpha	GSTA1	6	6p12	Tu et al., 1986; Board and Webb, 1987; Hayes et al., 1989; Rozen et al., 1992
GST A2–2	Alpha	GSTA2	6	6p12	Board and Webb, 1987; Rhoads et al., 1987; Hayes et al., 1989; Klöne et al., 1992; Röhrdanz et al., 1992; Suzuki et al., 1993
GST A3–3	Alpha	GSTA3	6	6p12	Suzuki et al., 1993; Board et al., 1998
GST A4–4	Alpha	GSTA4	6	6p12	Liu et al., 1998; Hubatsch et al., 1998; Board et al., 1998; Desmots et al., 1998
GST M1–1	Mu	GSTM1	1	1p13	Board, 1981; DeJong et al., 1988; Seidegård et al., 1988; Ross et al., 1993; Pearson et al., 1993; Zhong et al., 1992
GST M2–2	Mu	GSTM2	1	1p13	Vorachek et al., 1991; Taylor et al., 1991; Pearson et al., 1993
GST M3–3	Mu	GSTM3	1	1p13	Campbell et al., 1990; Pearson et al., 1993
GST M4–4	Mu	GSTM4	1	1p13	Taylor et al., 1991; Pearson et al., 1993; Comstock et al., 1993; Zhong et al., 1993b, Ross and Board, 1993
GST M5–5	Mu	GSTM5	1	1p13	Pearson et al., 1993; Takahashi et al., 1993
GST P1–1	Pi	GSTP1	11	11q13	Kano et al., 1987; Cowell et al., 1988; Moscow et al., 1988; Board et al., 1989; Morrow et al., 1989; Islam et al., 1989
GST T1–1	Theta	GSTT1	22	22q11.2	Meyer et al., 1991; Pemble et al., 1994; Webb et al., 1996, Coggan et al., 1998
GST T2–2	Theta	GSTT2	22	22q11.2	Tan et al., 1995; Coggan et al., 1998
GST K1–1	Kappa	GSTK1	nd	nd	Pemble et al., 1996
GST Z1–1	Zeta	GSTZ1	14	14q24.3	Board et al., 1997; Blackburn et al., 1998
GST O1–1	Omega	GSTO1	nd	nd	Board et al., 2000
MGST1	Membrane	MGST1	12	nd	DeJong et al., 1990
Leukotriene C$_4$ synthase	Membrane	LTC4S	5	5q35	Penrose et al., 1996

Notes

[a]Compilations of characteristic properties of GSTs, including substrate specificity profiles and differential sensitivities to inhibitors, have been published by Mannervik and Widersten (1995), Hayes and Pulford (1995), and Mannervik and Jemth (1999).

[b]The enzyme designations used are in agreement with the nomenclature proposed by Mannervik et al. (1992).

nd, not determined.

It has no known GST equivalent in human tissues, but is structurally related to another glutathione-linked enzyme, glyoxalase I (Cameron *et al.*, 1997; Bernat *et al.*, 1997).

All GST polymorphisms so far reported are limited to the soluble GSTs, and the following will therefore be restricted to this category.

Differential expression of the multiple forms of glutathione transferase

Tissue distribution

Studies of different organs in the rat demonstrated that the distribution of the multiple forms of GST varies from tissue to tissue (Mannervik *et al.*, 1983; Tu *et al.*, 1983). Every organ investigated has been found to contain GSTs, but in different amounts and with different representations of the distinct isoenzymes (Figure 15.2). It has also been demonstrated that within a given organ the isoenzyme distribution may vary from region to region. For example, both in rat (Rozell *et al.*, 1993) and human kidneys (Sundberg *et al.*, 1993), the proximal tubules express Alpha class GSTs, whereas distal tubules have low levels of these isoenzymes and are instead dominated by Mu and Pi class GSTs. Furthermore, adjacent epithelial cells in renal tubules showed a "mosaic expression", such that certain cells did not express the isoenzyme (e.g. GST M2-2) that was present in their neighbors (Rozell *et al.*, 1993). This observation was in contrast with the fact that all the neighboring cells showed a uniform presence of other forms of GST. Another spatial variation was noted in the partitioning of GSTs between cytoplasm and nucleoplasm, whereas the nucleolus appeared to be completely devoid of GSTs.

Human tissues also show a differential expression of the multiple forms of GST. Few tissues, if any, have identical isoenzyme profiles. In the liver, Alpha class enzymes are the predominant GSTs, in particular GST A1-1, which may represent 2–3% of the total cytosolic protein (van Ommen *et al.*, 1990; Rowe *et al.*, 1997). GST M1-1 is also a major hepatic form, in individuals expressing this isoenzyme. GST P1-1, which is present in most human tissues is not expressed in normal adult hepatocytes, and its presence in the liver appears to be restricted to epithelial cells such as those of the bile duct. The distribution of GSTs in normal human adult tissues is shown in Table 15.2.

Fetal expression

In contrast to the adult tissue, human fetal liver contains GST P1-1 as the major isoenzyme (Warholm *et al.*, 1981b; Guthenberg *et al.*, 1986). However, the isoenzyme pattern changes during fetal development such that the expression of GST P1-1 decreases precipitously at the end of the

prenatal period, whereas the expression of Alpha class GST remains high
during the fetal period, just as in the entire life period after birth (Strange
et al., 1989). In contrast, GST M1-1 evolves from low expression levels in

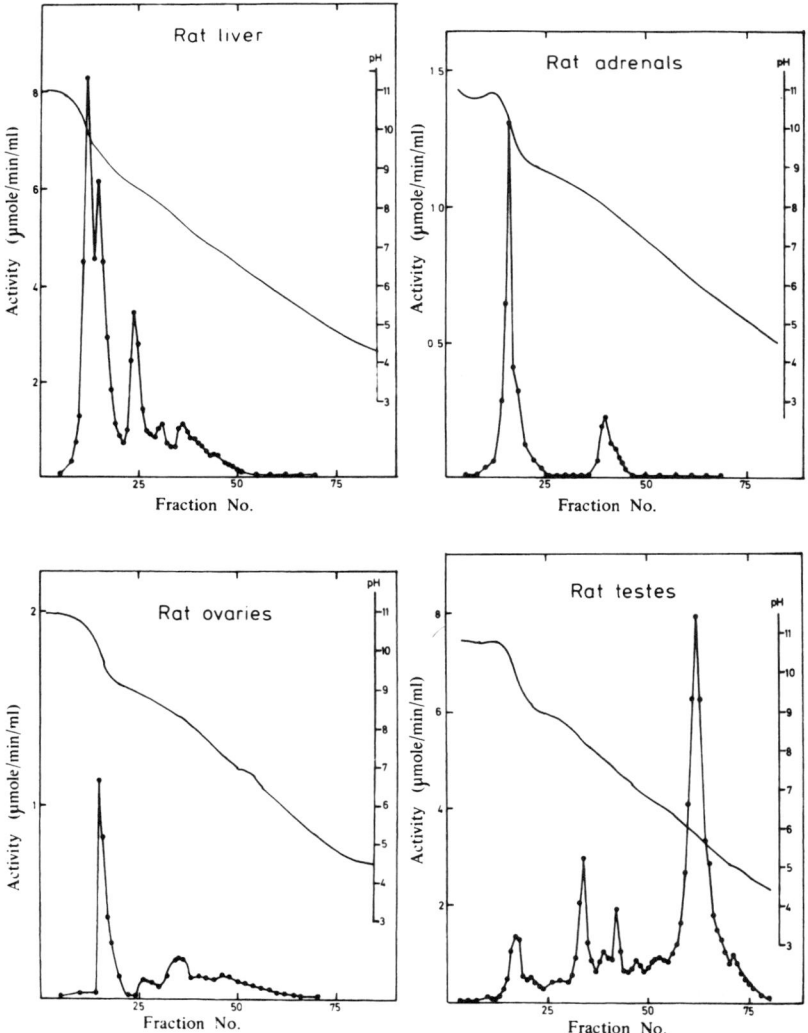

Figure 15.2 Differential expression of glutathione transferases in rat tissues. Cytosol
fractions of the tissues indicated were analyzed by isoelectric focusing followed
by activity measurements with 1-chloro-2,4-dinitrobenzene. The peaks obtained
at high pH values are primarily Alpha class GSTs. The several Mu class GSTs
have less basic or near-neutral isoelectric points, and rat GST P1-1 (prominent
in adrenal glands) has an isoelectric point of 7.0. The graphs have been reproduced from Mannervik *et al.* (1983) with permission from the publisher.

Table 15.2 Distribution of glutathione transferases in human adult tissues[a]

Tissue	Alpha			Mu					Pi	Theta		Unassigned[b]	Membrane
	A1–1	A2–2	A4–4	M1–1	M2–2	M3–3	M4–4	M5–5	P1–1	T1–1	T2–2		MGST1
Adipocytes									+				
Adrenal gland	+				+	+			+				+
Brain	+		+	+	+	+		+	+	+			
Brain cerebrum			+	+	+	+	+		+	+			
Breast				+									
Colon									+	+	+	+ (Basic)	+
Duodenum									+			+ (Basic)	
Erythrocytes									+			+ (Basic)	
Gall bladder									+			+ (Alpha)	
Heart/Aorta	+		+	+	+	+	+		+	+			+
Kidney	+		+	+	+	+			+	+		+(Basic)	+
Lens	+	+		+								+(Alpha)	+
Liver	+	+	+	+		+	+			+		+(Alpha, Mu)	+
Lung	+	+	+	+	+	+		+	+	+	+	+(Alpha, Mu)	+
Lymphocytes				+					+				+
Ovary									+			+(Alpha, Mu)	
Pancreas	+	+	+	+	+	+			+	+		+(Alpha)	+
Pituitary gland	+			+	+	+							+
Placenta									+				
Platelets									+				
Prostate			+	+		+			+	+		+(Alpha)	+
Retina									+			+(Basic)	
Skeletal muscle			+	+	+	+	+		+	+			+
Skin	+			+			+		+			+(Alpha)	
Small intestine	+		+	+		+			+	+			+
Spleen/Lymph nodes			+	+						+			+
Stomach									+			+(Alpha)	
Synovium						+			+				
Testis	+			+	+	+			+			+(Alpha)	+
Thymus									+			+(Alpha)	+
Urinary bladder			+									+(Alpha)	
Uterus									+			+(Neutral)	

Notes

[a]Data compiled from references cited in this chapter, in particular Rahilly et al., 1991; Hussey and Hayes, 1992; Singhal et al., 1994; Mannervik and Widersten, 1995; Juronen et al., 1996, Sherratt et al., 1997; Rowe et al., 1997; Estonius et al., 1999; de Bruin et al., 1999; Coles et al., 2000.

[b]Cannot be conclusively assigned, since they were found prior to identification of all isoenzymes currently known.

the early fetal period to a high expression level (in GSTM1-1-positive individuals) in the neonatal period. Isoenzyme distributions have also been studied in other fetal organs and differences from the adult tissues have been noted (Pacifici *et al.*, 1986; Faulder *et al.*, 1987). The distribution of GSTs identified in human fetal tissues is shown in Table 15.3.

Many of the published studies were conducted before the complexity of the GST superfamily had been fully recognized and clear distinctions among the isoenzymes now known to exist could not be made. Therefore, the GST isoenzyme distribution both in adult and fetal organs must still be regarded as incompletely known. Nevertheless, it is well established that tissues do differ from one another in their expression of GSTs, suggesting differential detoxication capacities and different sensitivities to toxic GST substrates.

Gender differences in glutathione transferase expression

Sexual dimorphisms in GST expression in rodents have been reported. In the mouse liver, expression of Pi class GST is under the control of testosterone, and the concentration of Pi class protein is approximately ten-fold higher in adult males than in females and prepubertal males (Hatayama *et al.*, 1986). Differences between male and female rats have also been reported, but the differences are less pronounced (Staffas *et al.*, 1992; Srivastava and Waxman, 1993; Meyer *et al.*, 1993).

Gender differences in the expression of GSTs have also been observed in humans. The expression of Mu class GST in the human colon differs between females and males (Singhal *et al.*, 1992). A Mu class GST with a p*I* value of 6.2 was identified in all females studied, but was not found in males. This gender difference requires further clarification. In addition, the activity of the Alpha class GST in the colon was approximately two-fold higher in males than in females. In another study, female skin was shown to contain approximately 1.6-fold higher GST levels as compared with male skin (Singhal *et al.*, 1993). Similarly, the expression of Alpha class GST in the olfactory mucosa was shown to be higher in females (Krishna *et al.*, 1995). GST P1-1 in plasma samples of blood donors was measured and, although plasma concentrations are low, 1.5-fold higher levels were observed in males (Mulder *et al.*, 1997). In contrast, no gender difference in the expression of Mu class GST and Pi class GST in lymphocytes was noted by van Lieshout and Peters (1998).

Differences in glutathione transferase expression as a function of age

Total GST activity in human erythrocytes was shown to be negatively correlated with increasing age (Ceballos-Picot *et al.*, 1992). The expression of Alpha class GST in the olfactory mucosa was shown to decrease with

Table 15.3 Distribution of glutathione transferases in human fetal tissues[a]

Tissue	Alpha			Mu						Pi	Theta		Membrane
	A1-1	A2-2	A4-4	Unassigned[b]	M1-1	M2-2	M3-3	M4-4	M5-5	P1-1	T1-1	T2-2	MGST1
Adrenal gland				+						+			
Brain	+									+			
Kidney	+			+	+					+			+
Liver	+				+[c]					+[d]			+
Spleen				+									
Lung	+									+			+

Notes

[a]Data compiled from Mannervik and Widersten, 1995; and Estonius et al., 1999.

[b]Cannot be conclusively assigned, since they were found prior to identification of all isoenzymes currently known.

[c]Increases during gestation.

[d]Decreases during gestation.

age, while no such trend was shown for GST P1-1 (Krishna *et al.*, 1995). In lymphocytes, the levels of Mu class GST and GST P1-1 were not correlated with age (van Lieshout and Peters, 1998). Alpha class GST could not be detected in the lymphocytes. In another study on healthy blood donors, the concentration of GST P1-1 in plasma was shown to increase with age (Mulder *et al.*, 1997). In view of the low GST levels in plasma, the observed increase may be a result of lysis of blood cells.

Interindividual variations in levels of glutathione transferase expression

A study of the expression of GSTs in human pancreas using high performance liquid chromatography (HPLC) for identification of the different subunits showed that the total GST expression level varied 7.3-fold between samples from different individuals (Coles *et al.*, 2000). The variation in expression of GSTs P1-1, A2-2, M3-3, A1-1 and M2-2 was between six- and 30-fold. The expression of GST A4-4 and a novel GST assigned to the Alpha class varied 50- to 100-fold between samples, which suggests that these GSTs are highly inducible. The samples were taken from a heterogeneous group (forty-three individuals) of different age, gender and ethnicity. However, in this study the phenotype appeared to be independent of age, gender and smoking status.

Factors affecting expression of glutathione transferases

GSTs are inducible, as are many other enzymes involved in the biotransformation of xenobiotics and reactive metabolites formed in the organism (Hayes and Pulford, 1995). GST induction is considered to be part of an adaptive response mechanism to chemical stress occurring widely in nature. The general opinion is that, besides providing protection against xenobiotics, GSTs are also involved in protection against oxidative stress (Mannervik, 1985; Ketterer, 1998). Many inducers of GSTs have in common that they can serve as acceptors in Michael addition reactions (e.g. addition of a nucleophile to alkenes with a carbon–carbon double bond conjugated to an electron-withdrawing group) or are metabolised to potential Michael acceptors or other electrophiles (Talalay *et al.*, 1988; Talalay and Spencer, 1990). Such reactive compounds may cause chemical stress in biological tissues and, therefore, the induction of xenobiotic-metabolising enzymes would represent an appropriate adaptive response. These inducers are also potential GST substrates, which are accordingly more rapidly metabolised as a consequence of the induction.

Induction of glutathione transferases in animals

Classical inducers of drug metabolism, such as phenobarbital and 3-methyl-cholanthrene, were found to afford a significant increase in the expression levels of hepatic GSTs (Fleischner *et al.*, 1972; Klaassen, 1975; Hales and Neims, 1977). Simultaneous administration of these inducers plus *trans*-stilbene oxide raised the level of GSTs in rat liver from 4.5% to 17.4% of the total cytosolic protein (Guthenberg *et al.*, 1980). Using the antioxidant 2(3)-*tert*-butyl-4-hydroxyanisole (BHA), known as a food additive, it was demonstrated that GST induction in rodents was tissue specific (Benson *et al.*, 1979). The fact that consumption of fruits and vegetables provides protection against cancer and other degenerative diseases (Block *et al.*, 1992; Steinmetz and Potter, 1996) has prompted research on the role of minor dietary constituents, including their possible function as inducers of detoxication enzymes (Wattenberg, 1983). For example, two potent GST inducers, cafestol palmitate and kahweol palmitate, were isolated from coffee beans (Wattenberg, 1983). In more detailed studies on the differential effects of cafestol palmitate in the mouse, it was demonstrated that Mu class GSTs in the liver were preferentially induced (Di Simplicio *et al.*, 1989). Thus, the effect of inducers has been shown to be both tissue-selective and isoenzyme-specific.

Studies of rodents have demonstrated that oltipraz, a synthetic 1,2-dithiole-3-thione derivative, is a potent inducer of phase II detoxication enzymes including GSTs (Kensler *et al.*, 1985; Ansher *et al.*, 1986; Rao *et al.*, 1991). Dietary administration of oltipraz was shown to produce a marked inhibition of aflatoxin B_1-induced hepatic tumorigenesis in rats (Liu *et al.*, 1988). In other animal cancer models, oltipraz has been found to inhibit chemically induced carcinogenesis in the bladder, colon, breast, stomach and skin (Benson, 1993).

Hormonal regulation of glutathione transferase expression

In addition to induction effected by xenobiotics or by products of oxidative metabolism, it has been demonstrated that GST gene expression is subject to hormonal control. Sex hormones may have profound effects on the GST levels (Hatayama *et al.*, 1986; Igarashi *et al.*, 1984), but other endocrine factors also play prominent roles. In the rat, adrenocorticotropic hormone (ACTH) appears to attenuate the expression of some GSTs, particularly in the adrenal gland, as evidenced by studies of hypophysectomised animals (Mankowitz *et al.*, 1990). Other hormones, including growth hormone, thyroxine, and cortisone, have similar effects on class Mu GSTs, with significant differences between males and females (Staffas *et al.*, 1992).

Insulin has been reported to increase the expression of human GST P1-1 through a *cis*-acting regulatory element in intron 1, while retinoic acid represses the transcription of the same *GSTP1* gene (Xia *et al.*, 1993). In contrast, Lo and Ali-Osman (1998) showed that retinoic acid induces transcription of an isolated *GSTP1* gene transfected into tumor cells.

Deletion of the retinoic acid response element abolished this response. This indicates that a complex mechanism exists for regulation of the *GSTP1* gene.

Induction of glutathione transferases in humans

Induction of GST expression in human cells and tissues definitely occurs (Morel *et al.*, 1993). Oral administration of oltipraz has been shown to elevate the concentrations of glutathione as well as GST in human lymphocytes (Gupta *et al.*, 1995). In exploratory studies, attempts are also being made at inducing GSTs in human subjects by dietary constituents, such as cruciferous vegetables. Healthy volunteers who consumed 300 g of Brussel sprouts per day for 3 weeks displayed a 1.4-fold increase in the plasma levels of Alpha class GST (Bogaards *et al.*, 1994). The inducing agent was not identified in this study, but Brussel sprouts contain significant amounts of allyl isothiocyanate and goitrin, substances that previously have been shown to induce rodent GST (Bogaards *et al.*, 1990). A particularly interesting isothiocyanate found in broccoli is sulforaphane (Zhang *et al.*, 1992), a potent inducer of GST expression, as well as an anticarcinogen in rodents (Zhang *et al.*, 1994; Fahey *et al.*, 1997). However, a difficulty in studies of GST induction in human subjects is the monitoring of the effects of the compounds tested as inducers. Blood samples and other accessible specimens may not be representative of the effects on the liver or other target organs. Furthermore, the human subjects may already be induced by dietary components, smoking or environmental factors. It is therefore not obvious what the proper non-induced control would be for human tissues.

It is not clear if elevated tissue levels of GSTs are desirable in the general population, because GST-catalysed reactions with some electrophiles may promote toxicity. However, it is a reasonable assumption that certain risk groups may benefit from GST induction. A prospective study of a Chinese population heavily exposed to dietary aflatoxin has been initiated, based on evidence that enzyme-mediated conjugation of the potent hepato-carcinogen is a major route of detoxication (Kensler *et al.*, 1999). The current approach is to induce GSTs by administration of oltipraz, originally an approved human drug for treatment of schistosomiasis.

Life-style effects on glutathione transferase levels

Viral infections

Epidemiologic and experimental evidence suggests that the risk of cervical cancer is related to both human papilloma virus (HPV) infection and cigarette smoking. GST M1-1 activity and mRNA levels in human GST M1-1 positive cervical keratinocytes transfected with HPV were measured and compared with those in the parental cells. GST M1-1 enzymatic activity was five- to seven-fold lower in the infected cells, and the corresponding mRNA level was only 6% of that of the parental cells, suggesting that viral infections attenuate the expression of GST M1-1 (Chen and Nirunsuksiri, 1999). A mouse model of chronic active hepatitis has demonstrated elevated levels of Alpha and Mu class GSTs associated with hepatocellular injury (Fernandes et al., 1996).

In relation to viral infections it should be noted that interferon has a differential effect on the expression of GSTs in mouse liver, including up-regulation of Pi class GST and down-regulation of all other GSTs investigated (Adams et al., 1987). Similarly, among other cytokines, interleukin-1β was found to up-regulate the expression of GST P1-1 and suppress the expression of Alpha and Mu class GSTs in rat hepatocytes (Maheo et al., 1997).

Obesity

Obesity has been shown to affect the expression of glutathione transferases in mice differently according to sex. Glutathione transferase activity was lower in obese male mice, whereas no difference was observed between lean and obese females (Roe et al., 1999).

Dietary habits

Dietary habits are known to affect the susceptibility to cancer (Ames et al., 1995; Beckman and Ames, 1998). A relationship between the protective effect of antioxidant micronutrients and GST expression was evidenced in a study where levels of DNA adducts with polycyclic aromatic hydro-carbons (PAHs) were measured in circulating mononuclear cells of cigarette smokers (Grinberg-Funes et al., 1994). The PAH-DNA adduct levels were shown to be negatively correlated to serum vitamin E and C concentrations, but only in individuals who were homozygously GSTM1 null. Similarly, another study involving lung cancer patients showed that the frequency of sister chromatid exchanges (SCE) was directly correlated with the GSTM1*O allele, but was inversely correlated with vitamin A and selenium intake (Cheng et al., 1995). Cruciferous vegetables are believed to prevent cancer by providing anticarcinogenic compounds, notably organic isothiocyanates. These compounds induce carcinogen-detoxicating enzymes including GSTs. However, since isothiocyanates are also substrates of GSTs (Zhang et al., 1995; Meyer et al., 1995; Kolm et al., 1995), they are conjugated to glutathione and excreted. A recent study (Lin et al., 1998a) showed that the protective effect of broccoli against colorectal adenomas was observed only in individuals carrying the GSTM1 null allele. In these subjects isothiocyanates were presumably less rapidly metabolised and reached higher tissue concentrations. Thus, sensitivity to DNA damage from exposure to cigarette smoke and environmental pollutants, as well as endogenous factors is dependent not only on GST genotype but also on dietary constituents.

Expression of glutathione transferases in tumors

Differences between normal and cancer cells

Cancer cells in general appear to have altered GST expression profiles as compared with the corresponding normal cells. In the rat, it was found that preneoplastic lesions in the liver caused by genotoxic agents led to the induction of GST P1-1, an enzyme not detectable in normal hepatocytes (Eriksson et al., 1983; Kitahara et al., 1984). Separation and quantitative analyses of GSTs from rat liver preneoplastic nodules demonstrated that in addition to the induction of GST P1-1, changes in the relative amounts of several other GSTs of other classes also occur (Jensson et al., 1985). Ascites cells of a rat hepatoma are completely dominated by GST P1-1 and essentially all of the other GSTs found in normal hepatocytes are undetectable (Tahir et al., 1989). It should also be noted that the presence of hepatoma cells in the ascites fluid induces the expression of GST P1-1 in liver (Tahir et al., 1989). The cause of this "bystander effect" has not yet been elucidated, but may be due to humoral factors derived from or elicited by the presence of hepatoma cells, or to an adaptive response to the burden of the ascites tumor.

The majority of human tumors, but far from all, overexpress GST P1-1. Many human cancer cell lines display high levels of the enzyme (Shea et al., 1988; Castro et al., 1990; Tew et al., 1996). However, the hepatoma cell line HepG2, like primary human liver tumors, expresses only low levels of GST P1-1, in contrast to hepatic neoplasias in the rat. Most normal human tissues express significant amounts of GST P1-1, and corresponding tumor tissues often have several-fold increased concentrations of the enzyme (Lewis et al., 1989; Kelley et al., 1994). Nevertheless, it should be noted that human prostate carcinoma tissue consistently appears to have completely down-regulated expression of GST P1-1, due to hypermethylation of the promoter region of its corresponding gene GSTP1 (Lee et al., 1994).

Cancer patients are known to differ in their response to chemotherapy, both with respect to the efficacy of the cytostatic drug on the tumor cells and with respect to the toxic side-effects on normal cells. Since alkylating cancer drugs serve as GST substrates, variability in GST expression may contribute to these differential effects. In order to probe this relationship, lymphocytes from GST M1-1 positive and GST M1-1 null individuals were exposed in vitro to 1,3-bis-(2-chloroethyl)-1-nitrosourea (BCNU) (Jungnelius et al., 1994). Mu class GSTs had been shown to contribute to

BCNU resistance in a rat glioma cell line (Smith *et al.*, 1989), but no significant effect of the lack of GST M1-1 expression was seen in the human lymphocytes (Jungnelius *et al.*, 1994). However, GST M3-3 is the most efficient GST catalysing the inactivation of BCNU (Berhane *et al.*, 1993), whereas human GST M1-1 has only a low activity with the drug.

Overexpression of glutathione transferases in drug resistant cells

GST concentrations are frequently elevated in cell lines selected for resistance to various cytostatic drugs. A mouse osteosarcoma cell line demonstrating multidrug resistance was found to express high levels of a Pi class GST (Dahllöf *et al.*, 1987), suggesting that this enzyme contributed to the resistance. Studies of other rodent GSTs indicated that they catalyse the inactivation of alkylating anticancer drugs (Buller *et al.*, 1987; Lewis *et al.*, 1988; Smith *et al.*, 1989). However, many of the cells that are resistant to nitrogen mustards show increased expression levels of class alpha GST (Tew *et al.*, 1994) and human breast tumor cells resistant to ethacrynic acid have increased levels of GST Mu (Hayes and Pulford, 1995). Nevertheless, it is not clear if the altered expression of GSTs is a cause or an effect of the emerging resistance phenotype.

Genetic polymorphisms

Known allelic variants

Four GSTs have well-established polymorphisms in the human population. They encompass GST M1-1, GST M3-3, GST T1-1, and GST P1-1. The enzymes GST M1-1 and GST T1-1 both have a frequently occurring null phenotype (Warholm *et al.*, 1980; Board, 1981; Pemble *et al.*, 1994). *GSTM1* and *GSTP1* have alleles with sequence variations. Table 15.4 summarises the allele designations of the known human GST polymorphisms, including the corresponding genotypes and the structural and functional consequences. In addition, sequence variations have been observed in the *GSTA2*, *GSTT1* and *GSTZ1* loci.

Mu class variants

Approximately half the human population is homozygous for the *GSTM1* null allele and consequently does not express the GST M1-1 protein. The gene appears to be absent in its entirety in deficient individuals (Seidegård *et al.*, 1988). *GSTM1* is located in the middle of a cluster of five Mu class genes, and unequal crossing over has been proposed as a mechanism for its elimination (Pearson *et al.*, 1993; Xu *et al.*, 1998a).

The expressed allelic GST M1-1 variants A and B differ in molecular charge, since the superficially located residue 173 is Lys in GST M1a-1a

Table 15.4 Allelic variants of human glutathione transferases

Protein	Allele designation	Characteristic	References
GST M1–1		Point mutation in exon 7;	
	GSTM1*A	amino acid 173 is Lys	DeJong et al., 1988
	GSTM1*B	amino acid 173 is Asn	Seidegård et al., 1988
	GSTM1*O	Deletion of the GSTM1 gene; lack of the enzyme	Seidegård et al., 1988
GST M3–3			Pearson et al., 1993
	GSTM3*A		
	GSTM3*B	Three-base deletion in intron 6; the deletion may influence recognition sites for transcription factors	Inskip et al., 1995; To-Figueras et al., 2000
GST P1–1		Point mutations in exons 5 and 6; amino acid 105 is part of the H-site	
	GSTP1*A	GSTP1 (Ile105/Ala114)	Kano et al., 1987; Cowell et al., 1988
	GSTP1*B	GSTP1 (Val105/Ala114)	Ahmad et al., 1990; Ali-Osman et al., 1997
	GSTP1*C	GSTP1 (Val105/Val114)	Board et al., 1989; Lo and Ali-Osman, 1997
	GSTP1*D	GSTP1 (Ile105/Val114)	Watson et al., 1998
GST T1–1			
	GSTT1		Pemble et al., 1994
	GSTT1*O	Deletion of the GSTT1 gene; lack of the enzyme	

and Asn in GST M1b-1b. This difference allows the allelic variants to be separated by electrophoretic and chromatographic methods. However, the amino acid substitution has no known consequences for the catalytic activity of the enzyme (Widersten *et al.*, 1991). In a study examining the potential association of the GSTM1 null phenotype with disease, it was observed that a small percentage of the subjects in a Saudi Arabian population displayed very high GST M1-1 activity with *trans*-stilbene oxide when compared with activities expected for heterozygosity or homozygosity of the *GSTM1* gene (Evans *et al.*, 1996). Genetic analysis revealed that this was due to a polymorphism in the form of gene duplication (McLellan *et al.*, 1997).

GST M3-3 has two alleles, *GSTM3*A* and *GSTM3*B*, where the B variant contains a 3-bp deletion in intron 6. This mutation in the non-coding region of the gene is believed to generate a recognition site for the transcription factor YY1 (Inskip *et al.*, 1995). YY1 regulates gene expression from intragenic sites and influences the transcription of many genes. In addition, putative binding sites for the heat-shock transcription factor (HSTF1) and nuclear factor for granulocyte/macrophage colony-stimulating factor gene promoter a (NF-GMa) have been identified in intron 6 close to the deletion (To-Figueras *et al.*, 2000). These findings suggest that GSTM3*A and GSTM3*B may be expressed at different levels and that the resultant GSTM3 phenotypes will confer different efficiencies in the metabolism of toxic substrates.

The expression of the Mu class enzymes GST M3-3 and GST M1-1 seems to be co-ordinated. Nakajima *et al.* (1995) reported that the expression of GST M3-3 in lung was lower in *GSTM1* null homozygotes compared with individuals with other *GSTM1* genotypes. A linkage between the presence of the GSTM3*B allele and the GSTM1*A allele was showed by Inskip *et al.* (1995) and was confirmed by To-Figueras *et al.* (2000). Their data suggest that individuals carrying the GSTM1*A allele have a reduced expression of GST M3-3. Thus, the *GSTM1/GSTM3* haplotype rather than only the *GSTM1* genotype should be studied when susceptibilities of different genotypes to diseases are assessed.

Pi class variants

In contrast to GST M1-1 forms A and B, allelic variants of GST P1-1 do have significant functional differences. Two sites in the coding DNA sequence of GST P1-1 are variable and are characterised by an A↔G transition at nucleotide 313 and a C↔T transition at nucleotide 341 of the cDNA. The resulting codon variations result in the amino acids Ile105 or Val105 and Ala114 or Val114. Consequently, the allelism of the human *GSTP1* locus comprises four different allelic variants designated GSTP1*A, GSTP1*B, GSTP1*C, and GSTP1*D (Kano *et al.*, 1987; Board *et al.*, 1989; Ahmad *et al.*, 1990; Ali-Osman *et al.*, 1997; Watson *et al.*, 1998) encoding GST P1a-1a (Ile105/Ala114), GST P1b-1b (Val105/Ala114), GST P1c-1c (Val105/Val114) and GST P1d-1d (Ile105/Val114), respectively. A guanine insertion in intron 1 of the GSTP1*C allele creates a potential site for 5′-cytosine methylation in the postulated insulin response element (Lo and Ali-Osman, 1997). Insulin has been shown to enhance the transcription of GST P1-1 and methylation may affect the expression level.

Theta class variants

The GSTT1 null phenotype is due to the deletion of the complete *GSTT1* gene (Pemble *et al.*, 1994). Sequence analysis of the cDNA for human GST T1-1 cloned independently in two different laboratories (Sherratt *et al.*, 1997; Jemth and Mannervik, 1997) showed variances from the previously published cDNA sequence (Pemble *et al.*, 1994). One of the nucleotide differences, a G→A substitution at codon 126, translates into an amino acid substitution of a Gly by Glu. Whether this sequence variation represents an allelic polymorphism in the human population has to be verified.

Alpha class variants

Three variants of *GSTA2* have been noted by comparison of isolated *GSTA2* genes (Röhrdanz *et al.*, 1992; Klöne *et al.*, 1992) and cDNA (Rhoads *et al.*, 1987). In the coding sequence, a G to C alteration changes amino acid Thr112 to Ser112 (counting the initiator Met as residue 1). The third observed variant has a Ser in position 112 and a change in the nucleotide sequence at position 695 from A to C, which results in Ala instead of Glu as amino acid residue 210 (Rhoads *et al.*, 1987; Röhrdanz *et al.*, 1992; Klöne *et al.*, 1992). Proteins corresponding to these three gene variants have been identified in samples from human pancreas (Coles *et al.*, 2000). The latter study showed that there are individuals who appear to be homozygous or heterozygous with respect to the three alternative forms, indicating that the variants are due to a real allelic variation at the *GSTA2* locus.

Zeta class variants

Human GST Z1-1 was recently characterised and a comparison of the expressed sequence tags (ESTs) encoding GST Z1-1 revealed sequence variations involving A and G at nucleotide positions 94 and 124. The A to G substitutions result in the replacement of Lys with Glu in position 32 and of Gly with Arg in position 42 in the amino acid sequence of the GST Z1 subunit (Board *et al.*, 1997). The three allelic variants have been denoted *GSTZ1*A* (A94/A124), *GSTZ1*B* (A94/G124) and *GSTZ1*C* (G94/G124). All three alleles have been shown to be present in a normal Caucasian population (Blackburn *et al.*, 1999).

In vitro studies of functional consequences of the glutathione transferase polymorphisms

Studies of purified allelic variants of glutathione transferase

Experiments with purified enzymes have been carried out in order to elucidate functional differences of allelic variants that may have significance for the assumed protective role of the GSTs. A comparison of the catalytic properties of GST M1a-1a and GST M1b-1b has been made with standard substrates, but no significant differences were detected (Widersten *et al.*, 1991). The surface location of the variant amino acid residue 173 in the

GST M1-1 molecule does not suggest effects on the catalytic functions of the two allelic variants.

In contrast, allelic variants of GST P1-1 involve the H-site residue 105, as well as residue 114 that follows α-helix 4, a helix that contributes to the H-site. These variant GSTs have been kinetically investigated both with standard substrates and with epoxides of mutagenic and carcinogenic PAHs. Significant differences in catalytic efficiencies have been demonstrated (Zimniak et al., 1994; Ali-Osman et al., 1997, Sundberg et al., 1998; Johansson et al., 1998; Hu et al., 1997, 1998) but their possible relationship to disease is unclear. Differences in the stability of the GST P1-1 variants have also been shown, although the results from different research groups are divergent. Stability differences may have toxicological relevance since GST P1-1 is a major component in many cells, including erythrocytes with a life span of 120 days.

Influence of glutathione transferase null phenotypes on susceptibility of isolated cells in vitro

At the cellular level, in vitro experiments involving cells of different GST genotypes have been performed. Potentially genotoxic agents that are GST substrates have been added to cells in vitro and the level of cytogenetic damage after exposure has been measured. For example, lymphocytes that lacked GST M1-1 were shown to be more prone to epoxide-induced sister chromatid exchange (SCE) when exposed to the GST M1-1 substrate trans-stilbene oxide (Wiencke et al., 1990). The results clearly show that epoxides, expected to be inactivated by GST M1-1-catalysed glutathione conjugation, give rise to significantly higher levels of chromosome damage in GST M1-1 null lymphocytes.

Hallier et al. (1993) found that three substrates of GST T1-1, methyl bromide, ethylene oxide and dichloromethane, when incubated with whole blood samples from conjugators and non-conjugators, all caused a marked increase of SCEs in the lymphocytes of the non-conjugators, but not in those of conjugators. In another study, the lack of the GSTT1 gene was shown to increase the genotoxic effect of the styrene metabolite, styrene-7,8-oxide, as monitored by SCEs (Ollikainen et al., 1998). Furthermore, the expression of human GST T1-1 in bacteria was shown to reduce the mutagenicity of 1,2-epoxy-3-(4-nitrophenoxy)propane (Thier et al., 1996). In contrast, the mutagenicity of ethylene dibromide and 1,2,3,4-diepoxy-butane (DEB) was increased. Such glutathione-dependent toxification of xenobiotics is well established for 1,2-dihaloalkanes and is due to formation of a reactive episulfonium derivative (Rannug et al., 1978; Guengerich, 1994). However, exposure of human lymphocyte cultures to DEB produced a considerably higher number of SCEs in lymphocytes that were GSTT1 null compared with GSTT1 positive lymphocytes, suggesting a protective role for GST T1-1 in detoxication of DEB in humans (Landi *et al.*, 1998).

Influence of glutathione transferase GST P1-1 variants on susceptibility of cells in vitro

Transfectants of HepG2 cells carrying cDNA encoding three allelic GST variants, GST P1a-1a, GST P1b-1b, and GST P1c-1c, or an empty vector, showed different levels of DNA modifications after exposure to (+)-*anti*-benzo[a]pyrene-7,8-diol 9,10-epoxide [(+)-*anti*-BPDE] (Hu *et al.*, 1999). The formation of (+)-*anti*-BPDE-DNA adducts was significantly reduced in transfectants containing cDNA encoding GST P1-1, and the expression of GST P1c-1c was shown to give the highest level of protection. This variant also displayed the highest k_{cat}/K_m value for (+)-*anti*-BPDE in measurements with the purified enzyme variants (Hu *et al.*, 1997).

Influence of glutathione transferase null phenotypes on lymphocytes exposed in human subjects

GST M1-1 is active towards certain epoxides of PAHs found in cigarette smoke and other combustion products. Smokers deficient in the *GSTM1* gene were shown to have increased SCE levels in their blood lymphocytes *in vivo* compared with *GSTM1* positive smokers (van Poppel *et al.*, 1993). In the absence of cigarette smoking, the *GSTM1* deletion did not affect the SCE frequency in peripheral lymphocytes of the individuals studied. A positive correlation between levels of PAH-DNA adducts and the *GSTM1* null genotype was found by Shields *et al.* (1993) and Rojas *et al.* (2000). Furthermore, Liu *et al.* (1991) showed that the presence of GST M1a-1a or GST M1b-1b in human liver cytosol inhibits the formation of adducts between aflatoxin B_1 and calf thymus DNA, in agreement with the high catalytic activity of GST M1-1 with aflatoxin B_1 *exo*-8,9-epoxide (Johnson *et al.*, 1997).

The biological consequences of homozygosity for the *GSTT1* null genotype in humans are difficult to predict, since this enzyme has both detoxication and toxification activities toward various environmental pollutants. GST T1-1 will detoxify monohalomethanes and ethylene oxide, but will enhance the toxicity of dichloromethane and other bifunctional agents (Pemble *et al.*, 1994; Guengerich, 1994; Anders and Dekant, 1998). Nevertheless, the *GSTT1* null genotype was shown to be associated with the background rate of SCEs (Schröder, 1995). Cells with the *GSTT1* null genotype displayed 7.55 SCEs/mitosis to compare with 7.26 SCEs/mitosis in *GSTT1* positive cells. Cells from smoking *GSTT1* null subjects exhibited the highest SCE rates (8.74 SCEs/mitosis). The *GSTT1* null genotype was also shown to be strongly correlated with SCEs induced by DEB (Wiencke *et al.*, 1995). A similar study involving both smokers and non-smokers showed the same correlation (Xu *et al.*, 1998b). DEB is a metabolite of the suspected human carcinogen 1,3-butadiene, which is used industrially in large amounts and also occurs in cigarette smoke. Chromosomal aberrations among workers exposed to 1,3-butadiene were significantly increased in workers lacking the *GSTT1* gene as compared with workers carrying the gene (Sorsa *et al.*, 1996).

A study investigating the influence of the *GSTT1* and *GSTM1* null genotypes on the level of ethylene oxide-protein adduct formation in humans showed that the adduct level was significantly increased in humans carrying the *GSTT1* null genotype, but only among non-smoking individuals (Müller *et al.*, 1998). The *GSTM1* null genotype was not correlated with adduct levels. This result is in accordance with the finding that ethylene oxide is a substrate for GST T1-1, but not for GST M1-1.

Differences in allele frequencies of glutathione transferases among different ethnic groups

The gene frequency of the different GST alleles varies among different ethnic groups. Reported allele frequencies of the known *GSTT1*, *GSTM1* and *GSTM3* polymorphisms of different ethnic or racial groups are compiled in Table 15.5. The distribution of the *GSTM1* and *GSTT1* null genotypes in different populations are illustrated in Figure 15.3 and Figure 15.4 respectively. Although the reported frequency of a GST allele in a certain population may vary considerably between different studies, it is clear that the *GSTM1* null genotype is less frequent in Africans (20-40%) compared with Caucasians and Orientals, in which approximately 50% of the population display the *GSTM1* null genotype. In Oceanian populations, the *GSTM1* null genotype is very frequent, with up to 100% of the Micronesian population being homozygous for the *GSTM1* null allele.

The *GSTT1* null genotype seems to be more frequent in Orientals (40–65%) and in Africans (20–40%) compared with Caucasians (10–20%).

Since the polymorphism at the *GSTP1* locus was discovered fairly recently, the data available for frequencies of the *GSTP1* alleles are not as comprehensive as for the *GSTM1* and *GSTT1* polymorphisms. The frequencies of the *GSTP1* allele variants reported for populations from different parts of the world are compiled in Table 15.6. The frequency of variants with Ile at position 105 varies from 58% in African Americans to 89% in Australian Aboriginals. The presence of a Val at position 114 is rare in all groups so far studied, but the frequency varies from 0% in Australian Aboriginals to 11% in Americans (ethnicity unspecified).

The recently discovered polymorphism in the *GSTZ1* gene has been investigated in a Caucasian population with frequencies of the alleles as

Table 15.5 Frequency of polymorphic GST alleles in different ethnic or racial groups

Population	GSTM1					GSTM3			GSTT1	
	AA (%)	AB (%)	BB (%)	+ (%)	− (%)	AA (%)	AB (%)	BB (%)	+ (%)	− (%)
Caucasian										
Europe										
Icelandic[a]									78	22
British[b,c,d,e,f,g,h,i]	26–28	4–6	12–16	42–58	42–58	74	21	5	80–86 84*	14–20 16*
French[j,k,l,h]				53 49*	47 51*					
North-West Mediterranean[m,n]	34	2	14	51	49	65	31	3	81	19
Portugese[o]				48	52					
German[p,q,r,s,t]	34	3	13	47–62	38–53				81–86	14–19
Norwegian[u]				53**	47**					
Swedish[v,w]				47	53				90	10
Finnish[x]				56	44					
Polish[y]				51	49					
Estonian[k]				50	50					
Turkish[z]									80	20
Australia[aa]				50	50				84	16
America										
USA[s,bb,cc,dd,ee,ff]				52–47 38*	48–53 62*				85–76 73*	15–24 27*
New England[cc]									84	16
Brazilian[gg]				45	55				81	19
American										
African American[cc,hh,dd,ee,s,bb]				59–77 59*	23–41 41*				78 71*	22 29*
North American[ii]				49	51				85	15
Mexican American[hh,cc]				60	40				88–90	10–12
African Brazilian[gg]				67	33				81	19
Amazonian Indian[gg]				80	20				89	11
Chilean[h]				79	21					
Jewish[s]				53	47					
Hispanic[s]				51–47	49–53					
Indian[s]				64	36					
Korean[s]				47	53					
Filipino[s]				41	59					
Japanese[s]				49	51					
Samoan[s]				12	88					

Table 15.5 (continued)

Population	GSTM1					GSTM3			GSTT1	
	AA (%)	AB (%)	BB (%)	+ (%)	− (%)	AA (%)	AB (%)	BB (%)	+ (%)	− (%)
African										
Egyptian[ii]				56	44				85	15
Zimbabwean[jj,kk]				76	24				74	26
Ghanaian[ll]				61	39					
Nigerian[j,mm]	71	6	1	78	22				62	38
Oceanian										
Micronesian[nn]				0	100					
Melanesian[nn]				20	80					
Polynesian[nn]				10	90					
Oriental										
Chinese[cc,s,oo,pp,ll]				59–37	41–63				36–49	51–64
Taiwanese[s]				55	45					
Japanese[qq,rr,ss]				39–52	44–48				56	44
Korean[cc]									40	60
Shanghaan[tt]				51	49				51	49
Malaysian[oo,uu]				36–38	62–64				62	38
Indian[oo,uu]				67–68	32–33				84	16

Notes
*Studies involving only females; ** Studies involving only males.
[a]Gudmundsdóttir and Eyfjörd, 1999; [b]Zhong et al., 1993a; [c]Heagerty et al., 1994; [d]Yengi et al., 1996; [e]Zhong et al., 1991; [f]Warwick et al., 1994; [g]Elexpuru-Camiruaga et al., 1995; [h]Quinônes et al., 1999; [i]Rollinson et al., 2000; [j]Zhao et al., 1994; [k]Mikelsaar et al., 1994; [l]Maugard et al., 1998; [m]To-Figueras et al., 1997; [n]To-Figueras et al., 2000; [o]Martins et al., 1998; [p]Bruhn et al., 1998; [q]Hengstler et al., 1998; [r]Brockmöller et al., 1993; [s]Lin et al., 1994; [t]Brockmöller et al., 1994; [u]Ryberg et al., 1997; [v]Warholm et al., 1995; [w]Alexandrie et al., 1994; [x]Hirvonen et al., 1993; [y]Gawronska-Szklarz et al., 1999; [z]Oke et al., 1998; [aa]Chenevix-Trench et al., 1995; [bb]Chen et al., 1996; [cc]Nelson et al., 1995; [dd]Bailey et al., 1998; [ee]Bell et al., 1993; [ff]Wiencke et al., 1997; [gg]Arruda et al., 1998; [hh]Kelsey et al., 1997; [ii]Abdel-Rahman et al., 1996; [jj]Mukanganyama et al., 1997; [kk]Masimirembwa et al., 1998; [ll]McGlynn et al., 1995; [mm]Rebbeck et al., 1997; [nn]Board et al., 1990; [oo]Lee et al., 1995; [pp]Lin et al., 1998b; [qq]Katoh et al., 1996; [rr]Nakachi et al., 1993; [ss]Harada et al., 1992; [tt]Shen et al., 1998; [uu]Zhao et al., 1995.

follows; 8% *GSTZ1*A*, 28% *GSTZ1*B*, and 64% *GSTZ1*C* (Blackburn et al., 1999).

The frequency of the *GSTM1* null allele has been obtained by electrophoretic phenotyping of liver samples and by measuring the GST activity with *trans*-stilbene oxide in mononuclear white blood cells (Board et al., 1990). However, phenotypic studies aimed at determining the presence or the absence of a GST allele do not always give the same results as genotyping studies. A higher reported frequency of the *GSTM1* null allele may be due to deficiencies in expression of the protein, even though DNA encoding GST M1-1 was present. Such discrepancies between genotype and phenotype should always be considered as a possibility. For a proper comparison of the frequencies of the GST alleles in different ethnic groups, the data compiled in Tables 15.5 and 15.6 were restricted to studies that made use of genotyping methods.

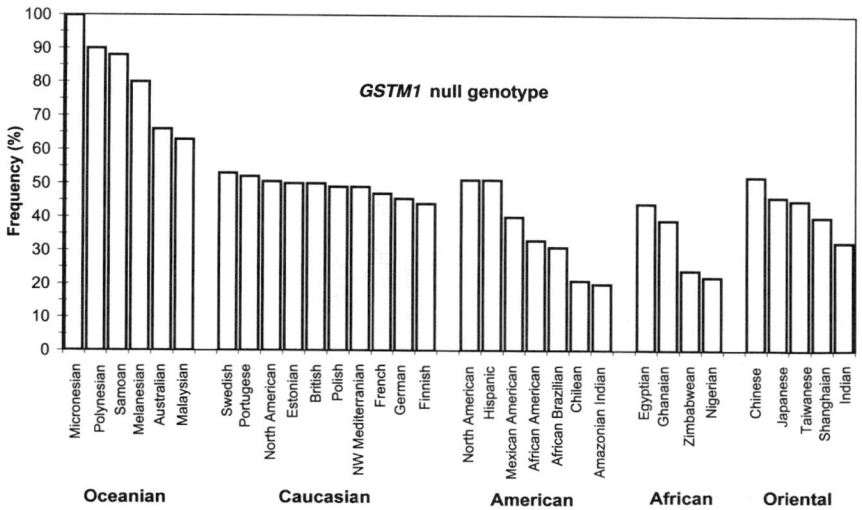

Figure 15.3 Distribution of the *GSTM1* null genotype in different populations. The frequency presented is a mean value in those cases where more than one frequency has been reported for a population. Only results from studies including both males and females are included in this graph. The graph is compiled from data presented in Table 15.5.

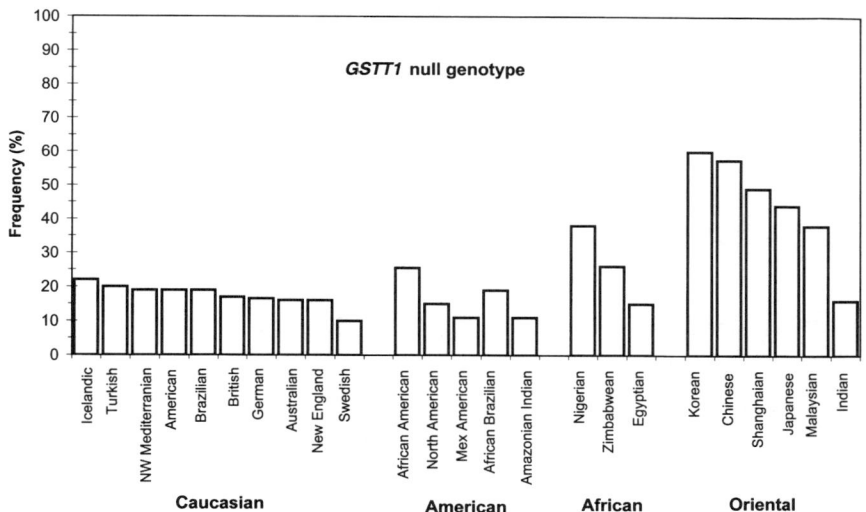

Figure 15.4 Distribution of the *GSTT1* null genotype in different populations. The frequency presented is a mean value in those cases where more than one frequency has been reported for a population. Only results from studies including both males and females are included in this graph. The graph is compiled from data presented in Table 15.5.

Table 15.6 Frequency of glutathione transferase P1-1 sequence variants and GSTP1 allele combinations in different ethnic or racial groups

Population	Residue subject to allelic variation										Frequency of GSTP1 allele combinations					
	Position 105		Position 114		Position 105			Position 114								
	Ile (%)	Val (%)	Ala (%)	Val (%)	Ile/Ile (%)	Ile/Val (%)	Val/Val (%)	Ala/Ala (%)	Ala/Val (%)	Val/Val (%)	AA (%)	AB (%)	AC (%)	BB (%)	BC (%)	CC (%)
Caucasian																
Europe																
English[a]	68	32			49	37	14									
Norwegian[b]**	71	29			52	39	9									
Swedish[c]**	70	30	94	6	44	47	9	87	13	0						
Scottish[d]	72	28			51	42	7									
German[e] NW	70	30			53	35	12									
Mediterranean[f]	69	31			48	41	11									
Australia[g,h]	66	34	93	7	40–41	48–51	9–11	85–87	13–15	0	41	39	10	7	3	0
USA[i]	67	33	91	9	42	51	7	82	18	0	51	28	9	5	0	7
American																
African[i]	70	30	89	11	51	37	12	84	9	7						
American[i]	58	42	97	3	35	46	19	95	5	0						
Oceanian																
Australian Aboriginal[h]	89	11	100	0	82	13	4	100	0	0						
Oriental																
Chinese[h,k]	76–81	19–24	99	1	61–65	31	4–8	98	2	0						
Japanese[l]	86	14			76	20	4									
Taiwanese[j]	82	18			67	30	3									
Indian[h]	73	27	91	9	50	45	5	85	13	2						

Notes

**Study involving only males.

[a]Rollinson et al., 2000; [b]Ryberg et al., 1997; [c]Carstensen et al., 1999; [d]Harries et al., 1997; [e]Matthias et al., 1997; [f]To-Figueras et al., 1999; [g]Menegon et al., 1998; [h]Harris et al., 1998; [i]Watson et al., 1998; [j]Ali-Osman 1997; [i]Lin et al., 1998b; [k]Katoh et al., 1999.

Epidemiology

Investigations of possible links between the absence of GST M1-1 and the development of diseases with electrophilic compounds as possible etiological factors were natural consequences of the discovery of the null phenotype and the characteristic substrate specificity of the enzyme (Warholm *et al.*, 1981a, 1983). Much interest was focused on the potential association between the *GSTM1* null genotype and lung cancer, since GST M1-1 is active with arene oxides of PAHs found in cigarette smoke and other combustion products. DNA-adduct formation following exposure to PAH has been found to be higher in cells of parenchymal lung tissue taken from GSTM1 null phenotype individuals (Shields *et al.*, 1993). GST P1-1 also has high catalytic efficiency with carcinogenic epoxides of PAHs (Robertson *et al.*, 1986; Sundberg *et al.*, 1997) and overexpression of GST P1-1 in a stably transfected human cell line was shown to protect DNA from damage induced by (+)-*anti*-BPDE (Fields *et al.*, 1998). Recent model studies on mice, in which both of the murine Pi class GST genes had been deleted, showed a significantly enhanced susceptibility to skin tumorigenesis induced by PAHs as evidenced by a 3.4-fold higher number of papillomas (Henderson *et al.*, 1998). This finding provides direct evidence that Pi class members, like other GSTs, play an important role in the cellular protection against carcinogenesis.

Associations between GST genotype and cancer

GSTM1 null, and alleles A and B

An early example of the attempts to correlate disease with GST deficiency was made by Seidegård *et al.* (1986). GST activity was measured with *trans*-stilbene oxide in leukocytes from lung cancer patients as well as from a control group. The study indicated an approximate 1.6-fold higher frequency of the GSTM1 null phenotype in individuals with lung cancer (65% GST M1-1 null) as compared with healthy controls (41% GST M1-1 null). It was later established that this enzyme assay is a proper measure of GST M1-1 activity (Seidegård *et al.*, 1987). Subsequent studies have not always showed a clear positive correlation between increased incidence of lung cancer and the GST M1-1 null phenotype. McWilliams *et al.* (1995) compiled the results of twelve studies of GSTM1 status and lung cancer risk involving a total of 1593 cases and 2135 controls. The results showed that deficiency of GST M1-1 is a moderate risk factor for development of lung cancer, with an odds ratio of 1.41. Discrepancies between different studies are not surprising, since the development of lung cancer is dependent on many factors. In addition, there are also other factors that should be taken into consideration in any attempt to determine the association between *GSTM1* genotypes and risk. The results of a study performed by

Tang *et al.* (1998) suggest that the effect of the *GSTM1* null genotype is greatest in female smokers, indicating that women are at higher risk of lung cancer than males, given equal smoking habits. This is supported by the observation that the levels of DNA adducts in lung tissue of females were higher than in males when adjusted for smoking habits (Ryberg *et al.*, 1994). It is clear that in addition to *GSTM1* null genotype, gender, age and smoking status influence the risk of getting cancer (Kihara *et al.*, 1995). These parameters should therefore be taken into consideration in any attempt to determine the association between cancer susceptibility and GST genotype.

It would appear that GST M1-1 can provide protection against some types of lung cancer, but not others. For instance, a study carried out in Japan, showed that 45% of the controls lacked the *GSTM1* gene. Among lung cancer patients, 54% of the subjects with adenocarcinoma were *GSTM1* null, whereas 63% of squamous and small cell carcinoma patients were *GSTM1* null (Kihara *et al.*, 1994). This indicates that *GSTM1*A* and *GSTM1*B* alleles protect preferentially against squamous and small cell carcinomas, but not against adenocarcinoma of the lung (Zhong *et al.*, 1991; Nazar-Stewart *et al.*, 1993; Hirvonen *et al.*, 1993). A difficulty in elucidating the association of a particular GST allele with risk in some cancers is that the relevant carcinogenic substrates of the enzymes are mostly unknown. In addition, the possible differential expression of GSTs in the various cell types in tissues such as the lung, makes correlation to the etiology of neoplasias uncertain.

The importance of combining alleles suspected to contribute to lung cancer susceptibility was evidenced in a study in Japan, where it was found that individuals at high risk had an increased frequency of a combination of homozygosity of the *GSTM1* null allele and a particular allele of the variant *CYP1A1* gene (Hayashi *et al.*, 1992). Ryberg *et al.* (1997), reported that the combined genotypes of *GSTM1* null and heterozygosity or homozygosity for *GSTP1* alleles with Val in position 105 significantly increases the risk of obtaining lung cancer. Kawajiri *et al.* (1996) reported an association of smoking-induced lung cancer susceptibility with *CYP1A1* and *GSTM1* polymorphisms combined with p53 mutations. In patients with non-small cell lung cancer, a susceptibility-conferring *CYP1A1* genotype combined with the *GSTM1* null genotype was correlated with a remarkably high frequency of mutations in the p53 gene. Also in gastric cancer patients an association between the *GSTM1* null genotype and p53 genomic instability has been found (Conde *et al.*, 1999).

The impact of the *GSTM1* null genotype on bladder cancer has been studied extensively. Although the frequency of the *GSTM1* null allele among bladder cancer patients compared with controls varies between different studies, a positive correlation between GST M1-1 deficiency and increased bladder cancer risk seems to exist (Daly *et al.*, 1993; Bell *et al.*,

1993; Brockmöller *et al.*, 1994). When restricted to smokers with bladder cancer, a significantly higher incidence of the *GSTM1* null genotype (71%) compared with controls (50%) was observed (Šalagovic *et al.*, 1999). Absence of GST M1-1 may also predispose an individual to stomach and colon cancer (Strange *et al.*, 1991; Zhong *et al.*, 1993a).

Skin cancer is another malignancy where the *GSTM1* null genotype may confer increased risk of disease. Heagerty *et al.* (1994) found that patients with two or more different types of skin tumors had an increased frequency of homozygosity for the *GSTM1* null allele. The same study showed that skin cancer patients with multiple basal cell carcinomas had a lower frequency of *GSTM1*A/GSTM1*B* heterozygosity, suggesting that having both *GSTM1*A* and *GSTM1*B* alleles may be an advantage.

In a single clinical trial, the GSTM1 null phenotype appeared to have a positive correlation with event-free survival in children with acute lymphoblastic leukaemia (Hall *et al.*, 1994) demonstrating that a null phenotype may be beneficial in certain instances. The possession of the *GSTM1*A* or *GSTM1*B* alleles was calculated to increase the risk of relapse approximately three-fold. The mechanism underlying this result is unclear.

GSTM3 alleles A and B

The *GSTM3*A* allele lacks the potential recognition motif for the transcription factor YY1 present in intron 6 of the *GSTM3*B* allele (Inskip *et al.*, 1995). The latter allele may also have altered interactions with two additional transcription factors, HSTF1 and NF-GMa, as judged from the presence of their binding motifs near the deletion in intron 6 (To-Figueras *et al.*, 2000). This means that *GSTM3*A* and *GSTM3*B* may be expressed at different levels and, if so, the different genotypes will confer different efficiencies in the metabolism of carcinogens. The available evidence suggests that the *GSTM3*B* allele is protective. In a study of the *GSTM3* genotype and the incidence of basal cell carcinoma, no association was found between homozygosity for the *GSTM3*A* allele alone and an increased number of tumors (Yengi *et al.*, 1996). However, the combination of homozygosity for *GSTM3*A*, skin type 1, *GSTM1* null or homozygosity for *CYP1A1m1* was shown to be associated with significantly increased tumor numbers, suggesting that homozygosity for *GSTM3*A* confers increased risk of multiple basal cell carcinoma. Similarly, homozygosity of *GSTM3*A* in combination with *GSTM1* null may predispose to lung cancer (To-Figueras *et al.*, 2000).

GSTT1 null

The biological consequences of the *GSTT1* null genotype are difficult to predict, since this enzyme has both detoxicating and toxifying properties, depending on the nature of the substrate. GST T1-1 will detoxicate mono-haloalkanes and ethylene oxide, but will toxify dichloromethane and other bifunctional alkylating agents (Hallier, 1993; Ketterer and Christodoulides, 1994). The tissue-specific expression of Theta class GSTs differs between rodents and humans (Hayes and Pulford, 1995). This complicates predictions based on animal models concerning health risks associated with the GSTT1 null phenotype. One of the differences is that GST T1-1 is expressed in human erythrocytes. The red blood cells have therefore been suggested to function as a detoxication sink in GST T1-1 positive individuals (Pemble *et al.*, 1994). If so, the erythrocytes will remove bifunctional alkylating agents from the circulation, preventing them from being transported to tissues where they, once activated, can cause genotoxicity. Support for this hypothesis was provided by a study showing that cultured lymphocytes of *GSTT1* null individuals exposed *in vitro* to DEB demonstrated a sixteen-fold increased frequency of SCE compared with lymphocytes with the *GSTT1* positive genotype (Wiencke *et al.*, 1995). However, few studies have reported a link between the *GSTT1* null genotype and cancer susceptibility. The frequency of the *GSTT1* null allele in a bladder cancer group was shown to be significantly higher in comparison with the control group (27% versus 17%) (Šalagovic *et al.*, 1999).

GSTP1 alleles A, B, C, and D

A case-control study of the correlation between the variability in position 105 and lung cancer showed that the lung cancer patients had a significantly higher frequency of the *GSTP1*B* and/or *GSTP1*C* genotypes (15.9%) and a lower frequency of the *GSTP1*A* and/or *GSTP1*D* genotypes (38.4%) than the controls (9.1% and 51.5%, respectively) (Ryberg *et al.*, 1997). The allelic variants B and C could not be distinguished, nor could A and D, since the codon in position 114 was not determined. Smoking lung cancer patients expressing GST P1-1 homozygous for Val in position 105 were shown to have significantly higher DNA adduct levels than patients homozygous for Ile in position 105. Similarly, the frequency of alleles encoding Val in position 105 was increased from 6.5% in controls to 19.7% in bladder cancer and to 18.7% in testicular cancer patients (Harries *et al.*, 1997). In contrast, prostate cancer patients were found to have a lower frequency (2.8%) of alleles containing Val in position 105.

Association between GST polymorphisms and other oxidative stress related diseases

GST M1-1 deficiency contributes to individual susceptibility to asbestos-induced pulmonary disease (Smith *et al.*, 1994). In a study investigating the correlation between GST polymorphisms and Parkinson's disease, the distribution of *GSTP1* genotypes was shown to differ significantly between a control group and patients who had been exposed to pesticides (Menegon *et al.*, 1998). The frequency of the *GSTP1*A/GSTP1*A* genotype was significantly lower in patients compared with controls, whereas the frequency of the *GSTP1*A/GSTP1*B, GSTP1*B/GSTP1*B* and *GSTP1*A/GSTP1*C* genotypes were increased in patients compared with controls. GST P1-1, which is expressed in the blood–brain barrier, may modulate the potency of neurotoxins and this may explain the susceptibility of some individuals to the Parkinsonism-inducing effects of pesticides.

Significance of the variability in expression of glutathione transferases

GSTs play a major role in the cellular defense against toxic electrophiles, the most important of which may derive from oxidative processes such as lipid peroxidation in the organism. Thus, there are not only known carcinogens such as PAHs and aflatoxin B_1 coming from exogenous sources, but also endogenously produced hydroperoxides, alkenals and quinones that may contribute to ageing and cause cellular damage and disease (Beckman and Ames, 1998). Many of these noxious chemical species are inactivated by reactions with glutathione (Berhane *et al.*, 1994), and deficiencies in the repertoire of GSTs would make tissues more vulnerable to toxic agents. Hydrogen peroxide, organic hydroperoxides and other reactive oxygen species are relevant to oxidative stress in general, inflammation, and a variety of other pathological states. Alkenals, in particular 4-hydroxynonenal, are important products of lipid peroxidation and these toxic compounds have been linked to, for example, atherosclerosis, cataract, and Alzheimer's disease (see references cited in Hubatsch *et al.*, 1998). Ortho-quinones are formed from catecholamines, and aminochrome, derived from dopamine, has been implied in the etiology of Parkinson's disease (Segura-Aguilar *et al.*, 1997). The catalytic efficiency with relevant alkenals is particularly high for GST A4-4 (Hubatsch *et al.*, 1998) and the activity with ortho-quinones is most prominent for GST M2-2 (Baez *et al.*, 1997). Deficiencies in these GSTs may therefore predispose to various degenerative diseases. However, polymorphisms in these enzymes have yet to be identified.

The fact that GSTs are part of a complex integrated detoxication system makes it difficult to demonstrate associations between GST polymorphisms and disease. There are several confounding factors that may modulate the sensitivity of the individual to toxic agents. Deletion of the gene for a particular GST inevitably leads to loss of functions associated with the corresponding protein. GST M1-1 has high catalytic efficiency with mutagenic and carcinogenic arene oxides (Warholm *et al.*, 1981a, 1983;

Sundberg et al., 1997) and the absence of this enzyme form may make an individual more susceptible to such genotoxic agents. Similarly, GST T1-1 is highly active with ethylene oxide (Föst et al., 1991), and the absence of this enzyme may also have toxicological consequences. However, the overall consequences of a gene deletion are not self-evident, since compensatory effects may exist in the organism. GSTs have overlapping substrate specificities, and overproduction of a less active isoenzyme may compensate for the missing enzyme form. Therefore, the entirety of the superfamily of GSTs should be considered, rather than just individual isoenzymes. Certain GST alleles influence the expression of other genes, as in the case of GSTM3 and GSTM1 (Inskip et al., 1995; To-Figueras et al., 2000). Further, although GST M1a-1a and GST M1b-1b have similar catalytic activities, some cancers seem to display a gene dosage effect with the GSTM1*A/GSTM1*B genotype conferring a reduced risk (Heagerty et al., 1994). The activity of the cytochrome P450 enzyme CYP1A2 was shown to be higher in individuals who possess the GSTM1 null allele compared with those expressing the GSTM1 alleles A and B (MacLeod et al., 1997). This suggests that there are consequential interactions of genes associated with different phases of the biotransformation of toxic agents.

It is clear that the GST expression profile influences the susceptibility of a cell to genotoxic compounds. However, life-style factors such as smoking and diet, as well as various environmental factors also affect the susceptibility of an individual to various diseases. For example, exposure to a noxious agent may not only cause a toxic challenge but also induce increased levels of GSTs involved in the cellular defense system. Detoxication enzymes other than GSTs, and especially phase I enzymes such as polymorphic enzymes belonging to the cytochrome P450 system, should also be taken into account in studies in which the susceptibility of individuals carrying a certain GST genotype to different diseases is analysed. The studies involving p53 mutations (Kawajiri et al., 1996) show that other factors such as tumor suppressors and oncogenes should also be considered in the assessment of cancer risk. For these various reasons it is not surprising that a phenotypic penetrance of a GST defect is often difficult to detect.

Methods for phenotyping and genotyping

Phenotyping

There are two principal approaches to the phenotyping of GSTs. The presence or absence of a particular isoenzyme in a tissue sample can be determined at the protein level, or the phenotype can be determined indirectly by measuring the activity with an isoenzyme specific substrate. In order to enable phenotyping without using isoenzyme specific substrates the multiple cytosolic GSTs have to be separated. Usually, high specificity or high-resolution techniques, or both, are required. Board (1981) described a method by which glutathione transferase isoenzymes in a tissue sample could be analysed using starch gel electrophoresis followed by a specific staining procedure detecting GST activity. Other analytical methods shown to be useful include sodium dodecyl sulfate-polyacrylamide gel electrophoresis (SDS-PAGE) (Hayes and Mantle, 1986b), isoelectric focusing (Warholm *et al.*, 1980; Hales *et al.*, 1978; Aceto *et al.*, 1989), reverse-phase HPLC (Ostlund Farrants *et al.*, 1987) and electrospray ionisation mass spectrometry (Yeh *et al.*, 1995; Rouimi *et al.*, 1995; Rowe *et al.*, 1997). GST isoenzymes can also be identified using immunoassays with either specific polyclonal antibodies specific for purified GSTs (Hao *et al.*, 1994), as well as for GST peptides (Rowe *et al.*, 1997), or monoclonal antibodies (Hayes, 1983; Hayes and Mantle, 1986a; Peters *et al.*, 1990).

GST M1-1

The deficiency of the *GSTM1* gene was first detected as the absence of a protein component in samples from some individuals compared with others using electrophoretic separations followed by determination of GST activity (Warholm *et al.*, 1980; Board, 1981). The phenotype of GST M1-1 can be determined in leukocytes as activity with the GST M1-1 specific substrate *trans*-stilbene oxide (Seidegård *et al.*, 1984). The low and high glutathione conjugation activities with *trans*-stilbene oxide identify absence and presence of the *GSTM1* gene, respectively. The assay may even be used to determine the number of active genes (McLellan *et al.*, 1997). The polymorphism was later studied by genotyping (Brockmöller *et al.*, 1992). Carriers of the GST M1-1 deficiency were identified by a specific radioimmunoassay (Hussey *et al.*, 1987), and a similar phenotyping assay using Western blotting and radioimmunoassay showed 100% concordance with a genetic assay based on restriction fragment length polymorphism (RFLP) analysis (Zhong *et al.*, 1991). The results of this phenotyping assay were in agreement with the earlier results of Seidegård *et al.* (1986). SDS-PAGE analysis of cytosolic GSTs followed by immunoblotting using anti-GST M1-1 antibodies was shown to be useful in identifying GST M1-1 null individuals (Rowe *et al.*, 1997). The charge difference between GST M1a-1a and GST M1b-1b makes it possible to determine the phenotypes GSTM1 A, GSTM1 B, and GSTM1 A,B using chromatofocusing (Strange *et al.*, 1992).

GST T1-1

Prior to the characterisation of human Theta class GSTs, erythrocytes were shown to metabolise methyl chloride to *S*-methylglutathione (Redford-Ellis and Gowenlock, 1971). Additional studies of halogenated alkanes such as methyl bromide and methyl iodide (Hallier *et al.*, 1990), methyl chloride

(Peter *et al.*, 1989), dichloromethane (Thier *et al.*, 1991) and epoxides like ethylene oxide (Föst *et al.*, 1991) further demonstrated an enzymatic conjugation with glutathione in human erythrocytes. Individual differences in the metabolism of these substances were reported (Peter *et al.*, 1989; Bogaards *et al.*, 1993; Hallier *et al.*, 1993, Warholm *et al.*, 1994; Ploemen *et al.*, 1995) and attributed to a polymorphism of the enzyme involved (Peter *et al.*, 1989). The enzyme was later identified as GST T1-1 (Pemble *et al.*, 1994). By measuring the enzyme activity of erythrocytes towards these substrates, individuals can be divided into one of three groups; non-conjugators, low conjugators and high conjugators. Individuals heterozygous for the *GSTT1* gene should exhibit the low conjugator phenotype, whereas homozygosity for the *GSTT1* gene should produce the high conjugator phenotype. Homozygosity for the *GSTT1* null allele results in the non-conjugator phenotype. Peter *et al.* (1989) incubated hemolysates with methyl chloride and studied the formation of *S*-methylglutathione using thin layer chromatography. About 60% of the blood samples showed a significant metabolic elimination of this substrate and the corresponding individuals were classed as conjugators, whereas 40% did not and were designated non-conjugators. Hallier *et al.* (1993) proposed a standard method for identification of conjugators and non-conjugators using the three GST T1-1 substrates methyl bromide, ethylene oxide and dichloromethane. The substrates were incubated *in vitro* with blood samples, and the disappearance of the substances, monitored by gas chromatography, was used as a measure of GST T1-1 activity. An alternative to determining the conjugator status is to use the substrate dichloromethane and photometrically measure the formation of formaldehyde, the final product of the metabolism of dichloromethane (Pemble *et al.*, 1994); this study also demonstrated a concordance between GSTT1 phenotype and genotype. An advantage of phenotyping assays in comparison with genotyping assays is that it is possible to determine the number of functional *GSTT1* alleles in a studied subject. Most importantly, the functional properties as such are the parameters governing the biotransformation of toxic compounds in the organism.

GST P1-1

GST P1-1 is the only abundant GST in erythrocytes that utilizes 1-chloro-2,4-dinitrobenzene (CDNB) as a substrate, and its activity can thus be measured directly in erythrocyte lysates (Board *et al.*, 1998). The activity of GST P1-1 with CDNB was investigated in normal lung tissue genotyped for the polymorphisms in amino acids 105 and 114. The CDNB conjugating activities were consistently lower in individuals with Val105 in the H-site in accordance with results from studies involving purified enzymes (Zimniak *et al.*, 1994; Ali-Osman *et al.*, 1997; Johansson *et al.*, 1998). A negative gene dosage effect between the number of alleles encoding Val in position 105 and CDNB activity was observed (Watson *et al.*, 1998).

Genotyping

New techniques in the area of DNA analysis are constantly evolving. The methods so far used in the analysis of GST genes (see below) need to be supplemented with rapid and sensitive screens for studies of large numbers of samples. Known polymorphisms can readily be identified by hybridisation, and methods for mutational analysis based on oligonucleotide microarray technologies are being developed (Collins, 1999; and other articles in that issue of *Nature Genetics*). A major change in experimental approaches is consequently forthcoming.

GSTM1

The low GST *trans*-stilbene oxide activity in approximately 50% of the population was shown to be associated with the absence of *Bam*HI and *Eco*RI restriction fragments in genomic DNA, suggesting that the *GSTM1* null genotype is due to the deletion of the *GSTM1* gene (Seidegård *et al.*, 1988). Comstock *et al.* (1990) and Mannervik *et al.* (1991) used polymerase chain reaction (PCR) with primers that amplified exons 4 and 5 and the intervening intron of the *GSTM1* gene. A PCR fragment is expected for individuals with one or two copies of the *GSTM1* gene and no fragment would be obtained when the *GSTM1* gene is homozygously deleted. Bell (1991) used a similar approach, and also included the β-globin gene as an internal control. The intensities of the β-globin and GSTM1 bands were measured with scanning laser densitometry, and the ratio between the bands was used to indicate hetero- or homozygosity. To identify the *GSTM1*A* and *GSTM1*B* alleles Fryer *et al.* (1993) made use of allele-specific PCR primers that by site-directed mutagenesis introduced a restriction site in DNA amplified from *GSTM1*A*, thereby allowing distinction of this allele from *GSTM1*B*. A PCR assay involving allele specific primers made it possible to identify the *GSTM1*A, *B, *A/*B* and *GSTM1* null genotypes in a single step (Yengi *et al.*, 1996). The "ultra-rapid" *trans*-stilbene oxide activity of individuals in a Saudi Arabian population was shown by RFLP analysis to be due to the presence of two *GSTM1* genes in tandem (McLellan *et al.*, 1997). The use of a quantitative multiplex PCR demonstrated that these individuals actually carry three active *GSTM1* genes (McLellan *et al.*, 1997).

GSTT1

Pemble *et al.* (1994) used PCR with specific primers and Southern blot analysis to demonstrate the presence of the *GSTT1* gene and concluded that the non-conjugator phenotype was due to a gene deletion. This conclusion was later verified in studies involving larger groups of individuals (Warholm *et al.*, 1995; Kempkes *et al.*, 1996).

The methods for genotyping of GSTs have been further improved. Multiplex PCR procedures for simultaneous analysis of the *GSTM1* and *GSTT1* polymorphisms have been designed (Abdel-Rahman *et al.*, 1996; Arand *et al.*, 1996). A method with high throughput and reproducibility using TaqMan probes has been developed for detecting the gene deletions of both *GSTM1* and *GSTT1* (Shi *et al.*, 1999).

GSTP1

The polymorphism of GST P1-1 in codons 105 and 114 was discovered by Board *et al.* (1989). An RFLP in the gene encoding GST P1-1 was detected with the restriction endonuclease *Bam*HI in Southern blot hybridization (Kumar *et al.*, 1994). Several PCR-based methods that identify individuals with amino acid variations at position 105 and 114 have been developed (Lo and Ali-Osman, 1997; Harries *et al.*, 1997, Harris *et al.*, 1998; Ali-Osman *et al.*, 1997). The amplified fragments containing the polymorphic locations are subjected to restriction analysis. Identifications of alleles are based on digestions with combinations of different restriction endonucleases, which are able to cut DNA of one allele but not DNA of the other one at the site of polymorphism. For example, variations at codon 105 can be detected using digestion of a PCR amplified fragment with *Alw*26I or *Mae*II. The *GSTP1* Val105 allele is cleaved, but not the Ile105 allele. The polymorphism at codon 114 can likewise be analysed by *Cac*8I or *Xcm*I digestion. The Ala114 allele is cleaved but the Val114 allele is not. The allele combinations in a sample can be determined except in the case where sequence variations are found in both codons 105 and 114. Thus, the allele combination AC cannot be distinguished from the combination BD.

GSTM3

The allelism in the *GSTM3* gene was identified using PCR of genomic DNA followed by sequencing (Inskip *et al.*, 1995). The nucleotide sequence revealed the presence of a three base deletion in intron 6 in some samples. The deletion in the allele denoted *GSTM3*B* creates an additional *Mnl*I recognition site, which makes it possible to detect the *GSTM3* polymorphism by making use of restriction endonuclease mapping.

Conclusions

Purified GSTs have unequivocally been shown to catalyse the inactivation (and in some cases the activation) of compounds strongly implicated in the etiology of various diseases. Variations in the expression of the relevant isoenzymes catalysing such reactions may therefore be predicted to alter biotransformation and the toxicity of those substrates. *In vitro* experiments lend strong support to the conclusion that cells lacking a particular GST are more susceptible to genotoxic effects of substrates inactivated by that same enzyme. Various GST deletions in animal models are currently being developed and may help to further clarify the effects at the organism level.

Acknowledgements

We gratefully acknowledge the help of colleagues in the area of glutathione transferase research for kindly helping us to access the relevant literature by providing reprints of their publications. The large number of publications in the subject area unfortunately has forced us to be selective in our citations. We thank Dr. Margareta Warholm, Institute of Environmental Medicine, Karolinska Institute, Stockholm, Sweden and Drs Gun Stenberg and Samantha Lien of our department for critically reviewing this chapter. Work from the authors' laboratory has been supported by the Swedish Cancer Society, the Swedish Natural Science Research Council, and Telik, Inc., South San Francisco, CA, USA. A.-S. J. is a recipient of a stipend from the Sven and Lilly Lawski Fund.

References

Abdel-Rahman, S. Z., El-Zein, R. A., Anwar, W. A. and Au, W. W. (1996) 'A multiplex PCR procedure for polymorphic analysis of GSTM1 and GSTT1 genes in population studies', *Cancer Lett.* **107**: 229–33.

Aceto, A., Di Ilio, C., Angelucci, S., Felaco, M. and Federici, G. (1989) 'Glutathione transferase isoenzymes from human testis', *Biochem. Pharmacol.* **38**: 3653–60.

Adams, D. J., Balkwill, F. R., Griffin, D. B., Hayes, J. D., Lewis, A. D. and Wolf, C.R. (1987) 'Induction and suppression of glutathione transferases by interferon in the mouse', *J. Biol. Chem.* **262**: 4888–92.

Ahmad, H., Wilson, D. E., Fritz, R. R., Singh, S. V., Medh, R. D., Nagle, G. T., Awasthi, Y. C. and Kurosky, A. (1990) 'Primary and secondary structural analyses of glutathione S-transferase π from human placenta', *Arch. Biochem. Biophys.* **278**: 398–408.

Alexandrie, A.-K., Ingelman-Sundberg, M., Seidegård, J., Tornling, G. and Rannug, A. (1994) 'Genetic susceptibility to lung cancer with special emphasis on CYP1A1 and GSTM1: a study on host factors in relation to age at onset, gender and histological cancer types', *Carcinogenesis* **15**: 1785–90.

Ali-Osman, F., Akande, O., Antoun, G., Mao, J.-X. and Buolamwini, J. (1997) 'Molecular cloning, characterization, and expression in *Escherichia coli* of full-length cDNAs of three human glutathone S-transferase Pi gene variants', *J. Biol. Chem.* **272**: 10004–12.

Ames, B. N., Gold, L. S. and Willett, W. C. (1995) 'The causes and prevention of cancer', *Proc. Natl. Acad. Sci. U.S.A.* **92**: 5258–65.

Anders, M. W. and Dekant, W. (1998) 'Glutathione-dependent bioactivation of haloalkenes', *Annu. Rev. Pharmacol. Toxicol.* **38**: 501–37.

Ansher, S. S., Dolan, P. and Bueding, E. (1986) 'Biochemical effects of dithiolthiones', *Food Chem. Toxicol.* **24**: 405–15.

Arand, M., Mühlbauer, R., Hengstler, J., Jäger, E., Fuchs, J., Winkler, L. and Oesch, F. (1996) 'A multiplex polymerase chain reaction protocol for the simultaneous analysis of the glutathione *S*-transferase GSTM1 and GSTT1 polymorphism', *Anal. Biochem.* **236**: 184–6.

Arca, P., Hardisson, C. and Suárez, J. E. (1990) 'Purification of a glutathione *S*-transferase that mediates fosfomycin resistance in bacteria', *Antimicrob. Agents Chemother.* **34**: 844–8.

Arca, P., Rico, M., Braña, A. F., Villar, C. J., Hardisson, C. and Suárez, J. E. (1988) 'Formation of an adduct between fosfomycin and glutathione: a new mechanism of antibiotic resistance in bacteria', *Antimicrob. Agents Chemother.* **32**: 1552–6.

Arruda, V. R., Grignolli, C. E., Goncalves, M. S., Soares, M. C., Menezes, R., Saad, S. T. O. And Costa, F. F. (1998) 'Prevalence of homozygosity for the deleted alleles of glutathione S-transferase mu (GSTM1) and theta (GSTT1) among distinct ethnic groups from Brazil: relevance to environmental carcinogenesis?', *Clin. Genet.* **54**: 210–14.

Askelöf, P., Guthenberg, C., Jakobson, I. and Mannervik, B. (1975) 'Purification and characterization of two glutathione *S*-aryltransferase activities from rat liver', *Biochem. J.* **147**: 513–22.

Bach, M. K., Brashler, J. R. and Morton, D. R. Jr. (1984) 'Solubilization and characterization of the leukotriene C$_4$ synthetase of rat basophil leukemia cells: A novel, particulate glutathione S-transferase', *Arch. Biochem. Biophys.* **230**: 455–65.

Baez, S., Segura-Aguilar, J., Widersten, M., Johansson, A.-S. and Mannervik, B. (1997) 'Glutathione transferases catalyse the detoxication of oxidized metabolites (*o*-quinones) of catecholamines and may serve as an antioxidant system preventing degenerative cellular processes', *Biochem. J.* **324**: 25–8.

Bailey, L. R., Roodi, N., Verrier, C. S., Yee, C. J., Dupont, W. D. and Parl, F. F. (1998) 'Breast cancer and *CYP1A1*, *GSTM1*, and *GSTT1* polymorphisms: evidence of a lack of association in Caucasians and African Americans', *Cancer Res.* **58**: 65–70.

Beckman, K. B. and Ames, B. N. (1998) 'The free radical theory of aging matures', *Physiol. Rev.* **78**: 547–81.

Bell, D. A. (1991) 'Detection of DNA sequence polymorphisms in carcinogen metabolism genes by polymerase chain reaction', *Environ. Mol. Mutagen.* **18**: 245–8.

Bell, D. A., Taylor, J. A., Paulson, D. F., Robertson, C. N., Mohler, J. L. and Lucier, G. W. (1993) 'Genetic risk and carcinogen exposure: a common inherited defect of the carcinogen-metabolism gene glutathione S-transferase M1 (GSTM1) that increases susceptibility to bladder cancer', *J. Natl. Cancer Inst.* **85**: 1159–64.

Benson A. B. (1993) 'Oltipraz: a laboratory and clinical review', *J. Cell Biochem. Suppl.* **17F**: 278–91.

Benson, A. M., Cha, Y.-N., Bueding, E., Heine, H. S. and Talalay, P. (1979)

'Elevation of extrahepatic glutathione S-transferase and epoxide hydratase activities by 2(3)-tert-butyl-4-hydroxyanisole', *Cancer Res.* **39**: 2971–7.

Berhane, K., Hao, X.-Y., Egyházi, S., Hansson, J., Ringborg, U. and Mannervik, B. (1993) 'Contribution of glutathione transferase M3-3 to 1,3-bis(2-chloroethyl)-1-nitrosourea resistance in a human non-small cell lung cancer cell line', *Cancer Res.* **53**: 4257–61.

Berhane, K., Widersten, M., Engström, Å., Kozarich, J. W. and Mannervik, B. (1994) 'Detoxication of base propenals and other α,β-unsaturated aldehyde products of radical reactions and lipid peroxidation by human glutathione transferases', *Proc. Natl. Acad. Sci. U.S.A.* **91**: 1480–4.

Bernat, B. A., Laughlin, L. T. and Armstrong, R. N. (1997) 'Fosfomycin resistance protein (FosA) is a manganese metalloglutathione transferase related to glyoxalase I and the extradiol dioxygenases', *Biochemistry* **36**: 3050–5.

Blackburn, A. C., McNiven, M., Webb, M. and Board, P. G. (1999) 'Detection of polymorphisms by expressed sequence tag (EST) database analysis: application to human glutathione transferase Zeta (GSTZ1) and analysis of the variants in cancer populations', *Proc. Amer. Assoc. Cancer Res.* **40**: 618.

Blackburn, A. C., Woollatt, E., Sutherland, G. R., Board, P. G. (1998) 'Characterization and chromosome location of the gene GSTZ1 encoding the human Zeta class glutathione transferase and maleylacetoacetate isomerase', *Cytogenet. Cell Genet.* **83**: 109–14.

Block, G., Patterson, B. and Subar, A. (1992) 'Fruit, vegetables and cancer prevention: a review of the epidemiologic evidence', *Nutr. Cancer* **18**: 1–29.

Board, P. G. (1981) 'Biochemical genetics of glutathione S-transferase in man', *Am. J. Hum. Genet.* **33**: 36–43.

Board, P. G. (1998) 'Identification of cDNAs encoding two human Alpha class glutathione transferases (GSTA3 and GSTA4) and the heterologous expression of GSTA4-4', *Biochem J.* **330**: 827–31.

Board, P. G., Baker, R. T., Chelvanayagam, G. and Jermiin, L. S. (1997) 'Zeta, a novel class of glutathione transferases in a range of species from plants to humans', *Biochem J.* **328**: 929–35.

Board, P. G., Coggan, M., Chelvanayagam, G., Easteal, S., Jermin, L. S., Schutte, G. K., Danley, D. E., Hoth, L. R., Griffor, M. C., Kamath, A. V., Rosner, M. H., Chrunyk, B. A., Perregaux, D. E., Gabel, C. A., Geoghegan, K. F. and Pandit, J. (2000) 'Identification, characterization and crystal structure of the Omega class glutathione transferases', *J. Biol. Chem.* **275**: 24798–806.

Board, P., Coggan, M., Johnston, P., Ross, V., Suzuki, T. and Webb, G. (1990) 'Genetic heterogeneity of the human glutathione transferases: A complex of gene families', *Pharmacol. Ther.* **48**: 357–69.

Board, P., Harris, M., Flanagan, J., Langton, L. and Coggan, M. (1998) 'Genetic heterogeneity of the structure and function of GSTT2 and GSTP1', *Chem. Biol. Interact.* **111–112**: 83-9.

Board, P. G. and Webb, G. C. (1987) 'Isolation of a cDNA clone and localization of human glutathione S-transferase 2 genes to chromosome band 6p12', *Proc. Natl. Acad. Sci. U.S.A.* **84**: 2377–81.

Board, P. G., Webb, G. C. and Coggan, M. (1989) 'Isolation of a cDNA clone and localization of the human glutathione S-transferase 3 genes to chromosome bands 11q13 and 12q13-14', *Ann. Hum. Genet.* **53**: 205–13.

Bogaards, J. J. P., van Ommen, B., Falke, H. E., Willems, M. I. and van Bladeren, P. J.

(1990) 'Glutathione S-transferase subunit induction patterns of Brussels sprouts, allyl isothiocyanate and goitrin in rat liver and small intestinal mucosa: a new approach for the identification of inducing xenobiotics', *Food Chem. Toxicol.* **28**: 81–8.

Bogaards, J. J. P., van Ommen, B. and van Bladeren, P. J. (1993) 'Interindividual differences in the *in vitro* conjugation of methylene chloride with glutathione by cytosolic glutathione S-transferase in 22 human liver samples', *Biochem. Pharmacol.* **45**: 2166–9.

Bogaards, J. J. P., Verhagen, H., Willems, M. I., van Poppel, G. and van Bladeren, P. J. (1994) 'Consumption of Brussels sprouts results in elevated alpha-class glutathione S-transferase levels in human blood plasma', *Carcinogenesis* **15**: 1073–5.

Booth, J., Boyland, E. and Sims, P. (1961) 'An enzyme from rat liver catalysing conjugations with glutathione', *Biochem. J.* **79**: 516–24.

Boyland, E. and Chasseaud, L. F. (1969) 'The role of glutathione and glutathione S-transferases in mercapturic acid biosynthesis', *Adv. Enzymol.* **32**: 173–219.

Brockmöller, J., Gross, D., Kerb, R., Drakoulis, N. and Roots, I. (1992) 'Correlation between *trans*-stilbene oxide-glutathione conjugation activity and the deletion mutation in the glutathione S-transferase class Mu gene detected by polymerase chain reaction', *Biochem. Pharmacol.* **43**: 647–50.

Brockmöller, J., Kerb, R., Drakoulis, N., Nitz, M. and Roots, I. (1993) 'Genotype and phenotype of glutathione S-transferase class μ isoenzymes μ and ψ in lung cancer patients and controls', *Cancer Res.* **53**: 1004–11.

Brockmöller, J., Kerb, R., Drakoulis, N., Staffeldt, B. and Roots, I. (1994) 'Glutathione S-transferase and its variants A and B as host factors of bladder cancer susceptibility: a case-control study', *Cancer Res.* **54**: 4103–11.

Bruhn, C., Brockmöller, J., Kerb, R., Roots, I. and Borchert, H.-H. (1998) 'Concordance between enzyme activity and genotype of glutathione S-transferase Theta (GSTT1)', *Biochem. Pharmacol.* **56**: 1189–93.

Buller, A. L., Clapper, M. L. and Tew, K. D. (1987) 'Glutathione S-transferases in nitrogen mustard-resistant and -sensitive cell lines', *Mol. Pharmacol.* **31**: 575–8.

Cameron, A. D., Olin, B., Ridderström, M., Mannervik, B. and Jones, T. A. (1997) 'Crystal structure of human glyoxalase I – evidence for gene duplication and 3D domain swapping', *EMBO J.* **16**: 3386–95.

Campbell, E., Takahashi, Y., Abramovitz, M., Peretz, M. and Listowsky I. (1990) 'A distinct human testis and brain μ-class glutathione S-transferase. Molecular cloning and characterization of a form present even in individuals lacking hepatic type μ isoenzymes', *J. Biol. Chem.* **265**: 9188–93.

Carstensen, U., Hou, S.-M., Alexandrie, A.-K., Högstedt, B., Tagesson, C., Warholm, M., Rannug, A., Lambert, B., Axmon, A. and Hagmar, L. (1999) 'Influence of genetic polymorphisms of biotransformation enzymes on gene mutations, strand breaks of deoxyribonucleic acid, and micronuclei in mononuclear blood cells and urinary 8-hydroxydeoxyguanosine in potroom workers exposed to polyaromatic hydrocarbons', *Scand. J. Work. Environ. Health* **25**: 351–60.

Castro, V. M., Söderström, M., Carlberg, I., Widersten, M., Platz, A. and Mannervik, B. (1990) 'Differences among human tumor cell lines in the expression of glutathione transferases and other glutathione-linked enzymes', *Carcinogenesis* **11**: 1569–76.

Ceballos-Picot, I., Trivier, J.-M., Nicole, A., Sinet, P.-M. and Thevenin, M. (1992)

'Age-correlated modifications of copper-zinc superoxide dismutase and glutathione-related enzyme activities in human erythrocytes', *Clin. Chem.* **38**: 66–70.

Chen, C. and Nirunsuksiri, W. (1999) 'Decreased expression of glutathione *S*-transferase M1 in HPV16-transfected human cervical keratinocytes in culture', *Carcinogenesis* **20**: 699–703.

Chen, C.-L., Liu, Q. and Relling, M. V. (1996) 'Simultaneous characterization of glutathione *S*-transferase M1 and T1 polymorphisms by polymerase chain reaction in American whites and blacks', *Pharmacogenetics* **6**: 187–91.

Chenevix-Trench, G., Young, J., Coggan, M. and Board, P. (1995) 'Glutathione *S*-transferase M1 and T1 polymorphisms: susceptibility to colon cancer and age of onset', *Carcinogenesis* **16**: 1655–7.

Cheng, T.-J., Christiani, D. C., Xu, X., Wain, J. C., Wiencke, J. K. and Kelsey, K. T. (1995) 'Glutathione *S*-transferase μ genotype, diet, and smoking as determinants of sister chromatide exchange frequency in lymphocytes.', *Cancer Epidemiol. Biomarkers Prev.* **4**: 535–42.

Coggan, M., Whitbread, L., Whittington, A. and Board, P. (1998) 'Structure and organization of the human Theta-class glutathione S-transferase and D-dopachrome tautomerase gene complex', *Biochem. J.* **334**: 617–23.

Coles, B. F., Anderson, K. E., Doerge, D. R., Churchwell, M. I., Lang, N. P. and Kadlubar, F. F. (2000) 'Quantitative analysis of interindividual variation of glutathione *S*-transferase expression in human pancreas and the ambiguity of correlating genotype with phenotype', *Cancer Res.* **60**: 573–9.

Collins, F.S. (1999) 'Microarrays and macroconsequences', *Nat. Genet.* **21** (Suppl. 2): 2, and other articles in the same issue of *Nature Genetics*.

Combes, B. and Stakelum, G. S. (1961) 'A liver enzyme that conjugates sulfobromophthalein sodium with glutathione', *J. Clin. Invest.* **40**: 981–8.

Comstock, K. E., Johnson, K. J., Rifenbery, D. and Henner, W. D. (1993) 'Isolation and analysis of the gene and cDNA for a human Mu class glutathione *S*-transferase, GSTM4', *J. Biol. Chem.* **268**: 16958–65.

Comstock, K. E., Sanderson, B. J. S., Claflin, G. and Henner, W. D. (1990) 'GST1 gene deletion determined by polymerase chain reaction', *Nucleic Acids Res.* **18**: 3670.

Conde, A. R., Martins, G., Saraiva, C., Rueff, J. and Monteiro, C. (1999) 'Association of p53 genomic instability with the glutathione *S*-transferase null genotype in gastric cancer in the Portugese population', *J. Clin. Pathol. Mol. Pathol.* **52**: 131–4.

Cowell, I. G., Dixon, K. H., Pemble, S. E., Ketterer, B. and Taylor, J. B. (1988) 'The structure of the human glutathione *S*-transferase π gene', *Biochem. J.* **255**: 79-83.

Dahllöf, B., Martinsson, T., Mannervik, B., Jensson, H. and Levan, G. (1987) 'Characterization of multidrug resistance in SEWA mouse tumor cells: increased glutathione transferase activity and reversal of resistance with verapamil', *Anti-cancer Res.* **7**: 65–70.

Daly, A. K., Thomas, D. J., Cooper, J., Pearson, W. R., Neal, D. E. and Idle, J. R. (1993) 'Homozygous deletion of gene for glutathione *S*-transferase M1 in bladder cancer', *BMJ* **307**: 481–2.

Daniel, V. (1993) 'Glutathione *S*-transferases: gene structure and regulation of expression', *Crit. Rev. Biochem. Mol. Biol.* **28**: 173–207.

Danielson, U. H. and Mannervik, B. (1985) 'Kinetic independence of the subunits of cytosolic glutathione transferase from the rat', *Biochem. J.* **231**: 263–7.

De Bruin, W. C. C., Wagenmans, M. J. M., Board, P. G. and Peters, W. H. M. (1999) 'Expression of glutathione S-transferase θ class isoenzymes in human colorectal and gastric cancers', *Carcinogenesis* 20: 1453–7.

DeJong, J. L., Chang, C.-M., Whang-Peng, J., Knutsen, T. and Tu, C.-P. D. (1988) 'The human liver glutathione S-transferase gene superfamily: expression and chromosome mapping of an Hb subunit cDNA', *Nucleic Acids Res.* 16: 8541–54.

DeJong, J. L., Mohandas, T. and Tu, C.-P. D. (1990) 'The gene for the microsomal glutathione S-transferase is on human chromosome 12', *Genomics* 6: 379-82.

Desmots, F., Rauch, C., Henry, C., Guillouzo, A. and Morel, F. (1998) 'Genomic organization, 5′-flanking region and chromosomal localization of the human glutathione transferase A4 gene', *Biochem. J.* 336: 437–42.

Di Simplicio, P., Jensson, H. and Mannervik, B. (1989) 'Effects of inducers of drug metabolism on basic hepatic forms of mouse glutathione transferase', *Biochem. J.* 263: 679–85.

Dunham, I., Shimizu, N., Roe, B. A. *et al.* (1999) 'The DNA sequence of human chromosome 22', *Nature (London)* 402: 489–95.

Elexpuru-Camiruaga, J., Buxton, N., Kandula, V., Dias, P. S., Campbell, D., McIntosh, J., Broome, J., Jones, P., Inskip, A., Alldersea, J., Fryer, A. A. and Strange, R. C. (1995) 'Susceptibility to astrocytoma and meningioma: influence of allelism at glutathione S-transferase (GSTT1 and GSTM1) and cytochrome P-450 (CYP2D6) loci', *Cancer Res.* 55: 4237–9.

Eriksson, L. C., Sharma, R. N., Roomi, M. W., Ho, R. K., Farber, E. and Murray, R. K. (1983) 'A characteristic electrophoretic pattern of cytosolic polypeptides from hepatocyte nodules generated during liver carcinogenesis in several models', *Biochem. Biophys. Res. Commun.* 117: 740–5.

Estonius, M., Forsberg, L., Danielsson, O., Weinander, R., Kelner, M. J. and Morgenstern, R. (1999) 'Distribution of microsomal glutathione transferase 1 in mammalian tissues – a predominant alternate first exon in human tissues', *Eur. J. Biochem.* 260: 409–13.

Evans, D. A. P., Seidegård, J., Narayanan, N. (1996) 'The GSTM1 genetic polymorphism in healthy Saudi Arabians and Filipinos, and Saudi Arabians with coronary atherosclerosis', *Pharmacogenetics* 6: 365–7.

Fahey, J. W., Zhang, Y. and Talalay, P. (1997) 'Broccoli sprouts: an exceptionally rich source of inducers of enzymes that protect against chemical carcinogens', *Proc. Natl. Acad. Sci. U.S.A.* 94: 10367–72.

Faulder, C. G., Hirrell, P. A., Hume, R. and Strange, R. C. (1987) 'Studies of the development of basic, neutral and acidic isoenzymes of glutathione S-transferase in human liver, adrenal, kidney and spleen', *Biochem. J.* 241: 221–8.

Fernandes, C. L., Dong, J. H., Roebuck, B. D., Chisari, F. V., Montali, J. A., Schmidt, D. E. Jr. and Prochaska, H. J. (1996) 'Elevations of hepatic quinone reductase, glutathione, and α- and μ-class glutathione S-transferase isoforms in mice with chronic hepatitis: a compensatory response to injury', *Arch. Biochem. Biophys.* 331: 104–16.

Fields, W. R., Morrow, C. S., Doss, A. J., Sundberg, K., Jernström, B. and Townsend, A. J. (1998) 'Overexpression of stably transfected human glutathione S-transferase P1-1 protects against DNA damage by benzo[a]pyrene diol-epoxide in human T47D cells', *Mol. Pharmacol.* 54: 298–304.

Fleischner, G., Robbins, J. and Arias, I. M. (1972) 'Immunological studies of Y protein. A major cytoplasmic organic anion-binding protein in rat liver', *J. Clin. Invest.* 51: 677–84.

Föst, U., Hallier, E., Ottenwälder, H., Bolt, H. M. and Peter, H. (1991) 'Distribution of ethylene oxide in human blood and its implications for biomonitoring', *Hum. Exp. Toxicol.* 10: 25–31.

Fryer, A. A., Zhao, L., Alldersea, J., Pearson, W. R. and Strange, R. C. (1993) 'Use of site-directed mutagenesis of allele-specific PCR primers to identify the GSTM1 A, GSTM1 B, GSTM1 A,B and GSTM1 null polymorphisms at the glutathione S-transferase, GSTM1 locus', *Biochem. J.* 295: 313–15.

Gawronska-Szklarz, B., Wójcicki, M., Kuprianowicz, A., Kedzierska, K., Kedzierski, M., Górnik, W. and Pawlik, A. (1999) 'CYP2D6 and GSTM1 genotypes in a Polish population', *Eur. J. Clin. Pharmacol.* 55: 389–92.

Grinberg-Funes, R. A., Singh, V. N., Perera, F. P., Bell, D. A., Young, T. L., Dickey, C., Wang, L. W., Santella, R. M. (1994) 'Polycyclic aromatic hydrocarbon-DNA adducts in smokers and their relationship to micronutrient levels and the glutathione-S-transferase M1 genotype', *Carcinogenesis* 15: 2449–54.

Gudmundsdóttir, K. and Eyfjörd, J. E. (1999) 'GST polymorphism in Icelandic breast cancer patients', *Proc. Amer. Assoc. Cancer Res.* 40: 608.

Guengerich, F. P. (1994) 'Metabolism and genotoxicity of dihaloalkanes', *Adv. Pharmacol.* 27: 211–36.

Gupta, E., Olopade, O. I., Ratain, M. J., Mick, R., Baker, T. M., Berezin, F. K., Benson III, A. B. and Dolan, M. E. (1995) 'Pharmacokinetics and pharmaco-dynamics of oltipraz as a chemopreventive agent', *Clin. Cancer Res.* 1: 1133–8.

Gustafsson, A. and Mannervik, B. (1999) 'Benzoic acid derivatives induce recovery of catalytic activity in the partially inactive Met208Lys mutant of human glutathione transferase A1-1', *J. Mol. Biol.* 288: 787–800.

Guthenberg, C., Morgenstern, R., DePierre, J. W. and Mannervik, B. (1980) 'Induction of glutathione *S*-transferases A, B and C in rat liver cytosol by *trans*-stilbene oxide', *Biochim. Biophys. Acta* 631: 1–10.

Guthenberg, C., Warholm, M., Rane, A. and Mannervik, B. (1986) 'Two distinct forms of glutathione transferase from human foetal liver. Purification and comparison with isoenzymes isolated from adult liver and placenta', *Biochem. J.* 235: 741–5.

Habig, W. H., Pabst, M. J. and Jakoby, W. B. (1974) 'Glutathione *S*-transferases. The first enzymatic step in mercapturic acid formation', *J. Biol. Chem.* 249: 7130–9.

Hales, B. F. and Neims, A. H. (1977) 'Induction of rat hepatic glutathione *S*-transferase B by phenobarbital and 3-methylcholantrene', *Biochem. Pharmacol.* 26: 555–6.

Hales, B. F., Jaeger, V. and Neims, A. H. (1978) 'Isoelectric focusing of glutathione *S*-transferases from rat liver and kidney', *Biochem. J.* 175: 937–43.

Hall, A. G., Autzen, P., Cattan, A. R., Malcolm, A. J., Cole, M., Kernahan, J. and Reid, M. M. (1994) 'Expression of μ class glutathione *S*-transferase correlates with event-free survival in childhood acute lymphoblastic leukemia', *Cancer Res.* 54: 5251–4.

Hallier, E., Deutschmann, S., Reichel, C., Bolt, H. M. and Peter, H. (1990) 'A comparative investigation of the metabolism of methyl bromide and methyl iodide in human erythrocytes', *Int. Arch. Occup. Environ. Health* 62: 221–5.

Hallier, E., Langhof, T., Dannappel, D., Leutbecher, M., Schröder, K., Goergens, H. W., Müller, A. and Bolt, H. M. (1993) 'Polymorphism of glutathione conjugation of methyl bromide, ethylene oxide and dichloromethane in human blood: influence on the induction of sister chromatid exchanges (SCE) in lymphocytes', *Arch. Toxicol.* **67**: 173–8.

Hao, X.-Y., Castro, V. M., Bergh, J., Sundström, B. and Mannervik, B. (1994) 'Isoenzyme-specific quantitative immunoassays for cytosolic glutathione transferases and measurement of the enzymes in blood plasma from cancer patients and in tumor cell lines', *Biochim. Biophys. Acta* **1225**: 223–30.

Harada, S., Misawa, S., Nakamura, T., Tanaka, N., Ueno, E. and Nozoe, M. (1992) 'Detection of GST1 gene deletion by the polymerase chain reaction and its possible correlation with stomach cancer in Japanese', *Hum. Genet.* **90**: 62–4.

Harries, L. W., Stubbins, M. J., Forman, D., Howard, G. C. W. and Wolf, C. R. (1997) 'Identification of genetic polymorphisms at the glutathione S-tranferase Pi locus and association with susceptibility to bladder, testicular and prostate cancer', *Carcinogenesis* **18**: 641–4.

Harris, M. J., Coggan, M., Langton, L., Wilson, S. R. and Board, P. G. (1998) 'Polymorphism of the Pi class glutathione S-transferase in normal populations and cancer patients', *Pharmacogenetics* **8**: 27–31.

Hatayama, I., Satoh, K. and Sato, K. (1986) 'Developmental and hormonal regulation of the major form of hepatic glutathione S-transferase in male mice', *Biochem. Biophys. Res. Commun.* **140**: 581–8.

Hayashi, S., Watanabe, J. and Kawajiri, K. (1992) 'High susceptibility to lung cancer analyzed in terms of combined genotypes of P450IA1 and Mu-class glutathione S-transferase genes', *Jpn. J. Cancer Res.* **83**: 866–70.

Hayes, J. D. (1983) 'Rat liver glutathione S-transferases. A study of the structure of the basic YbYb-containing enzymes', *Biochem. J.* **213**: 625–33.

Hayes, J. D., Kerr, L. A. and Cronshaw, A. D. (1989) 'Evidence that glutathione S-transferases B_1B_1 and B_2B_2 are the products of separate genes and that their expression in human liver is subject to inter-individual variation. Molecular relationships between the B_1 and B_2 subunits and other Alpha class glutathione S-transferases', *Biochem J.* **264**: 437–45.

Hayes, J. D. and Mantle, T. J. (1986a) 'Use of immuno-blot techniques to discriminate between the glutathione S-transferase Yf, Yk, Ya, Yn/Yb and Yc subunits and to study their distribution in extrahepatic tissues. Evidence for three immunochemically distinct groups of transferase in the rat', *Biochem. J.* **233**: 779–88.

Hayes, J. D. and Mantle, T. J. (1986b) 'Anomalous electrophoretic behaviour of the glutathione S-transferase Ya and Yk subunits isolated from man and rodents. A potential pitfall for nomenclature', *Biochem. J.* **237**: 731–40.

Hayes, J. D. and Pulford, D. J. (1995) 'The glutathione S-transferase supergene family: regulation of GST and the contribution of the isoenzymes to cancer chemoprotection and drug resistance', *Crit. Rev. Biochem. Mol. Biol.* **30**: 445–600.

Heagerty, A. H. M., Fitzgerald, D., Smith, A., Bowers, B., Jones, P., Fryer, A. A., Zhao, L., Alldersea, J. and Strange, R. C. (1994) 'Glutathione S-transferase GSTM1 phenotypes and protection against cutaneous tumours', *Lancet* **343**: 266–8.

Henderson, C. J., Smith, A. G., Ure, J., Brown, K., Bacon, E. J. and Wolf, C. R. (1998) 'Increased skin tumorigenesis in mice lacking pi class glutathione S-transferases', *Proc. Natl. Acad. Sci. U.S.A.* **95**: 5275–80.

Hengstler, J. G., Kett, A., Arand, M., Oesch-Bartlomowicz, B., Oesch, F., Pilch, H. and Tanner, B. (1998) 'Glutathione S-transferase T1 and M1 gene defects in ovarian carcinoma', *Cancer Lett.* **130**: 43–8.

Hirvonen, A., Husgafvel-Pursiainen, K., Anttila, S. and Vainio, H. (1993) 'The *GSTM1* null genotype as a potential risk modifier for squamous cell carcinoma of the lung', *Carcinogenesis* **14**: 1479–81.

Hu, X., Herzog, C., Zimniak, P. and Singh, S. V. (1999) 'Differential protection against benzo[a]pyrene-7,8-dihydrodiol-9,10-epoxide-induced DNA damage in HepG2 cells stably transfected with allelic variants of π class human glutathione S-transferase', *Cancer Res.* **59**: 2358–62.

Hu, X., Xia, H., Srivastava, S. K., Pal, A., Awasthi, Y. C., Zimniak, P. and Singh, S. V. (1998) 'Catalytic efficiencies of allelic variants of human glutathione S-transferase P1-1 toward carcinogenic *anti*-diol epoxides of benzo[c]phenanthrene and benzo[g]chrysene', *Cancer Res.* **58**: 5340–3.

Hu, X., Xia, H., Srivastava, S. K., Herzog, C., Awasthi, Y. C., Ji, X., Zimniak, P. and Singh, S. V. (1997) 'Activity of four allelic forms of glutathione S-transferase hGSTP1-1 for diol epoxides of polycyclic aromatic hydrocarbons', *Biochem. Biophys. Res. Commun.* **238**: 397–402.

Hubatsch, I., Ridderström, M. and Mannervik, B. (1998) 'Human glutathione transferase A4-4: an Alpha class enzyme with high catalytic efficiency in the conjugation of 4-hydroxynonenal and other genotoxic products of lipid peroxidation', *Biochem. J.* **330**: 175–9.

Hussey, A. J. and Hayes, J. D. (1992) 'Characterization of a human class-Theta glutathione S-transferase with activity towards 1-menaphthyl sulphate', *Biochem. J.* **286**: 929–35.

Hussey, A. J., Hayes, J. D. and Beckett, G. J. (1987) 'The polymorphic expression of neutral glutathione S-transferase in human mononuclear leucocytes as measured by specific radioimmunoassay', *Biochem. Pharmacol.* **36**: 4013–15.

Igarashi, T., Satoh, T., Ono, S., Iwashita, K., Hosokawa, M., Ueno, K. and Kitagawa, H. (1984) 'Effect of steroidal sex hormones on the sex-related differences in the hepatic activities of γ-glutamyltranspeptidase, glutathione S-transferase and glutathione peroxidase in rats', *Res. Commun. Chem. Pathol. Pharmacol.* **45**: 225–32.

Inskip, A., Elexperu-Camiruaga, J., Buxton, N., Dias, P. S., MacIntosh, J., Campbell, D., Jones P. W., Yengi, L., Talbot, J. A., Strange, R. C. and Fryer, A. A. (1995) 'Identification of polymorphism at the glutathione S-transferase, GSTM3 locus: evidence for linkage with *GSTM1*A*', *Biochem J.* **312**: 713–16.

Islam, M. Q., Platz, A., Szpirer, J., Szpirer, C., Levan, G. and Mannervik, B. (1989) 'Chromosomal localization of human glutathione transferase genes of classes alpha, mu and pi', *Hum. Genet.* **82**: 338–42.

Jakobsson, P.-J., Morgenstern, R., Mancini, J., Ford-Hutchinson, A. and Persson, B. (1999a) 'Common structural features of *MAPEG* – A widespread superfamily of membrane associated proteins with highly divergent functions in eicosanoid and glutathione metabolism', *Protein Sci.* **8**: 689–92.

Jakobsson, P.-J., Thorén, S., Morgenstern, R. and Samuelsson, B. (1999b) 'Identification of human prostaglandin E synthase: A microsomal, glutathione-dependent, inducible enzyme, constituting a potential novel drug target', *Proc. Natl. Acad. Sci. U.S.A.* **96**: 7220–5.

Jakschik, B. A., Harper, T. and Murphy, R. C. (1982) 'Leukotriene C_4 and D_4 formation by particulate enzymes', *J. Biol. Chem.* **257**: 5346–9.

Jemth, P. and Mannervik, B. (1997) 'Kinetic characterization of recombinant human glutathione transferase T1-1, a polymorphic detoxication enzyme', *Arch. Biochem. Biophys.* **348**: 247–54.

Jensson, H., Eriksson, L. C. and Mannervik, B. (1985) 'Selective expression of glutathione transferase isoenzymes in chemically induced preneoplastic rat heptocyte nodules', *FEBS Lett.* **187**: 115–20.

Johansson, A.-S., Stenberg, G., Widersten, M. and Mannervik, B. (1998) 'Structure-activity relationships and thermal stability of human glutathione transferase P1-1 governed by the H-site residue 105', *J. Mol. Biol.* **278**: 687–98.

Johnson, W. W., Ueng, Y.-F., Widersten, M., Mannervik, B., Hayes, J. D., Sherratt, P. J., Ketterer, B. and Guengerich, F. P. (1997) 'Conjugation of highly reactive aflatoxin B_1 *exo*-8,9-epoxide catalyzed by rat and human glutathione transferases: estimation of kinetic parameters', *Biochemistry* **36**: 3056–60.

Jungnelius, U., Ridderström, M., Hansson, J., Ringborg, U. and Mannervik, B. (1994) 'Similar toxic effect of 1,3-bis(chloroethyl)-1-nitrosourea on lymphocytes from human subjects differing in the expression of glutathione transferase M1-1', *Biochem. Pharmacol.* **47**: 1777–80.

Juronen, E., Tasa, G., Uusküla, M., Pooga, M. and Mikelsaar, A.-V. (1996) 'Purification, characterization and tissue distribution of human class Theta glutathione S-transferase T1-1', *Biochem. Mol. Biol. Int.* **39**: 21–9.

Kamisaka, K., Habig, W. H., Ketley, J. N., Arias, I. M. and Jakoby, W. B. (1975) 'Multiple forms of human glutathione *S*-transferase and their affinity for bilirubin', *Eur. J. Biochem.* **60**: 153–61.

Kano, T., Sakai, M. and Muramatsu, M. (1987) 'Structure and expression of a human class π glutathione *S*-transferase messenger RNA', *Cancer Res.* **47**: 5626–30.

Katoh, T., Kaneko, S., Takasawa, S., Nagata, N., Inatomi, H., Ikemura, K., Itoh, H., Matsumoto, T., Kawamoto, T. and Bell, D. A. (1999) 'Human glutathione *S*-transferase P1 polymorphism and susceptibility to smoking related epithelial cancer; oral, lung, gastric, colorectal and urothelial cancer', *Pharmacogenetics* **9**: 165–9.

Katoh, T., Nagata, N., Kuroda, Y., Itoh, H., Kawahara, A., Kuroki, N., Ookuma, R. and Bell, D. A. (1996) 'Glutathione *S*-transferase M1 (GSTM1) and T1 (GSTT1) genetic polymorphism and susceptibility to gastric and colorectal adenocarcinoma', *Carcinogenesis* **17**: 1855–9.

Kawajiri, K., Eguchi, H., Nakachi, K., Sekiya, T., Yamamoto, M. (1996) 'Association of *CYP1A1* germ line polymorphisms with mutations of the *p53* gene in lung cancer', *Cancer Res.* **56**: 72–6.

Kelley, M. K., Engqvist-Goldstein, Å., Montali, J. A., Wheatley, J. B. and Schmidt, D. E., Jr. and Kauvar, L. M. (1994) 'Variability of glutathione S-transferase isoenzyme patterns in matched normal and cancer breast tissue', *Biochem. J.* **304**: 843–8.

Kelsey, K. T., Spitz, M. R., Zuo, Z.-F. and Wiencke, J. K. (1997) 'Polymorphisms in the glutathione S-transferase class *mu* and *theta* genes interact and increase susceptibility to lung cancer in minority populations (Texas, United States)', *Cancer Causes Control* **8**: 554–9.

Kempkes, M., Wiebel, F. A., Golka, K., Heitmann, P. and Bolt, H. M. (1996) 'Comparative genotyping and phenotyping of glutathione S-transferase GSTT1', *Arch. Toxicol.* **70**: 306–9.

Kensler, T. W., Egner, P. A., Trush, M. A., Bueding, E. and Groopman, J. D. (1985) 'Modification of aflatoxin B1 binding to DNA *in vivo* in rats fed phenolic antioxidants, ethoxyquin and a dithiolthione', *Carcinogenesis* **6**: 759–63.

Kensler, T. W., Groopman, J. D., Sutter, T. R., Curphey, T. J. and Roebuck, B. D. (1999) 'Development of cancer chemopreventive agents: Oltipraz as a paradigm', *Chem. Res. Toxicol.* **12**: 113–26.

Ketterer, B. (1998) 'Glutathione S-transferases and prevention of cellular free radical damage', *Free Radical Res.* **28**: 647–58.

Ketterer, B. and Christodoulides, L. G. (1994) 'Enzymology of cytosolic glutathione S-transferases', *Adv. Pharmacol.* **27**: 37–69.

Kihara, M., Kihara, M. and Noda, K. (1994) 'Lung cancer risk of *GSTM1* null genotype is dependent on the extent of tobacco smoke exposure', *Carcinogenesis* **15**: 415–18.

Kihara, M., Noda, K. and Kihara, M. (1995) 'Distribution of *GSTM1* null genotype in relation to gender, age and smoking status in Japanese lung cancer patients', *Pharmacogenetics* **5** (Suppl.): 74–9.

Kitahara, A., Satoh, K., Nishimura, K., Ishikawa, T., Ruike, K., Sato, K., Tsuda, H. and Ito, N. (1984) 'Changes in molecular forms of rat hepatic glutathione S-transferase during chemical hepatocarcinogenesis', *Cancer Res.* **44**: 2698–703.

Klaassen, C. D. (1975) 'Biliary excretion of drugs: role of ligandin in newborn immaturity and in the action of microsomal enzyme inducers', *J. Pharmacol. Exp. Ther.* **195**: 311–19.

Klöne, A., Hussnätter, R. and Sies, H. (1992) 'Cloning, sequencing and characterization of the human Alpha glutathione S-transferase gene corresponding to the cDNA clone pGTH2', *Biochem. J.* **285**: 925–8.

Kolm, R. H., Danielson, U. H., Zhang, Y., Talalay, P. and Mannervik, B. (1995) 'Isothiocyanates as substrates for human glutathione transferases: structure-activity studies', *Biochem. J.* **311**: 453–9.

Krishna, N. S. R., Getchell, T. V., Dhooper N., Awasthi Y. C. and Getchell, M. L. (1995) 'Age- and gender-related trends in the expression of glutathione S-transferases in human nasal mucosa', *Ann. Otol. Rhinol. Laryngol.* **104**: 812–22.

Kumar, A., Das, B. C. and Sharma, J. K. (1994) '*Bam*HI restriction fragment length polymorphism (RFLP) at the human GST3 gene locus', *Hum. Genet.* **94**: 107–8.

Landi, S., Norppa, H., Frenzilli, G., Cipollini, G., Ponzanelli, I., Barale, R. and Hirvonen, A. (1998) 'Individual sensitivity to cytogenetic effects of 1,2:3,4-diepoxybutane in cultured human lymphocytes: influence of glutathione S-transferase M1, P1 and T1 genotypes', *Pharmacogenetics* **8**: 461–71.

Lee, W.-H., Morton, R. A., Epstein, J. I., Brooks, J. D., CampbelL, P. A., Bova, G. S., Hsieh, W.-S., Isaacs, W. B. and Nelson, W. G. (1994) 'Cytidine methylation of regulatory sequences near the π-class glutathione S-transferase gene accompanies human prostatic carcinogenesis', *Proc. Natl. Acad. Sci. U.S.A.* **91**: 11733–7.

Lee, E. J., Wong, J. Y., Yeoh, P. N. And Gong, N. H. (1995) 'Glutathione S-transferase-θ (*GSTT1*) genetic polymorphism among Chinese, Malays and Indians in Singapore', *Pharmacogenetics* 5: 332–4.

Lewis, A. D., Forrester, L. M., Hayes, J. D., Wareing, C. J., Carmichael, J., Harris, A. L., Mooghen, M. and Wolf, C. R. (1989) 'Glutathione S-transferase iso-enzymes in human tumours and tumour derived cell lines', *Br. J. Cancer* 60: 327–31.

Lewis, A. D., Hickson, I. D., Robson, C. N., Harris, A. L., Hayes, J. D., Griffiths, S. A., Manson, M. M., Hall, A. E., Moss, J. E. and Wolf, C. R. (1988) 'Amplification and increased expression of alpha class glutathione S-transferase-encoding genes associated with resistance to nitrogen mustards', *Proc. Natl. Acad. Sci. U.S.A.* 85: 8511–15.

Lin, H. J., Han, C.-Y., Bernstein, D. A., Hsiao, W., Lin, B. K. and Hardy, S. (1994) 'Ethnic distribution of the glutathione transferase Mu 1-1 (*GSTM1*) null genotype in 1473 individuals and application to bladder cancer susceptibility', *Carcinogenesis* 15: 1077–81.

Lin, H. J., Probst-Hensch, N. M., Louie, A. D., Kau, I. H., Witte, J. S., Ingles, S. A., Frankl, H. D., Lee, E. R. and Haile, R. W. (1998a) 'Glutathione transferase null genotype, broccoli, and lower prevalence of colorectal adenomas', *Cancer Epidemiol. Biomarkers Prev.* 7: 647–52.

Lin, D.-X., Tang, Y.-M., Peng, Q., Lu, S.-X., Ambrosone, C. B. and Kadlubar, F. F. (1998b) 'Susceptibility to esophageal cancer and genetic polymorphisms in glutathione S-transferases T1, P1 and M1 and cytochrome P450 2E1', *Cancer Epidemiol. Biomarkers Prev.* 7: 1013–18.

Liu, S., Stoesz, S. P. and Pickett, C. B. (1998) 'Identification of a novel human glutathione S-transferase using bioinformatics', *Arch. Biochem. Biophys.* 352: 306–13.

Liu, Y.-L., Roebuck, B. D., Yager, J. D., Groopman, J. D. and Kensler, T. W. (1988) 'Protection by 5-(2-pyrazinyl)-4-methyl-1,2-dithiol-3-thione (oltipraz) against the hepatotoxicity of aflatoxin B1 in the rat', *Toxicol. Appl. Pharmacol.* 93: 442–51.

Liu, Y. H., Taylor, J., Linko, P., Lucier, G. W. and Thompson, C. L. (1991) 'Glutathione S-transferase μ in human lymphocyte and liver: role in modulating formation of carcinogen-derived DNA adducts', *Carcinogenesis* 12: 2269–75.

Lo, H.-W. and Ali-Osman, F. (1997) 'Genomic cloning of *hGSTP1*C*, an allelic human Pi class glutathione S-transferase gene variant and functional charac-terization of its retinoic acid response elements', *J. Biol. Chem.* 272: 32743–9.

Lo, H.-W. and Ali-Osman, F. (1998) 'Structure of the human allelic glutathione S-transferase-π gene variant, *hGSTP1*C*, cloned from a glioblastoma multiforme cell line', *Chem.-Biol. Interact.* 111–112: 91–102.

MacLeod, S., Sinha, R., Kadlubar, F. F. and Lang, N. P. (1997) 'Polymorphisms of *CYP1A1* and *GSTM1* influence the in vivo function of CYP1A2', *Mutat. Res.* 376: 135–42.

McGlynn, K. A., Rosvold, E. A., Lustbader, E. D., Hu, Y., Clapper, M. L., Zhou, T., Wild, C. P., Xia, X.-L., Baffoe-Bonnie, A., Ofori-Adjei, D., Chen, G.-C., London, W. T., Shen, F.-M. and Buetow, K. H. (1995) 'Susceptibility to hepatocellular carcinoma is associated with genetic variation in the enzymatic detoxification of aflatoxin B$_1$', *Proc. Natl. Acad. Sci. U.S.A.* 92: 2384–7.

McLellan, R. A., Oscarson, M., Alexandrie, A.-K., Seidegård, J., Price Evans, D. A.

P., Rannug, A. and Ingelman-Sundberg, M. (1997) 'Characterization of a human glutathione S-transferase μ cluster containing a duplicated GSTM1 gene that causes ultrarapid enzyme activity', *Mol. Pharmacol.* **52**: 958–65.

McWilliams, J. E., Sanderson, B. J. S., Harris, E. L., Richert-Boe, K. E. and Henner, W. D. (1995) 'Glutathione S-transferase M1 (GSTM1) deficiency and lung cancer risk', *Cancer Epidemiol. Biomarkers. Prev.* **4**: 589–94.

Maheo, K., Antras-Ferry, J., Morel, F., Langouët, S. and Guillouzo, A. (1997) 'Modulation of glutathione S-transferase subunits A2, M1, and P1 expression by interleukin-1β in rat hepatocytes in primary culture', *J. Biol. Chem.* **26**: 16125–32.

Mankowitz, L., Castro, V. M., Mannervik, B., Rydström, J. and DePierre, J. W. (1990) 'Increase in the amount of glutathione transferase 4-4 in the rat adrenal gland after hypophysectomy and down-regulation by subsequent treatment with adrenocorticotropic hormone', *Biochem. J.* **265**: 147–54.

Mannervik, B. (1985) 'The isoenzymes of glutathione transferase', *Adv. Enzymol. Rel. Areas Mol. Biol.* **57**: 357–417.

Mannervik, B., Ålin, P., Guthenberg, C., Jensson, H., Tahir, M. K., Warholm, M. and Jörnvall, H. (1985) 'Identification of three classes of cytosolic glutathione transferase common to several mammalian species: correlation between structural data and enzymatic properties', *Proc. Natl. Acad. Sci. U.S.A.* **82**: 7202–6.

Mannervik, B., Awasthi, Y. C., Board, P. G., Hayes, J. D., Di Ilio, C., Ketterer, B., Listowsky, I., Morgenstern, R., Muramatsu, M., Pearson, W. R., Pickett, C. B., Sato, K., Widersten, M. and Wolf, C. R. (1992) 'Nomenclature for human glutathione transferases', *Biochem. J.* **282**: 305–6.

Mannervik, B., Berhane, K., Castro V. M., Olin, B., Ridderström, M., Vignani, R., Kozarich, J. W. and Ringborg, U. (1991) 'Glutathione-linked enzymes in normal and tumor cells and their role in resistance against genotoxic agents', in L. Ernster, H. Esumi, Y. Fujii, H. V. Gelboin, R. Kato and T. Sugimura (eds), *Xenobiotics and Cancer* London: Taylor & Francis Ltd, pp. 253–62

Mannervik, B., Guthenberg, C., Jakobson, I. and Warholm, M. (1978) 'Glutathione conjugation: reaction mechanism of glutathione S-transferase A', in A. Aitio (ed.), *Conjugation Reactions in Drug Biotransformation*, Amsterdam: Elsevier/ North-Holland Biomedical Press, pp. 101–10.

Mannervik, B., Guthenberg, C., Jensson, H., Warholm, M. and Ålin, P. (1983) 'Isozymes of glutathione S-transferases in rat and human tissues', in A. Larsson, S. Orrenius, A. Holmgren and B. Mannervik (eds), *Functions of Glutathione: Biochemical, Physiological, Toxicological, and Clinical aspects*, New York: Raven Press, pp. 75–88.

Mannervik, B. and Jemth, P. (1999) 'Measurement of glutathione transferases", in M. D. Maines, L. G. Costa, D. J. Reed, S. Sassa, and I. G. Sipes (eds), *Current Protocols in Toxicology*, New York: John Wiley & Sons, pp. 6.4.1–6.4.10.

Mannervik, B. and Jensson, H. (1982) 'Binary combinations of four protein subunits with different catalytic specificities explain the relationship between six basic glutathione S-transferases in rat liver cytosol', *J. Biol. Chem.* **257**: 9909–12.

Mannervik, B. and Widersten, M. (1995) 'Human glutathione transferases: classification, tissue distribution, structure and functional properties', in G. M. Pacifici, and G. N. Fracchia (eds), *Advances in Drug Metabolism in Man*, Luxembourg: Commission of the European Communities, pp. 407–59.

Martins, G., Alves, M., Dias, J., Santos, R., Costa Neves, B., Mafra, M., Martins,

A. P., Ramos, S., Mexia, J., Quina, M., Rueff, J. and Monteiro, C. (1998) 'Glutathione S-transferase μ polymorphism and gastric cancer in the Portugese population', *Biomarkers* 3: 441–7.

Masimirembwa, C. M., Dandara, C., Sommers, D. K., Snyman, J. R. and Hasler, J. A. (1998) 'Genetic polymorphism of cytochrome P4501A1, microsomal epoxide hydrolase, and glutathione S-transferases M1 and T1 in Zimbabweans and Venda of Southern Africa', *Pharmacogenetics* 8: 83–5.

Matthias, C., Bockmühl, U., Jahnke, V., Harries, L. W., Wolf, C. R., Jones, P. W., Alldersea, J., Worall S. F., Hand, P., Fryer, A. A. and Strange, R. C. (1998) 'The glutathione S-transferase *GSTP1* polymorphism: effects on susceptibility to oral/pharyngeal and laryngeal carcinomas', *Pharmacogenetics* 8: 1–6.

Maugard, C. M., Charrier, J. and Bignon, Y.-J. (1998) 'Allelic deletion at glutathione S-transferase M1 locus and its association with breast cancer susceptibility', *Chem.-Biol. Interact.* **111–112**: 365–75.

Menegon, A., Board, P. G., Blackburn, A. C., Mellick, G. D. and Le Couteur, D. G. (1998) 'Parkinson's disease, pesticides, and glutathione transferase polymorphisms', *Lancet* **352**: 1344–6.

Meyer, D. J., Coles, B., Pemble, S. E., Gilmore, K. S., Fraser, G. M. and Ketterer, B. (1991) 'Theta, a new class of glutathione transferases purified from rat and man', *Biochem. J.* **274**: 409–14.

Meyer, D. J., Crease, D. J. and Ketterer, B. (1995) 'Forward and reverse catalysis and product sequestration by human glutathione S-transferases in the reaction of GSH with dietary aralkyl isothiocyanates', *Biochem. J.* **306**: 565–9.

Meyer, D. J., Harris, J. M., Gilmore, K. S., Coles, B., Kensler, T. W. and Ketterer, B. (1993) 'Quantitation of tissue-specific and sex-specific induction of rat GSH transferase subunits by dietary 1,2-dithiole-3-thiones', *Carcinogenesis* **14**: 567–72.

Mikelsaar, A.-V., Tasa, G., Pärlist, P. and Uusküla, M. (1994) 'Human glutathione S-transferase GSTM1 genetic polymorphism in Estonia', *Hum. Hered.* **44**: 248–51.

Morel, F., Fardel, O., Meyer, D. J., Langouet, S., Gilmore, K. S., Meunier, B., Tu, C. P. D., Kensler, T. W., Ketterer, B. and Guillouzo, A. (1993) 'Preferential increase of glutathione-S-transferase class-α transcripts in cultured human hepatocytes by phenobarbital, 3-methylcholanthrene and dithiolethiones', *Cancer Res.* **53**: 231–4.

Morgenstern, R. and DePierre, J. W. (1983) 'Microsomal glutathione transferase. Purification in unactivated form and further characterization of the activation process, substrate specificity and amino acid composition', *Eur. J. Biochem.* **134**: 591–7.

Morgenstern, R., DePierre, J. W. and Ernster, L. (1979) 'Activation of microsomal glutathione S-transferase by sulfhydryl reagents', *Biochem. Biophys. Res. Commun.* **87**: 657–63.

Morgenstern, R., Lundqvist, G., Andersson, G., Balk, L. and DePierre, J. W. (1984) 'The distribution of microsomal glutathione transferase among different organelles, different organs, and different organisms', *Biochem. Pharmacol.* **33**: 3609–14.

Morrow, C. S., Cowan, K. H. and Goldsmith, M. E. (1989) 'Structure of the human genomic glutathione S-transferase-π gene', *Gene* **75**: 3–11.

Moscow, J. A., Townsend, A. J., Goldsmith, M. E., Whang-Peng, J., Vickers, P. J., Poisson, R., Legault-Poisson, S., Myers, C. E. and Cowan, K. H. (1988)

'Isolation of the human anionic glutathione S-transferase cDNA and the relation of its gene expression to estrogen-receptor content in primary breast cancer', *Proc. Natl. Acad. Sci. U.S.A.* **85**: 6518–22.

Mukanganyama, S., Masimirembwa, C. M., Naik, Y. S. and Hasler, J. A. (1997) 'Phenotyping of the glutathione S-transferase M1 polymorphism in Zimbabweans and the effects of chloroquine on blood glutathione S-transferases M1 and A', *Clin. Chim. Acta.* **265**: 145–55.

Mulder, T. P. J., Peters, W. H. M., Wobbes, T., Witteman, B. J. M. and Jansen, J. B. M. J. (1997) 'Measurement of glutathione S-transferase P1-1 in plasma. Pitfalls and significance of screening and follow-up of patients with gastrointestinal carcinoma', *Cancer* **80**: 873–80.

Müller, M., Krämer, A., Angerer, J. and Hallier, E. (1998) 'Ethylene oxide-protein adduct formation in humans: influence of glutathione-S-transferase polymorphisms', *Int. Arch. Occup. Environ. Health* **71**: 499–502.

Nakachi, K., Imai, K., Hayashi, S. and Kawajiri, K. (1993) 'Polymorphisms of the *CYP1A1* and glutathione S-transferase genes associated with susceptibility to lung cancer in relation to cigarette dose in a Japanese population', *Cancer Res.* **53**: 2994–9.

Nakajima, T., Elovaara, E., Anttila, S., Hirvonen, A., Camus, A.-M., Hayes, J. D., Ketterer, B. and Vainio, H. (1995) 'Expression and polymorphism of glutathione S-transferase in human lungs: risk factors in smoking-related lung cancer', *Carcinogenesis* **16**: 707–11.

Nazar-Stewart, V., Motulsky, A. G., Eaton, D. L., White, E., Hornung, S. K., Leng, Z.-T., Stapleton, P. and Weiss, N. S. (1993) 'The glutathione S-transferase μ polymorphism as a marker for susceptibility to lung carcinoma', *Cancer Res.* **53**: 2313–8.

Nelson, H. H., Wiencke, J. K., Christiani, D. C., Cheng, T. J., Zuo, Z.-F., Schwartz, B. S., Lee, B.-K., Spitz, M. R., Wang, M., Xu, X. and Kelsey, K. T. (1995) 'Ethnic differences in the prevalence of the homozygous deleted genotype of glutathione S-transferase theta', *Carcinogenesis* **16**: 1243–5.

Oke, B., Akbas, F., Aydin, M. and Berkkan, H. (1998) 'GSTT1 null genotype frequency in a Turkish population', *Arch. Toxicol.* **72**: 454-5.

Ollikainen, T., Hirvonen, A. and Norppa, H. (1998) 'Influence of *GSTT1* genotype on sister chromatid exchange induction by styrene-7,8-oxide in cultured human lymphocytes', *Environ. Mol. Mutagen.* **31**: 311–15.

Ostlund Farrants, A.-K., Meyer, D. J., Coles, B., Southan, C., Aitken, A., Johnson, P. J. and Ketterer, B. (1987) 'The separation of glutathione transferase subunits by using reverse-phase high-pressure liquid chromatography', *Biochem. J.* **245**: 423–8.

Pacifici, G. M., Warholm, M., Guthenberg, C., Mannervik, B. and Rane, A. (1986) 'Organ distribution of glutathione transferase isoenzymes in the human fetus: differences between liver and extrahepatic tissues', *Biochem. Pharmacol.* **35**: 1616–19.

Pearson, W. R., Vorachek, W. R., Xu, S., Berger, R., Hart, I., Vannais, D. and Patterson, D. (1993) 'Identification of class-mu glutathione transferase genes *GSTM1-GSTM5* on human chromosome *1p13*', *Am. J. Hum. Genet.* **53**: 220–3.

Pemble, S., Schröder, K. R., Spencer, S. R., Meyer, D. J., Hallier, E., Bolt, H. M., Ketterer, B. and Taylor, J. B. (1994) 'Human glutathione S-transferase theta

(GSTT1): cDNA cloning and the characterization of a genetic polymorphism', *Biochem. J.* **300**: 271–6.

Pemble, S. E., Wardle, A. F. and Taylor, J. B. (1996) 'Glutathione S-transferase class Kappa: characterization by the cloning of rat mitochondrial GST and identification of a human homologue', *Biochem. J.* **319**: 749–54.

Penrose, J. F., Spector, J., Baldasaro, M., Xu, K., Boyce, J., Arm, J. P., Austen, K. F. and Lam, B. K. (1996) 'Molecular cloning of the gene for human leukotriene C_4 synthase', *J. Biol. Chem.* **271**: 11356–61.

Peter, H., Deutschmann, S., Reichel, C. and Hallier, E. (1989) 'Metabolism of methyl chloride by human erythrocytes', *Arch. Toxicol.* **63**: 351–5.

Peters, W. H. M., Kock, L., Nagengast, F. M. and Roelofs, H. M. J. (1990) 'Immunodetection with a monoclonal antibody of glutathione S-transferase Mu in patients with and without carcinomas', *Biochem. Pharmacol.* **39**: 591– 7.

Ploemen, J. H. T. M., Wormhoudt, L. W., van Ommen, B., Commandeur, J. N. M., Vermeulen, N. P. E. and van Bladeren, P. J. (1995) 'Polymorphism in the glutathione conjugation activity of human erythrocytes towards ethylene dibromide and 1,2-epoxy-3-(p-nitrophenoxy)-propane', *Biochim. Biophys. Acta* **1243**: 469–76.

Quiñónes, L., Berthou, F., Varela, N., Simon, B., Gil, L. and Lucas, D. (1999) 'Ethnic susceptibility to lung cancer: differences in *CYP2E1, CYP1A1* and *GSTM1* genetic polymorphisms between French Caucasian and Chilean populations', *Cancer Lett.* **141**: 167–71.

Rahilly, M., Carder, P. J., al Nafussi, A. and Harrison, D. J. (1991) 'Distribution of glutathione S-transferase isoenzymes in human ovary', *J. Reprod. Fertil.* **93**: 303–11.

Rannug, U., Sundvall, A. and Ramel, C. (1978) 'The mutagenic effect of 1,2-dichloroethane on *Salmonella Typhimurium* I. Activation through conjugation with glutathione in vitro', *Chem.-Biol. Interact.* **20**: 1–16.

Rao, C. V., Nayini, J. and Reddy, B. S. (1991) 'Effect of oltipraz [5-(2-pyrazinyl)-4-methyl-1,2-dithiol-3-thione] on azoxymethane-induced biochemical changes related to early colon carcinogenesis in male F344 rats', *Proc. Soc. Exp. Biol. Med.* **197**: 77–84.

Rebbeck, T. R. (1997) 'Molecular epidemiology of the human glutathione S-transferase genotypes GSTM1 and GSTT1 in cancer susceptibility', *Cancer Epidemiol. Biomarkers Prev.* **6**: 733–43.

Redford-Ellis, M. and Gowenlock, A. H. (1971) 'Studies on the reaction of chloromethane with human blood', *Acta Pharmacol. Toxicol. (Copenhagen)* **30**: 36–48.

Rhoads, D. M., Zarlengo, R. P. and Tu, C.-P. D. (1987) 'The basic glutathione S-transferases from human livers are products of separate genes', *Biochem. Biophys. Res. Commun.* **145**: 474–81.

Robertson, I. G. C., Guthenberg, C., Mannervik, B., and Jernström, B. (1986) 'Differences in stereoselectivity and catalytic efficiency of three human glutathione transferases in the conjugation of glutathione with 7β,8α-dihydroxy-9α,10α-oxy-7,8,9,10-tetrahydrobenzo(a)pyrene', *Cancer Res.* **46**: 2220–4.

Roe, A. L., Howard, G., Blouin, R., Snawder, J. E. (1999) 'Characterization of cytochrome P450 and glutathione S-transferase activity and expression in male and female *ob/ob* mice', *Int. J. Obesity* **23**: 48–53.

Röhrdanz, E., Nguyen, T. And Pickett, C. B. (1992) 'Isolation and characterization of the human glutathione S-transferase A2 subunit gene', *Arch. Biochem. Biophys.* **298**: 747–52.

Rojas, M. Cascorbi, I., Alexandrov, K., Kriek, E., Auburtin, G., Mayer, L., Kopp-Schneider, A., Roots, I. and Bartsch, H. (2000) 'Modulation of benzo[a]pyrene diolepoxide–DNA adduct levels in human white blood cells by *CYP1A1*, *GSTM1* and *GSTT1* polymorphism', *Carcinogenesis* **21**: 35–41.

Rollinson, S., Roddam, P., Kane, E., Roman, E., Cartwright, R., Jack, A. and Morgan, G. J. (2000) 'Polymorphic variation within the glutathione S-transferase genes and risk of adult acute leukemia', *Carcinogenesis* **21**: 43–7.

Ross, V. L. and Board, P. G. (1993) 'Molecular cloning and heterologous expression of an alternatively spliced human Mu class glutathione S-transferase transcript', *Biochem. J.* **294**: 373–80.

Ross, V. L., Board, P. G. and Webb, G. C. (1993) 'Chromosomal mapping of the human Mu class glutathione S-transferases to 1p13', *Genomics* **18**: 87–91.

Rouimi, P., Debrauwer, L. and Tulliez, J. (1995) 'Electrospray ionization-mass spectrometry as a tool for characterization of glutathione S-transferase isozymes', *Anal. Biochem.* **229**: 304–12.

Rowe, J. D., Nieves, E. and Listowsky, I. (1997) 'Subunit diversity and tissue distribution of human glutathione S-transferases: interpretations based on electrospray ionization-MS and peptide sequence-specific antisera', *Biochem. J.* **325**: 481–6.

Rozen, F., Nguyen, T. and Pickett, C. B. (1992) 'Isolation and characterization of a human glutathione S-transferase Ha₁ subunit gene', *Arch. Biochem. Biophys.* **292**: 589–93.

Rozell, B., Hansson, H.-A., Guthenberg, C., Tahir, M. K. and Mannervik, B. (1993) 'Glutathione transferases of classes α, μ and π show selective expression in different regions of rat kidney', *Xenobiotica* **23**: 835–49.

Rushmore, T. H. and Pickett, C. B. (1993) 'Glutathione S-transferases, structure, regulation, and therapeutic implications', *J. Biol. Chem.* **268**: 11475–8.

Ryberg, D., Hewer, A., Phillips, D. H. and Haugen, A. (1994) 'Different susceptibility to smoking-induced DNA damage among male and female lung cancer patients', *Cancer Res.* **54**: 5801–3.

Ryberg, D., Skaug, V., Hewer, A., Phillips, D. H., Harries, L. W., Wolf, C. R., Øgreid, D., Ulvik, A., Vu, P. and Haugen, A. (1997) 'Genotypes of glutathione transferase M1 and P1 and their significance for lung DNA adduct levels and cancer risk', *Carcinogenesis* **18**: 1285–9.

Šalagovic, J., Kalina, I., Habalová, V., Hrivnák, M., Valansky, L. and Biroš, E. (1999) 'The role of human glutathione S-transferases M1 and T1 in individual susceptibility to bladder cancer', *Physiol. Res.* **48**: 465–71.

Schmidt-Krey, I., Murata, K., Hirai, T., Mitsouka, K., Cheng, Y., Morgenstern, R., Fujiyoshi, Y. and Hebert, H. (1999) 'The projection structure of the membrane protein microsomal glutathione transferase at 3 Å resolution as determined from two-dimensional hexagonal crystals', *J. Mol. Biol.* **288**: 243–53.

Schröder, K. R., Wiebel, F. A., Reich, S., Dannappel, D., Bolt, H. M., Hallier, E. (1995) 'Glutathione-S-transferase (GST) theta polymorphism influences background SCE rate', *Arch. Toxicol.* **69**: 505–7.

Segura-Aguilar, J., Baez, S., Widersten, M., Welch, C. J. and Mannervik, B. (1997)

'Human class Mu glutathione transferases, in particular isoenzyme M2-2, catalyze detoxication of the dopamine metabolite aminochrome', *J. Biol. Chem.* **272**: 5727–31.

Seidegård, J., DePierre, J. W., Birberg, W., Pilotti, Å. and Pero, R. W. (1984) 'Characterization of soluble glutathione transferase activity in resting mononuclear leukocytes from human blood', *Biochem. Pharmacol.* **33**: 3053– 8.

Seidegård, J., Guthenberg, C., Pero, R. W. and Mannervik, B. (1987) 'The *trans*-stilbene oxide-active glutathione transferase in human mononuclear leucocytes is identical with the hepatic glutathione transferase μ', *Biochem. J.* **246**: 783–5.

Seidegård, J., Pero, R. W., Miller, D. G. and Beattie, E. J. (1986) 'A glutathione transferase in human leukocytes as a marker for the susceptibility to lung cancer', *Carcinogenesis* **7**: 751–3.

Seidegård, J., Vorachek, W. R., Pero, R. W. and Pearson, W. R. (1988) 'Hereditary differences in the expression of the human glutathione transferase active on *trans*-stilbene oxide are due to a gene deletion', *Proc. Natl. Acad. Sci. U.S.A.* **85**: 7293–7.

Shea, T. C., Kelley, S. L. and Henner, W. D. (1988) 'Identification of an anionic form of glutathione transferase present in many human tumors and human tumor cell lines', *Cancer Res.* **48**: 527–33.

Shen, J., Lin, G., Yuan, W., Tan, J., Bolt, H. M. and Thier, R. (1998) 'Glutathione transferase T1 and M1 genotype polymorphism in the normal population of Shanghai', *Arch. Toxicol.* **72**: 456–8.

Sherratt, P. J., Pulford, D. J., Harrison, D. J., Green, T. and Hayes, J. D. (1997) 'Evidence that human class Theta glutathione S-transferase T1-1 can catalyse the activation of dichloromethane, a liver and lung carcinogen in the mouse. Comparison of the tissue distribution of GST T1-1 with that of classes Alpha, Mu and Pi GST in human', *Biochem. J.* **326**: 837–46.

Shi, M. M., Myrand, S. P., Bleavins, M. R., de la Iglesia, F. A. (1999) 'High-throughput genotyping method for glutathione S-transferase T1 and M1 gene deletions using TaqMan probes', *Res. Commun. Mol. Pathol. Pharmacol.* **103**: 3–15.

Shields, P. G., Bowman, E. D., Harrington, A. M., Doan, V. T. and Weston, A. (1993) 'Polycyclic aromatic hydrocarbon-DNA adducts in human lung and cancer susceptibility genes', *Cancer Res.* **53**: 3486–92.

Shows, T. B., McAlpine, P. J., Boucheix, C. *et al.* (1987) 'Guidelines for human gene nomenclature. An international system for human gene nomenclature (ISGN, 1987)', *Cytogenet. Cell Genet.* **46**: 11–28.

Singhal, S. S., Saxena, M., Awasthi, S., Ahmad, H., Sharma, R. and Awasthi, Y. C. (1992) 'Gender related differences in the expression and characteristics of glutathione S-transferases of human colon', *Biochim. Biophys. Acta* **1171**: 19–26.

Singhal, S. S., Saxena, M., Awasthi, S., Mukhtar, H., Zaidi, S. I. A., Ahmad, H. and Awasthi, Y. C. (1993) 'Glutathione S-transferases of human skin: qualititative and quantitative differences in men and women', *Biochim. Biophys. Acta* **1163**: 266–72.

Singhal, S. S., Zimniak, P., Sharma, R., Srivastava, S. K., Awasthi, S. and Awasthi, Y. C. (1994) 'A novel glutathione S-transferase isozyme similar to GST 8-8 of rat and mGSTA4-4 (GST 5.7) of mouse is selectively expressed in human tissues', *Biochim. Biophys. Acta* **1204**: 279-86.

Smith, C. M., Kelsey, K. T., Wiencke, J. K., Leyden, K., Levin, S. and Christiani, D. C. (1994) 'Inherited glutathione-S-transferase deficiency is a risk factor for pulmonary asbestosis', *Cancer Epidemiol. Biomarkers Prev.* **3**: 471–7.

Smith, M. T., Evans, C. G., Doane-Setzer, P., Castro, V. M., Tahir, M. K. and Mannervik, B. (1989) 'Denitrosation of 1,3-bis(2-chloroethyl)-1-nitrosourea by class Mu glutathione transferases and its role in cellular resistance in rat brain tumor cells', *Cancer. Res.* **49**: 2621–5.

Söderström, M., Hammarström, S. and Mannervik, B. (1988) 'Leukotriene C synthase in mouse mastocytoma cells. An enzyme distinct from cytosolic and microsomal glutathione transferases', *Biochem. J.* **250**: 713–18.

Söderström, M., Mannervik, B., Garkov, V. and Hammarström, S. (1992) 'On the nature of leukotriene C_4 synthase in human platelets', *Arch. Biochem. Biophys.* **294**: 70–4.

Sorsa, M., Osterman-Golkar, S., Peltonen, K., Saarikoski, S. T. and Sram, R. (1996) 'Assessment of exposure to butadiene in the process industry', *Toxicology* **113**: 77–83.

Srivastava, P. K. and Waxman, D. J. (1993) 'Sex-dependent expression and growth hormone regulation of class Alpha and class Mu glutathione S-transferase mRNAs in adult rat liver', *Biochem. J.* **294**: 159–65.

Staffas, L., Mankowitz, L., Söderström, M., Blanck, A., Porsch-Hällström, I., Sundberg, C., Mannervik, B., Olin, B., Rydström, J. and DePierre, J. W. (1992) 'Further characterization of hormonal regulation of glutathione transferase in rat liver and adrenal glands. Sex differences and demonstration that growth hormone regulates the hepatic levels', *Biochem. J.* **286**: 65–72.

Steinmetz, K. A. and Potter, J. D. (1996) 'Vegetables, fruit, and cancer prevention: a review', *J. Am. Diet. Assoc.* **96**: 1027–39.

Stockman, P. K., Beckett, G. J. and Hayes, J. D. (1985) 'Identification of a basic hybrid glutathione S-transferase from human liver. Glutathione S-transferase δ is composed of two distinct subunits (B1 and B2)', *Biochem. J.* **227**: 457–65.

Strange, R. C., Fryer, A. A., Matharoo, B., Zhao, L., Broome, J., Campbell, D. A., Jones, P., Pastor, I. C. and Singh, R. V. P. (1992) 'The human glutathione S-transferases: comparison of isoenzyme expression in normal and astrocytoma brain', *Biochim. Biophys. Acta* **1139**: 222–8.

Strange, R. C., Howie, A. F., Hume, R., Matharoo, B., Bell, J., Hiley, C., Jones, P. and Beckett, G. J. (1989) 'The developmental expression of alpha-, mu- and pi-class glutathione S-transferases in human liver', *Biochim. Biophys. Acta* **993**: 186–90.

Strange, R. C., Matharoo, B., Faulder, G. C., Jones, P., Cotton, W., Elder, J. B. and Deakin, M. (1991) 'The human glutathione S-transferases: a case-control study of the incidence of the GST1 0 phenotype in patients with adenocarcinoma', *Carcinogenesis* **12**: 25–8.

Sundberg, A. G. M., Nilsson, R., Appelkvist, E.-L. and Dallner, G. (1993) 'Immuno-histochemical localization of α and π class glutathione transferases in normal human tissues', *Pharmacol. Toxicol.* **72**: 321–31.

Sundberg, K., Johansson, A.-S., Stenberg, G., Widersten, M., Seidel, A., Mannervik, B. and Jernström, B. (1998) 'Differences in the catalytic efficiencies of allelic variants of glutathione transferase P1-1 towards carcinogenic diol epoxides of polycyclic aromatic hydrocarbons', *Carcinogenesis* **19**: 433–6.

Sundberg, K., Widersten, M., Seidel, A., Mannervik, B. and Jernström, B. (1997) 'Glutathione conjugation of bay- and fjord-region diol epoxides of polycyclic aromatic hydrocarbons by glutathione transferases M1-1 and P1-1', *Chem. Res. Toxicol.* **10**: 1221–7.

Suzuki, T., Johnston, P. N. and Board, P. G. (1993) 'Structure and organization of the human Alpha class glutathione *S*-transferase genes and related pseudogenes', *Genomics* **18**: 680–6.

Tahir, M. K., Guthenberg, C. and Mannervik, B. (1989) 'Glutathione transferases in rat hepatoma cells. Effects of ascites cells on the isoenzyme pattern in liver and induction of glutathione transferases in the tumour cells', *Biochem. J.* **257**: 215–20.

Tahir, M. K. and Mannervik, B. (1986) 'Simple inhibition studies for distinction between homodimeric and heterodimeric isoenzymes of glutathione transferase', *J. Biol. Chem.* **261**: 1048–51.

Takahashi, Y., Campbell, E. A., Hirata, Y., Takayama, T. and Listowsky, I. (1993) 'A basis for differentiating among the multiple human Mu-glutathione *S*-transferases and molecular cloning of brain *GSTM5*', *J. Biol. Chem.* **268**: 8893–9.

Talalay, P., De Long, M. J. and Prochaska, H. J. (1988) 'Identification of a common chemical signal regulating the induction of enzymes that protect against chemical carcinogenesis', *Proc. Natl. Acad. Sci. U.S.A.* **85**: 8261–5.

Talalay, P. and Spencer, S. R. (1990) 'Regulation of the induction of glutathione transferases and NAD(P)H:quinone reductase by glutathione transferase substrates', in J. D. Hayes, C. B. Pickett, and T. J., Mantle (eds), *Glutathione S-Transferases and Drug Resistance*, London: Taylor and Francis, London, pp. 176–85.

Tan, K. L., Webb, G. C., Baker, R. T. and Board, P. G. (1995) 'Molecular cloning of a cDNA and chromosomal localization of a human Theta-class glutathione *S*-transferase gene (*GSTT2*) to chromosome 22', *Genomics* **25**: 381–7.

Tang, D. L., Rundle, A., Warburton, D., Santella, R. M., Tsai, W.-Y., Chiamprasert, S., Hsu, Y. Z. and Perera, F. P. (1998) 'Associations between both genetic and environmental biomarkers and lung cancer: evidence of a greater risk of lung cancer in women smokers', *Carcinogenesis* **19**: 1949–53.

Taylor, J. B., Oliver, J., Sherrington, R. and Pemble, S. E. (1991) 'Structure of human glutathione *S*-transferase class Mu genes', *Biochem. J.* **274**: 587–93.

Tew, K. D. (1994) 'Glutathione-associated enzymes in anticancer drug resistance', *Cancer Res.* **54**: 4313–20.

Tew, K. D., Monks, A., Barone, L., Rosser, D., Akerman, G., Montali, J. A., Wheatley, J. B. And Schmidt, Jr., D. E. (1996) 'Glutathione-associated enzymes in the human cell lines of the National Cancer Institute drug screening program', *Mol. Pharmacol.* **50**: 149–59.

Thier, R., Foest, U., Deutschmann, S., Schroeder, K. R., Westphal, G., Hallier, E. and Peter, H. (1991) 'Distribution of methylene chloride in human blood', *Arch. Toxicol. Suppl.* **14**: 254–8.

Thier, R., Pemble, S. E., Kramer, H., Taylor, J. B., Guengerich, F. P. and Ketterer, B. (1996) 'Human glutathione S-transferase T1-1 enhances mutagenicity of 1,2-dibromoethane, dibromomethane and 1,2,3,4-diepoxybutane in *Salmonella typhimurium*', *Carcinogenesis* **17**: 163–6.

To-Figueras, J., Gené, M., Gómez-Catalán, J., Galán, M. C., Fuentes, M., Ramón,

J. M., Rodamilans, M., Huguet, E. and Corbella, J. (1997) 'Glutathione *S*-transferase M1 (GSTM1) and T1 (GSTT1) polymorphisms and lung cancer risk among Northwestern Mediterraneans', *Carcinogenesis* **18**: 1529–33.

To-Figueras, J., Géne, M., Gómez-Catalán, J., Piqué, E., Borrego, N., Carrasco, J. L., Ramón, J. and Corbella, J. (1999) 'Genetic polymorphism of glutathione *S*-transferase P1 gene and lung cancer risk', *Cancer Causes Control* **10**: 65–70.

To-Figueras, J., Géne, M., Gómez-Catalán, J., Piqué, E., Borrego, N., Marfany, G., Gonzalez-Duarte, R. and Corbella, J. (2000) 'Polymorphism of glutathione *S*-transferase M3: interaction with glutathione *S*-transferase M1 and lung cancer susceptibility', *Biomarkers* **5**: 73–80.

Tsuchida, S., Maki, T. and Sato, K. (1990) 'Purification and characterization of glutathione transferases with an activity towards nitroglycerin from human aorta and heart. Multiplicity of the human class Mu forms', *J. Biol. Chem.* **265**: 7150–7.

Tu, C.-P. D. and Qian, B. (1986) 'Human liver glutathione S-transferases: complete primary sequence of an Ha subunit cDNA', *Biochem. Biophys. Res. Commun.* **141**: 229–37.

Tu, C.-P. D., Weiss, M. J., Li, N. and Reddy, C. C. (1983) 'Tissue-specific expression of the rat glutathione *S*-transferases', *J. Biol. Chem.* **258**: 4659–62.

van Lieshout, E. M. M. and Peters, W. H. M. (1998) 'Age and gender dependent levels of glutathione and glutathione *S*-transferases in human lymphocytes', *Carcinogenesis* **19**: 1873–5.

van Ommen, B., Bogaards, J. J. P., Peters, W. H. M., Blaauboer, B. and van Bladeren, P. J. (1990) 'Quantification of human hepatic glutathione *S*-transferases', *Biochem. J.* **269**: 609–13.

van Poppel, G., Verhagen, H., van 't Veer P., van Bladeren P. J. (1993) 'Markers for cytogenetic damage in smokers: associations with plasma antioxidants and glutathione *S*-transferase μ', *Cancer Epidemiol. Biomarkers Prev.* **2**: 441–7.

Vorachek, W. R., Pearson, W. R. and Rule, G. S. (1991) 'Cloning, expression, and characterization of a class-mu glutathione transferase from human muscle, the product of the *GST4* locus', *Proc. Natl. Acad. Sci. U.S.A.* **88**: 4443–7.

Warholm, M., Alexandrie, A.-K., Högberg, J., Sigvardsson, K. And Rannug, A. (1994) 'Polymorphic distribution of glutathione transferase activity with methyl chloride in human blood', *Pharmacogenetics* **4**: 307–11.

Warholm, M., Guthenberg, C., Mannervik, B, von Bahr, C. and Glaumann, H. (1980) 'Identification of a new glutathione *S*-transferase in human liver', *Acta Chem. Scand.* **B34**: 607–10.

Warholm, M., Guthenberg, C., Mannervik, B., Pacifici, G. M. and Rane, A. (1981b) 'Glutathione *S*-transferases in human fetal liver', *Acta Chem. Scand.* **B35**: 225–7.

Warholm, M., Guthenberg, C., Mannervik, B. and von Bahr, C. (1981a) 'Purification of a new glutathione *S*-transferase (transferase μ) from human liver having high activity with benzo(a)pyrene-4,5-oxide', *Biochem. Biophys. Res. Commun.* **98**: 512–19.

Warholm, M., Guthenberg, C. and Mannervik, B. (1983) 'Molecular and catalytic properties of glutathione transferase μ from human liver: an enzyme efficiently conjugating epoxides', *Biochemistry* **22**: 3610–17.

Warholm, M., Rane, A., Alexandrie, A.-K., Monaghan, G. and Rannug, A. (1995)

'Genotypic and phenotypic determination of polymorphic glutathione transferase T1 in a Swedish population', *Pharmacogenetics* 5: 252–4.

Warwick, A., Sarhanis, P., Redman, C., Pemble, S., Taylor, J. B., Ketterer, B., Jones, P. Alldersea, J., Gilford, J., Yengi, L., Fryer, A. and Strange, R. C. (1994) 'Theta class glutathione S-transferase GSTT1 genotypes and susceptibility to cervical neoplasia: interactions with GSTM1, CYP2D6 and smoking', *Carcinogenesis* 15: 2841–5.

Watson, M. A., Stewart, R. K., Smith, G. B. J., Massey, T. E. and Bell, D. A. (1998) 'Human glutathione S-transferase P1 polymorphisms: relationship to lung tissue enzyme activity and population frequency distribution', *Carcinogenesis* 19: 275–80.

Wattenberg, L. W. (1983) 'Inhibition of neoplasia by minor dietary constituents', *Cancer Res.* 43 (Suppl.): 2448–53.

Webb, G., Vaska, V., Coggan, M. and Board, P. (1996) 'Chromosomal localization of the gene for the human Theta class glutathione transferase (GSTT1)', *Genomics* 33: 121–3.

Widersten, M., Pearson, W. R., Engström, Å. and Mannervik, B. (1991) 'Heterologous expression of the allelic variant Mu-class glutathione transferases μ and ψ', *Biochem. J.* 276: 519–24.

Wiencke, J. K., Kelsey, K. T., Lamela, R. A. and Toscano Jr., W. A. (1990) 'Human glutathione S-transferase deficiency as a marker of susceptibility to epoxide-induced cytogenetic damage', *Cancer Res.* 50: 1585–90.

Wiencke, J. K., Pemble, S., Ketterer, B. and Kelsey, K. T. (1995) 'Gene deletion of glutathione S-tranferase θ: correlation with induced genetic damage and potential role in endogenous mutagenesis', *Cancer Epidemiol. Biomarkers Prev.* 4: 253–9.

Wiencke, J. K., Wrensch, M. R., Miike, R., Zuo, Z. and Kelsey, K. T. (1997) 'Population-based study of glutathione S-transferase mu gene deletion in adult glioma cases and controls', *Carcinogenesis* 18: 1431–3.

Yeh, H. I., Hsieh, C.-H., Wang, L.-Y., Tsai, S.-P., Hsu, H.-Y. and Tam, M. F. (1995) 'Mass spectrometric analysis of rat liver cytosolic glutathione S-transferases: modifications are limited to N-terminal processing', *Biochem J.* 308: 69–75.

Yengi, L., Inskip, A., Gilford, J., Alldersea, J., Bailey, L., Smith, A., Lear, J. T., Heagherty, A. H., Bowers, B., Hand, P., Hayes, J. D., Jones, P. W., Strange, R. C. and Fryer, A. A. (1996) 'Polymorphism at the glutathione S-transferase locus GSTM3: interactions with cytochrome P450 and glutathione S-transferase genotypes as risk factors for multiple cutaneous basal cell carcinoma', *Cancer Res.* 56: 1974–7.

Yoshimoto, T., Soberman, R. J., Lewis, R. A. and Austen, K. F. (1985) 'Isolation and characterization of leukotriene C_4 synthetase of rat basophilic leukemia cells', *Proc. Natl. Acad. Sci. U.S.A.* 82: 8399–403.

Xia, C., Taylor, J. B., Spencer, S. R. and Ketterer, B. (1993) 'The human glutathione S-transferase P1-1 gene: modulation of expression by retinoic acid and insulin', *Biochem. J.* 292: 845–50.

Xu, S., Wang, Y., Roe, B. and Pearson, W. R. (1998a) 'Characterization of the human class Mu glutathione S-transferase gene cluster and the GSTM1 deletion', *J. Biol. Chem.* 273: 3517–27.

Xu, X., Wiencke, J. K., Niu, T., Wang, M., Watanabe, H., Kelsey, K. T. and Christiani, D. C. (1998b) 'Benzene exposure, glutathione S-transferase Theta homozygous deletion, and sister chromatid exchanges', *Am. J. Industr. Med.* **33**: 157–63.

Zhang, Y., Kensler, T. W., Cho, C.-G., Posner, G. H. and Talalay, P. (1994) 'Anticarcinogenic activities of sulforaphane and structurally related synthetic norbornyl isothiocyanates', *Proc. Natl. Acad. Sci. U.S.A.* **91**: 3147–50.

Zhang, Y. Kolm, R. H., Mannervik, B. and Talalay, P. (1995) 'Reversible conjugation of isothiocyanates with glutathione catalyzed by human glutathione transferases', *Biochem. Biophys. Res. Commun.* **206**: 748–55.

Zhang, Y., Talalay, P., Cho, C.-G. and Posner, G. H. (1992) 'A major inducer of anticarcinogenic protective enzymes from broccoli: Isolation and elucidation of structure', *Proc. Natl. Acad. Sci. U.S.A.* **89**: 2399–403.

Zhao, L., Alldersea, J., Fryer, A., Tighe, A., Ollier, B., Thomson, W., Jones, P. and Strange, R. (1994) 'Polymorphism at the glutathione S-transferase GSTM1 locus: a study of the frequencies of the GSTM1 A, B, A/B and null phenotypes in Nigerians', *Clin. Chim. Acta* **225**: 85–8.

Zhao, B., Lee, E. J. D., Wong, J. Y. Y., Yeoh, P. N. and Gong, N. H. (1995) 'Frequency of mutant *CYP1A1*, *NAT2* and *GSTM1* alleles in normal Indians and Malays', *Pharmacogenetics* **5**: 275–80.

Zhong. S., Howie, A. F., Ketterer, B., Taylor, J., Hayes, J. D., Beckett, G. J., Wathen, C. G., Wolf, C. R. and Spurr, N. K. (1991) 'Glutathione S-transferase mu locus: use of genotyping and phenotyping assays to assess association with lung cancer susceptibility', *Carcinogenesis* **12**: 1533–7.

Zhong, S., Spurr, N. K., Hayes, J. D., Wolf, C. R. (1993b) 'Deduced amino acid sequence, gene structure and chromosomal location of a novel human class Mu glutathione S-transferase', GSTM4. *Biochem J.* **291**: 41–50.

Zhong, S., Wolf, C. R. and Spurr, N. K. (1992) 'Chromosomal assignment and linkage analysis of the human glutathione S-transferase μ gene (GSTM1) using intron specific polymerase chain reaction', *Hum. Genet.* **90**: 435–9.

Zhong, S., Wyllie, A. H., Barnes, D., Wolf, C. R., Spurr, N. K. (1993a) 'Relationship between the GSTM1 genetic polymorphism and susceptibility to bladder, breast and colon cancer', *Carcinogenesis* **14**: 1821–4.

Zimniak, P., Nanduri, B., Pikula, S., Bandorowicz-Pikula, J., Singhal, S. S., Srivastava, S. K., Awasthi, S. and Awasthi, Y. C. (1994) 'Naturally occurring human glutahione S-transferase GSTP1-1 isoforms with isoleucine and valine in position 104 differ in enzymic properties', *Eur. J. Biochem.* **224**: 893–9.

Index

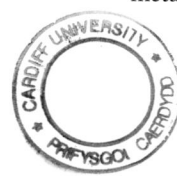